Medicinal Chemistry

Second Revised Edition

Medicinal Chemistry

Second Revised Edition

Prof. Rama Rao Nadendla
M.Pharm, Ph.D. FIC
Dean, Faculty of Pharmacy,
Acharya Nagarjuna University.
and
Principal,
Chalapathi Institute of Pharmaceutical Sciences,
Chalapathi Nagar, Lam, Guntur-34.

PharmaMed Press
An imprint of Pharma Book Syndicate
A Unit of BSP Books Pvt. Ltd.
4-4-309/316, Giriraj Lane,
Sultan Bazar, Hyderabad - 500 095.

Medicinal Chemistry, ***Second Revised Edition, by Prof. Rama Rao Nadendla***

Published by

PharmaMed Press

An imprint of Pharma Book Syndicate

A Unit of BSP Books Pvt. Ltd.

4-4-309/316, Giriraj Lane, Sultan Bazar, Hyderabad - 500 095.

Phone: 040-23445600, 23445688; Fax: 91+40-23445611

E-mail: info@pharmamedpress.com

ISBN: 978-93-8681-971-0 (HB)

Dedicated to,

Masterji of Shri Ram Chandra Mission

CONTENTS

Chapter 8

Penicillins

Chapter 9

Cephalosporins

Chapter 10

Aminoglycosides

Chapter 11

Tetracyclines

Chapter 12

Macrolides

Chapter 13

Polypeptide and miscellaneous group of antibiotics

Chapter 14

Urinary antiseptics

Chapter 15

Anti-tubercular drugs

Chapter 16

Antileprotic drugs

Chapter 17

Antimalarials

Chapter 18

Anti-protozoal drugs

Chapter 19

Anthelmentics

Chapter 20

Antifungal agents

Chapter 21

Antiviral agents

Chapter 22

Anticancer drugs

Chapter 23

Gastrointestinal agents

Chapter 24

Cardiovascular agents

Chapter 25

Coagulants and anticoagulants

Chapter 26

Diagnostic agents

Chapter 27

Chemistry of vitamins

Chapter 28

Steroids

PREFACE TO SECOND EDITION

The first edition of the book "Medicinal Chemistry" was written in simple and comprehensible style to meet the specific needs of pharmacy students. The first edition was popular and reached wider readership. Constructive suggestions received from students, teachers and colleagues have been considered for preparing this second edition. Some chapters like Quantitative structure activity relationships, drug design, sulfonamides, aminoglycosides, antiviral agents, anticancer drugs, steroids and steroidal drugs were thoroughly revised.

The second edition of Medicinal Chemistry comprises of 28 chapters. Introduction to medicinal chemistry, general principles of drug action and physicochemical properties of organic medicinal agents are explained in chapter 1, 2 and 3 respectively. Chapter 4, 5 and 6 explain quantitative structure activity relationship studies, drug design and combinatorial chemistry respectively. Chapter 7 to 28 explain chemistry, properties, mechanism of action, structure activity relationship studies, synthetic techniques and therapeutic uses of various classes of drugs.

I wish to recall my gratitude to members of Chalapathi Educational Society (Sri Y. V. Anjaneyulu, President), Guntur, staff members of Chalapathi Institute of Pharmaceutical Sciences, Guntur for their kind cooperation. I am also wish to acknowledge indebtedness to all who have assisted with the completion of the book. The cooperation of publishers, M/s Pharma Book Syndicate is very much appreciated in bringing out this book. The contribution that I received by sustained cooperation of my wife and daughter can't be ignored.

I have made every effort to avoid printing errors. However, despite best efforts, some might have crept in inadvertently. I shall be oblished if these are brought to my notice. Constructive suggestions, comments and criticism on the subject matter of the book will be gratefully acknowledged, as they will certainly help to improve future editions of the book.

It is hoped that both students and teachers of pharmacy, science and scientists will receive the book favorably as an effective textbook. This book is dedicated to my Masterji (Pujya Shri Parthasarathi Rajagopalachariji) of Shri Ram Chandra Mission.

-Author

PREFACE TO FIRST EDITION

Medicinal Chemistry has been designed to cater the needs of B. Pharmacy and Science students and teachers of Medicinal Chemistry. It meets the requirements of AICTE, New Delhi and various Indian Universities for B. Pharmacy Course. An attempt has been made to present a complete, authoritative and easily understandable medicinal chemistry text for pharmacy, medical, and other health science students. Postgraduate students will also find it useful for refreshing their basics.

This book comprises of 28 chapters. Chapter 1 explains Introduction of medicinal chemistry. Chapter 2 describes principles of drug action and physicochemical properties of organic medicinal substances are explained in Chapter 3. Chapter 4, 5 and 6 explain quantitative structure activity relationship studies, drug design and combinatorial chemistry respectively. Chapter 7 to 28 explain chemistry, properties, mechanism of action, structure activity relationship studies, synthetic techniques and therapeutic uses of various classes of drugs.

I wish to recall my gratitude to members of Chalapathi Educational Society, Guntur, staff members of Chalapathi Institute of Pharmaceutical Sciences, Guntur for their kind cooperation. I am also wish to acknowledge indebtedness to all who have assisted with the completion of the book. The cooperation of publishers, M/s Pharma Book Syndicate is very much appreciated in bringing out this book. The contribution that I received by sustained cooperation of my wife and daughter can't be ignored.

I have made every effort to avoid printing errors. However, despite best efforts, some might have crept in inadvertently. I shall be oblished if these are brought to my notice. Constructive suggestions, comments and criticism on the subject matter of the book will be gratefully acknowledged, as they will certainly help to improve future editions of the book.

It is hoped that both students and teachers of pharmacy, science and scientists will receive the book favorably as an effective textbook. This book is dedicated to my Masterji (Pujya Shri Parthasarathi Rajagopalachariji) of Shri Ram Chandra Mission.

-Author

1

INTRODUCTION TO MEDICINAL CHEMISTRY

The subject of medicinal chemistry explains the design and production of compounds that can be used for the prevention, treatment or cure of human and animal diseases. Medicinal chemistry includes the study of already existing drugs, of their biological properties and their structure activity relationships.

Medicinal chemistry was defined by IUPAC specified commission as, "it concerns the discovery, the development, the identification and the interpretation of the mode of action of biologically active compounds at the molecular level".

Medicinal chemistry covers the following stages :

(i) In the first stage new active substances or drugs are identified and prepared from natural sources, organic chemical reactions or biotechnological processes. They are known as lead molecules.

(ii) The second stage is optimization of lead structure to improve potency, selectivity and lessen toxicity.

(iii) Third stage is development stage involves optimization of synthetic route for bulk production and modification of pharmacokinetic and pharmaceutical properties of active substance to render it chemically useful.

Medicinal chemistry is the application of chemical research techniques to the synthesis of pharmaceuticals. During the early stages of medicinal chemistry development, scientists were primarily concerned with the isolation of medicinal agents found in plants. Today, scientists in this field are also equally concerned with the creation of new synthetic drug compounds. Medicinal chemistry is almost always geared towards drug discovery and development.

Medicinal chemists apply their chemistry training to the process of synthesizing new pharmaceuticals. They also work on improving the process by which other pharmaceuticals are made. Most chemists work with a team of scientists from different disciplines, including biologists, toxicologists, pharmacologists, theoretical chemists, microbiologists, and biopharmacists. Together this team uses sophisticated analytical techniques to synthesize and test new drug products and to develop the most cost-effective and environmentally friendly means of production.

The focus on development of new synthetic drug compounds has resulted in the incorporation of many other disciplines, such as biochemistry and molecular biology into medicinal chemistry. These areas include biology, computer-aided design, X-ray crystallography, metabolism and pharmacokinetics, legal and regulatory affairs, clinical, franchise management, pharmaceutics, and process research chemistry.

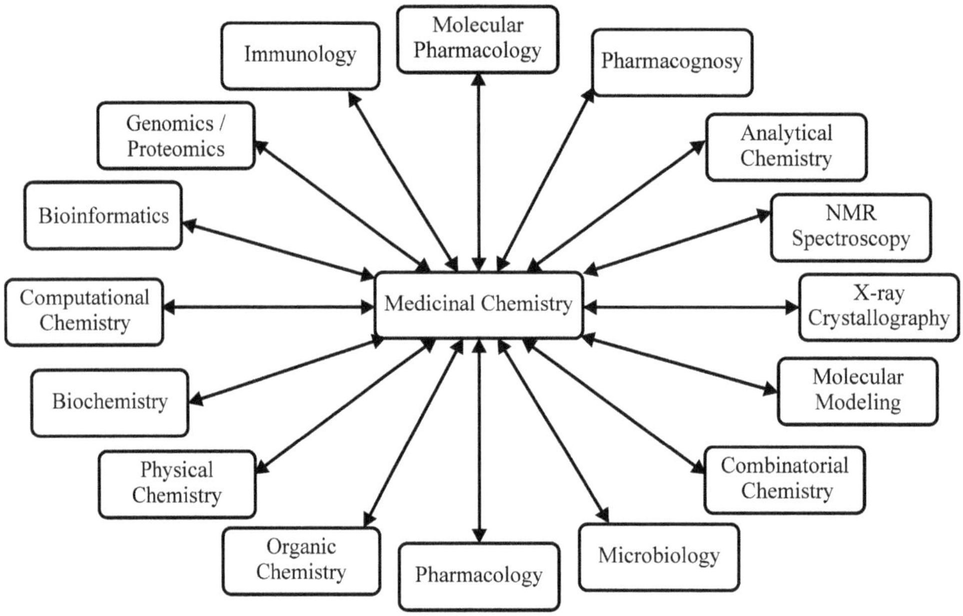

Modern Medicinal Chemistry

Chronology of drug introductions

8000 BC : Prehistoric medicine

It is difficult to imagine anything other than modern medical treatments but for thousands of years humans have become ill and for the same amount of time people have tried to cure them. Our ideas about medicines in prehistoric times come from archaeologists who have excavated and explored ancient sites. Their findings reveal a very different world to the one we experience today.

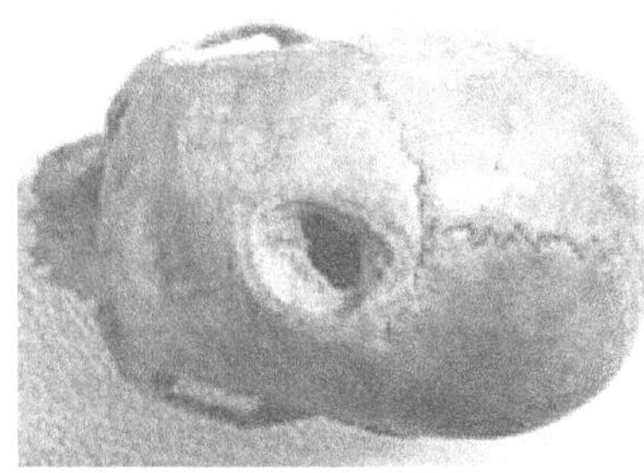

Trepanning: An ancient human skull viewed from above. Note the large hole!

Cave paintings and symbolic artefacts found by archaeologists suggest the earliest humans believed in spirits and supernatural forces. One form of primitive surgery seems quite shocking. Ancient skulls have been found with a hole bored into them. This appears to have been a deliberate operation and carried out whilst the person was still alive. We can only speculate as to the reason for this operation, called trepanning, but it may have been to allow the evil spirits to leave a sick person.

2000 BC : Egyptian medicines

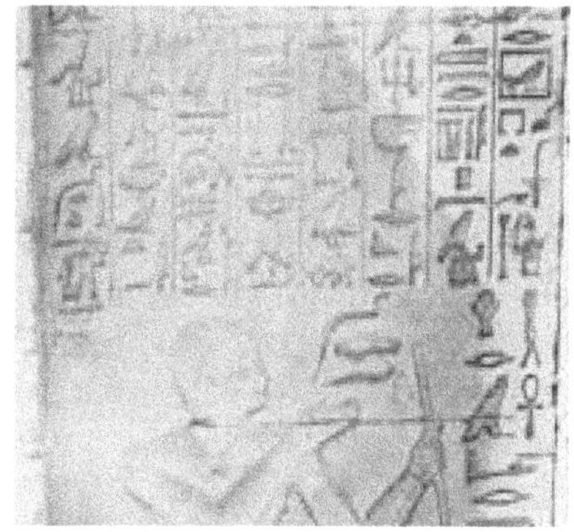

Egyptian hieroglyphs: like this one, show medical procedures. *Wellcome Library, London*

The ancient Egyptians built pyramids to bury their pharaohs and worshipped gods who ruled every aspect of their lives. The goddess Sekhmet was believed to cause or cure diseases and priests played a large part in Egyptian medicine. Archaelogists have found documents, written on a type of paper called papyrus, that describe medical techniques similar to those used today. The Egyptians used compression on a wound to stop bleeding and had specialists in obstetrics and gynecology who were the forerunners of modern midwives.

Their pharmacists prepared prescriptions of ointments, lotions, inhalers and pills by processing plant materials that were used to treat specific illnesses. Records show that they used many preparations including opium, cannabis, linseed oil and senna. Many modern drugs have originated from the study and isolation of active ingredients from plants with healing properties.

450 BC to 300 AD: Greeks and Romans

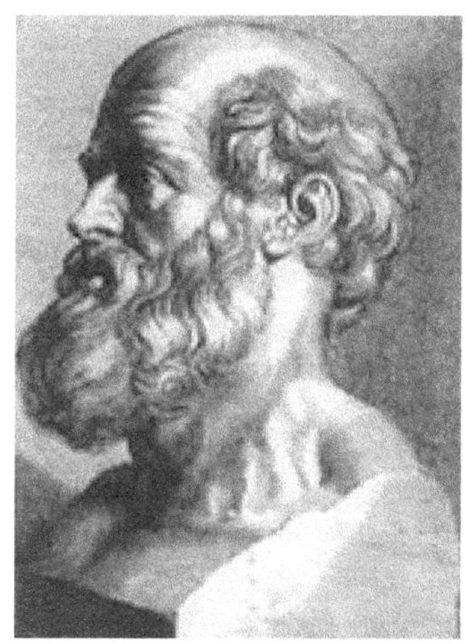

Hippocrates: famed for the Hippocratic oath.

Greece was home to one of the earliest civilizations. writing, mathematics, philosophy and the arts all flourished. The Greeks believed in many different gods but they also tried to understand their world in a much more scientific way.

Possibly the most famous name in medicine belongs to the Greek philosopher Hippocrates. He is seen as the father of modern medicine and gives his name to the hippocratic oath that doctors take.

The Romans realized that there was a link between dirt and disease. To improve public health, they built aqueducts to supply clean drinking water and sewers to remove wastes safely. Improved personal hygiene helped to reduce disease and Roman baths were places to socialize as well as stay clean.

500 - 1400 AD: The middle ages

The fall of the Roman Empire meant that many of their public hygiene practices were soon lost. The middle ages in Europe saw most people without access to clean drinking water, regular bathing or a sewage system. This meant that health conditions were often worse than during the Roman occupation of earlier centuries. Most people were farmers and food was not as plentiful as today. Starvation and disease were common.

Medicine in the middle ages was dominated by religion. Sickness was believed to be a punishment from God for sins committed and the only way to cure someone was to pray for their forgiveness. Doctors in the middle ages were usually priests or other religious scholars. Hospitals often sprang up in monasteries and other religious establishments. The patients were given food and comforted by religious nursing staff but little else was done to cure their illness.

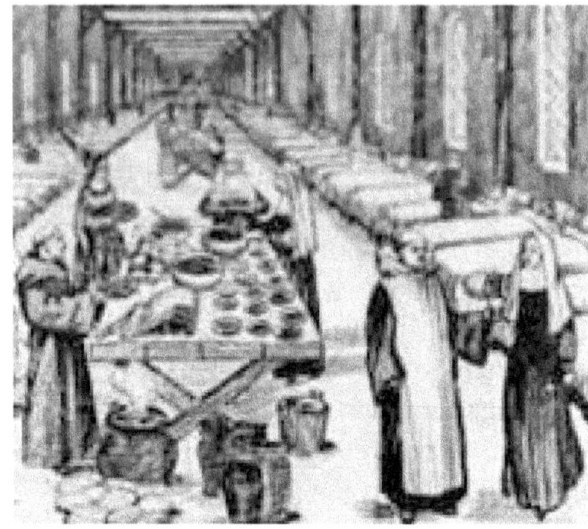

A medieval hospital: Patients were given food and cared for by monks and nuns. *Wellcome Library, London*

Traditional cures, using herbal remedies and potions were seen as witchcraft and outlawed by the church. Laws stated that only trained and registered people could practice medicine. Schools and universities began to educate wealthy individuals in religion, the arts, law and medicine. Generally men, and occasionally a few women, were trained and allowed to become physicians. As universities developed, more and more came from a non-religious background and eventually it was not necessary to be a cleric to practice medicine.

Surgery was a crude practice during the middle ages but operations such as amputations, setting broken bones, replacing dislocations and binding wounds were relatively common. Opium was sometimes used as an anesthetic while wounds were cleaned with wine to prevent infections.

During the middle ages, the only treatments were superstitious remedies, prayer, herbal medicines and recipes for clearing the air of miasma or poison. The plague was considered to be a punishment from God and so public health was not considered to be important.

700 - 1500 AD: Arabic medicines

For many centuries after the fall of the Roman Empire, the Arabic world was the centre of scientific and medical knowledge. Texts from Greece and Rome were translated into Arabic and studied by Islamic scholars. They developed and refined Hippocrate's theories and Islamic physicians began to use the regulation of diet, exercise and the prescription of medicinal herbs in the treatment of their patients. Arabic pharmacists became skilled in the formulation of medicines from plants and minerals. Even though they did not know about microbes, they used alcohol to clean wounds which healed better and did not become infected.

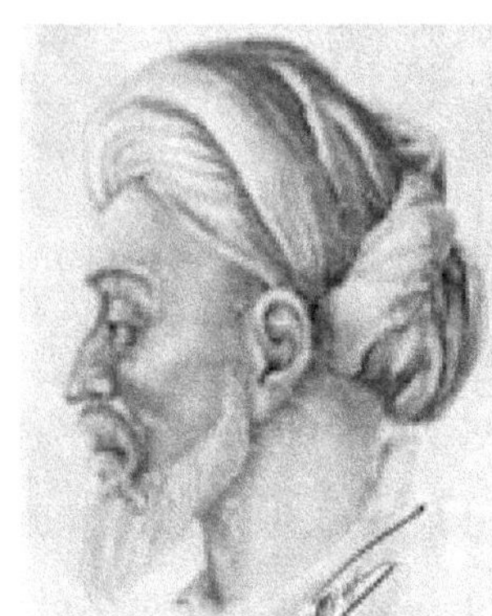

The Arab Physician and scholar **Ibn Sina** (or Avicenna). *Wellcome Library, London*

Records show that Arabic doctors performed many different surgical operations including the removal of varicose veins, kidney stones and the replacement of dislocated limbs. They used sponges soaked in narcotic drugs which were placed over the patient's nose as early anesthetics.

1700 - 1900: Eighteenth and nineteenth centuries

The industrial revolution of the eighteenth and nineteenth centuries saw a massive change in the way people lived and how this affected their health. People moved from small villages and an agricultural lifestyle to live in towns and cities that sprang up around the new factories, where they could work. People lived in dirty, overcrowded conditions with poor sanitation and dirty drinking water. Many died from diseases such as cholera, tuberculosis, measles and pneumonia infections that could spread quickly and easily in these conditions. Two of the big medical advances of this time were: vaccinations, X-rays.

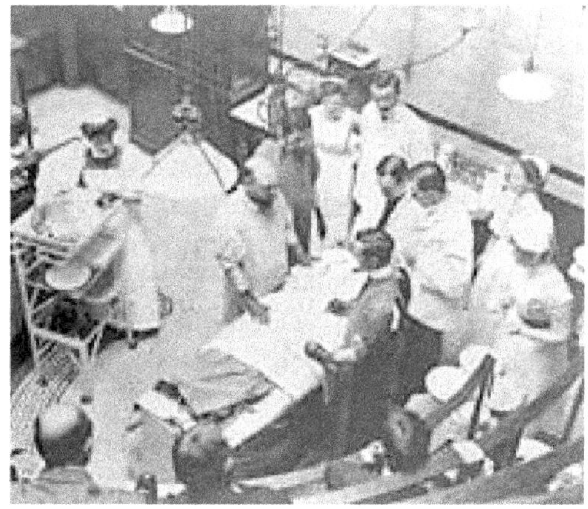

Operating theatres: In 1900 were not the sterile environments

Edward Jenner pioneered the earliest vaccinations and discoveries by Louis Pasteur and Robert Koch led to the understanding that infections were caused by certain bacteria or germs. The study of microbes, or microbiology, was born and the increased knowledge of pathogenic microbes led to the development of new medicines to tackle infectious diseases. The pharmaceutical industry was born.

The ideas of an earlier physician,Thomas Sydenham, were applied and this led to a great advance in the treatment of patients. He recognized the importance of detailed observation, record-keeping and the influence of the environment on the health of the patient.

1900 - 2000: The twentieth century

In 1901, the average life expectancy in the United Kingdom was 47 years. By the year 2000 it had risen to 77 years. New medicines, improved air quality and better public hygiene has contributed to this 64 percent increase in the life-expectancy. The twentieth century has seen some major advances in healthcare. These have included the development of:

Penicillin : The discovery and development of antibiotics by Fleming, Florey and Chain.

Insulin : Banting and best's work to show that insulin can be used to treat diabetes.

Other medicines : Pharmaceutical laboratories around the world are constantly producing new treatments for diseases.

Development of various classes of drugs

Anesthetics

In the first century AD the Greek physician Dioscorides (40-90 AD) described the use of wine of mandragora to produce sleep. Early Arab writings also mention anesthesia by inhalation. Guy de Chauliac (1300-1368) employed compression of the nerve trunk in the 1300s, and Ambroise Pare did the same in the 1500s. Priestly discovered nitrous oxide in 1772, and in 1800 Humphrey Davy discovered the gas's anesthetic properties when inhaled. Davy's student, Michael Faraday, showed in 1818 that inhalation of ether had the same effect. Henry Hill Hickman (1800-1830) experimented with both carbon dioxide and nitrous oxide on animals to carry out painless surgery in the early 1820s. Boston dentist William T.G. Morton arranged the first public demonstration of ether-anesthetized surgery in 1846. In 1842, Crawford W.Long, a physician of Georgia, flashed with the possibility of using ether as an agent to relieve pain. Queen Victoria's use of chloroform for her own labors in 1853 and 1857 firmly established the procedure as standard in childbirth. In 1922 ethylene was added to the list of general anesthetics. In 1929 at the university of Toronto, Lucas and Henderson used cyclopropane as general anesthetics. This gas gives deep surgical anesthesia in concentrations of 15 percent compared with 90 percent with nitrous oxide or 80 to 90 percent of ethylene.

Carl Koller demonstrated the use of cocaine as a local anesthetic in 1884. The addictive cocaine was replaced by synthetics beginning with Novocaine in 1904. The German doctor August Bier refined the technique in 1898, and Rudolph Matas of New Orleans introduced it to the United States in 1899. By the 1920s the use of spinal anesthesia was widespread in the United States. Robert Boyle first attempted intravenous anesthesia and the renowned architect. The idea, however, was abandoned until about 1874, when Pierre Ore used chloral hydrate intravenously on a dog and then, in 1875, on a human patient. Once barbiturates were discovered in the early 1900s, and especially after improved substances were developed in the 1920s, the use of intravenous anesthetics became firmly established.

Non-steroidal anti-inflammatory agents

In 1874 Thomas John Maclagan introduced salicylic acid as an antiseptic tablet for internal use. In 1876 he observed antirheumatic activity for salicylic acid. In 1886, Eahn and Hepp reported acetanilide as an antipyretic. Shortly after the introduction of acetanilide Hinsberg introduced phenacetin (somewhat less toxic). In 1893 paracetamol (a metabolite of phenacetin) was introduced but its superiority over phenacetin was recognized after 60 years. In 1837 Charles Gergardt synthesized acetylsalicylic acid. Twenty one non-steroidal anti-inflammatory drugs (NSAIDs) approved by 1990.

Cardiovascular drugs

In 1775 William Withesing reported foxglove as medicine. Oswald Schmiedberg managed to produce digitoxin (1882-1911). Albert Arnaud (1853-1915) extracted Ouabain from Acocanthera roots and bark and strophanthin from strophanthus. Amylnitrate had been synthesized in 1844 by Balard at the Sorborne. In 1878 Antoine Jesome Balard synthesized nitroglycerine.

The use of quinidine as anti-arrhythmic agent was established in 1920. In 1936 Frederick Mantz of clevelant proved procaine as superior anti-arrhythmic agent than cocaine or piperocaine.

Antibiotics

Gramicidin, the first natural antibiotic extracted from soil bacteria in 1939. It arrests the growth of *staphylococcus* but highly toxic. The modern history of antibiotics began with the observation in 1928 by British bacteriologist Alexander Flemming. He found that *Penicillium notatum* produced a substance which has bacteriostatic action. In mid-1950s, penicillin is available orally to the public without prescription. Penicillin was first obtained as pure crystals by Wintersteiner in 1943. In 1957, Sheeran synthesized phenoxymethyl penicillin or penicillin V. In 1940, Selman Waksman isolated and purificd actinomycin from *Actinomyces griseus* (Later named *Streptomyces griseus*). In 1942 Walksman introduced streptomycin. In 1952, Walksman was awarded the Noble prize in Physiology or medicine for his discovery of streptomycin. During the following years, a succession of antitubercular drugs appeared. These were important because with streptomycin monotherapy, resistant mutants began to appear within few years, P-aminosalicylic acid (1949), isoniazid (1952), pyrazinamide (1954), cycloserine (1955), ethambutol (1962) were introduced as antitubercular drugs. The discovery of rifampicin in 1967 was considered one of the greatest achievements in the history of chemotherapy against tuberculosis. Chloramphenicol was first isolated from cultures of *streptomyces venezuelae* an organism from a soil sample collected from venezuela (1948). During the immediate past war years, microbiologists conducted an extensive global search for novel antibiotic producing organisms. In 1945 G. Brotzn cultivated *cephalosporium acremonium* from sea water near a sewage outlet on the coast of Sardinia. Cephosporin C was structurally related to penicillins, but exhibited resistance to penicillinase. In 1964, cephalothin and cephaloridine were marketed as broad spectrum injectable antibiotics. Cyclosporin was one of the several antifungal antibodies isolated from certain varieties of fungi imperfecti in 1969.

Antitubercular drugs

Tuberculosis was one of the major causes of death until the beginning of the twentieth century. Half of the patients with active pulmonary tuberculosis died within two years, a quarter recovered and a quarter became chronic positive cases. In 1943 the Swedish researcher Lehmann discovered the anti-tuberculous action of para-aminosalicylic acid (PAS). In 1946 the development of streptomycin led to a true revolution in treatment (Selman Waksman, Nobel Prize 1952). In 1952 isoniazid (INH) was discovered as a tuberculostatic. Rifampicin then followed in 1970.

Antiseptics

The concept of antiseptics was introduced in 1750 by Sir John Pringle. In 1815 the antiseptic properties of coal tar were recognized. Mercury benzoate, carbolate and salicylate were introduced in the late 1880s. These were water insoluble and later water soluble compounds were introduced one after the other.

Antihistaminic drugs

In 1910, it was shown that histamine was formed by putrefaction of proteins containing the amino acid histidine. In 1942 Boret and Stanb introduced *phenbenzamine*. Boret introduced mepyramine in 1944 followed by tripelennamine, diphenhydramine, triprolidine and cyclizine. The early antihistamines were unable to antagonize the release of gastric acid caused by the action of histamine. In 1976 cimetidine was introduced into clinical practice. Ten years later it and the closely related ranitidine had become the two best selling drugs in the world.

Antiepileptic drugs

The original first generation antiepileptic drug, a bromide salt appeared in 1857. In 1912 phenobarbitone came into use for epilepsy. Tracy J. Putnam and Houstan H. Merritt introduced phenytoin as an antiepilepic drug in 1938. In early 1960s, carbamazepine and valproic acid and its derivatives were introduced to treat epilepsy. In mid-1990s a series of novel antiepileptic drugs were approved (felbamate, lamotrigine, gabapentin etc.).

Diuretics

In 1925 chlorothiazide, thiazide and diuril were introduced. In 1962 Mersalyl and ethacrynic acid were identified. Potassium sparing diuretics, triamterene was found in 1963.

Anticancer agents

Many anticancer drugs are extracted from plants. More than 1600 genera have been examined in recent decades (vincristine, vinblastine, taxol etc.). Taxol introduced into the market in January 1993 by Bristol-Myers. Besides natural products, synthetic anticancer drugs flourished in various directions. The first agents were nitrogen mustards, among which 2-2′-2″-trichloro triethylamine was the prototype first studied by Louis Goodman and Alfred Gitroan. Antimetabolites in cancer treatment were discovered by George Hitchings and Gertrude Elion (6-mercaptopurine, azathioprine, allopurinol. etc). Daunorubicin was isolated from *S.Pencautius* in 1962. In 1972 the National Cancer Institute introduced cisplatin into clinical trials.

2

GENERAL PRINCIPLES OF DRUG ACTION

Definition of drugs

A very broad definition of a drug would include "all chemicals other than food that affect living processes." If the affect helps the body, the drug is a medicine. However, if a drug causes a harmful effect on the body, the drug is a poison. The same chemical can be a medicine and a poison depending on conditions of use and the person using it.

Another definition would be "medicinal agents used for diagnosis, prevention, treatment of symptoms, and cure of diseases." Contraceptives would be outside of this definition unless pregnancy was considered as a disease. All drugs have the potential for producing more than one response. Some unavoidable adverse drugs responses which are appearing at therapeutic doses are termed side effects. In contrast, adverse drug effects appearing at extreme drug doses are described as toxic effects.

Classification of drugs

Drugs can be classified according to various criteria:

1. **By Origin - sources of drugs**

   Drugs may be obtained from 1. Plants 2. Animals, 3. Minerals or 4. Microorganisms. The drugs may also be semisynthetic or synthetic compounds. The sources of drugs are summarized as follows:

   (i) Synthetic: Most of the drugs in use today are synthetic in orgin. Such drugs are chemically pure and it is easy to maintain supply line. E.g., Aspirin, paracetamol.

   (ii) Natural: There are number of natural sources. They are:

   (a) *Plants*: A number of plant based drugs such as vincristine, taxol, digoxin, quinine, reserpine, ergotamine, ephedrine, colchicine etc are still a part of standard therapy. Most of these don't have any synthetic substitutes. Several other plant products are used in formulations that are sold across the counter in several countries.

(b) ***Animals :*** Some modern drugs continue to be derived from animal sources because the synthesis of such chemicals is very cumbersome and expensive. E.g., Gonadotropins, heparin, insulin, thyroid extracts and enzymes.

(c) ***Micro organisms :*** Following the accidental discovery of penicillin from a mould in 1928 and its successful use in chemotheraphy in 1940, a large number of antibiotics have been discovered from a variety of soil fungi and some bacteria. These drugs form the most important group of chemotherapeutic agents used against infective diseases. E.g., Penicillin, streptomycin and tetracycline.

(d) ***Minerals :*** Minerals or mineral-containing medicated springs have been in use. E.g., Several such hot water springs with medicinal value are popular in India. E.g., Rajgrin (Bihar), Sahashradhara (Dehradun). Minerals of medicinal value are iron, calcium, magnesium, aluminium, sodium and potassium etc.

(iii) **Semi-synthetic :** In some cases, especially with complex molecules, the synthesis of a drug may be very difficult or expensive and uneconomical. At the same time, the ones derived from natural sources may be impure. In these cases semisynthetic processes are used. E.g., 6-Aminopenicillanic acid is obtained from the fungus *Penicillium chrysogenum.*

(iv) **Biosynthetic:** Several drugs are complex polypeptides. It is difficult to obtain these drugs in pure form from natural sources and it is difficult as well as very expensive to synthesize them in the laboratory. E.g., Biosynthetic human insulin, interferon, erythropoietin and hepatitis vaccine.

Amongst all these, synthetic drugs are used most widely because of their cheapness, ease of quality control, mass production and therapeutic efficacy. Chemical processes prepare the synthetic drugs. E.g., Chloroquine, acetylsalicylic acid, chlorpromazine and ephedrine etc.

2. By Therapeutic Use

These drugs mainly affect the normal dynamic processes of the body. They are:

(i) Anti-arrhythmics
(ii) Antianginals
(iii) Vasodialators
(iv) Anti-hypertensives
(v) Cardiotonics
(vi) Hypocholesteramic agents
(vii) Antiallergenic agents
(viii) Drugs acting on gastro intestinal tract (GIT)
(ix) Drugs influence renal function
(x) Drugs acting on central nervous system
(xi) Drugs acting on peripheral nervous system

3. **By site of drug action**

   For instance alcohol is a depressant drug because of its central nervous system (CNS) depressant action. This system is limited when a drug has an effect at several body sites (e.g., The CNS stimulant cocaine also has local anesthetic (pain reducing) effects).

4. **By chemical structure**

   Drugs are classified according to the chemical moiety or functional group. They may be further sub classified as:
   (i) Hydrocarbons
   (ii) Halogenated compounds
   (iii) Alcohols
   (iv) Carboxylic acids
   (v) Phenols
   (vi) Nitro compounds
   (vii) Amides
   (viii) Amines
   (ix) Sulphonamides, sulphones, stilbenes, thioureas, ureides etc.

Characteristics of different routes of drug administration

Drugs can be administered by various routes. The choice of appropriate route in a given situation depends both on drug as well as patient related factors. Drugs may be administered locally or systematically. The drugs administered through systemic routes is intended to be absorbed into blood and distributed all over.

1. **Oral/swallowed**

   Oral ingestion is the oldest and commonest mode of drug administration. Both solid dosage forms and liquid dosage forms can be given orally. Most drugs in this route of administration are absorbed in small intestine. Full stomach delays absorption (e.g., Alcohol). Several drugs may subject to first-pass metabolism by liver due to which the drugs may undergo extensive metabolism before reaching target receptors. It is safer, more convenient, noninvasive, often painless.

2. **Oral/sublingual**

   The tablet or pellet containing the drug is placed under the tongue or crushed in the mouth and spread over the buccal mucosa. In this mode of administration fast systemic absorption is observed which, bypass gastrointestinal tract. It avoids absorption and first-pass metabolism in the liver and is useful for those likely to vomit from swallowed medication.

3. **Rectal**

   Here, the drugs are absorbed directly from the rectum. It partially avoids first-pass metabolism by liver and also for those likely to vomit and loss the swallowed medication. Certain irritant and unpleasant drugs can be put into rectum as suppositories or retention enema for systemic effect. E.g., Aminophylline, indomethacin, paraldehyde, diazepam, ergotamine and few other drugs are some times given rectally.

4. Epithelial

In this technique drugs are absorbed through the skin. This route is useful for those likely to vomit (e.g. Nicotine patch). Highly lipid soluble drugs can be applied over the skin for slow and prolonged absorption. The liver is also bypassed by this route of administration. The drug can be incorporated in an ointment and applied over specified area of skin.

5. Inhalation

Volatile oils and gases are given by inhalation E.g., General anesthetics, amylnitrite. The drugs enter the bloodstream very rapidly from the lungs. Here no absorption or first-pass metabolism problems. This route is potentially dangerous because it is so fast and direct.

6. Parentral route

Parentral administration refers to administration by injection into tissue fluid or blood without having to cross the intestinal mucosa. This route can be employed even in unconscoius, uncooperative or vomiting patient. The important parenteral routes are subcutaneous, (SC); intramuscular, (IM); intravenous, (IV). The rate of absorption depends on blood flow through injection site. SC or IM exert effects more quickly than oral administration. IV is the fastest route and most certain, in terms of obtaining desired concentration of drug in blood plasma.

Sites of drug action

1. Enzyme inhibition

Drugs act within the cell by modifying normal biochemical reactions. Enzyme inhibition may be reversible or non-reversible; competitive or non-competitive. Antimetabolites may be used which mimic natural metabolites. Gene functions may be suppressed.

2. Drug-receptor interactions

Drugs act on the cell membrane by physical and/or chemical interactions. This is usually through specific drug receptor sites known to be located on the membrane. A receptor is the specific chemical constituents of the cell with which a drug interacts to produce its pharmacological effects. Some receptor sites have been identified with specific parts of proteins and nucleic acids. In most cases, the chemical nature of the receptor site remains obscure.

3. Non-specific interactions

Drugs act exclusively by physical means outside the cells. These sites include external surfaces of skin and gastrointestinal tract. Drugs also act outside of the cell membranes by chemical interactions. Neutralization of stomach acid by antacids is a good example.

Mode of drug action

It is important to distinguish between actions of drug and their effects. Actions of drugs are the biochemical physiological mechanisms by which the chemical produces a response in living organisms. The effect is the observable consequence of a drug action. For example, the action of penicillin is to interfere with cell wall synthesis in bacteria and the effect is the death of the bacteria.

One major problem of pharmacology is that no drug produces a single effect. The primary effect is the desired therapeutic effect. Secondary effects are all other effects beside the desired effect, which may be either beneficial or harmful. Drugs are chosen to exploit differences between normal metabolic processes and any abnormalities, which may be present. Since the differences may not be very great, drugs may be nonspecific in action and alter normal functions as well as the undesirable ones. This leads to undesirable side effects.

The biological effects observed after a drug has been administered are the result of an interaction between the chemical and some part of the organism. Mechanisms of drug action can be viewed from different perspectives, namely, the site of action and the general nature of the drug-cell interaction.

1. Killing foreign organisms

Chemotherapeutic agents act by killing or weakening foreign organisms such as bacteria, worms, and viruses. The main principle of action is selective toxicity, i.e., the drug must be more toxic to the parasite than to the host.

2. Stimulation and depression

Drugs act by stimulating or depressing normal physiological functions. Stimulation increases the rate of activity while depression reduces the rate of activity.

3. Irritation

It is a non-specific action of a drug that can occur in all the body tissues. Certain drugs act by causing irritation. E.g., Drugs like senna and castor oil show their laxative effects by their irritant action on gastrointestinal tract.

4. Replacement

Drugs serve as replacement of essential body chemicals that are either absent or present in less than required quantity due to disease. E.g., Insulin is used in diabetes. Levodopa therapy in Parkinson's disease.

Mechanism of drug action

A drug acts by virtue of its various properties like physical, chemical, physiological etc. The fundamental mechanisms of drug action can be distinguished into following categories:

1. Physical properties

A physical property of the drug is responsible for its action.

For example,

(i) **Taste:** Bitter taste drugs increase the flow of hydrochloric acid reflexly in the stomach. E.g., Quasia, chirata.

(ii) **Mass :** By increasing the bulk of drug in intestine produce laxative effect E.g., Isapgol

(iii) **Absorption:** Certain drugs like kaolin absorb water on to its surface and thereby reduce gastric motility.

(iv) **Radioactivity:** The radioactive substances are commonly used to treat cancer. E.g., I^{131}.

2. Chemical properties

The drugs react extracellularly according to simple chemical reactions like neutralization, chelation, oxidation etc.

For example,

(i) Aluminium hydroxide neutralizes acid in stomach.

(ii) Toxic heavy metals can be eliminated by chelating agents like EDTA, BAL, penicillamine etc.

(iii) Oxidizing agents are germicidal.

3. Through enzymes

Enzymes are very important targets of drug action because almost all biological reactions are carried out under the influence of enzymes. Drugs may either increase or decrease enzymatic reactions.

For example,

(i) Adrenaline stimulates adenyl cyclase.

(ii) Pyridoxine acts as a cofactor and increases decarboxylase activity

(iii) Allopurinol competes with hypoxanthine for xanthine oxidase.

(iv) Physostigmine and neostigmine compete with acetylcholine for cholinesterase.

4. Through receptors

A large number of drugs act through specific macromolecular components of the cell, which regulate critical functions like enzymatic activity, permeability, structural features, template function etc. These macromolecules, which bind and interact with the drugs, are called receptors.

Drug receptor interactions

1. Introduction

The concept of proteins as drug targets is not novel and was suggested at the end of the nineteenth and the beginning of the twentieth centuries. Ehrlich and Langley both contributed the idea that compounds display biological activity by binding to cellular constituents (Ehrlich: 'corpora non agunt, nisi fixata', which tells us that 'agents do not work, unless bound') that were soon named 'receptors' (Langley: 'receptive substances'). One could consider that every protein that acts as the molecular target for a certain drug should be called a receptor. A receptor is a component of a cell or organism that interacts with a drug and initiates the chain of biochemical events leading to the drug's observed effects.

2. Drug-receptor complex nomenclature

(i) Agonist - a drug that activates a receptor:

- Agonists can differ in both affinity and efficacy for the receptor.
- High efficacy agonists are full agonists because they elicit maximal effects
- Low efficacy agonists are partial agonists because they cannot elicit a maximal effect at receptors even at high concentrations (false transmitters).
- Direct agonists act on receptors, while indirect agonists facillitate the actions of the endogenous agonist (the neurotransmitter, itself).

(ii) Antagonist - a drug that does not activate the receptor:

- Antagonists also prevent the activation of the receptor by an agonist, thus antagonists are essentially zero efficacy drugs.
- Competitive antagonists bind to the same binding site as the agonist and therefore compete with the agonist for that binding site.
- Noncompetitive antagonists have a different binding site to the agonist and therefore do not compete with the agonist. Some noncompetitive antagonists have a binding site within the ion channel associated with the receptor complex.

3. Chemical nature of receptors

For many years, receptors remained hypothetical structures, until in the 1970s the development of radioactive ligand led to the visualization and quantification of binding sites for drugs in tissues or isolated cells. Nowadays, detailed structural information (X-ray, NMR) of a variety of receptor proteins is known and this has led to the development of detailed insights in the molecular processes involved in drug-receptor interactions.

Receptors are no longer hypothetical. Hundreds of receptor proteins have been isolated, purified, cloned, and their primary amino acid sequence has been established. It has been possible to study the receptor by binding assay, biochemical characterization, immunological characterization and molecular biological characterization.

Most of the receptors like regulatory enzymes (dihydrofolate reductase enzyme), acetylcholinesterase transport proteins and structural proteins (Tubulin) are proteineous in nature and some are glycoproteins (G-protein coupled receptors) or nucleic acids.

4. Types of receptors

However, the overall structure of receptor proteins is often not so divergent, suggesting that signal transmission via receptor proteins is governed by a limited number of basic mechanisms that are utilized in an extremely efficient way. One distinguishes four super-families of receptor proteins, which cover most of the relevant receptor proteins. These four receptor families are:

(i) **Ligand-gated ion channels:** Ligand-gated ion channels, which are membrane-bound receptors, directly linked to an ion channel. They are also known as ionotropic receptors. Examples include the nicotine acetylcholine receptor, glutamate receptor and the GABA-A receptor.

(ii) **G-protein coupled receptors:** G-protein coupled receptors, which are membrane-bound receptors coupled to G-proteins. After activation of the G-proteins a variety of biochemical signal transduction pathways can be activated. Many chemical messengers, like hormones and various neurotransmitters, act through G-protein coupled receptors. They are also known as metabotropic receptors or 7-transmembrane receptors. E.g., Muscarinic acetylcholine receptors and adrenergic receptors.

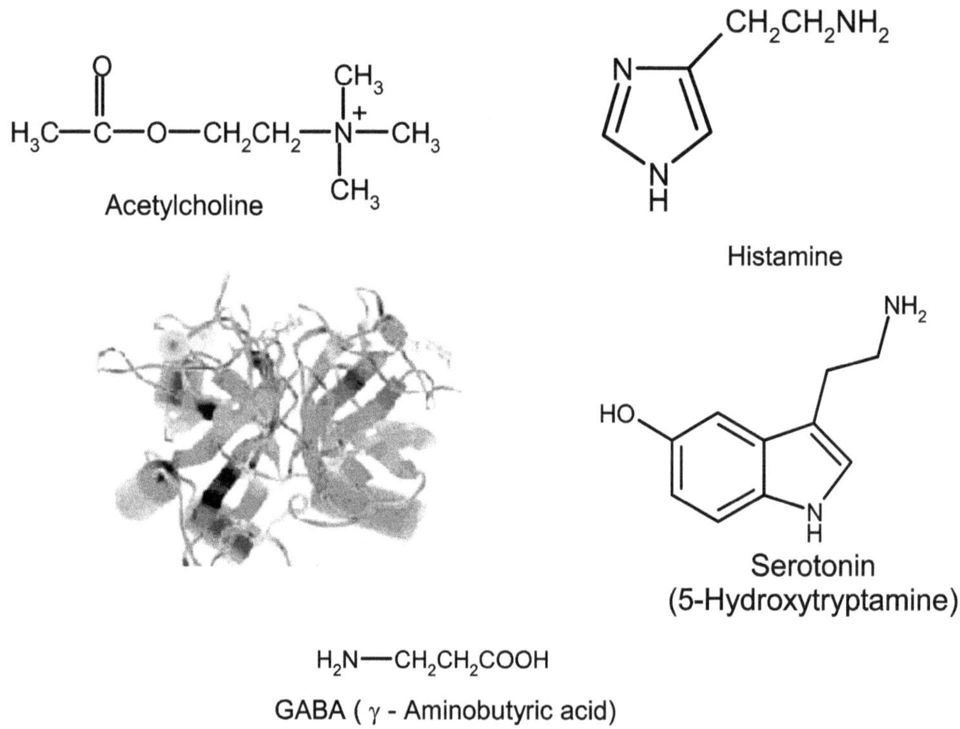

Figure 2.1 Structures of selected ligands for G-protein coupled receptors.

(iii) **Tyrosine kinase-linked receptors:** Tyrosine kinase-linked receptors, are membrane bound receptors and contain an intrinsic enzymatic function (tyrosine kinase activity) in their intracellular domain. Upon activation by ligand like insulin, the receptor is activated and is able to phosphorylate tyrosine residues of other intracellular proteins. Protein phosphorylation is one of the underlying mechanisms of the regulation of protein function. E.g., Receptors for insulin and various cytokines and growth factors.

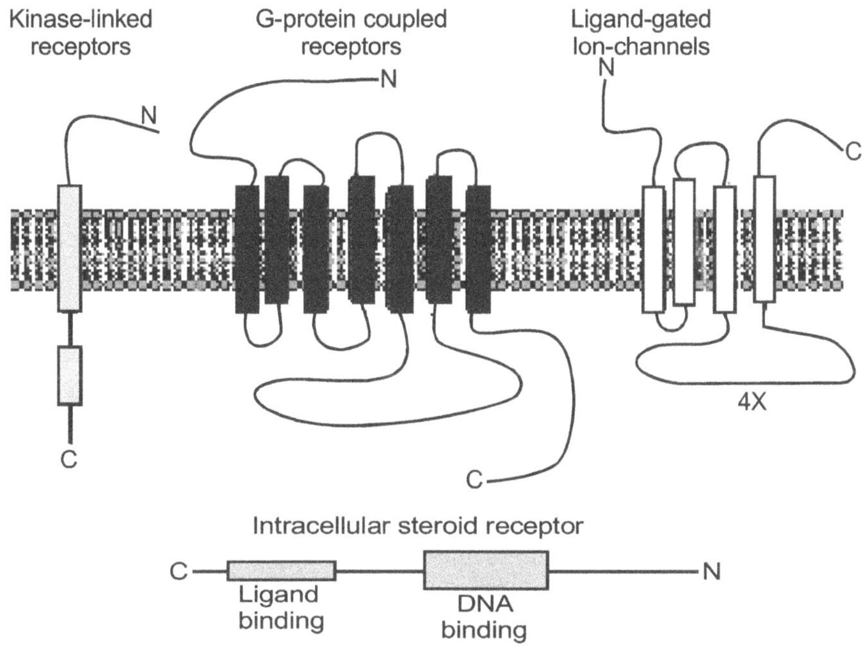

Figure 2.2 Schematic representation of the four major classes of receptor proteins. Except for the steroid receptors, the receptor proteins are localized in the cell membrane. The ligand-gated ion channels are made up of an assembly of 4-5 subunits, which each contain four transmembrane domains.

(iv) **Intracellular receptors regulating gene transcription:** Intracellular receptors regulating gene transcription, which are located in the cytosol. Upon binding of the appropriate chemical signal, e.g., Steroid hormones, the activated receptors translate to the nucleus and initiate gene transcription. These are known as nuclear receptors: E.g., Receptors for steroid hormones, thyroid hormone and vitamin D.

5. Drug-receptor Interactions

The vast majority of drugs show a remarkably high correlation of structure and specificity to produce pharmacological effects. A minimum three-point attachment of a drug to a receptor site is required. In most cases a rather specific chemical structure is required for the receptor site and a complementary drug structure. Slight changes in the molecular structure of the drug may drastically change specificity. To initiate a biological response, the drug must form bond with the receptor surface. Different types of binding forces that may exist in drug-receptor interactions are as follows:

(i) **Covalent interaction (bond) :** These chemical forces may result in a temporary binding of the drug to the receptor. Frequently, a covalent bond is firm and described as essentially "irreversible" under biological conditions. Since by definition the drug-receptor interaction is reversible, covalent bond formation is rather rare except in a rather toxic situation. Examples:

(a) A covalent bond is formed between the activated form of phenoxybenzamine (a receptor antagonist) and the alpha adrenergic-receptor.

(b) Antineoplastic or antibiotic drugs act mainly through the formation of covalent bonds.

(c) The DNA-alkylating chemotherapy agents are chemically highly reactive, forming covalent bonds with DNA functional groups. Such covalently modified DNA may be incompatible with successful tumor cell division.

(ii) **Ionic interactions:** Since many drugs contain acid or amine functional groups, which are ionized at physiological pH. Ionic bonds are formed by the attraction of opposite charges in the receptor site with the ionized groups of the drug molecule. They are strong electrostatic interactions (5-10 kcal/mol) and are responsible for relative orientation of the drug to its binding site. Electrostatic interactions tend to be much more common than the covalent bonding in drug-receptor interactions. Attraction between ions of opposite charges is inversely proportional to the square of the distance between them. Strong electrostatic interactions occur between permanently charged ionic molecules. The overall contribution ($D^+ R^- \leftrightarrow DR$) of ionic interactions may be overemphasized due to desolvation. Ionic bonds have a relatively high stability.

For example, in acetylcholine molecule, the positively charged quaternary nitrogen may be attracted to the negatively charged ionized carboxyl group present in the receptor site.

(iii) **Hydrogen bonding interactions (non-ionic/neutral):** Polar-polar interactions are the attraction of opposite charges. The drug-receptor reaction is essentially an exchange of the hydrogen bond between a drug molecule, surrounding water, and the receptor site. The hydrogen bond strength is distance dependent may range from 0.5 – 7 kcal/mol, depending on the binding environment. The Vander Waals interaction forces have the following characteristic features :

(a) Interactions at a close range.

(b) The Vander Waals interaction forces occur less frequently than hydrophobic forces.

(c) Interactions are much weaker (~0.5-1 kcal/mol) than other electrostatic interactions.

(d) Close contacts (attractive forces) over a large surface area i.e. at the interface of ligand and binding site, may contribute to binding. E.g., Many drugs contain hydroxyl, amino, carboxyl and carbonyl groups. They can form hydrogen bonds with the complimentary groups present on the receptor surface.

(e) Hydrophobic/lipophilic Interactions: Finally hydrophobic bonds are formed between non-polar hydrocarbon groups on the drug and those in the receptor site. These bonds are not very specific but the interactions do occur to exclude water molecules. Most of the drug molecules have a non-polar portion (alkyl or aryl groups) which may combine with nonpolar portion of the receptor site through hydrophobic forces. Hydrophobic interactions are generally weak, but important. Hydrophobic interactions are probably significant in driving interactions:

- Between lipophilic drugs and the lipid component of biological membranes.
- Between drugs and relatively non polar (not charged) receptor regions.

6. Receptor site theories

After attachment of drug molecule to a receptor site, a drug may either initiate a response or prevent a response from occurring.

This concept can be easily understood if one considers the 'lock-and-key' principle for ligand– receptor interaction (Fig. 2.3). Only keys (ligands) that fulfil all criteria for fitting into the lock (receptor) can open the door (produce an effect). Some keys can fit in the lock, but not perfectly. Consequently, they cannot open the door yet, by fitting into the lock, these keys prevent the original key from fitting into the lock and opening the door. The concept of receptor antagonism is extremely important in medicinal chemistry and is very often the underlying mechanism of drug action. E.g., To prevent the constriction of airway smooth muscle in asthmatic conditions one can administer receptor antagonists that prevent the actions of the signaling molecules causing muscle contraction (e.g., histamine and leukotriene antagonists).

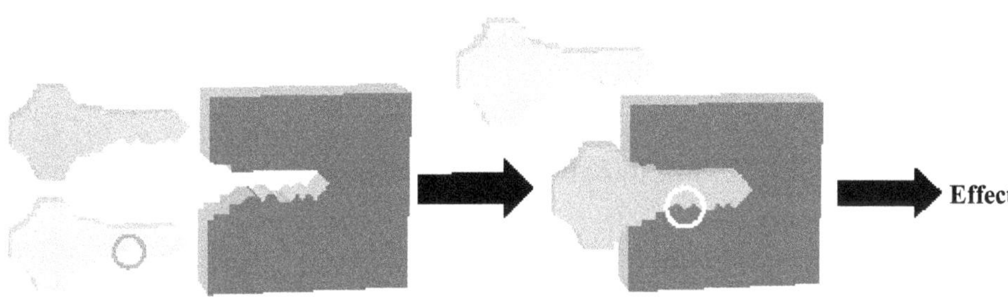

Figure 2.3 Lock-and-key principle for receptor-ligand interactions. Only one of the keys (ligands) fits perfectly into the lock (receptor) and will be able to open the lock (give a response). The small difference between the two keys is indicated by the circle. The 'imperfect' key will fit in the lock, but is not able to open the lock. By sitting in the lock the imperfect key prevents the perfect key getting into the lock. One could regard an antagonist as an imperfect key and a receptor agonist as the perfect key.

(i) Occupation theory:

In fact, similar mathematical models have been applied to the receptor– ligand interaction. Clark's occupation theory was the first model that could describe the observations of drug action in isolated tissues. In this theory the receptor–ligand interaction is considered to be a bimolecular interaction, in which the receptor–ligand complex is responsible for the generation of the biological effect. Clark assumed that the effects of a drug were proportional to the fraction of receptors occupied by the drug. Consequently, for a maximal effect the drug has to occupy all receptors. In Clark's theory, the agonist (A) interacts in a reversible way with the receptor (R) and the formed complex (AR) gives rise to the effect:

$$A + R \Leftrightarrow AR \rightarrow \text{effect}$$

In equilibrium, the rate of the forward reaction of an agonist A reversibly bound to its receptor R is proportional to the concentration of A and R, and the proportionality constant is denoted by K_1:

$$\text{Rate of dissociation} = K_1 [A] [R]$$

Similarly, the rate of the backward reaction, in which the agonist–receptor complex dissociates again, is proportional to the concentration of the AR complex:

$$\text{Rate of dissociation} = K_2 [AR]$$

In equilibrium the rate of the forward reaction equals the rate at which existing AR complexes dissociate i.e., $K_1 [A] [R] = K_2 [AR]$. In other words, within a certain period of time the same number of molecules A will bind to and dissociate from the receptor. In equilibrium the dissociation constant K can be described as follows:

$$K = \frac{K_1}{K_2} = \frac{[A][R]}{[AR]}$$

(ii) Rate theory: Rate theory was proposed by Paton and Rang in 1965. According to this theory the most important factor in determining drug action is the rate at which drug receptor combination takes place. The rate theory can be explained by the formula :

$$\text{Rate of receptor occupation} : \frac{K_2}{1 + \frac{K_1}{[A]}}$$

(iii) Induced-fit theory: This theory states that after combination, the substrate induces a change in confirmation of the enzyme, leading to an enzymatically active orientation of groups. E.g., Acetylcholine may interact with the regulating protein and alter the normal forces.

3

Physicochemical and Stereochemical Properties of Organic Medicinal Agents

At the most fundamental level, the ability of a chemical compound to elicit a pharmacologic/therapeutic effect is influenced by various physical and chemical (*physicochemical*) properties of the chemical substance on the biomolecule(s). Among the most pharmacologically influential physicochemical and stereochemical properties of organic medicinal agents (OMAs) are:

(i) Solubility
(ii) Partition coefficient
(iii) Dissociation constants pK_a
(iv) Ionization of drugs
(v) Hydrogen bonding
(vi) Molar refractivity (MR)
(vii) Drug shape
(viii) Complexation
(ix) Surface activity
(x) Protein binding
(xi) Bioisosterism

(I) Solubility

The solubility of a substance at a given temperature is defined as the concentration of the dissolved solute, which is in equilibrium with the solid solute. Solubility depends on the nature of solute and solvent as well as temperature, pressure, and pH. The solubility of a substance is the ratio of these rate constants at equilibrium in a given solution.

$$K_{solubility} = \frac{k_{solution}}{k_{solid}}$$

The solubility of an organic medicinal agent may be expressed in terms of its affinity/philicity or repulsion/phobicity for either an aqueous (hydro) or organic (lipo) solvent.

- Hydrophilic .... water loving
- Lipophobic .... lipid hating
- Lipophilic .... lipid loving
- Hydrophobic .... water hating

The atoms and molecules of all organic substances are held together by various types of bonds (e.g., London forces, hydrogen bonds, dipole-dipole etc). These forces are intricately involved in solubility because it is the solvent-solvent, solute-solute, and solvent-solute interactions that govern solubility.

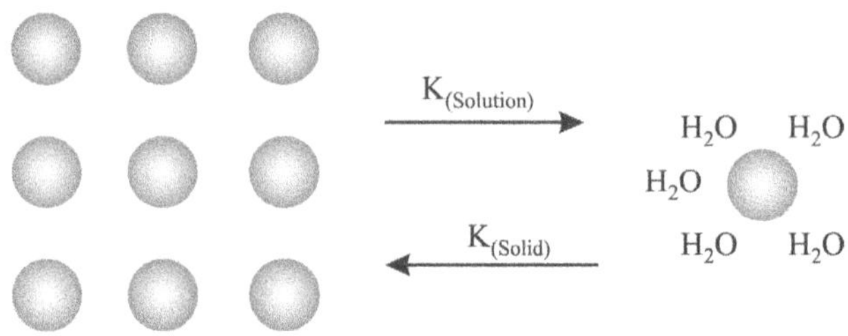

The most important intermolecular attractive forces (bonds) that are involved in the solubilization process are:

1. Van der Waal's attraction

They are weakest intermolecular forces (0.5-1.0 kcal/mole) which occurs between nonpolar groups (e.g., Hydrocarbons). They are highly distance and temperature dependent.

2. Dipole-dipole bonding

These forces occur when electronegative elements are attached to carbon. They are stronger (1.0 to 10 kcal/mole) and occur electrostatically between electron deficient and electron rich atoms (dipoles). Hydrogen bonding is a specific example of this bonding and serves as a prime contributor to hydrophilicity.

3. Ionic bonding

Ionic bond is electrostatic attraction between cations and anions. These ionic attractions are common in inorganic compounds and salts of organic molecules and are relatively strong (5 kcal/mole).

4. Ion-dipole bonding

Ion-Dipole bonding is electrostatic between a cation/anion and a dipole. It is relatively strong (1-5 kcal/mole) and is low temperature and distance dependence. Ion-Dipole bonding is an important interaction between OMAs and H_2O.

The solubility of a drug is a very important physicochemical property governing transfer of OMA's through the biological membrane barriers. Solubility of an OMA is a function of the presence of both lipophilic and hydrophilic features within its structure, which serve to determine the extent of interaction of the OMA with lipid and/or aqueous phases.

Methods to improve solubility of drugs

Structural modifications:

(i) One method to increase solubility of a drug is to alter the structure of the molecule. The addition of polar groups like carboxylic acids, ketones and amines can increase solubility by increasing hydrogen bonding and the interaction with water.

(ii) Another structural modification can be to reduce intramolecular forces. An example of structure modification to enhance solubility by this latter method is methyl dopa (solubility ~10 mg/ml) and methyl dopate (solubility 10-300 mg/ml depending on pH). The addition of the ethyl ester to methyl dopa reduces the intramolecular hydrogen bond between the carboxylic acid and primary amine. Therefore, this addition reduces the melting point and increases solubility.

(iii) ***Use of cosolvents*:** Another method to increase solubility is the use of co-solvents. The use of cosolvents can increase the solubility by several orders of magnitude. Some of the commonly used cosolvents in drug formulation are propylene glycol, polyethylene glycols, ethanol and sorbitol. The addition of a co-solvent can increase solubility of hydrophobic molecules by reducing the dielectric constant of the solvent. Some problems with the use of cosolvents are precipitation of the drug with dilution of solvent mixture and tissue damage or pain upon injection. (This dilution occurs after administration of the drug into the body.)

(iv) ***Employing surfactants*:** Surfactants can also be used to enhance solubility. A surfactant or surface active agent is amphiprotic, means it has polar end (the circular head) and a nonpolar end (the tail). When a surfactant is placed in water it will form micelles. A nonpolar drug will partition into the hydrophobic core of the micelle and the polar tails will solubilize the complex.

(v) ***Complexation*:** There are many types of complexing agents. Complexation relies on relatively weak forces such as London forces, hydrogen bonding and hydrophobic interactions. As the concentration of complexing agent is increased, the solubility increases up to a point. In some cases however, the complex can precipitate out of solution as the concentration of complexing agent is increased.

Importance of solubility

1. The concept of solubility is important to pharmacist because it governs the preparation of liquid dosage forms and the drug must be in solution before it is absorbed by the body to elicit the biological activity.
2. Drugs must be in solution to interact with receptors. Drugs have some degree of solubility in both aqueous and lipid compartments. In order for a chemical compound to dissolve in a particular solvent/medium the compound must exhibit attractive forces between itself and molecules of the solvent. Hence, it is possible to estimate the solubility properties of an OMA (hydrophilic vs. lipophilic) by examining the structure of the OMA and noting whether its structural features promote affinity for aqueous or lipid media.

(II) Partition coefficient

Partition coefficient influences the absorption and transport of drugs in body compartments. The ability of a drug to partition into a lipid phase when an aqueous phase is also present, this is also referred as lipophilicity, which can be best characterized by determining partition coefficient. It can be defined as the equilibrium constant of drug concentrations for "unionizable" molecules in the two phases:

$$P = \frac{[\text{drug}]_{\text{lipid}}}{[\text{drug}]_{\text{water}}}$$

and for "ionizable" molecules (acids, bases, salts), where alpha is the degree of ionization in aqueous solution. It is basically a constitutive property.

$$P = \frac{[\text{drug}]_{\text{lipid}}}{(1-\alpha)[\text{drug}]_{\text{water}}}$$

Thus, partition coefficient is described as:

$$\text{Drug}_{\text{W(aqueous)}} \xrightarrow{\text{PC}} \text{Drug}_{\text{O(organic)}}$$

Partition coefficient thoroughly influence drug transport characteristics; the way the drugs reaches the site of action from the site of application (e.g., injection site, gastrointestinal tract, and so forth). Since the blood distributes drugs, they must penetrate and traverse many cells to reach the site of action. Hence, the partition coefficient will determine to which tissues a given compound can reach. Naturally, the partition coefficient is one of the several physicochemical parameters influencing drug transport and distribution, which itself is (only) one aspect of drug activity. The contribution of each functional group, their structural arrangement help to determine the lipophilic or hydrophilic character of the drug molecule and hence its partitioning. Partitioning coefficient is one of the most widely used properties in QSAR studies.

For example,

Compound	Lipid/water partition coefficient
Ethanol	0.03
Morphine	0.40
Barbitone	1.40
Phenobarbitone	5.90

Phenobarbitone has a high lipid/water partition coefficient of 5.9. Thiopentone sodium has a chloroform/water partition coefficient of about 100, so it is highly soluble in lipid. Hence thiopentone sodium is used as ultra-short acting barbiturate.

Partition coefficient measurement

Since partition coefficients are difficult to measure in living systems, they are usually determined *invitro* using 1-octanol (n-octanol) as the lipid phase and a phosphate buffer of pH 7.4 as the aqueous phase. This permits standardized measurements of partition coefficients. Because it is a ratio, P is dimensionless, and its logarithm (log P) is widely used as the measure of lipophilicity.

1. **Log P by shake flask:** The shake flask method is the oldest and most tedious way of measuring log P values. The ultraviolet (UV) absorbance of an aqueous solution is measured before and after being shaken with a known volume of octanol. The method is messy and smelly but is the only method that can be used in case of very low log P values. One advantage of this method is that the appearance of compound in the octanol may be checked against the disappearance from the aqueous phase to see if any surface effects have occurred. The experiment must be performed over 3 days or more to ensure equilibrium is reached, although the actual time taken in doing the experiment is about 12 hours.
2. **Log P by high performance liquid chromatography (HPLC) :** HPLC may be used to estimate log P values. Compounds with known log P's are injected onto a C-18 reverse phase HPLC column to create a calibration curve. Unknown compounds are then injected to predict log P. Strictly this technique is only valid for neutral molecules. Charged molecules have far more complex retention behavior than simple molecules.

   The chromatographic methods suffer the disadvantage that the retention time is linearly related to the partition coefficient, i.e., for a doubling of the log P, there is a ten fold increase in the retention. This often requires different length columns to be used, short ones for high log P values and long ones for low values.

Relationship between Log P and biological activity

The partition coefficient is also a very useful parameter that may be used in combination with the pK_a to predict the distribution of drug in biological system. Factors such as absorption, excretion and penetration of the CNS may be related to the log P value of a drug and in certain cases predictions can be made. Drugs should be designed with the lowest possible log P, to reduce toxicity, non-specific binding, increase ease of formulation and bioavailability (Drugs should also be as low molecular weight as possible to lower the risk of allergic reactions).

Relationships between log P and activity are often found in series where structural modifications have not significantly affected the pK_a values. Hansch in 1964 showed that these relationships were often parabolic hence the relationship often leads to an optimum value for the log P for a desired activity or selective distribution. Relationships of the following type are generated using regression analysis to correlate observed biological data with measured partition coefficients.

$$\text{Activity} = m \log P + k^1 \text{ (linear)}$$

$$\text{Activity} = m \log P - c(\log P)2 - k\text{(parabolic)}$$

$$\text{Activity} = m \log P - c(b\log P + 1) - k \text{ (rectilinear)}$$

(where m, k and c are constants)

The best way of relating log P, pK_a and other physicochemical data to biological activity is using multivariate techniques such as Principal Components Analysis (PCA) and Partial Least Squares Regression (PLSR).

(III) Dissociation constants (pK_a)

The dissociation constant is one of the most important characteristic features of a pharmaceutical compound. It is important to understand how it is calculated, and its significance. The majority of drugs are weak acids or weak bases and like acetic acid or like ammonia, they react with water to form conjugate pairs. The pK_a or 'Dissociation constant' is a measure of the strength of an acid or a base and is sometimes called the acidity constant or the ionization constant. It is a numeric representation of the relative proton transfer for that substance, or the likelihood of that compound donating a proton. It is calculated in the same manner as the equilibrium constant.

$$\underset{\text{}}{\text{Drug-Weak Acid}} + \underset{\text{(base)}}{\text{Water}} \rightleftharpoons \underset{\text{conjugate acid}}{H_3O^+} + \underset{\text{conjugate base}}{\text{Drug}}$$

$$\underset{\text{}}{\text{Drug-Weak Base}} + \underset{\text{(acid)}}{\text{Water}} \rightleftharpoons \underset{\text{conjugate base}}{OH^-} + \underset{\text{conjugate acid}}{\text{Drug}}$$

Let's consider equation for the protolysis of water by an acidic drug.

$$HA + H_2O \rightleftharpoons H_3O^+ + A^-$$

At equilibrium, the velocity of the reaction proceeding to the ionized components (k_1) is equal to the velocity of the reaction resulting in the unionized HA and H_2O (k_2).

$$(k_1) = [HA][H_2O]$$

$$(k_2) = [H_3O^+][A^-]$$

Weakly acidic and basic drugs ionize only slightly in the presence of water. If that being the case, the concentration of water in the above equation may be taken as a constant, by rearranging the equation to yield:

$$K_a = k_{eq}\,[H_2O] = K_{eq}\,(55.53) = \frac{[H_3o^+][A^-]}{[HA]}$$

where 55.53 is the number of moles of water per liter at 25°C.

This value K_a gives us numeric value to express the degree to which a compound ionizes, or dissociates, in an aqueous solution. This dissociation constant is an important characteristic of drug molecules, and provides a tool to anticipate some of the "behaviors" of that compound. Dissociation constants are determined by experimental data, and are unique to each molecule. Conductivity, freezing point depression, pH of solution, and spectrophotometric data may be used to determine a compound's dissociation constant.

E.g., Acetaminophen is an acidic drug with a K_a of 1.2×10^{-10}, and is thus much less likely to ionize in aqueous solution than aspirin (acetyl salicylic acid), which has a K_a of 3.27×10^{-4}.

Often, it is cumbersome to deal with exponential forms, so pK_a may be used to describe the tendency of a weak acid to ionize. The following equation should be used to calculate the pK_a of a substance.

$$pK_a = -\log\ [A^-][H_3O^+]/[HA]$$

Relationship to pK_a and acid strength

For almost all the drugs, the dissociation constants are reported as pK_a, regardless of whether the drug is a weak acid or a weak base. For acids, K_a refers to the ability of the acid to give out the proton. Therefore, the higher the tendency of an acid to give out the proton, the stronger the acid (or the lower the pK_a value). For bases, K_a refers to the ability of the conjugated acid form of the base to give out the proton. Therefore, the higher the conjugated acid's (of the base) tendency to give out the proton (the lower the pK_a value), the weaker the original base. In other words, the conjugated acid of a stronger base has a lesser tendency to give out the proton because a strong base attracts the proton more than a weak base does.

Let's look at some examples of acidic and basic drugs:

Acidic drugs:

$$HA + H_2O \rightleftharpoons H_3O^+ + A^-$$

	K_a	K_b*	pK_a	pK_b*
Penicillin V	2.0×10^{-3}	5.4×10^{-12}	2.7	11.3
Acetylsalicylic Acid	3.3×10^{-4}	3.1×10^{-11}	3.5	10.5
Ascorbic Acid	5.0×10^{-5}	2.0×10^{-10}	4.3	9.7
Zidovudine	2.0×10^{-10}	5.0×10^{-5}	9.7	4.3

Basic drugs:

$$A + H_2O \rightleftharpoons HA^+ + OH^-$$

	K_a	K_b*	pK_a	pK_b*
Caffeine	2.5×10^{-4}	4.0×10^{-11}	3.6	10.4
Zalcitabine	6.3×10^{-5}	1.6×10^{-10}	4.2	9.8
Theophylline	3.4×10^{-6}	1.6×10^{-9}	5.2	8.8
Morphine	7.4×10^{-7}	7.4×10^{-7}	7.9	6.1
Erythromycin	2.0×10^{-9}	6.3×10^{-6}	8.8	5.2

Importance of pK_a : The ratio of ionized over unionized form affects drug's solubility, permeability, binding, and other characteristics. pK_a and log P measurements are useful parameters in understanding the behaviour of drug molecules.

(IV) Ionization of drugs

The accumulation of an ionized drug in a compartment of the body is known as "ion trapping". The ionization of a drug is dependent on its pK_a and the pH. The pK_a is the negative log of K_a. The K_a is the acidification constant of a compound, its tendency to release a proton. The ratio of ionized/ non ionized drug may be determined by use of the Henderson- Hasselbalch relationship,

$$\text{pH-p}K_a = \log([A^-]/[HA])$$
$$= \log([\text{ionized}]/[\text{non ionized}]) \text{ for acids}$$
$$\text{pH-p}K_a = \log([B]/[HB^+])$$
$$= \log([\text{non ionized}]/[\text{ionized}]) \text{ for bases}$$

fraction non ionized = $[HA]/([HA] + [A^-]) = 1/ 1 + ([A^-]/ [HA])) = 1/(1 + antilog(pH - pK_a))$

This may be used to derive an Effective Partition Coefficient:

Effective Partition Coefficient = (fraction non ionized) × (partition coefficient)

An example of this is given below to illustrate the penetration of weak acid thiopental into the cerebrospinal fluid. The pK_a of thiopental is 7.6, and its partition coefficient non-ionized is 3.3. The pH of cerebrospinal fluid is 7.4.

The ratio of ionized/ non-ionized is antilog (– 0.2) = 0.63. Therefore the fraction non-ionized is 1/1.63, and the effective partition coefficient is 2.013

Since its pK_a is 7.6, pH values below this favor the formation of protonated, unionized drug, and increase its lipophilicity and membrane permeability.

Importance of ionization of drugs

1. The lower the pH relative to the pK_a: Greater fraction of protonated drug (protonated drug may be charged or uncharged)
2. Weak acid at acid pH: More lipid-soluble because it is uncharged, the uncharged form more readily passes through biological membranes.
    - Note that a weak acid at acid pH will pick up a proton and become uncharged
    - $RCOO^- + H^+ \rightarrow RCOOH$
3. Weak base at alkaline pH: More lipid-soluble because it is uncharged, the uncharged form more readily passes through biological membranes.
    - Note that a weak base at more alkaline pH will lose a proton.
    - $RNH_3^+ \rightarrow RNH_2 + H^+$

(V) Hydrogen bonding

The hydrogen bond is a special type of dipole-dipole interaction between the hydrogen atom in a polar bond such as N-H, O-H, or F-H and an electronegative atom O, N, or F atom. This interaction is written as A-H….B-H. A & B represent O, N or F. A-H is one molecule (or) part of a molecule and B is a part of another molecule; and the dotted line represents the hydrogen bond. These three atoms usually lie along the straight line, but the angle A-H-B or A-H-A can deviate as much as 30° from linearity.

E.g : Hydrogen bonding in NH_3, H_2O and HF

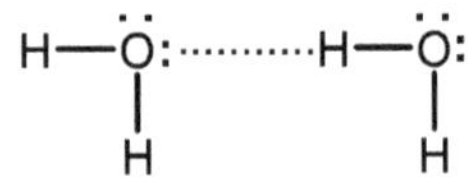

H_2O-H_2O

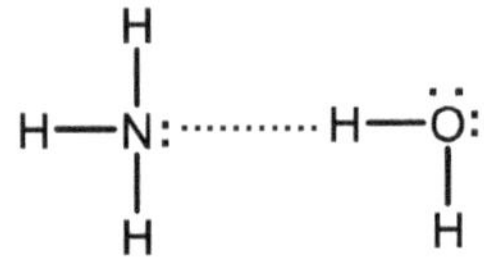

NH_3-H_2O

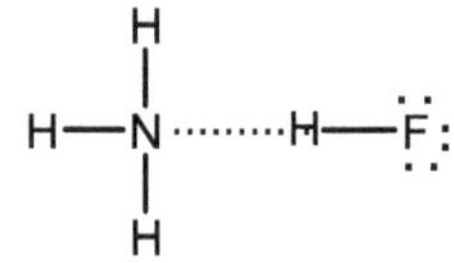

NH_3-HF

Generally the hydrogen bonding is classified into two types

1. Intermolecular hydrogen bonding,
2. Intramolecular hydrogen bonding.

1. Intermolecular hydrogen bonding

In this type, hydrogen bonding occurs between two or more than two molecules of the same or different compound and results in the formation of polymeric aggregate.

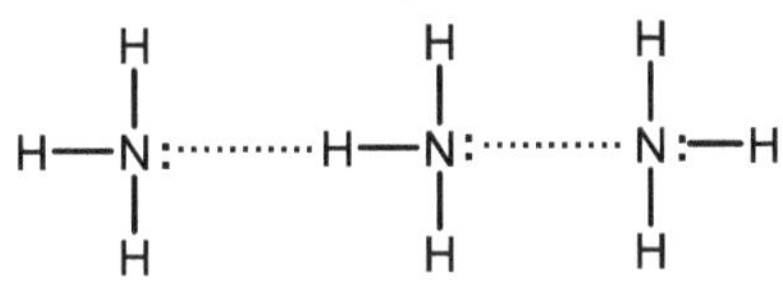

Hydrogen bonding ammonia

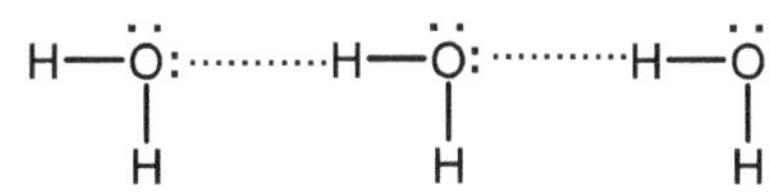

Hydrogen bonding in water

Intermolecular hydrogen bonding increases the boiling point of the compound and also its solubility in water. The increase in boiling point is due to association of several molecules of the compound. As a result the effective molecular weight of the compound increases and hence more energy (large amount of heat) is required to dissociate the molecules for vaporization. The molecules that are able to develop intermolecular hydrogen bonding posses more solubility in water. E.g., Ethanol shows higher boiling point and higher solubility in water than dimethyl ether even though both have the same molecular weight.

	Molecular weight	**Boiling point**
Ethanol (C_2H_6O)	46	78°C
Dimethyl ether (C_2H_6O)	46	-25°C
Diethyl ether ($C_4H_{10}O$)	74	61°C
1-Butanol ($C_4H_{10}O$)	74	118°C

2. Intramolecular hydrogen bonding

In this type, hydrogen bonding occurs within two atoms of the same molecule. This type of hydrogen bonding is commonly known as chelation and frequently occurs in organic compounds. Sometimes intramolecular hydrogen bonding develops a six or five-membered ring. E.g.,

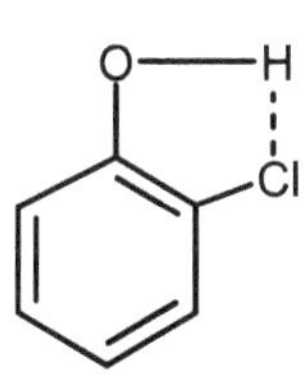

Hydrogen bonding in o-Chlorophenol

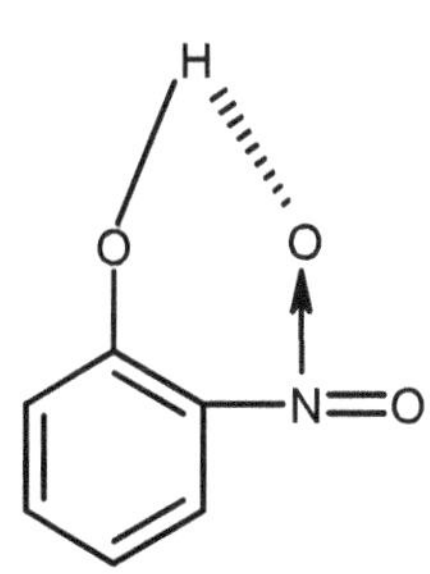

Hydrogen bonding in *o*-Nitro phenol

Intramolecular hydrogen bonding decreases the boiling point of the compound and also its solubility in water. This is because of the fact that the chelation between the ortho substituted groups restricts the possibility of intermolecular hydrogen bonding with water and thus prevents association of the molecules, which would have raised the melting point, boiling point. Chelation is not possible in the corresponding *meta* and *para* isomers because the two groups are far away from each other. Hence in such cases, intermolecular hydrogen bonding takes place, which in turn increases the boiling point. Thus we can explain the low melting point and boiling point of the *ortho* isomers of hydroxy, nitro and carbonyl compounds than the corresponding *meta* and *para* isomers.

o-Nitrophenol — Boiling point

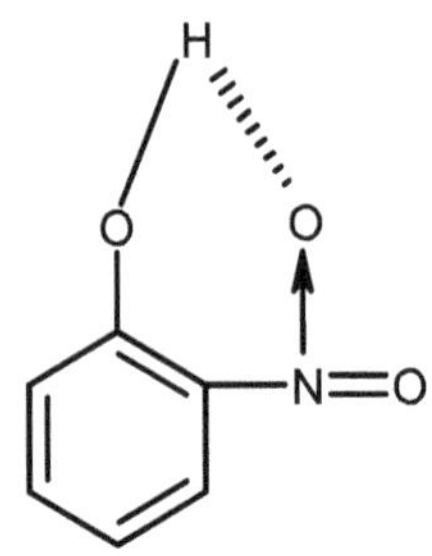

215 °C

Hydrogen bonding in *o*-Nitro phenol

p-Nitrophenol — Boiling point

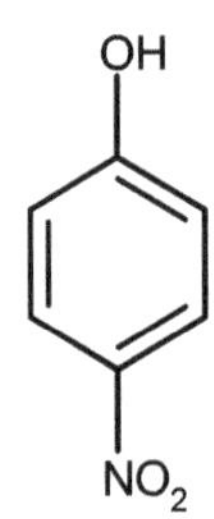

279 °C

m-Nitrophenol

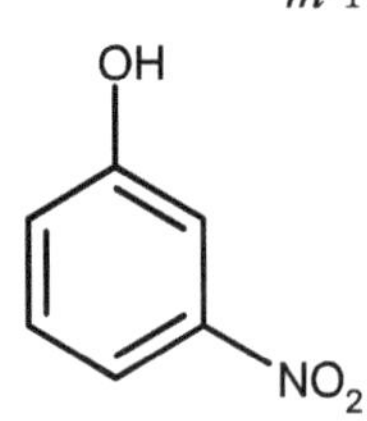

279 °C

Effects of hydrogen bonding

Almost all physical properties are affected by hydrogen bonding. Here only those properties that prominently alter boiling point, melting point, water solubility etc., are discussed. In addition to physical properties several chemical properties like acid character, basic character, properties of carbonyl group are also affected by hydrogen bonding.

(i) **Boiling and melting points:** Intermolecular hydrogen bonding increases the boiling point of the compound due to association of several molecules of the same compound. As a result the intermolecular forces are increased and hence more energy (large amount of heat) is required to dissociate the molecules for vaporization. Intramolecular hydrogen bonding decreases the boiling point of the compound because of the fact that the chelation between the groups of same molecule restricts the possibility of intermolecular hydrogen bonding and thus prevents association of the molecules, which would have raised the melting point and boiling point.

(ii) **Water solubility:** Solubility of a substance increases tremendeously when hydrogen bonding is possible between the solvent and the solute. E.g., Methanol and ethanol are highly soluble in water due to hydrogen bonding between molecules.

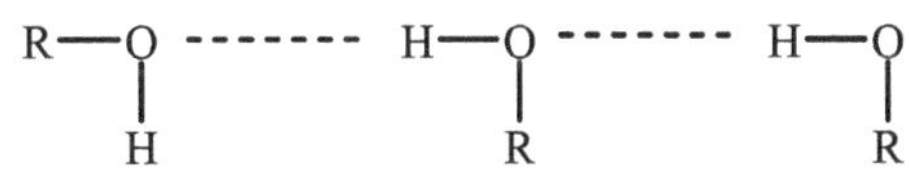

The high solubility of polyhydric phenols and sugars may be attributed to the fact that these compounds make available greater number of –OH groups for hydrogen bonding.

(iii) **Strength of acids:** Any structural feature that contributes for the greater stability of anion in comparison to free acid will shift the ionization equilibrium to the right. Thus if the anion of acid were stabilized due to intramolecular hydrogen bonding, there would be marked increase in the strength of acid. E.g., The ionization constant of salicylic acid is higher than the other two isomers and is 17 times more acidic than benzoic acid.

(iv) **Spectroscopic properties:** The hydrogen bonding shifts the position of bands in infrared and NMR spectra of organic compounds. E.g., Infrared spectrum of ethyl alcohol in vapour phase shows absorption band at 3700 cm^{-1} due to free hydroxyl group. In solution this band is completely replaced by a broad band around 3500 cm^{-1} which is characteristic of hydrogen bonded hydroxyl groups.

(v) **On surface tension and viscosity:** The compounds, which possess hydrogen bonding, are found to have higher surface tension and viscosity. Glycerol, glycol, sulphuric acid, sugar syrup, phosphoric acid, etc., are viscous liquids due to extensive hydrogen bonding between their molecule. Due to more number of hydroxyl (OH) groups, the extent of hydrogen bonding is more in glycerol. So, it is more viscous than glycol.

(vi) **Biological products:** The three dimensional structures of proteins and nucleic acids are due to hydrogen bonding. In α-helices, hydrogen bonds extend from the hydrogen atoms of polar N - H units in peptide group to oxygen atoms of polar carbonyl units.

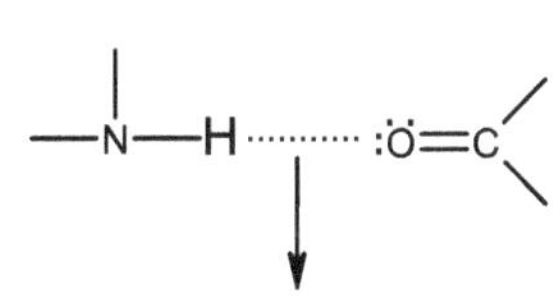

Hydrogen bonding

Hydrogen bonds are extremely important in the chemistry of the genetic code. As we will study later, the double strands of Deoxyribonucleic acid (DNA) are held together by hydrogen bonds. The replication of DNA depends on hydrogen bonds which selectively connect specific base pairs, as there are several steps by which the genetic message determines the specific order of amino acids in a protein.

(vii) **Drug-receptor interactions:** Hydrogen bonding is also a secondary binding force in drug-receptor interactions.

(V) Molar refractivity (MR)

The molar refractivity is the molar volume corrected by the refractive index. It represents size and polarizability of a fragment or a molecule. Originally it was proposed by Pauling and Pressman as a parameter for the correlation of dispersion forces involved in the binding of haptens to antibodies. But now it is determined from the refractive index 'n', the molecular weight 'MW' and the density of a crystal 'd'.

A smaller MR for the same molecular weight indicates stronger interactions in the crystal (larger density indicates that the packing is better due to stronger interactions).

$$MR = \frac{(n^2 - 1)}{(n^2 + 1)} \times \frac{MW}{d}$$

(VII) Drug shape

The shape of the drug is an important factor in defining the nature of the drug-receptor interaction. The three-dimensional shape of the drug is thought to interact with a complementary structural binding region of the receptor, typically a protein. The specific nature of the interaction defines whether the drug acts as an agonist promoting a change in cellular function or as an antagonist, which blocks the receptor usually resulting in biological effect.

For example, let's consider acetylcholine or a synthetic analogue bethanechol (urecholine). Interaction of these molecules with receptor (nicotinic or muscarinic cholinergic receptor) causes a physiological response i.e., a decrease in heartbeats for instance. By contrast, a muscarinic antagonist such as atropine may bind even more tightly than acetylcholine to muscarinic receptor but causes no direct effect. However, following administration of antagonist a biological response may be observed as a result of receptor blockade.

(VIII) Complexation

Complexes or coordination compounds result from a donor-acceptor mechanism (donating-accepting electron or, rather, an electron pair) or Lewis acid-base reaction (donating-accepting protons). Any nonmetallic atom or ion, whether free or contained in a neutral molecule or in an ionic compound, that can donate an electron pair, may serve as the donor. The acceptor, or constituent that accept a share in the pair of electrons, can be a metal ion or sometimes also a neutral molecule. In addition to "coordinate covalence" (i.e., bonds formed by the classical electron donor-acceptor mechanism), intramolecular forces can also be involved in the formation of complexes.

Complexes may be divided broadly into two classes depending on whether the acceptor compound is a metal ion or an organic molecule:

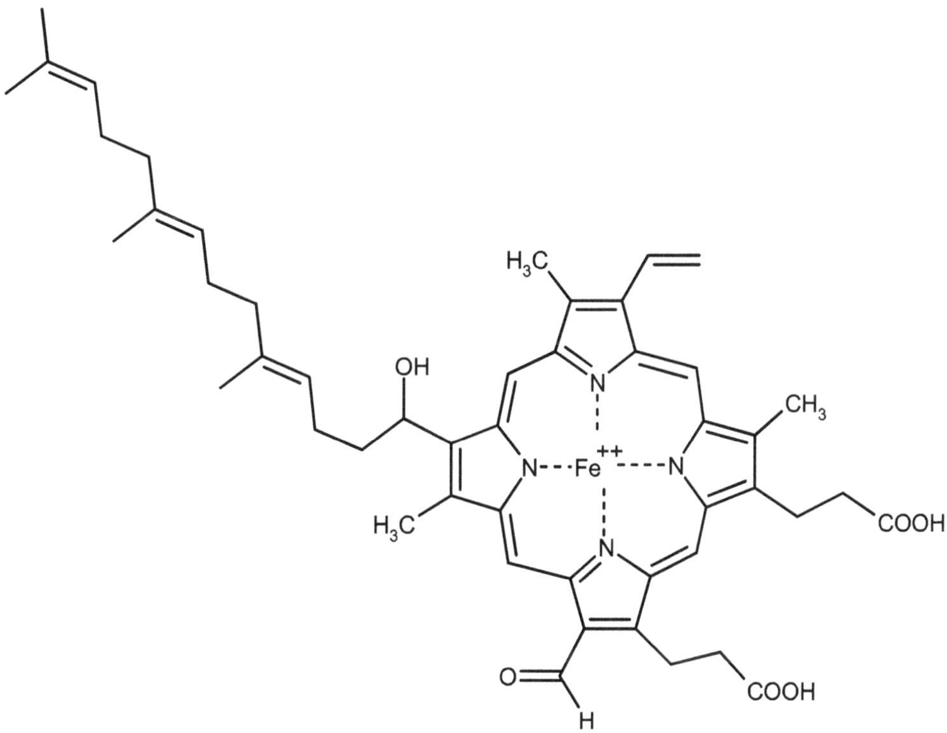

Hema (Found in cytochrome oxidase)

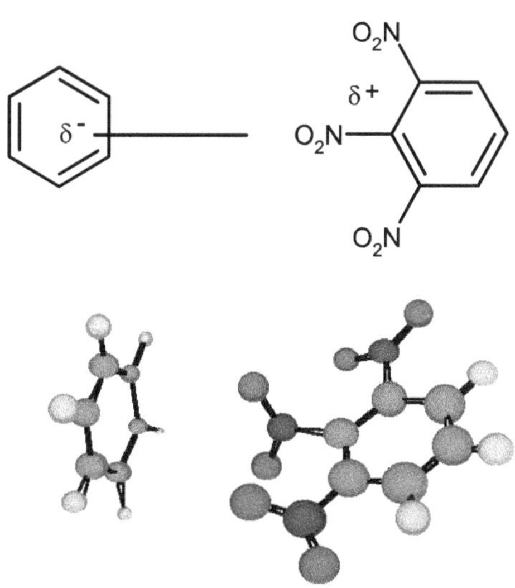

A third class, the inclusion complexes, involve the entrapment of one compound in the molecular framework of another:

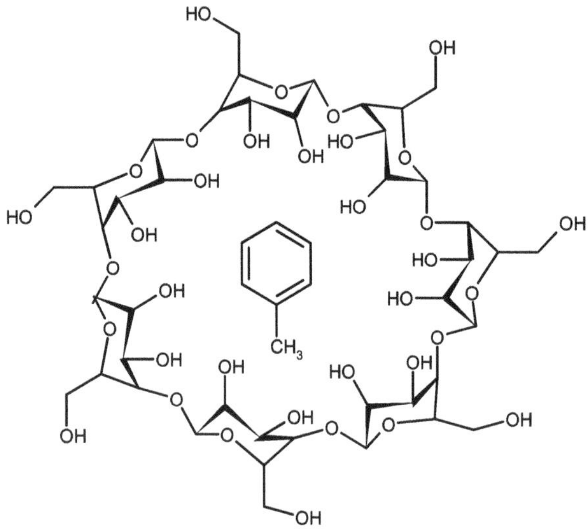

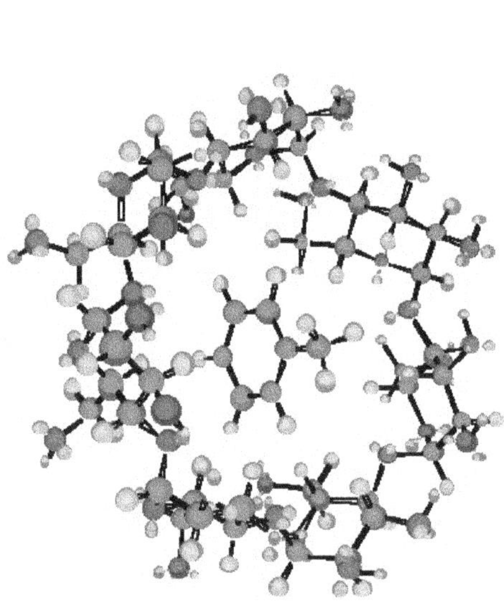

The compounds that are obtained by donating electrons to metal ion with the formation of a ring structure are called Chelates. The compounds capable of forming a ring structure with a metal atom are termed as ligands. Most of the metals are capable of forming Chelates or complexes (if the metal is not in a ring, the compound is called a metal complex), but the chelating property is restricted to atoms like N, O and S, which are electron donating.

Applications of chelation

The phenomenon of chelation is significantly involved in biological system and to some extent in explaining drug action.

1. Dimercaprol is a chelating agent. It is an effective antidote for organic arsenical lewsite, but can also be used for poisoning due to antimony, gold and mercury.
2. Penicillamine is an effective antidote for the treatment of copper poisoning because it forms water soluble chelate with copper and other metal ions.
3. 8-Hydroxyquinoline and its analogues act as antibacterial and antifungal agents by complexing with iron or copper.

(IX) Surface activity

A surfactant is briefly defined as a material that can greatly reduce the surface tension of water when used in very low concentrations. This molecule is made up of water soluble (hydrophilic) and a water insoluble (hydrophobic) components.

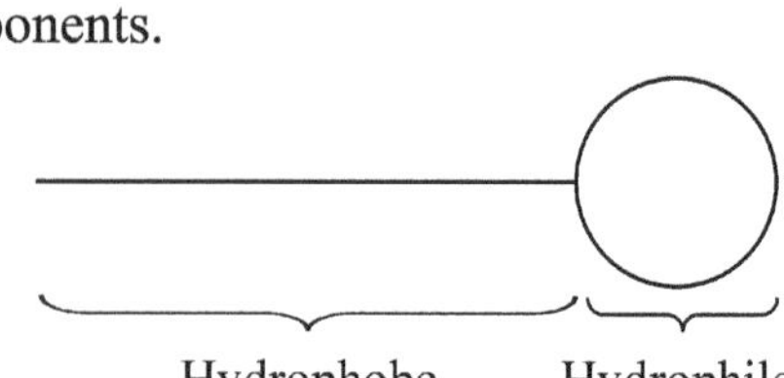

The hydrophobe is usually the equivalent of an eight to eighteen carbon, hydrocarbon, and can be aliphatic, aromatic, or a mixture of both. The sources of hydrophobes are normally natural fats and oils, petroleum fractions, relatively short synthetic polymers, or relatively high molecular weight synthetic alcohols. The hydrophilic groups give the primary classification to surfactants, and are anionic, cationic and non-ionic in nature. The anionic hydrophiles are the carboxylates (soaps), sulphates, sulphonates and phosphates. The cationic hydrophiles are some form of an amine product. The non-ionic hydrophiles associate with water at the ether oxygens of a polyethylene glycol chain. In each case, the hydrophilic end of the surfactant is strongly attracted to the water molecules and the force of attraction between the hydrophobe and water is only slight. As a result, the surfactant molecules align themselves at the surface and internally so that the hydrophile end is towards the water and the hydrophobe is squeezed away from the water.

Because of this characteristic behaviour of surfactants to orient at surfaces and to form micelles, all surfactants perform certain basic functions. Foaming agents, emulsifiers, and dispersants are surfactants, which suspend respectively, a gas, an immiscible liquid, or a solid in water or some other liquid.

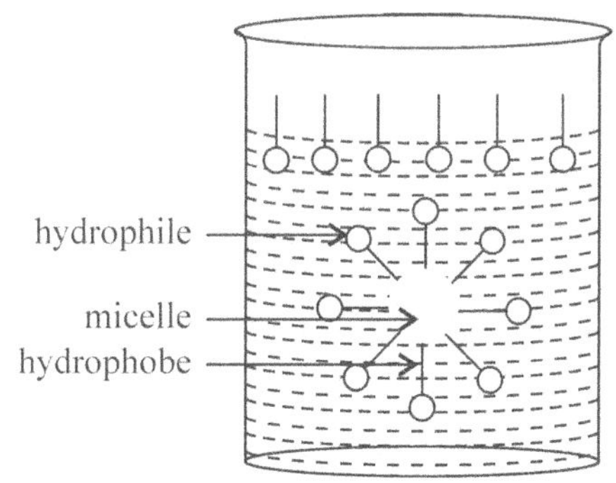

1. The bactericidal activity of cationic quaternary ammonium compounds such as benzalkonium chloride, cetrimide, cetylpyridinium chloride, etc., is explained through their surface activity property.
2. The anthelmentic activity of hexylresorcinols is explained by their surface activity property.
3. Steroidal hormones and barbiturates have surface activity properties.
4. Phenol and cresol act as disinfectants by denaturing the proteins of biological membranes.

(X) Protein binding

Depending upon whether the drug is a weak or strong acid or base, or is neutral, it can bind to a single blood protein, to multiple proteins (e.g., Serum albumin, acid-glycoprotein (AGP) or lipoproteins). The most significant protein involved in the binding of drugs is albumin, which comprises more than half of all blood proteins. Albumin can interact with acidic or basic drugs in the plasma by van der Waals dispersion forces, hydrophobic bonding, hydrogen bonding, and ionic interactions. AGP interacts mainly with basic entities whereas lipoproteins bind to both basic and neutral drugs. Protein binding, whether covalent or non-specific, is strongly influenced by inter-molecular electrostatic interactions. Zeta potential is a function of the particle surface charge density, and can be used as a measure of the strength of these electrostatic interactions. Protein binding values (% fraction bound) are normally given as the percentage of the total plasma concentration of a drug that is bound to all plasma proteins. In most cases, binding to plasma proteins is reversible, and the concentration of the free and bound species of the drug at equilibrium may be expressed as:

$$\text{Free drug } [D_f] + \text{Free protein } [P_f] \rightleftharpoons \text{Drug/Protein complex } [DP]$$

The total plasma concentration of the drug is expressed as the sum of the percent of free drug and the percent bound.

Total plasma concentration $[D_t] = [D_f] + [DP]$

Binding measurements are made *invitro*, at multiple drug plasma concentration levels in the clinically achievable range. A single (average) value result of such measurements indicates a relatively constant bound-to-free ratio over the range of plasma concentrations examined. In situations like where drug binding is concentration dependent, two values are given, representing the percent bound values for the upper and lower limits of the range of concentrations examined. Only single activity values, indicating an average, were used in the generation of this model. The protein samples used in binding studies are taken from healthy individuals because there are several disease states that can affect the protein binding of drugs. Examples include hepatic diseases that alter the concentration of albumin in the plasma and uremia that can cause changes in the binding affinity of some drugs.

Importance

The extent to which a drug is bound to plasma proteins can affect the distribution of the drug in several ways.

The drug/protein complex does not pass through phospholipid bilayers, including capillary membranes, glomerular membranes in the nephrons, and the blood brain barrier.

Bound drugs are also less available to the enzymes involved in first-pass metabolism. After the metabolic and excretory processes have cleared much of the free drug, the reversible drug/protein complex serves as a depot to replenish the concentration *in vivo*.

For these reasons, drugs with high protein binding activity values tend to have a greater half-life compared to those with lower values. The prolonged activity resulting from these factors may be desirable, or may promote the emergence of undesirable side effects

The fraction of the drug which is bound to the protein is incapable of crossing cell membranes and interacting with receptors. It is the fraction which is free in the plasma water which has biological activity. Drugs may interact with one another at the level of plasma protein binding and some drugs may displace others from their binding sites. In this event, although the total concentration of the drug in the plasma is unaltered, its unbound concentration rises. The potency of the drug may rise as a consequence. This may have important toxic and therapeutic consequences in some cases.

(XI) Bioisosterism

I. Langmuir introduced the term isosterism in 1919 and postulated that two molecules or ions or radicals having the same number and arrangement of electrons are called isosteres. Accordingly the isosters should be isoelectric i.e., they should possess same total charge.

   For example,

   (i) CO and NO_2

(ii) CO_2 and N_2O
(iii) N_3 and NCO^-
(iv) CH_2N_2 and $CH_2 = CO$

The widespread application of the concept of isosterism is to modify (or) improve biological activity that has been risen to the term bioisosterism. Bioisosteres are components or groups that possess nearly equal molecular shapes and volumes, approximately with the same distribution of electrons, and which exhibit similar physical properties. Bioisosteres, however, are substituents or groups that do not necessarily have the same size or volume, but have a similarity in chemical or physical properties, produce broadly similar biological properties. Traditionally bioisosteres have been classified into two groups. They are:

1. Classical bioisosteres

Classical replacement is "like for like" in terms of number of atoms, valency, degree of unsaturation, and aromaticity and then only becomes a bioisosteric replacement if biological activity is retained. The classical bioisosteres may be univalent atoms and groups [(a).–CH_3, –NH_2, –OH, –F, –Cl; (b). –Cl, –NH_2 –SH; (c). –Br, –I, –propyl and (d) *tert*-butyl] bivalent atoms and groups [(a). –CH_2–, –NH, –O–, –S–, –Se–; (b). –$COCH_2$–, CONH–, –COO–, –COS–], trivalent atoms and groups [(a). –CH=, –N= and (b). –P=, –AS=], tetravalent atoms and groups [(a). >C<, >Si< and (b). =C=, =N^+=, =P^+=] or ring equivalents [(a). benzene, thiophene; (b). benzene, pyridine; (c). tetrahydrofuran, tetrahydrothiophene, cyclopentane, pyrrolidine].

(i) **Fluorine vs. hydrogen replacement:** The substitution of hydrogen by fluorine is one of the most commonly employed monovalent isosteric replacements. The antineoplastic agent 5-fluorouracil represents a classical example of how fluorine substitution of a normal enzyme substrate can result in a derivative, which can alter the enzymatic processes.

(ii) **Divalent replacements involving double bonds:** The replacement of C=S with C=O in tolrestat (1), an aldose reductase inhibitor currently under study in human subjects for the treatment of diabetic neuropathy, resulted in oxo-tolrestat(2) which retained activity both *invitro* and *invivo*.

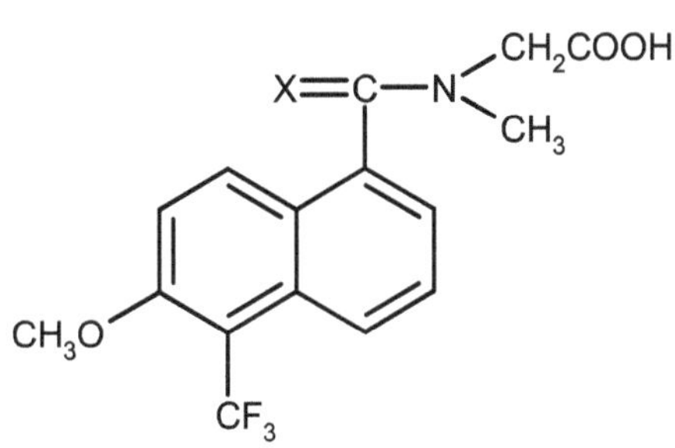

1 X = S

2 X = O

Tolrestat

(iii) Trivalent ring equivalents: The trivalent substitution of –CH= with –N= is commonly used in modern drug design, trivalent ring subsitution of –CH= with –N= in the antibacterial agent norfloxacin resulted in enoxacin which is also in clinical use for its antibacterial activity.

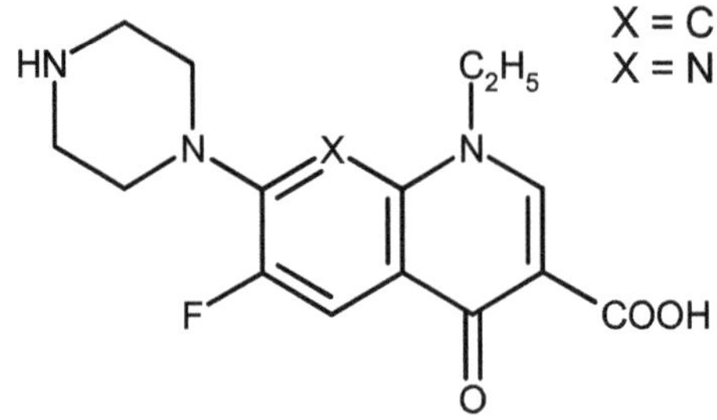

X = C Norfloxacin
X = N Enoxacin

2. Non-classical bioisosteres

The non classical bioisosters comprise groups which are structurally similar but do not meet the electronic and steric requirements in the rigorous sense. These isosters retain the activity by mimicking the spatial arrangements, electronic properties or physico chemical property of the molecule like pka.

For Example,

(i) Attempts to increase the duration of action artilyperfeasive of agents by preventing their metabolism has resulted in potent and selective agents.

They are albuterol (3-CH_2OH), soterenol(3-$NHSO_2CH_2$) and carbuterol (3-NH $CONH_2$).

Isoproterenol (3-OH) is the prototype of the β-adrenergic agonists and is widely used as bronchodialator; however it is not a β_2-selective agent.

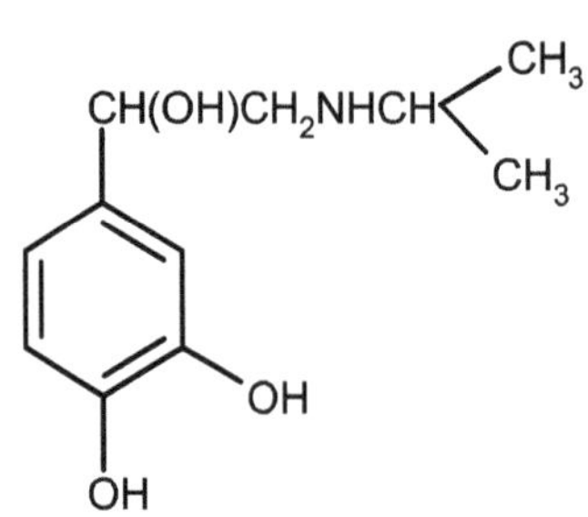

Isoproterenol

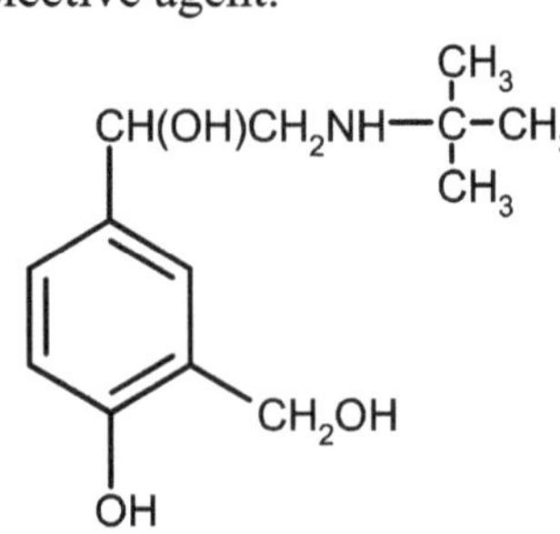

Albuterol

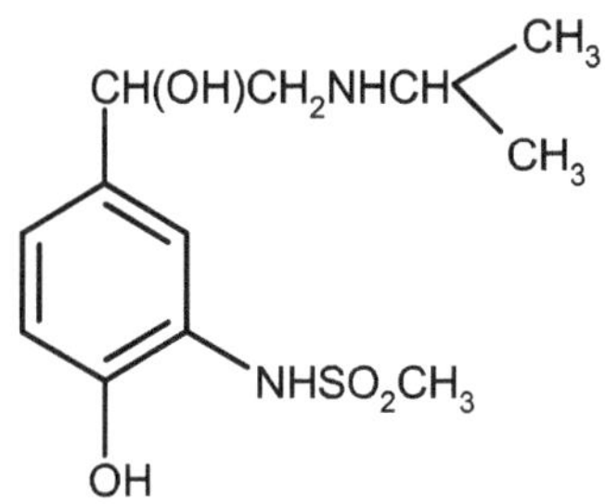

Soterenol

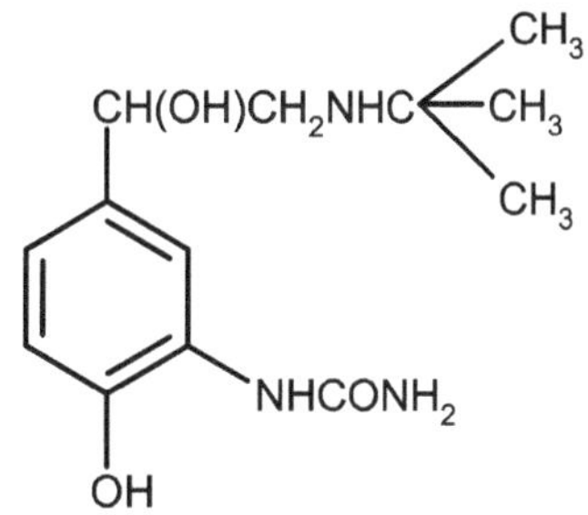

Carbuterol

Isoproterenol is rapidly metabolized by catechol-*o*-methyltransferase (COMT) which catalyzes the methylation of the m-hydroxy group. But albuterol and soterenol are not susceptible to metabolism by COMT.

(ii) Peptide bonds and peptide fragments have been replaced with a wide variety of structural moieties in attempts to convert peptides into chemically stable and orally available molecules. Bioisosteres of the amide bond are:

-CONH-, NHCN-, CH_2NHCO-, -COCH_2-, -NHCONH-, -CH_2NH-, NHCO_2-, NHCOS-, CO_2-, NHSO_2-, -CH(OH)CH_2, etc.

(iii) In search for improved antihyperlipidemic agents, the tetrazolyl analogue of nicotinic acid was found to be three times as active in lowering blood cholesterol.

Bioisosterism represents one approach used by the medicinal chemists for the rational modification of lead compounds into safer and more clinically effective agents. Thus bioisosterism has numerous advantageous and applications in resolving biological problems effectively.

4

QUANTITATIVE STUCTURE-ACTIVITY RELATIONSHIP

Introduction

Many important properties of biomolecules are dependent on the macroscopic properties of the molecules from which it is made up. Sometimes a single residue change in a peptide sequence or a single atomic change in a small organic molecule will profoundly affect the biological properties. Quantifying the effect of structural modification in a molecule in relation to biological activity is the basic principle property of quantitative structure-activity relationships (QSAR). Computationally intensive methods such as molecular dynamics or *ab initio* molecular orbital methods can often study structure-property relationships. Quantitative structure-activity relationship (QSAR) is the name usually applied to methods which correlate molecular structure to some kind of *in vitro* or *in vivo* biological property. When this approach is applied to modeling of toxicological data, it is termed quantitative structure-toxicity relationships (QSTR). When applied to modeling of physicochemical properties it is called quantitative structure-property relationships (QSPR). Quantitative structure-activity relationship and structure property relationship (QSAR/QSPR) studies are of great importance in discovery and development of lead compounds.

QSAR parameters

QSAR is essentially a computerized statistical method, which tries to explain the observed variance in the biological effect of certain classes of compounds as a function of molecular changes caused by the substituents. Thus it is a scientific empiricism in drug design to ensure that every drug synthesized and pharmacologically tested should be as meaningful as possible. The aim of quantitative structure-activity relationship (QSAR) techniques is to develop correlation between any property or form of activity, frequently biological activity, and the properties, usually physicochemical properties, of a set of molecules, in particular substituent properties. The biological activity of a drug is a function of chemical features i.e., Lipophilicity, electronic and steric properties of the substituents and the skeleton of a drug molecule. Ideally the activities and properties are connected by some known mathematical function, **(F)**.

Biological activity = F (Physicochemical properties)

Biological activity can be any measure like C, K_i, IC_{50}, ED_{50} and K_m. Physicochemical properties can be broadly classified into three general types: Electronic, steric and hydrophobic.

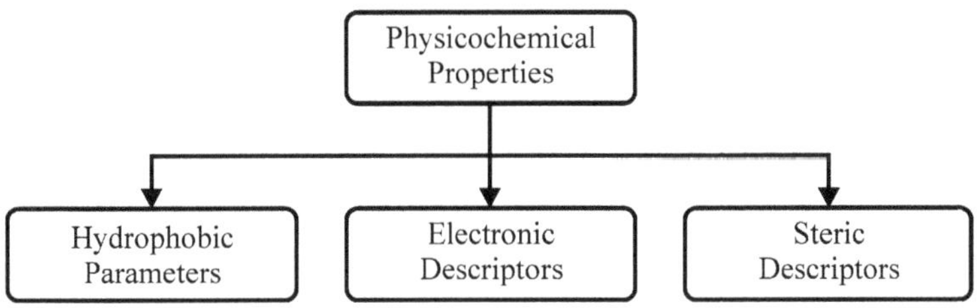

Parameter	Symbol
Hydrophobic parameters	
Partition coefficient	$\log P$
Hydrophobic fragmental constant	f, f'
Distribution coefficient	$\log D$
Apparent partition coefficient (fixed pH)	$\log P'$, $\log P_{app}$
Capacity factor in HPLC	$\log k$, $\log k_w$
Solubility parameter	$\log S$
Electronic descriptors	
Hammett constants	σ^- (sigma)
Taft's inductive (polar) constants	$I\ \sigma^+$
Swain and Lupton field parameter	F
Swain and Lupton resonance parameter	R
Ionization constant	pK_a Δpk_a
Chemical shifts (^{13}C and ^{1}H)	σ
Steric descriptors	
Taft's steric parameter	E_s
Molar volume	MV
Molecular weight	MW
Van der Waals radius	r
Van der Waals volume	V_w
Molar refractivity	MR
Parachor	P_r
STERMOL parameters	L, B_i

QSAR methods

QSAR method involves following steps:

1. In the first step convert molecular structures into mathematical descriptors
2. Select the best descriptors from a larger set of accessible, relevant descriptors.
3. Mapping the molecular descriptors into the properties, preferably using a model-free mapping system. These relationships are often complex, unknown and non-linear.
4. Validate the models.

Generation of descriptors

There are several methods for generating molecular descriptors. The molecular descriptors may be fragment descriptors or whole molecular descriptors. The fragment descriptors used in QSAR studies are hydrophobic constant, molar refractivity, Hammett constants and several other less well known constants.

The hydrophobic constant is related to the difference between the log of the partition coefficient of an unsubstituted molecule and that of a molecule with given substituent. It measures polar/non-polar character of the substituent.

Molar refractivity is the measure of size and polarizability of substituents and is derived from the Lorentz-Lorenz equation and is a function of refractive index, density and molecular weight.

Hammett constant shall be illustrated by the following examples: Louis Hammett (1894-1987), correlated electronic properties of organic acids and bases with their equilibrium constants and reactivity. Consider the dissociation of benzoic acid:

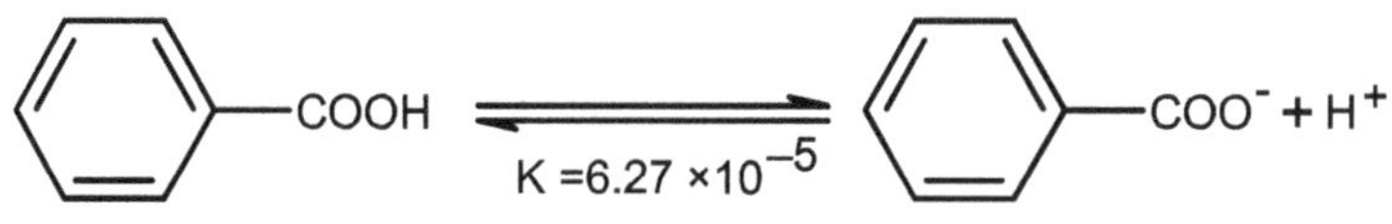

Hammett observed that adding substituents to the aromatic ring of benzoic acid influence quantitative effect on the dissociation constant. For example,

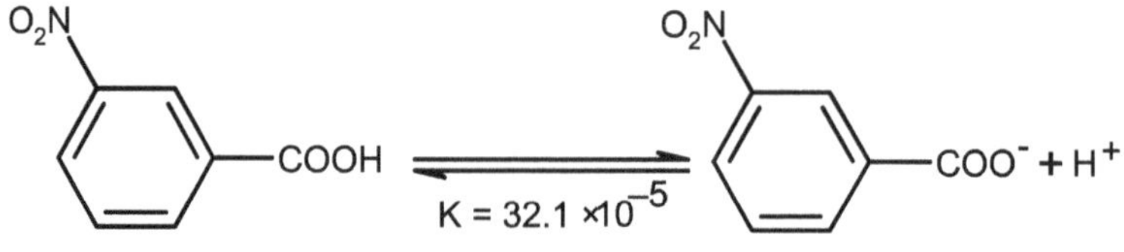

a nitro group in the meta position increases the dissociation constant, because the nitro group is electron-withdrawing, thereby stabilizing the negative charge that develops.

Consider now the effect of a nitro group in the para position:

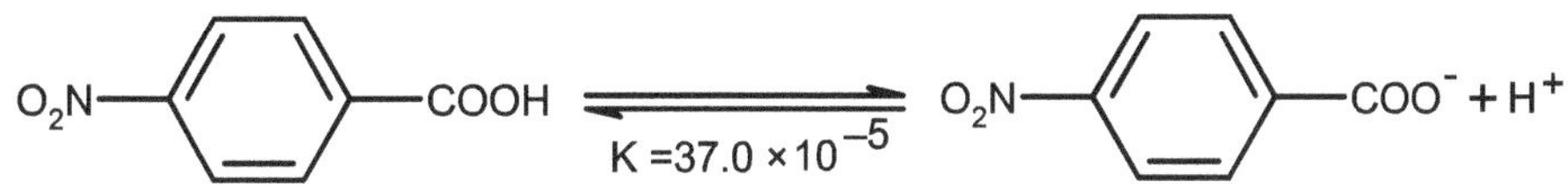

The equilibrium constant is even larger than for the nitro group in the meta position, indicating even greater electron-withdrawal. Now consider the case in which an ethyl group is in para position:

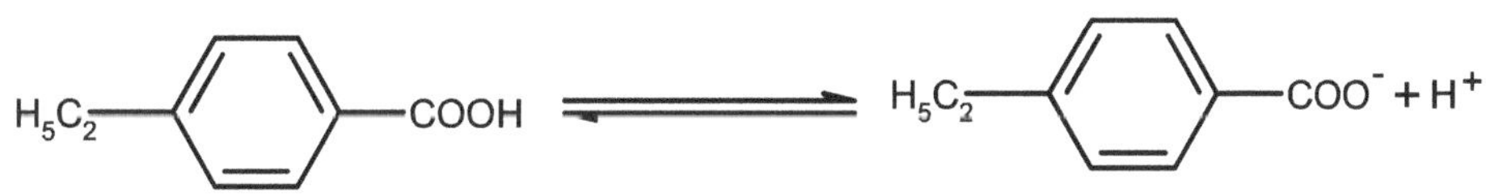

In this case, the dissociation constant is lower than the unsubstituted compound, indicating that the ethyl group is electron-donating, thereby destabilizing the negative charge that arises upon dissociation. Hammett also observed that substituents have a similar effect on the dissociation of other organic acids and bases. Consider the dissociation of phenylacetic acids:

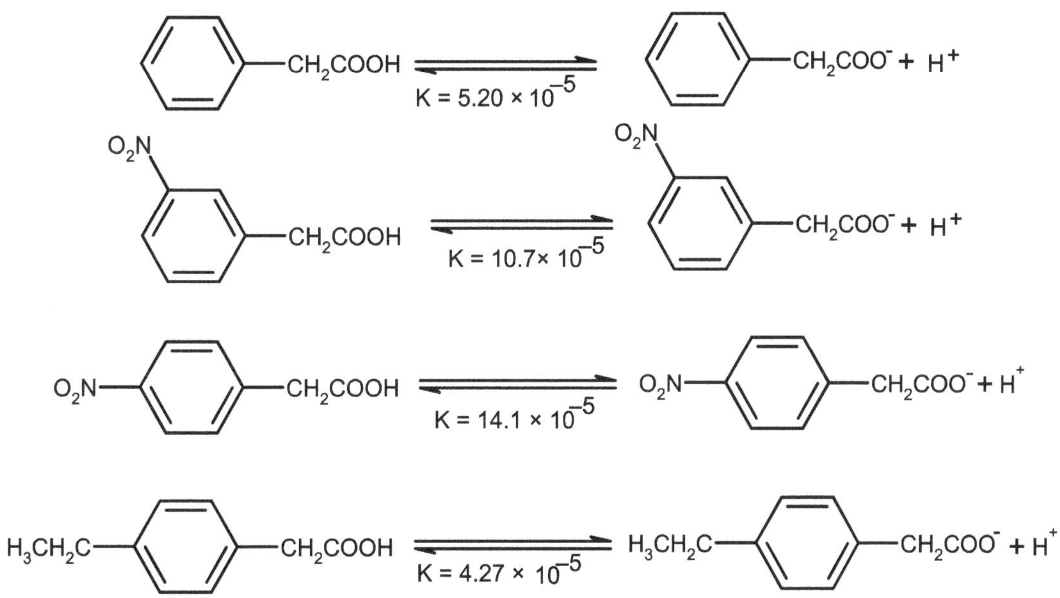

Electron-withdrawal by the nitro group increases dissociation, with the effect being less for the *meta* than for the *para* substituent, just as it was observed with benzoic acid. The electron-donating ethyl group decreases the equilibrium constant, as would be expected. Data for this equilibrium typically are graphed as illustrated below:

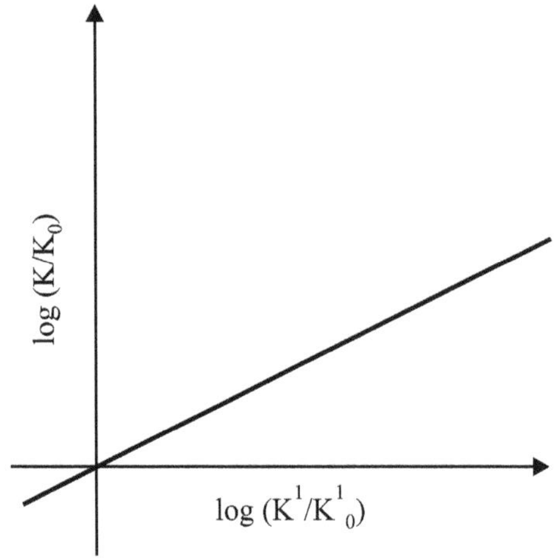

Figure 4.1 Linear free energy relationship. K_0 or K_0^1 represent equilibrium constants for unsubstituted compounds and K or K^1, for substituted compounds. Values for the abscissa are calculated from the dissociation constants of unsubstituted and substituted benzoic acid. Values for the ordinate are obtained from another organic acid or base with identical patterns of substitution, in this case phenylacetic acid.

Because this relationship is linear, the following equation can be written:

$$\log\frac{K}{K_0} = \rho\log\frac{K^1}{K_0^1}$$

Where ρ is the slope of the line. The values for the abscissa in Figure 4.1 are always those for benzoic acid and are given the symbol,. Therefore, the equation can be written as:

$$\log\frac{K}{K_0} = \rho\sigma,$$

the slope of the line, is a proportionality constant pertaining to a given equilibrium. It relates the effect of substituents on that equilibrium to the effect of those substituents on the benzoic acid equilibrium. That is, if the effect of substituents is proportionally greater than the benzoic acid equilibrium, then > 1; if the effect is less than the benzoic acid equilibrium, < 1. The magnitude gives the relative strength of the electron-withdrawing or electron-donating properties of the substituents. It is positive if the substituent is electron-withdrawing and negative if it is electron-donating.

These relationships as developed by Hammett are termed linear free energy relationships. Recall the equation relating free energy to an equilibrium constant:

$$\Delta G = -RT \ln K$$

That is, the free energy is proportional to the logarithm of the equilibrium constant. These linear free energy relationships are termed "extrathermodynamic". Although they can be stated in terms of thermodynamic parameters, no thermodynamic principle states that the relationships should be true.

Some illustrative values for substituents in the meta and para positions are given below :

Substituent	σ_m	σ_p
–H	0.0	0.0
$–NO_2$	0.71	0.78
–Cl	0.37	0.23
$–OCH_3$	0.12	– 0.27

By definition, σ_m and σ_p values for hydrogen is 0. The positive values for the nitro group indicate that it is electron-withdrawing. In understanding the magnitudes of the values for the nitro group in *meta* vs. *para* positions, consider the mechanisms of electron withdrawal or donation. For a nitro group in the *meta* position, electron-withdrawal is due to an inductive effect produced by the electronegativity of the constituent atoms. If only induction were operative, one would expect the electron-withdrawing effect of a nitro group in the *para* position to be less than in the *meta* position. The larger value for a *para*-substituted nitro group results from the combination of both inductive and resonance effects. For chlorine, the electronegativity of the atom produces an inductive electron-withdrawing effect, with the magnitude of the effect in the *para* position being less than in the *meta* position. For chlorine, only the inductive effect is possible. The methoxy group can be electron-donating or -withdrawing depending on the position of substitution. In the meta position, the electronegativity of the oxygen produces an inductive electron-withdrawing effect. In the *para* position, only a small inductive effect would be expected. Moreover, an electron-donating resonance effect occurs for the methoxy group in the *para* position, giving an overall electron-donating effect. Tables of values for numerous substituents have been given above. In some cases, the sigma values are generally applicable to many different equilibria. In other cases, sigma values have been derived for specific equilibria, which is particularly true when one considers sigma values for ortho substituents. Consider the substituted benzoic acid.

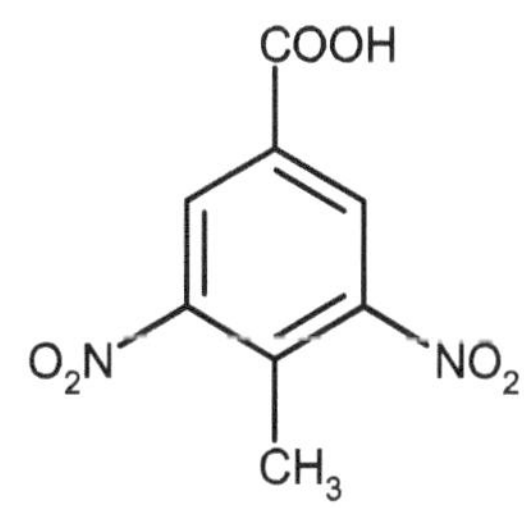

4-Methyl-3,5 - Dinitor benzole acid

In given compound σ value for nitrogroup is 0.71, σ value for methyl group is – 0.13, the calculated pK_a value is 2.91, which coincides favourably with the experimental value of 2.97.

The second example illustrates the applicability of Hammett's electronic descriptors in a QSAR relating the inhibition of bacterial growth by a series of sulphonamides,

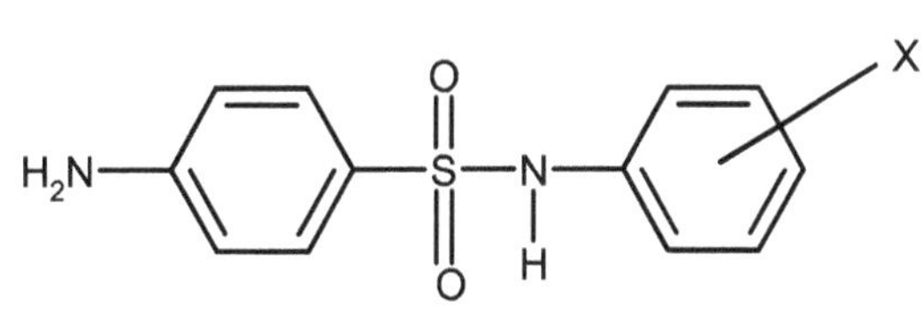

where X represents various substituents. A QSAR was developed based on the values of the substituents,

$$\log\left(\frac{1}{C}\right) = 1.05\sigma - 1.28$$

where C is the minimum concentration of compound that inhibited growth of E. coli. From this relationship, we see that electron-withdrawing substituents favour inhibition of growth.

$$\log\left(\frac{1}{C}\right) = k_1\pi + k_2\sigma + k_3$$

The Hammett substituent parameter is

$$p = \log\left(\frac{P_x}{P_H}\right)$$

One interpretation to account for this term is that many membranes must be traversed for compounds to get to the target site, and those with greatest hydrophobicity will become localized in the membranes they encounter initially. Thus, an optimum hydrophobicity may be found in some test systems.

QSAR attempts to find consistent relationships between the variations in the values of molecular properties and the biological activity for a series of compounds so that these "rules" can be used to evaluate new chemical entities (NCE's).

Free and wilson approach: An alternative approach to Hammett constant is Free and Wilson approach. Free and Wilson used a series of substituent constants which related biological activity to the presence of a specific functional group at a specific location on the parent molecule. The relationship between biological activity and the presence or absence of a substituent was then expressed by the following equation:

$$\text{Activity} = A + G_{ij} X_{ij}$$

where A was defined as the average biological activity for the series, G_{ij} the contribution to activity of a functional group **i** in the jth position and X_{ij} the presence (1.0) or absence (0.0) of the functional group **i** in the jth position.

Whole molecular descriptors: Some of the earlier molecular descriptors were molecular size and lipophilicity, properties such as the molecular weight or molecular volume and log of octanol-water partition coefficient (log *P*). Octanol-water partition coefficient, referred to as log *P* is a frequently used parameter in organic synthetic chemistry. However, the practical applications of log *P* are much broader. For neutral compounds, log *P* serves as a quantitative descriptor of lipophilicity, one of the key determinants of pharmacokinetic properties. Log *P* is commonly used in QSAR studies and drug design, since this property is related to drug absorption, bioavailability, metabolism, and toxicity. This parameter is also used in many environmental studies to determine the environmental fate of chemicals.

Hansch analysis: The linear equation which describes the relationship between activity and this parameter set was the Hansch equation

$$\log(1/[C]) = A(\log P) - B(\log P)^2 + C(E_s) + D + E + \ldots\ldots$$

Multiple linear regression analysis was used to derive the values of the coefficients. In general, Hansch type studies were performed on compounds, which contain a common template (usually a rigid one such as an aromatic ring), with structural variation limited to functional group changes at specific sites.

Hansch utilized this approach in his analysis of 256 compound 4, 6-diamino-1, 2-dihydro -2,3-dimethyl-1-(X-phenyl)-s-triazines was active against tumor dihydrofolate reductase. It was demonstrated that for 244 compounds, activity could be correlated to the presence of hydrophobic groups at third and fourth positions of the N-phenyl ring. The parameters used to derive this correlation were the hydrophobic constant (f) and molar refractivity constant (MR) for meta and para substituents on the N-phenyl ring and six indicator variables I_1-I_6 which were used to indicate the presence (a value of 1) or absence (a value of 0) of specific structural features. The equation which was formulated from these data using the method of least squares.

Topliss analysis: In 1972, John Topliss published a paper, with detailed methodology to automate the Hansch approach. The method assumed that the lead compound of interest contained at least one phenyl ring, which could serve as the template for functional group modifications. The first modification to the template was preparation of the para-chloro derivative to examine lipophilicity. Additional substitution patterns were then made sequentially in an attempt to explore and optimize the relationship between activity and the hydrophobic and electronic character of the molecule. While the Topliss approach is easy to follow, it has several drawbacks. The primary problems are that the procedure is not applicable to all types of studies and that there is a high degree of risk associated with its use (it essentially ignores the possibility of interactions between substituents as it changes one substituent at a time).

Descriptor selection: To build a good QSAR model, a minimal set of information-rich descriptors is required. The earliest method of variable selection used step wise regression. Variable selection involves choosing descriptors containing relevant information, either by experience, variable reduction methods or intelligent selection methods.

Another widely used variable reduction method is principal component analysis (PCA). This involves creating a smaller set of new orthogonal descriptors and using these to generate QSAR models. An alternative approach is to use Bayesian statistics to rank input descriptors according to relevance to the model, effectively removing uninformative descriptors. This method is known as automatic relevance determination (ARD). It has the advantage that it is a non-linear process, which has sound statistical basis.

Structure activity mapping

Many methods have been used to map molecular description to properties. Regression was the majorly used one. Regression methods attempt to fit a specific function with free parameters to a set of data. They usually do this using some gradient descent method such as least squares, which finds the best set of free parameters that minimize the sum of the squares of the errors between the measured values of the dependent variables, and those calculated by the fitted function.

In the last decade, neural networks have emerged as the most useful way to overcome many of these shortcomings. Neural networks are regression methods, which automatically learn the functional relationships between molecular structure and properties without any subjective input from the researcher. The class of neural network most often used for empirical structure-property modeling, the back-propagation neural network learns in similar way to the brain by example.

An alternative method of mapping structure with properties includes recursive partitioning, Gaussian process, radial basis functions (RBF) and other types of neural networks. The support vectors machine (SVM), a classification algorithm widely used in pattern recognition, is showing considerable promise in finding good QSAR models in a very computationally efficient manner.

Validation and testing

It is important to know how predictive a model is, once derived to show whether a structure-property mapping method has overfitted the data. Several methods have been developed to estimate the validity or predictivity of the derived structure-property model. The most common method is leave -one-out cross-validation. This involves leaving each molecule out of the training set in turn, then creating a model using the remainder of the training set. The property of the omitted molecule is predicted using the model derived from all of the other molecules.

Applications

QSAR has been applied extensively and successively over several decades to find predictive models for activity of bioactive agents. It is applied to areas related to discovery and subsequent development of bioactive agents. It is also employed to distinguish drug from non-drug like molecules, drug resistance, toxicity production, physicochemical properties prediction (e.g., Hydrophilicity, lipophilicity), gastrointestinal absorption, activity of peptides, data mining, drug metabolism, and prediction of other pharmacokinetic and ADME properties.

Case study

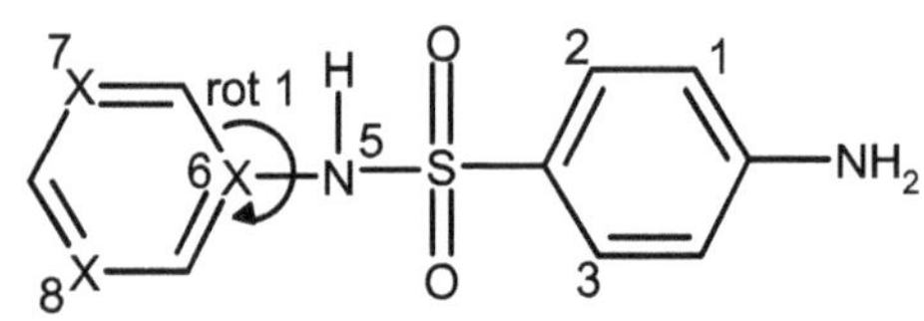

Sulphones and sulphanilamides, have been shown to inhibit dihydropteroate synthetase (DHPS) isolated from *Pneumocystis carinii*. In order to develop a pharmacophoric model for this inhibition, quantitative structure-activity relationships (QSAR's) for sulpha drugs active against DHPS have been studied. Accurate 50% inhibitory concentrations were collected for 44 analogs, and other parameters, such as partition coefficients and molar refractivity, were calculated. Conventional multiple regression analysis of these data did not provide acceptable QSAR. However, three-dimensional QSAR provided by comparative molecular field analysis did give excellent results. Upon removal of poorly correlated analogs, a data set of 36 analogs, all having a common $NHSO_2$ group, provided a cross-validated r^2 value of 0.699 and conventional r^2 value of 0.964. Hence the resulting pharmacophore model should be useful for understanding and predicting the binding of DHPS by new sulpha drugs.

Advantages of QSAR

- Quantifying the relationship between structure and activity provides an understanding of the effect of structure on activity, which may not be straightforward when large amounts of data are generated.
- There is also the potential to make predictions leading to the synthesis of novel analogues. Interpolation is readily justified, but great care must be taken not to use extrapolation outside the range of the data set.
- The results can be used to help understand interactions between functional groups in the molecules of greatest activity, with those of their target. To do this it is important to interpret any derived QSAR in terms of the fundamental chemistry of the set of analogues, including any outliers.

Disadvantages of QSAR

- False correlations may arise by relying entirely on biological data, which, by its nature, is subject to considerable experimental error.
- Frequently, experiments upon which QSAR analysis depend, lack design in the strict sense of experimental design. Therefore the data collected may not reflect the complete property space. Consequently, many QSAR results cannot be used to confidently predict the most likely compounds of best activity.

Various physicochemical parameters are known to be cross-correlated. Therefore only variables or their combinations that have little covariance should be used in a QSAR analysis; similar considerations apply when correlations are sought for different sets of biological data.

5

DRUG DESIGN

Introduction

Drugs are the substances that exert some kind of physiological or biochemical effects on our bodies. They may be single compounds or mixtures, and their effects may be beneficial or harmful. In the beginning, plants and other natural products were the source of most medicinal substances. For example, the foxglove plant can be used to treat congestive heart failure. As the science of medicinal chemistry evolved, it was discovered that foxglove contains digoxin and other cardiotonic glycosides which are responsible for the therapeutic effect. Other medicines, which came into existence, are mostly due to accidental observations and discoveries. E.g., Penicillin. Alexander Fleming noticed that some of his bacterial cultures were ruined because of contamination with mold. Wherever the mold grew, the bacteria were apparently killed. It was found that the mold (Penicillium) produces a substance called penicillin, which kills many kinds of bacteria. Later, antibiotics such as streptomycin, neomycin, gentamicin, erythromycin, and the tetracyclines were isolated from various sources. Chemical modification of known drugs can often lead to improved drugs. Naturally occurring penicillin G is broken down by bacterial beta-lactamases. Addition of two $-OCH_3$ groups produce methicillin, which is resistant to lactamase.

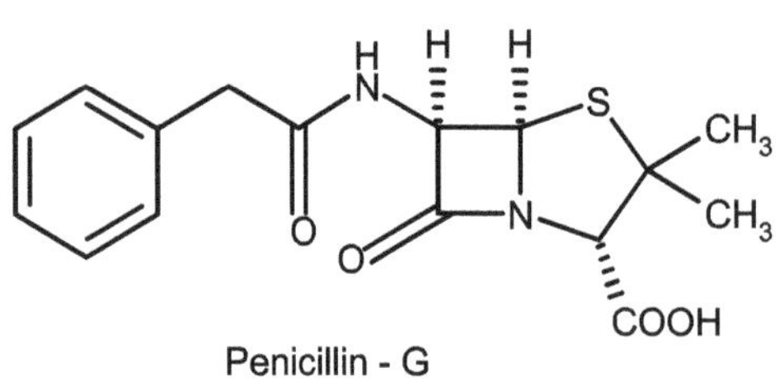

Penicillin - G

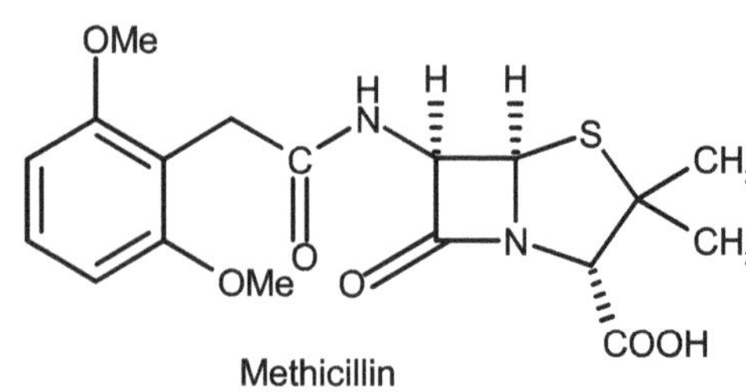

Methicillin

With the advent of scientific technologies and molecular biology, the discovery of drugs entered into a novel approach known as drug design. It is the approach of finding drugs by design, based on what the drug is targeting. Typically a drug target is a key molecule involved in a particular metabolic or signaling pathway that is specific to a disease condition or pathological state. Drugs may be so designed that they effectively bind to the active region and inhibit this key molecule. However these drugs would also have to be designed in such a way, as not to affect any other important molecules that may be similar in appearance to the key molecules. The structure of the drug molecule that can specifically interact with the biomolecules can be attempted using computational tools. These tools can allow a drug molecule to be constructed based on the structure of biomolecule using knowledge of its structure and the nature of its active site. E.g., Ritonavir – a HIV protease inhibitor was developed by studying the nature of the enzyme and its active site with which the drug binds. In order to be successful in the drug design, a new drug must satisfy the following criteria:

- Must be safe to be used in therapy
- Must be effective for the intended use
- Must be stable (chemically and metabolically)
- Must have good solubility profile
- Must be synthetically feasible
- Must be novel in its properties

The development of a new therapeutic drug is a complex, lengthy and expensive process. It can take from 10-15 years and over £500 000 000 to bring a drug from concept to market. This includes 2-4 years of pre-clinical development, 3-6 years of clinical development and additional time for dealing with the regulatory authorities.

Methodology for drug design

The following steps are involved in development of a new drug :

1. Lead finding

A lead is chemical compound, which shows the biological activity and is not the same as drug. Lead generation is an important step in drug discovery process. During lead generation researchers develop tests, called assays, to screen libraries of leads against targets to evaluate their therapeutic value. There are number of ways of discovering new leads :

- Isolation of active substances from natural products,
  E.g., Penicillin, quinine
- Modification of natural products,
  E.g., Thienamycin
- Broad screening of known synthetic substances,
  E.g., Sulphonamides
- Derivation and application of quantitative structure-activity relationship studies,
  E.g., Cephalosporin
- Mechanism based molecular design,
  E.g., Carbonic anhydrase inhibitors
- Chemical intuition,
  E.g., Enalapril

2. Lead optimization

Lead optimization is a complex, multistep process of refining the chemical structure of a compound to improve its drug characteristics with the goal of producing a preclinical drug candidate. Researchers focus on a number of considerations in optimizing a drug candidate, including the following drug characteristics:

- *Potency* : The amount of a drug required to effectively treat the disease.
- *Selectivity* : The extent to which a drug interacts only with the target; the greater the selectivity, the lower the probability of harmful side effects.
- *Toxicity* : The presence and significance of any harmful side effects.
- *Metabolism* : How rapidly the drug works and how long it stays effective, and
- *Formulation* : How the drug is administered to patients, for example, orally or by injection.

3. Receptor-based drug design

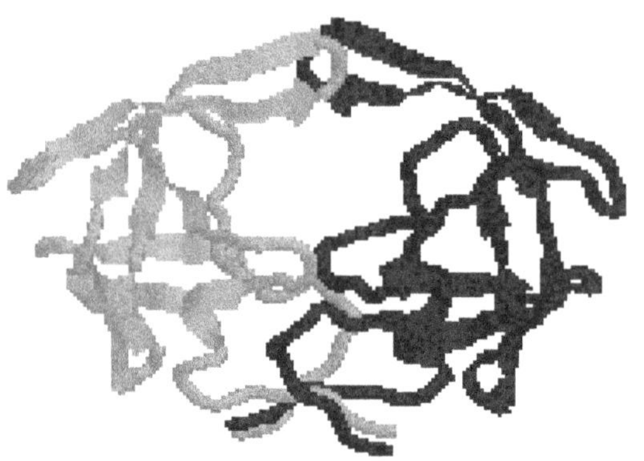

X-Ray crystallographic structure of HIV-1 Protease

The *receptor* is the target (usually a protein) to which a drug molecule binds in order to cause a biological effect. Emil Fischer (in 1894) proposed the analogy that a drug molecule is like a key, which fits into a lock. The specificity of a drug molecule for its target is like the specificity of a key for its lock; if you make similar keys, they may also "fit" into the "lock." Ehrlich coined the term “receptor” in 1909 to describe the target. The structure of the target can be identified and characterized by X-ray crystallographies and NMR spectroscopy studies. For example, in 1988 the role of the HIV protease was established, and its amino acid sequence was determined. It was shown to have considerable homology to Rous sarcoma virus protease. In 1989 the structure of HIV protease was determined by X-ray crystallography, and the homology-modeled structure was shown to be essentially correct. NMR spectroscopy can provide information about the three-dimensional (3-D) structure of proteins. The 3-D structure will guide the design of ligands.

X-ray crystallographic structure of HIV-1 protease. The protein is a dimer; one subunit is shown in gray, and the other black. The large open space (top center) is the active site.

4. Proteins as cellular targets of medicinal drugs

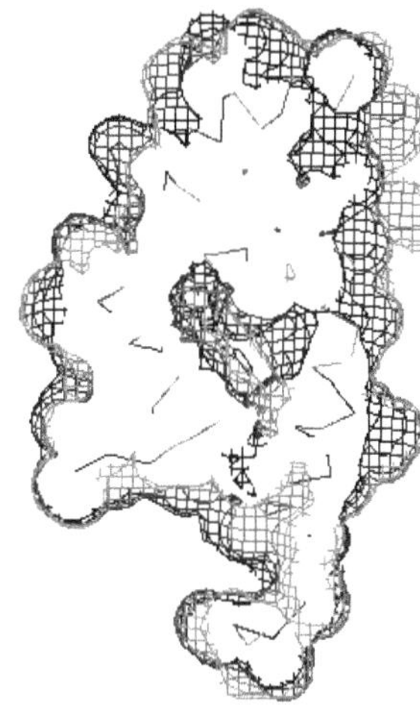

The cellular targets (or receptors) of many drugs used for medical treatment are proteins. By binding to the receptor, drugs either enhance or inhibit its activity. Basically there are two major groups of receptor proteins: proteins that "float" around in the cytoplasm of the cell, and proteins that are incorporated into the cell membrane. In the latter case, a drug does not even need to enter the cell, it can bind simply to an extracellular binding site of the protein and control intracellular reactions from the outside.

5. Ligand-based drug design

Many receptors are not readily amenable to receptor-based drug design. For example, many important receptors are membrane-bound proteins, which are difficult to isolate. In such cases, a lead compound or active ligand must be found, and then the structure of the ligand guides the drug design process. This case may be illustrated with the story of the discovery of sildenafil, better known under the trade name Viagra.

The figure below shows the structures of cyclic guanacin monophosphate (cGMP) and sildenafil. It is likely that the SO_2 group of sildenafil mimics the phosphate in cGMP. It is possible to superimpose these two structures with quite good matching of gross shape, in such a way that the SO_2 group aligns roughly with the phosphate, and the 4-piperidone rings (six-membered ring with N at one end and C=O at the other) roughly superimpose. The match isn't perfect. An inhibitor doesn't have to bind in exactly the same way as substrate. It just has to bind tightly enough so that it inhibits substrate from getting in. Remember that the natural substrate should bind reasonably well, but not too tightly or it will never release the drug, it's the transition state which should bind most tightly. This is why many drugs are designed to look like transition states.

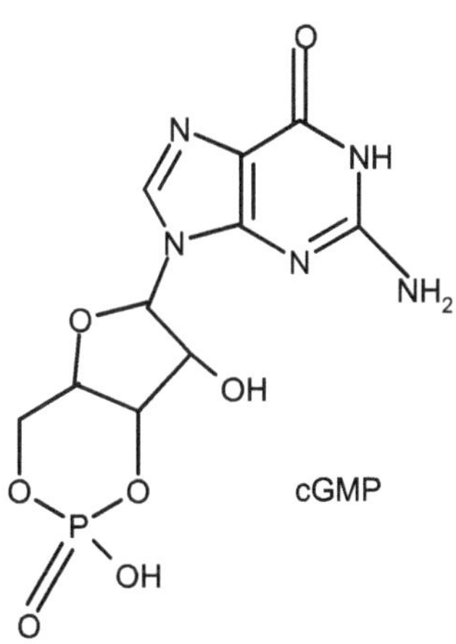

cGMP

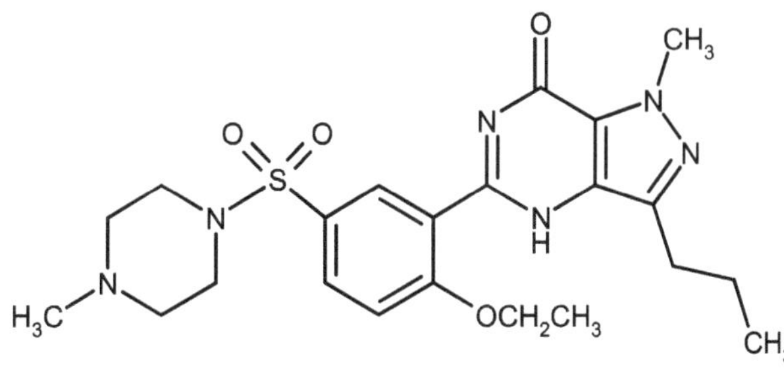

Sidenafil

6. Drug specificity and side effects

An important criterion to determine the medicinal value of a drug is specificity, the physiological effect of the drug should be as clearly defined as possible. It has to specifically bind to the target protein in order to minimize undesired side-effects. The idea that molecules can interact in a highly specific manner has a long history in medicinal chemistry. A century ago Fischer and Ehrlich already used a "lock-and-key" analogy. Undesired side-effects however, are not always an indication for insufficient specificity of drugs as these effects might also result from a reaction of our body to the desired and therefore successful regulation of the malfunctioning biochemical process.

The molecular basis of drug specificity

On the molecular level, specificity includes two more or less independent mechanisms: First the drug has to bind to its receptor site with a suitable affinity (better binding means lower doses) and second it has to either stimulate or inhibit certain functions of the receptor protein in order to regulate its activity. Both mechanisms are mediated by a variety of interactions between the drug and its receptor site. Usually tens of thousands of compounds have to be screened to find a promising new drug and only very few of these candidates will make their way through the final clinical tests. Looking for help from powerful computers seems straightforward.

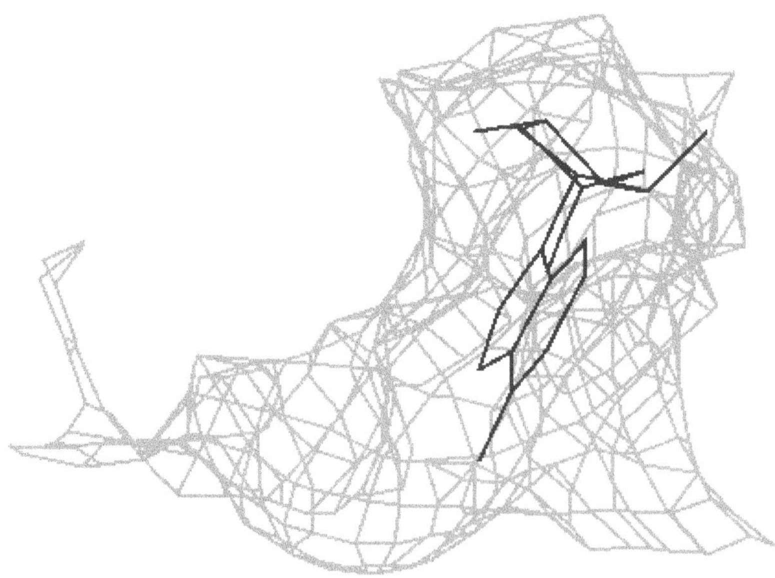

6

COMBINATORIAL CHEMISTRY

Introduction

Combinatorial Chemistry is a new sub field of chemistry with the goal of synthesizing very large number of chemical entities by condensing a small number of reagents together in all combinations. It is a time and cost effective technology.

Combinatorial chemistry is defined as "the systematic and repetitive, covalent connection of a set of different building blocks of varying structures to each other to yield a large array of diverse molecular entities. It is also referred as matrix chemistry".

Combinatorial synthesis

$$A + B \longrightarrow AB$$

Orthodox Synthesis

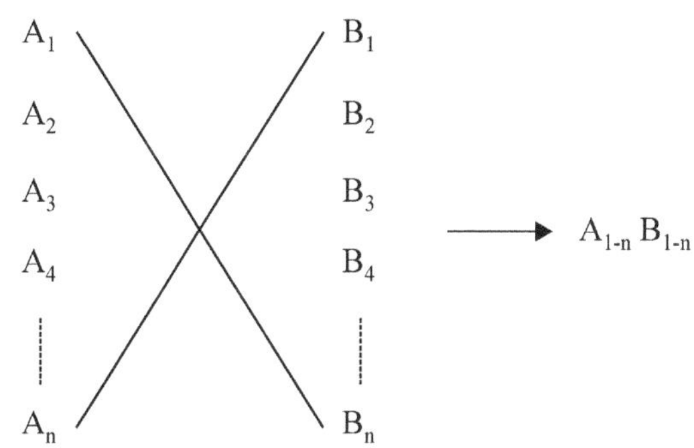

Combinatorial Synthesis

The idea of combinatorial synthesis is to form large libraries of molecules instead of synthesizing compounds one by one, as has been done traditionally. Traditionally, the new chemical entities were prepared one at a time. This generally takes six years under the best conditions to prepare a chemical library.

Combinatorial chemistry involves the systematic synthesis of all possible combinations of a set of chemical building blocks into new chemical compounds, according to a specified chemical reaction sequence. This provides the rapid production of hundreds, or thousands of diverse molecules. Thus a combinatorial approach involves the generation of large number of compounds; a "library", which incorporates this diversity. In this regard, naturally occurring proteins and peptides are the result of nature's ongoing experiment in combinatorial libraries.

For example in the following figure A_1combines with B_1 to give the product A_1B_1. Supposing if one were to combine "n" numbers of variants of B_1 such as B_2, B_3.......B_n with A to get A_1B_1, A_2B_2,.....A_nB_n, then by traditional medicinal chemistry approach it is possible, but it can be prepared only one by one. Obviously one by one synthesis of a large number of compounds rendered the drug discovery process tedious, time consuming and expensive as well.

Combinatorial Chemistry on the other hand can produce the same products A_1B_1, A_1B_2,.....A_1B_n, all at the same time as individual compounds by bringing A_1 with B_1 and its variants parallel and hence saves time. Further if one has to make variations simultaneously in A also, such as A_2, A_3...A_n, then the situation is still handleable by combinatorial chemistry and as a result the library is bound to have more diversity.

The following key steps are involved in the generation of combinatorial library:

1. Creation of chemical library.
2. Screening of the library components and
3. Determination of the chemical structures of active compounds.

1. Creation of chemical library

The following methods are employed for creation of combinatorial chemical libraries. They are :

(i) Solid phase method: Since Merrifield pioneered solid phase synthesis back in 1963, which earns him a Nobel Prize, the subject, has changed radically. Merrifield's Solid Phase synthesis concept, first developed for biopolymer, has spread in every field where organic synthesis is involved. Many laboratories and companies focused on the development of technologies and chemistry suitable to SPS. This resulted in the spectacular outburst of combinatorial chemistry, which profoundly changed the approach for new drugs, new catalyst or new natural discovery.

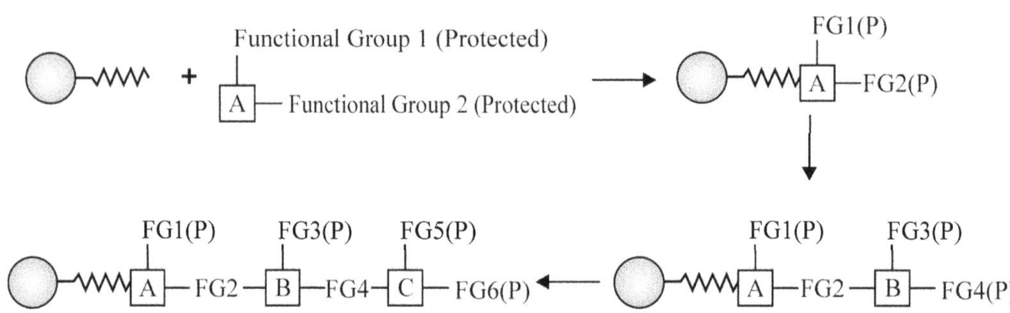

The use of solid support for organic synthesis relies on three interconnected requirements:

(a) A cross linked insoluble polymeric material that is inert to the condition of synthesis;

(b) Some means of linking the substrate to this solid phase that permits selective cleavage of some or all of the product from the solid support during synthesis for analysis of the extent of reaction(s), and ultimately to give the final product's of interest.

(c) A chemical protection strategy to allow selective protection and deprotection of reactive groups.

Merrifield developed a series of chemical reactions that can be used to synthesize proteins. The direction of synthesis is opposite to that used in the cell. The intended carboxy terminal amino acid is anchored to a solid support. Then, the next amino acid is coupled to the first one. In order to prevent further chain growth at this point, the amino acid, which is added, has its amino group blocked. After the coupling step, the block is removed from the primary amino group and the coupling reaction is repeated with the next amino acid. The process continues until the peptide or protein is completed. Then, the molecule is cleaved from the solid support and any groups protecting amino acid side chains are removed. Finally, the peptide or protein is purified to remove partial products and products containing errors.

Combinatorial synthesis on solid supports is usually carried out using by either the parallel synthesis or the Furka split mix procedures.

(ii) Solution phase method : Combinatorial synthesis in solution can be used to produce libraries that consist of single compounds or mixtures using traditional organic chemistry. Single compound libraries are prepared using the parallel synthesis technique. Libraries of mixtures are formed by separately reacting each of the members of a set of similar compound with the same mixture of all the members of the second set of the compounds.

Two groups have recently disclosed solution libraries prepared in mixtures. In each case the groups from Glaxo and Pirrung have synthesized dimeric compounds using amide, ester or carbamate bond-forming reactions. Every library compound was prepared twice in mixtures of different composition. Testing of all these mixtures allows identification of likely active compounds without the need to resynthesize every compound in an active mixture.

In an example 40 acid chlorides were reacted with 40 amines or alcohols to gives amides or ester respectively in two sets. In the first set, each acid chloride (A) was reacted with a stoichiometric amount of an equimolar mixture of all 40 nucleophiles (N_{1-40}). In the second set each amine or alcohol (N) was reacted with an equimolar mixture of the acid chlorides (A_{1-40}). The 80 mixtures of 40 components each were screened against a wide variety of pharmacological targets, and a positive result from any sample identified half of the structure of a likely active dimeric compound. Weak leads against the neurokinin-3-receptor 1 and matrix metallo proteinase - 1 and 2 were detected.

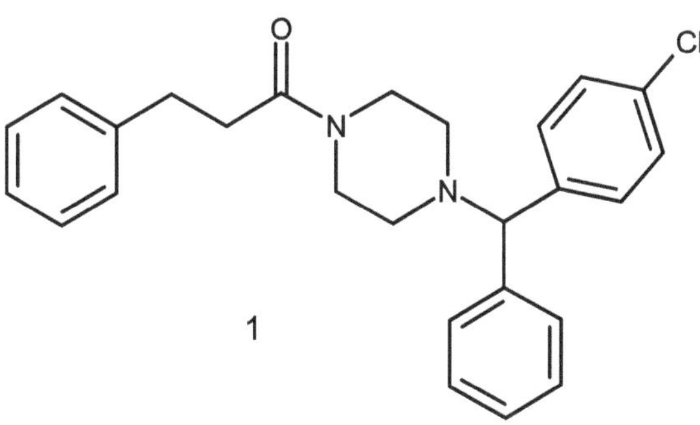

1

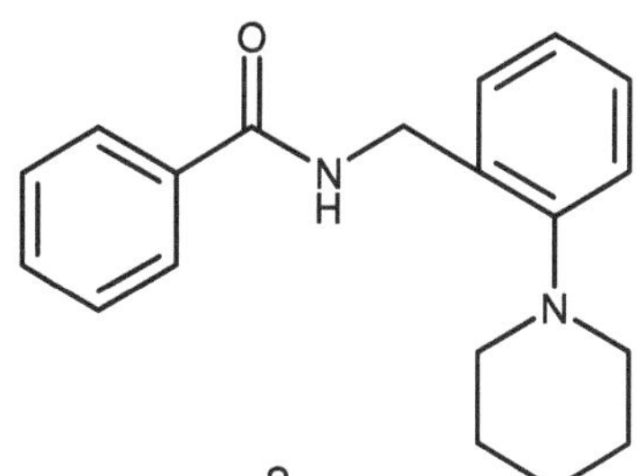

2

The main problem with preparing libraries using solution chemistry is the difficulty of removing unwanted impurities at each step in the synthesis.

2. Screening of library components

A reliable high throughput assay is essential to successfully screen a combinatorial library. Both solid phase and solution phase assays have been developed for the combinatorial libraries.

In the solid phase assays the ligands are still attached to the solid support. These assays are of two types. They are:

(i) Direct binding of molecular target to the bead–bound ligand, this binding can be detected by direct visualization or by using a reporter group such as an enzyme, a radio nuclide.

(ii) Detection of functional properties of the bead–bound ligand such as identifying phosphorylation or proteolytic substrates.

There are two general approaches to screen compound library with solution phase assays. They are:

(i) The 96 – well two-stage releasable assays.

(ii) The *insitu* releasable solution phase assay with immobilized beads.

In both of these approaches, ligands are attached to the solid support *via* cleavable linkers. The ligands are then released from each bead into solution phase when the biological assays take place. The released drug can subsequently identified and isolated for structure determination.

3. Determination of the chemical structures of active compounds

The ultimate goal of producing combinatorial libraries is to discover compounds that have some desired behavior and associated with this behavior to serve as a drug. A major challenge in developing a library of compounds is identification of chemical species responsible. Primarily three methods are used for structural determination of active compounds. They are (i) Parallel iterative deconvolution (ii) Positional screening and (iii) Encoding.

Parallel iterative deconvolution: In this approach pools of compounds are prepared such that each separate pool has defined building blocks. The optimal building blocks at the defined positions is selected by determining which pool has the greatest biological activity. Each pool is evaluated for biological activities in order to select the optimal building block at the additional define position.

Positional screening: It involves the screening of separate, single defined position of synthetic combinatorial libraries and to individually identify the most important functionalities at each position of diversity within a library. The structure of individual compounds can be determined from such a screening since each compound is present in only one mixture of each sub-library.

Encoding: This method employs a readable chemical tag that is simultaneously attached to the individual bead for each step in the synthesis of the actual molecule on the bead. The identity of active compounds are determined by analysis of tags cleaved either by UV irradiation of a photolabile linker followed by gas chromatography (GC) or by acid hydrolysis followed by GC.

Applications of combinatorial chemistry

The following are various applications of combinatorial chemistry:

1. Finding the right combination of drug molecules

Combinatorial chemistry enables drug researchers to generate quickly as many as several million structurally related molecules. E.g., Select 30 structurally related compounds that all contain an amino group ($-NH_2$). Next choose a second set of 30 compounds that all possess carboxylic acid ($-COOH$). Then under appropriate conditions mix and match every amine with every carboxylic acid to form new molecules called amides ($-CONH$). The reaction of each of the 30 amines with each of the 30 carboxylic acids gives a total of 30×30 or 900 different combinations.

2. Combinatorial chemistry provides fresh and promising leads for medicinal chemistry

The recent emergence of combinatorial chemistry has greatly advanced the development of active lead compounds like anti-neoplastic compounds, antimicrobial compounds, antiepileptic drugs, benzodiazepine derivates having different biological activity. E.g., Benzodiazepine derivatives derived through combinatorial synthesis showed some other important biological activities (Opioid receptor antagonist, HIV antagonist) in addition to potent psychotic activities.

3. Synthesis of small molecular libraries

Combinatorial chemistry began with synthesis of large libraries like peptides and oligonucleotides. In recent years combinatorial research has shifted to synthesis of small libraries having the molecular weight of 500 daltons or less due to poor oral bioavailability. E.g., Synthesis of 1, 4-benzodiazepine library.

4. Applications of antibody libraries obtained by combinatorial chemistry

Antibody combinatorial libraries have been developed to treat a series of human viral disease such as HIV-1, RSV and herpes simplex viruses 1 and 2 infections.

5. Development of enzyme inhibitors by combinatorial chemistry

Various enzyme inhibitors like acetyl cholinesterase enzyme inhibitors (Carbamates, Tetrahydroacridines) were developed by combinatorial methods.

6. Combinatorial chemistry has been developed as a tool for lead optimization

Lead molecules were optimized by combinatorial chemistry. E.g., Optimization of leukotriene D_4 antagonist.

7. Qualitative and quantitative characterization of drug database through combinatorial libraries

The objective of this work is to provide both qualitative and quantitative characterization of known drugs, which will help to generate drug-like libraries. In this work comprehensive medicinal chemistry database and seven different subsets belonging to different classes of drug molecules (CNS active drugs, cardiovascular, cancer, inflammation and infection disease state drugs) are analyzed.

7

SULPHONAMIDES OR SULPHA DRUGS

Chemotherapy

The term chemotherapy was coined in 1913 by Pul Ehrlich, the father of modern chemotherapy. The term chemotherapy means chemical therapy or chemical treatment. The goal of chemotherapeutic treatment is to selectively attenuate or destroy pathogenic microorganisms or cells with minimal side effects to the host. These targeted cells or organisms may be bacteria, viruses, protozoans, fungi, helminths, or tumor cells. Modern chemotherapy started with the discovery of Trypan Red I dye that Ehrlich used effectively against tripanosomiasis (sleeping sickness). In 1935 Domagk healed his daughter from a streptococcal infection using the dye prontosil. In 1936, Ernest Fourneau of the Pasteur Institute in Paris demonstrated that prontosil breaks down in the human body to produce sulfanilamide, the active agent against streptococci.

$$\text{Prontosil} \xrightarrow{\textit{in vivo}} \text{Sulphanilamide}$$

History

Prontosil is a red dye that the company Bayer thought it would work like other common dyes.

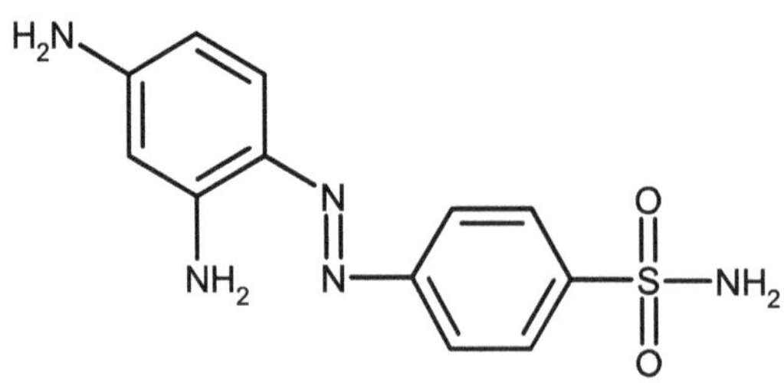

Prontosil

They hoped that prontosil would be taken up by bacteria, and not by humans, like other gram stains were known to do. They guessed that this stain would serve as a poison and kill the targeted bacteria. German scientist Domagk began working with the compound Prontosil, and found that it, like other azo dyes had actions against streptococci and other infections. He also found that while the compound prontosil worked well in mice (*in vivo*), it had no activity on isolated bacterial cells (*in vitro*). French scientists, Trefouel and Bovet, grew interested in Domagk's work and investigated further. They took the urine of a patient that received prontosil, and were able to isolate the active substance known as sulfanilamide.

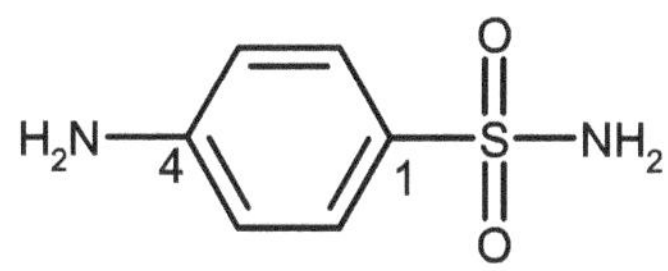

Sulphanilamide

It turned out that when a patient received prontosil, the drug was metabolized (or changed) by that person into the active form known as sulfanilamide. With this discovery the world now knew about prodrugs, a drug that gets changed into its active form once administered to the patient.

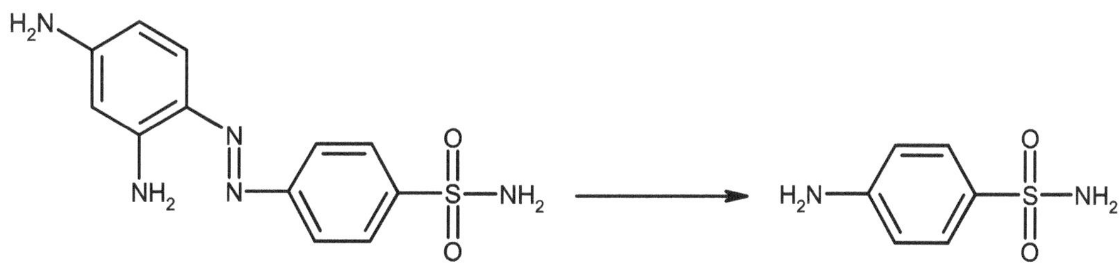

Prontosil Sulphanilamide

This discovery led to further investigation into the uses of sulphonamides, leading to the development of sulphonylureas as hypoglycemic agents and carbonic anhydrase inhibitor as diuretic. Sulphonamides have been an important part of our antibacterial history. Since the 1930's over 4500 different sulphonamides have been synthesized.

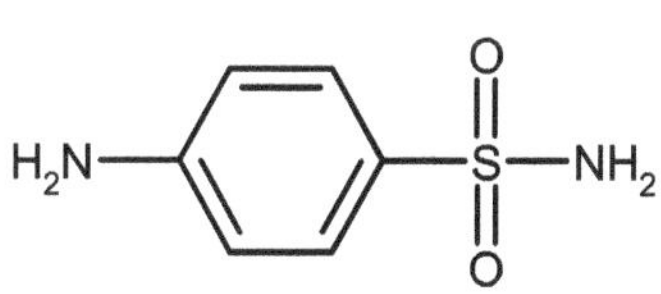

Sulfanilamide

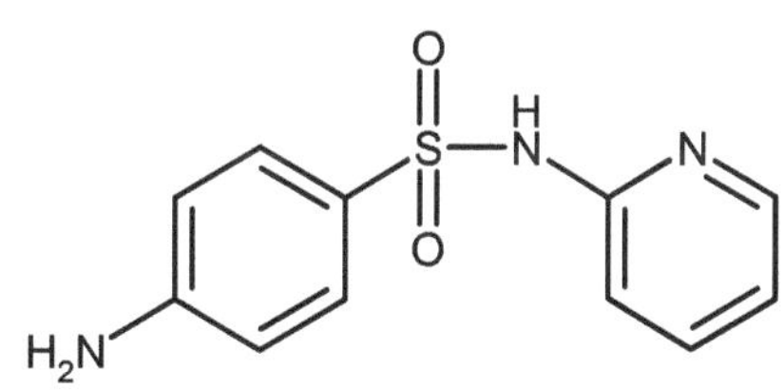

Sulfapyridine

Mechanism of action

1. The basic structure of sulphonamides resembles the structure of para-amino benzoic acid (PABA). PABA is a vitamin to bacteria, which require it for the synthesis of folic acid. Because of their structural similarity to PABA, the sulphonamides compete with this substrate for the bacterial enzyme (dihydropteroate synthetase). Thus sulphonamides inhibit synthesis of folic acid.

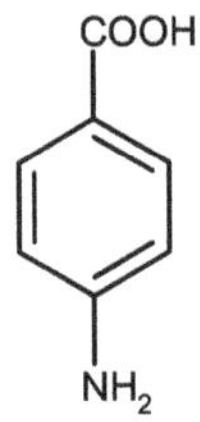

p-Amino benzoic acid

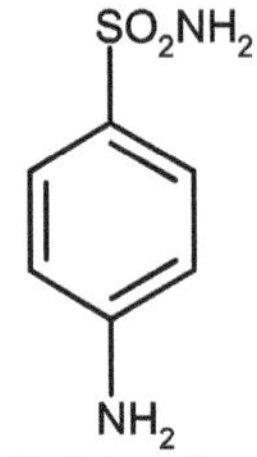

Sulphanilamide

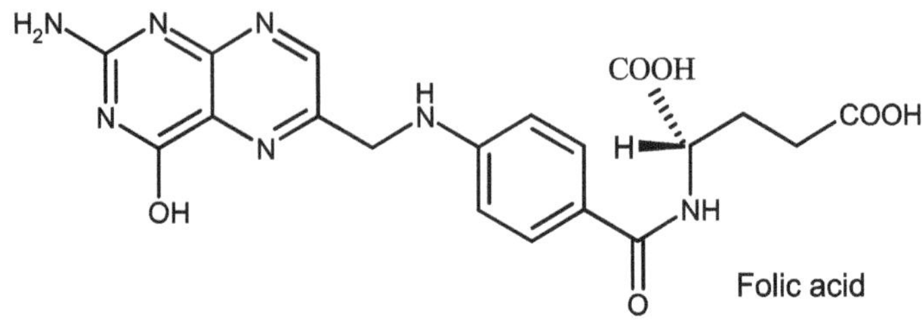

Folic acid

The depletion of folic acid in bacteria leads to a decrease in thymidylate. Thymidylate (thymine) is a DNA base. Without this thymine being produced the bacteria's DNA synthesis is stopped, inhibiting the growth of the bacteria in the patients body. The reason for this is incorporation of incorporate of the sulphonamide into the active site of dihydropteroate synthetase (DHPS) in place of PABA. Thus, ultimately inhibiting the synthesis of folic acid in bacteria.

2. Sulphonamides are bacteriostatic with slow onset of action.
3. Toxicity is selective for bacteria because human cells must take up folic acid (a vitamin) rather than synthesizing it. Most bacteria cannot take up exogenous folic acid.
4. Antibacterial spectrum is broad, but resistance is common.

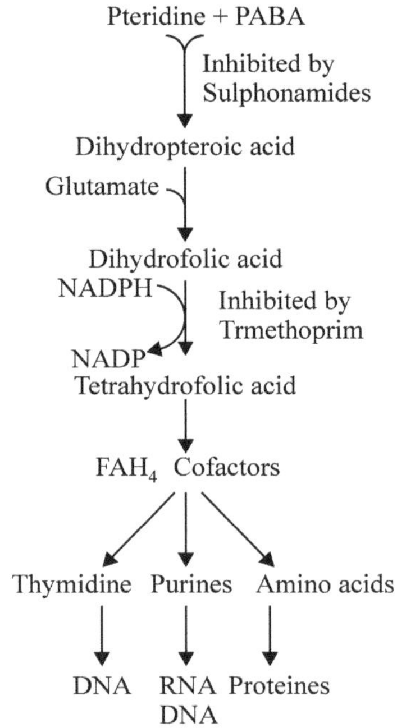

Figure 7.1 Folic acid (FAH_4) metabolism is inhibited by sulphonamides and trimethoprim.

Classification

Sulphonamides are classified according to their utility as follows :

1. Sulphonamides used for the treatment of systemic infections

They are usually administered orally and are further subdivided according to their duration of action.

(i) **Short acting sulphonamides :** Sulphanilamide, sulphadiazine, sulphadimidine, sulphamerazine, sulphamethizole etc.,

(ii) **Intermediate acting sulphonamides :** Sulphamethoxazole, sulphaphenazole etc.,

(iii) **Long acting sulphonamides :** Sulphamethoxypyridazine, sulphadimethoxine etc.,

(iv) **Ultra long acting:** Sulphadoxine etc.,

2. Sulphonamides used for the treatment of local gastrointestinal infection

Sulphaguanidine, succinylsulphathiazole, phthalyl sulphathiazole etc.

SAR of sulphonamides

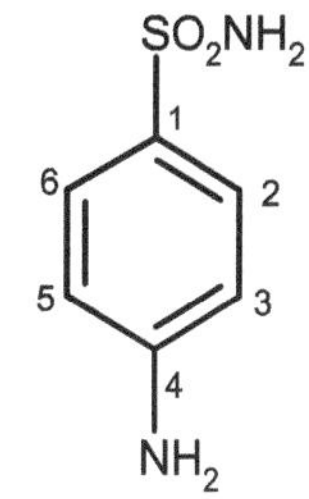

Sulphanilamide

1. Sulphonamides consist of a benzene ring, an amine moiety (–NH_2), and a sulphonamide group (–SO_2NH_2). Most of the sulphonamides are relatively insoluble in water but their sodium salts are readily soluble.
2. The amino and sulphonamido groups must be para to one another in order to possess antibacterial properties.
3. The *p*-amino group must be un-substituted and only mono-substitution (i.e., substituting a different functional group in place of one of the hydrogens) is allowed on the sulphonamide group.
4. A final requirement for sulphonamides is that the amino group possesses a pK_a of 4.7 and the sulphonamide moiety possesses a pK_a of 6.5. The basis for these requirements is to mimic the structure of PABA and subsequently produce antibacterial effects.
5. Mono-substitution on the sulphonamide group is the basis for pharmacokinetic variation within this class of antibacterials. The addition of different functional groups manipulate the properties of the drug. For instance sulphamethoxazole has a pK_a of 6.1, however, the half-life of sulphamethoxazole is 11 hours whereas the half-life of sulphadoxine is 150 hours. It appears that functional groups that impart beneficial antibacterial effects are those that lower the sulphonamide pK_a, specially electron withdrawing groups and heterocyclic rings.

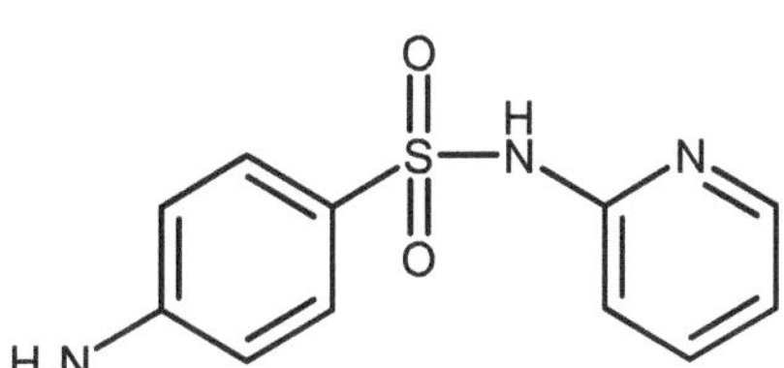

Sulfapyridine
Pneumonia 1938

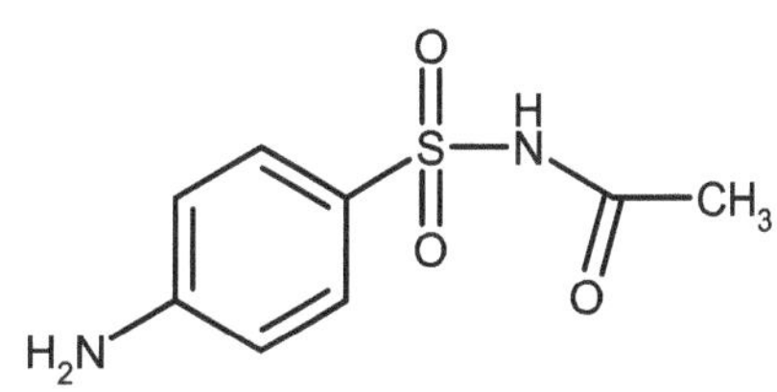

Sulfacetamide
1941 - 1st drug against urinary tract infections

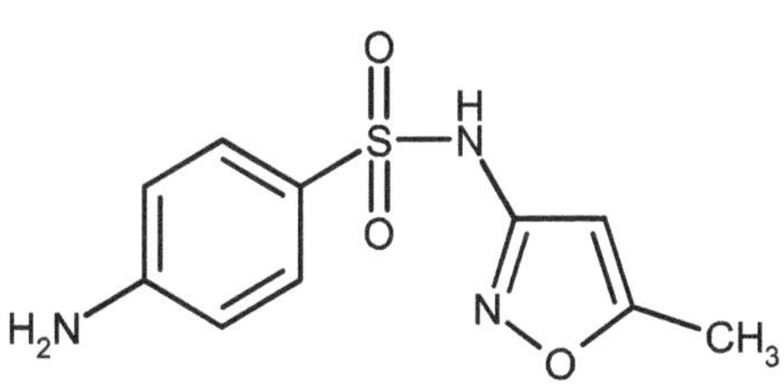

Sulfamethoxazole

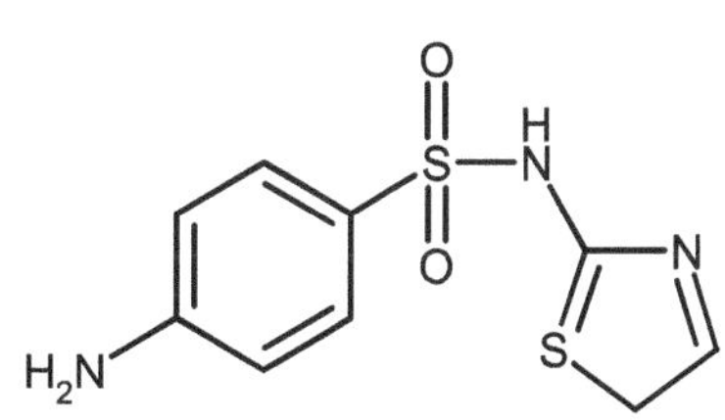

Sulfathiazole

Crystalluria

Sulphonamides are good antibacterial agents. Sulphonamides and their metabolites are excreted entirely in urine. They cause severe renal damage by crystallizing in kidneys. The pK_a of sulphonamide group is 10.4 and 50% of these drugs are ionized at pH 10.4. If the pH is above pK_a the sulphonamides are insoluble and nonionised in kidneys. Hence to overcome crystalluria semisynthetic penicillins possess lower pK_a values because of strong electron withdrawing group (heterocyclic ring) at N-1. These drugs donate proton and thus pK_a values are lowered.

Sulphanilamide

Sulphanilamide is prepared from sulphanilic acid by following chemical reactions :

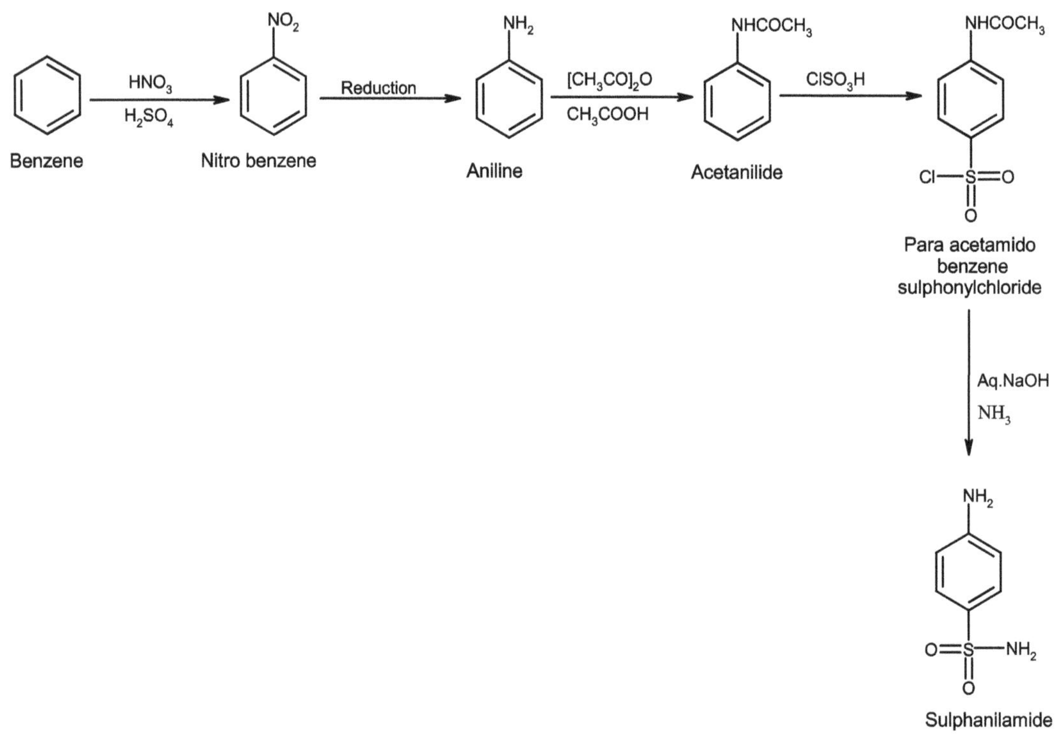

Sulfadiazine

Sulphadiazine is short acting sulphonamide. Chemically it is 4-amino-N-2-pyrimidinyl benzene sulphonamide. It is prepared by condensing 2-aminopyrimidine with *p*-acetamido benzene sulphonyl chloride and alkaline hydrolysis.

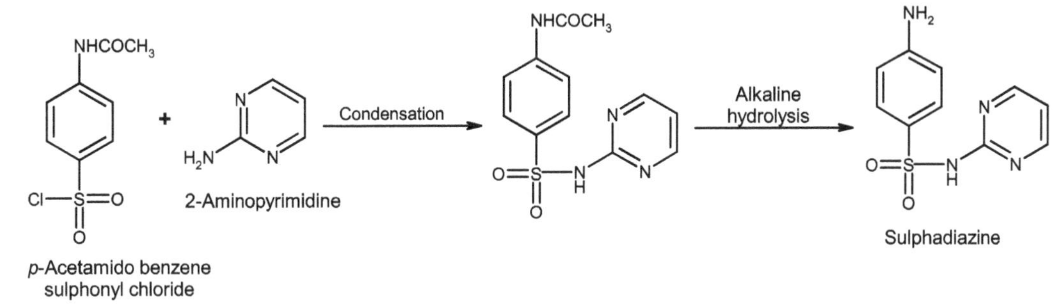

Properties

Sulphadiazine occurs as white or slightly yellow crystalline powder. It is sparingly soluble in water but freely soluble in dilute mineral acids, alkali solutions and in ammonia water.

Sulphathiazole

Sulphathiazole is 4-amino-N-(thiazol-2-yl) benzene sulphonamide. It is prepared by condensing *P*-acetamido benzene sulphonyl chloride with 2-amino thiazole followed by hydrolysis of products. Sulphathiazole is used topically to treat skin and vaginal infections.

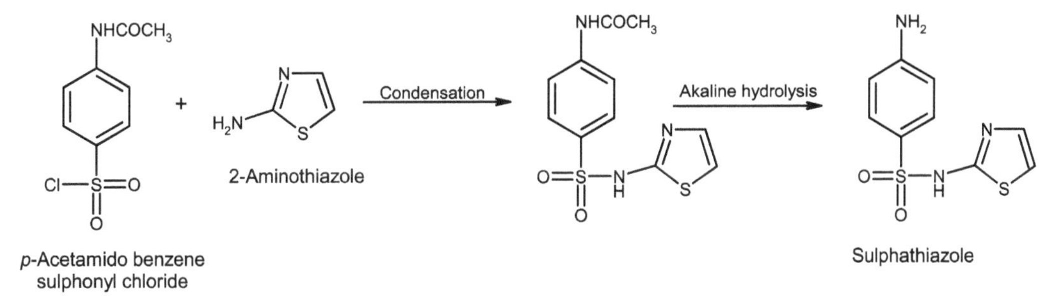

Sulphamethoxazole

Sulphamethoxazole is 4-amino-N-[-5methyl-3-isoxazolyl] benzene sulphonamide. It is synthesized from 4-acetyl amino benzenesulphonyl chloride by the following chemical reactions.

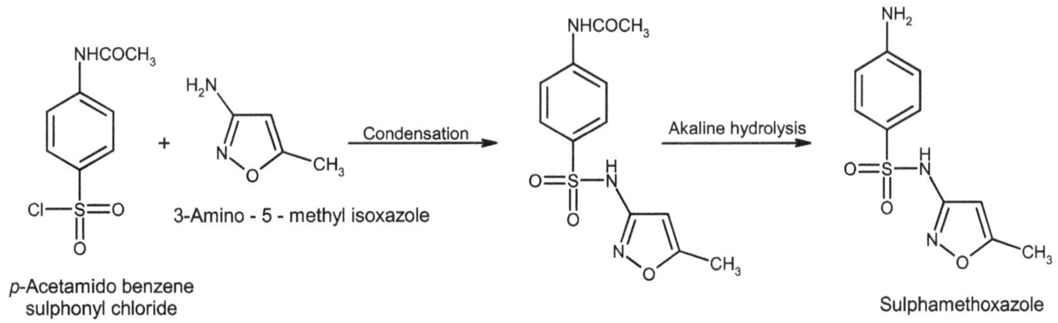

1. The use of sulphamethoxazole has been limited because of increasing incidents of resistant organisms. It is mainly used to treat acute, uncomplicated urinary tract infections caused by *Escherichia coli.*
2. Cotrimoxazole contains sulpamethoxazole and trimethoprim in 5:1 proportions to produce bactericidal or bacteristatic action against wide range of gram-positive and gram-negative organisms. It is also used to treat respiratory and gastrointestinal tract infections.

Sulphaphenazole

H-Amino-N-(1-phenyl-1-H-pyrozol-5-yl) benzene sulphanamide

Sulphaphenazole is administered orally. It is prepared by the following chemical reaction.

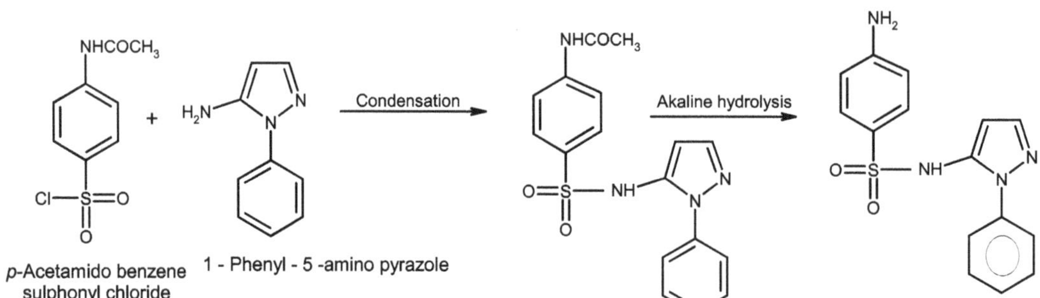

Sulphadimethoxine

Sulphadimethoxine is 4-amino-N-(2,6-dimethoxy-4-pyrimidinyl) benzene-sulphonamide.

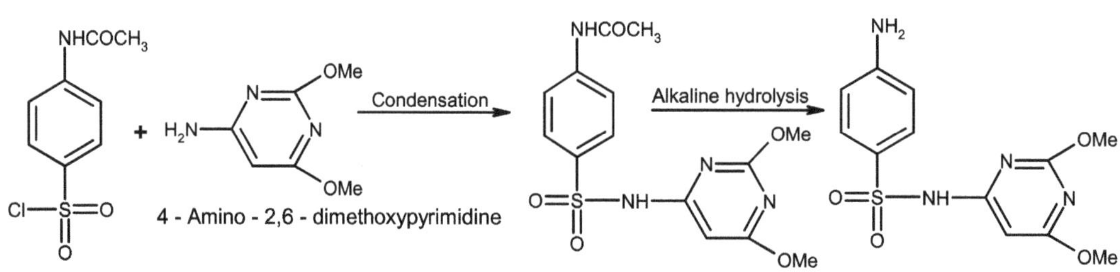

Properties

It occurs as a white, odorless, crystalline powder. It is slightly solube in alcohol and dissolves in dilute mineral acids and in solutions of alkali hydroxides and carbonates

Uses

Sulphadimethoxine is a long acting sulphonamide and is readily absorbed from the gastro-intestinal tract. Sulphadimethoxine is indicated for the treatment of a wide range of respiratory, genitor urinary tract, enteric, and soft tissue infections. A fixed dose combination of 20 parts sulphadoxine and one part of pyrimethamine is given in the treatment of falciparum malaria resistant to other agents.

Sulphaguanidine

Sulphaguanidine is 4-amino-N-(diaminomethylene) benzene sulphonamide. Sulphaguanidine is prepared by condensing p-acetyl amino benzene sulphonylchloride with guanidine followed by hydrolysis of the intermediate products.

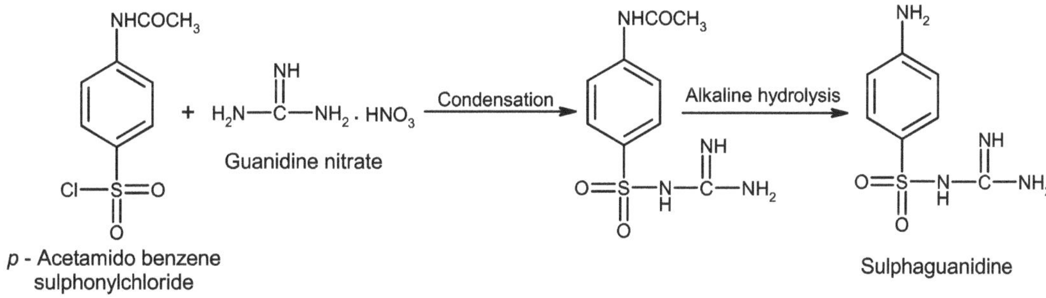

Properties

It is available as colourless crystalline powder. It is sparingly soluble in alcohol (or) acetone and freely soluble in mineral acids. It is insoluble in NaOH solutions at normal temperature.

Uses

It used in combination with other drugs to treat gastrointestinal infections, skin infections and throat infections.

Phthalylsulphathiazole

Phthalylsulphathiazole can be considered as a derivative of sulphathiazole in which the hydrogen of the amino group in position 4 has been substituted by aliphatic acid residue. Phthalylsulphathiazole is 4[1]-(thiazol-2-ylsulphamoyl) phthalanilic acid. It is prepared by condensation of sulphathiazole with phthalic anhydride.

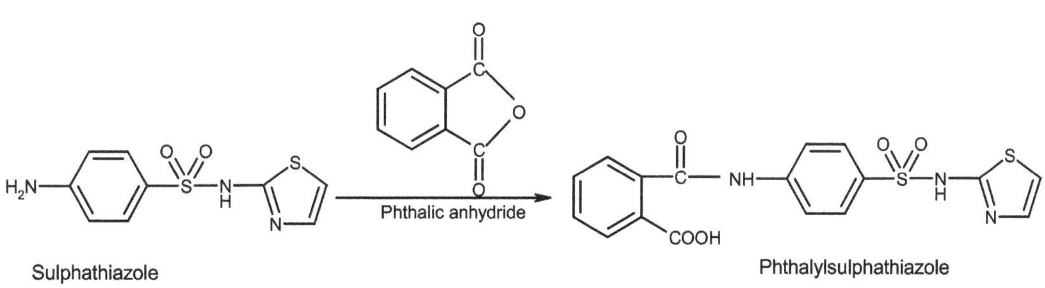

Phthalylsulphathiazole is highly effective with respect to the intestinal flora. The drug is mainly retained in the intestine, where the active sulphonamide part of the molecule is detached and exhibits its antibacterial action.

Succinylsulphathiazole

Succinylsulphathiazole is 4-(N-thiazol-2-ylsulphamoyl) succinalic acid. Succinylsulphathiazole is obtained by refluxing succinic anhydride with sulphathiazole in alcohol.

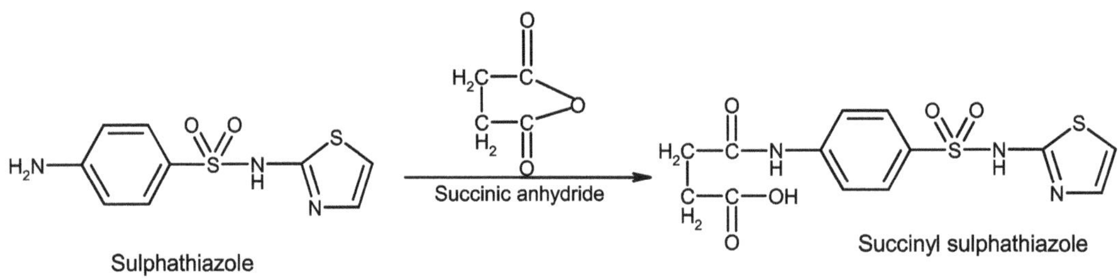

Properties

It is a white or slightly yellowish crystalline powder. It evolves pungent fumes on heating to melting point. It is soluble in solutions of alkali hydroxides and in solutions of sodium bicarbonate with the evolution of CO_2. It is sparingly soluble in alcohol and in acetone and is insoluble in chloroform and ether.

Uses

Succinylsulphathiazole has been used as antibacterial especially in enteric infections.

Sulphacetamide

Sulphacetamide is an acetyl derivative of sulphanilamide. It is prepared by acetylation and followed by selective alkaline hydrolysis.

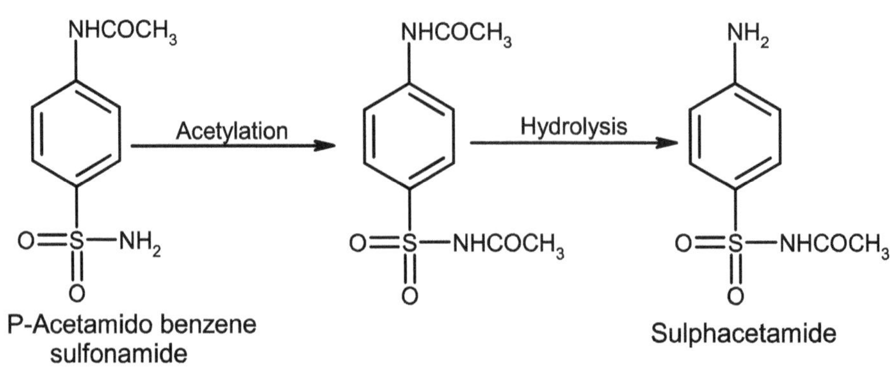

Sulphacetamide occurs as sodium salt. Sulphacetamide sodium dissolves in water. The solutions of sulphacetamide are slightly alkaline. It is used in the form of injection or eyedrops or eye ointments to treat eye infections.

Sulphasalazine

Sulphasalazine is 2-Hydroxy-5- ((E) 2-{4-[pyridin-2-yl) sulphamoyl) phenyl} diazen-1-yl] benzoic acid. Sulphasalazine is poorly absorbed into the small intestine and breaks into sulphapyridine and 5-aminosalicylic acid by the bacteria.

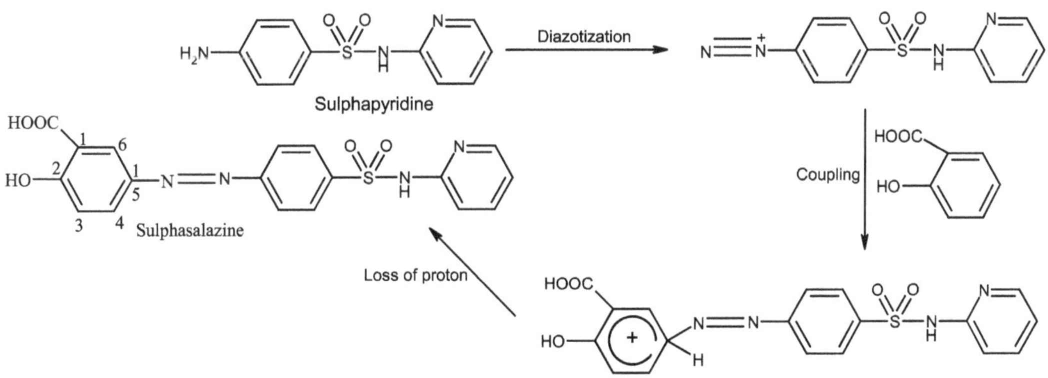

Sulphasalazine is a prodrug, i.e., it is not active in its ingested form. It is broken down by bacteria in the colon into two products: 5-aminosalicylic acid (5-ASA) and sulfapyridine. It is known that 5ASA has therapeutic effect. In the colon, the products created by the breakdown of sulphasalazine work as anti-inflammatory agents for treating inflammation of the colon. The beneficial effect of sulphasalazine is believed to be due to a local effect on the bowel, although there may also be a beneficial systemic immune-suppressant effect as well. Following oral administration, 33 percent of the sulphasalazine is absorbed, all of the sulphapyridine is absorbed, and about 33 percent of the 5-ASA is absorbed.

Uses

Sulphasalazine is believed to reduce inflammation, tissue damage, and diarrhoea. Sulphasalazine is used to treat ulcerative colitis and to maintain remission. Sulphasalazine may also be used to treat Crohn's disease in some cases.

Trimethoprim-sulphamethoxazole

Trimethoprim-sulphamethoxazole combination (1:5) is usually given orally but I.V. administration is reserved for more svere conditions.

Chemistry

Trimethoprim is structurally similar to dihydrofolic acid, a cofactor necessary for synthesis of purines, thymidine and methionine. Sulphamethoxazole is a sulphonamide.

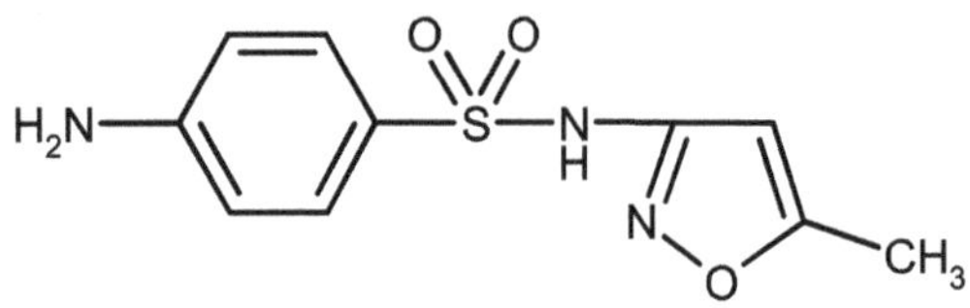

Sulphamethoxazole

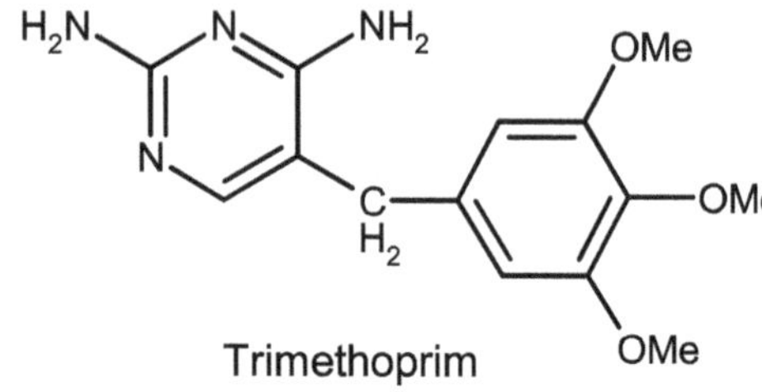

Trimethoprim

5-(3, 4, 5 – Trimethexybenzyl) Pyrimidine-2, 4 - diamine

Mechanism of action

(a) This combination inhibits two steps in the synthesis of tetrahydrofolic acid (see figure 7.2). Inhibiting two steps makes this combination more effective than either drug alone (i.e., synergistic), or any sulphonamide alone. Dihydrofolic acid competes with trimethoprim for the dihydrofolate reductase. Blockade of dihydrofolate synthesis by a sulphonamide enhances the effect of trimethoprim.

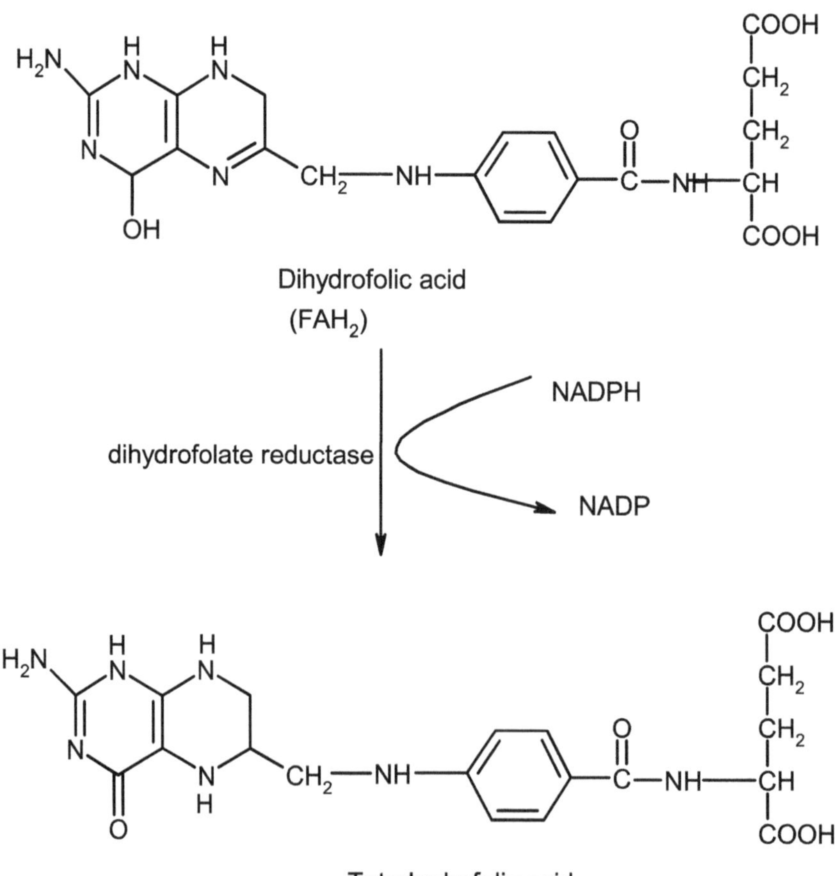

Tetrahydrofolic acid

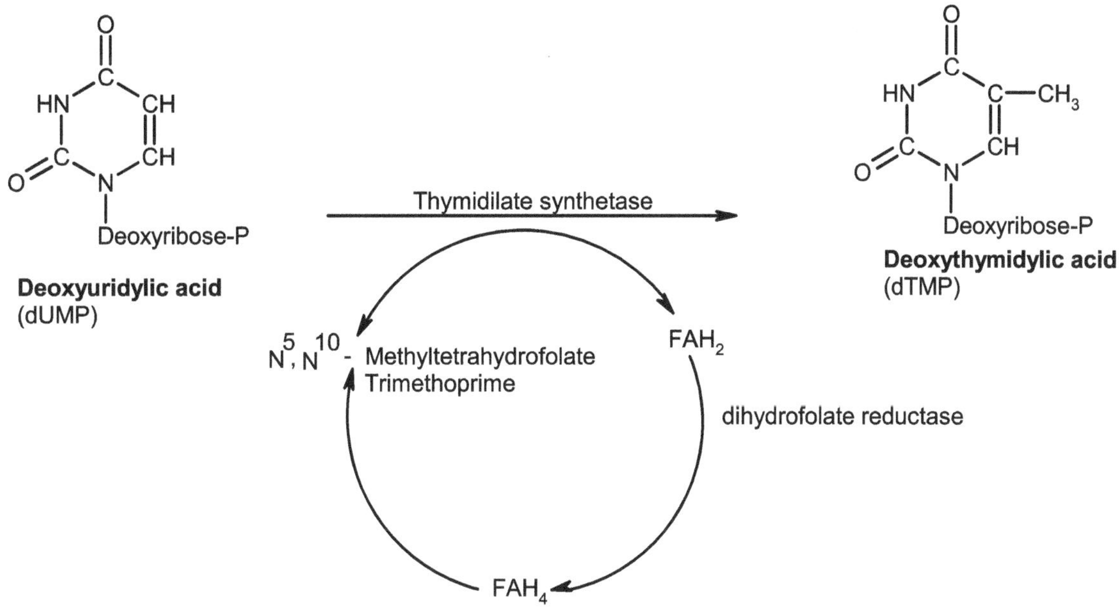

Figure 7.2

(b) The combination of sulphamethoxazole and trimethoprim possess broad spectrum of antimicrobial properties and is bactericidal in urine and blood in part because it depletes folic acid supplies needed for the thymidylate synthetase reaction.

Clinical uses : Sulphamethoxazole-trimethoprsim combination has been used to treat :

(a) Urinary tract infections
(b) Otitis media - both acute and chronic infections
(c) traveler's diarrhea
(d) *Pneumocystis carinii* pneumonia and
(e) Shigelosis.

8

PENICILLINS

History of antimicrobial therapy

At the beginning of the twentieth century, Paul Ehrlich, one of the pioneers in research on anti-infectives, studied the interaction of different substances with infectious protozoans and bacteria. Ehrlich used chemicals for his *in vitro* experiments, and thus, this therapy of infectious diseases is known as chemotherapy. In the early 1930s, Bayer researcher Gerhard Domagk, discovered a substance called prontosil, which was effective in treatment of bacterial infections *in vivo*.

Prontosil was safe enough to be used clinically and it was the first effective chemotherapeutic agent against infectious disease in humans. A short time later, it was discovered that prontosil was a prodrug, which had to be hydrolyzed in the organism to become effective. The active metabolite was identified as sulphanilamide, the first synthetic sulphonamide introduced to the market in 1936.

In 1929, Alexander Fleming coincidentally found that penicillin moulds inhibit the growth of bacteria *in vitro*. Florey, an English researcher, first used penicillin for therapy in humans in 1940. Today, synthetic penicillins and other members of the group of beta-lactam antibiotics, such as cephalosporins (discovered in1960), are still among the most important chemotherapeutic agents.

Research for new substances to fight bacterial and protozoal infections rapidly went on. Streptomycin (1944), the first aminoglycoside, chloramphenicol (1947), the first broad spectrum anti-infective, and chlortetracycline (1948) are examples of this rapid development. The area of quinolones began with the introduction of nalidixic acid in 1962 for treatment of kidney infections in humans.

Summary

Early 20th century	PAUL EHRLICH pioneers "chemotherapy"
1929	ALEXANDER FLEMING demonstrates inhibition of bacterial growth with penicillin moulds
Early 1930s	GERHARD DOMAGK discovers "prontosil" a prodrug to sulphanilamide
1936	Sulphanilamide, the first synthetic sulphonamide in human medicine
1940	First therapeutic use of "penicillin" by Florey
1944	Streptomycin
1947	Chloramphenicol, the first broad-spectrum antibiotic
1948	Chlortetracycline

1960	Cephalosporines
1962	GEORGE Y. LESHER discovers nalidixic acid during chloroquine synthesis
1970s	New 4-quinolones (pipemidic acid, oxolinic acid, cinoxacin)
1980	Norfloxacin, the first fluoroquinolone
1980	Enrofloxacin synthesized by Grohe and Peterson

β-Lactam antibiotics

β-Lactam antibiotics are a broad class of antibiotics which contain a β-lactam nucleus in its molecular structure. A beta-lactam (β-lactam) or penam is a lactam with a heteroatomic ring structure, consisting of three carbon atoms and one nitrogen atom.

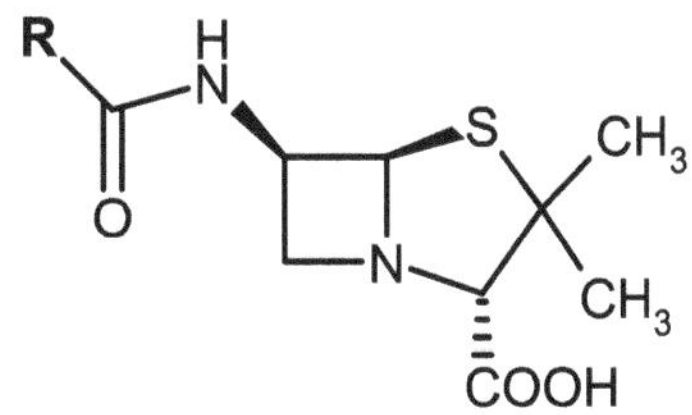

Penicillin nucleus (Beta lactam is the square at the center).

They are the most widely used antibiotics, which include penicillin derivatives, cephalosporins, monobactams, carbapenems and β-lactamase inhibitors. Traditionally, β-lactam antibiotics were mainly active against Gram-positive bacteria. The development of broad-spectrum β-lactam antibiotics (active against various Gram-negative organisms) has increased the usefulness of the β-lactam antibiotics. There are five relevant ring systems which appear in active beta lactams, including the **penam, penem, carbapenem, cefem and monobactam** ring structures (shown below). Following numbering is given according to chemical abstracts which are further given by bridged heterocycles nomenclature.

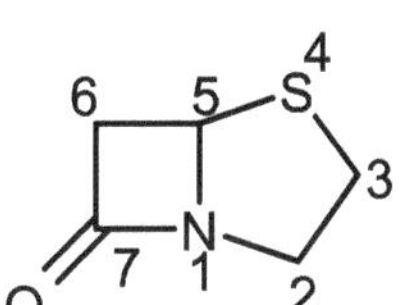

Penam
(4-Thia-1-azabicyclo[3.2.0] heptane-7-one)

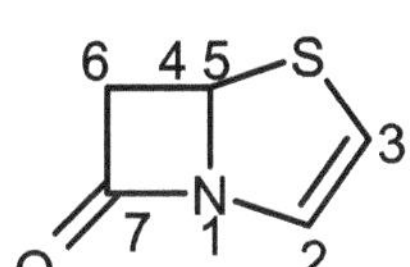

Penem
(4-Thia-1-azabicyclo[3.2.0] hept-2-ene-7-one)

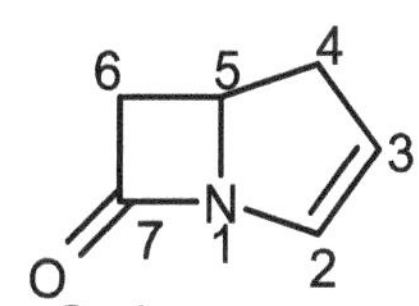

Carbapenem
(1-Azabicyclo[3.2.0] hept-2-ene-7-one)

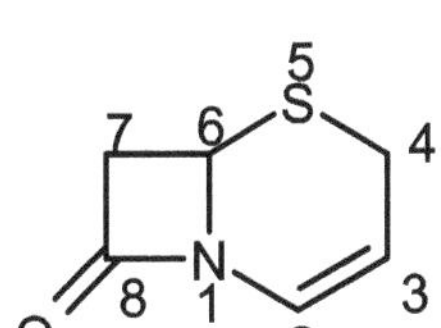

Cephem
(5-Thia-1-azabicyclo[4.2.0] oct-2-ene-8-one)

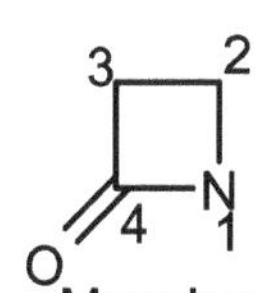

Monobactam
(1-Azacyclobutan-4-one)

Mode of action

β-Lactam antibiotics are bactericidal, and they target the synthesis of the peptidoglycan layer of the bacterial cell wall. Since peptidoglycan is only present in prokaryotic cells, toxicity to the eukaryotic cells of the patient is low. Peptidoglycan is a major component of the bacterial cell wall and is essential for the stability of the cell wall of both gram-positive and gram-negative bacteria. The peptidoglycan layer is a highly cross-linked crystal lattice structure formed from linear chains of backbone formed by alternating β-1,4-*N*-acetylglucosamines and *N*-acetylmuramic acids (amino sugars). The biosynthesis of

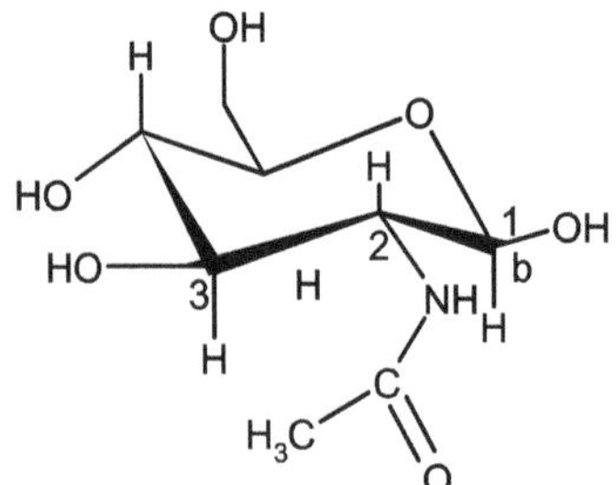

N-Acetyl glucosamine(NAG)

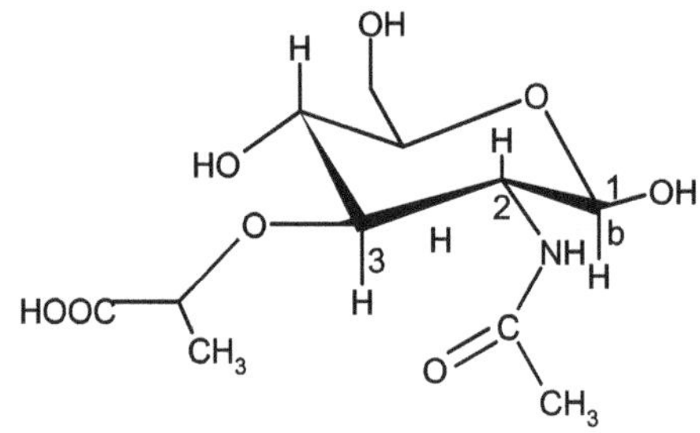

N-Acatylmuramic acid(NAM)

peptidoglycan may be considered in three stages. In the first stage uridine diphosphate-acetylmuramylpentapeptide is formed in cytoplasm. In the second stage uridine diphosphate-acetylmuramylpentapeptide and uridine diphosphate-acetylglucosamine are linked to form a long polymer. The final stage is transpeptidation involves cross-linking (cross-links are covalent bonds linking one polymer chain to another) of one polymer chain into another. The final transpeptidation step in the synthesis of the peptidoglycan is facilitated by transpeptidases known as penicillin binding proteins (PBPs). β-Lactam antibiotics are analogues of D-alanyl-D-alanine the terminal amino acid residues on the precursor NAM/NAG-peptide subunits of the nascent peptidoglycan layer. The structural similarity between β-lactam antibiotics and D-alanyl-D-alanine facilitates their binding to the active site of penicillin binding proteins (PBPs). The β-lactam nucleus of the molecule irreversibly binds to the PBP active site. This irreversible inhibition of the PBPs prevents the final cross-linking (transpeptidation) of the nascent peptidoglycan layer, disrupting cell wall synthesis. Inhibition of PBPs may also lead to the activation of autolytic enzymes in the bacterial cell wall.

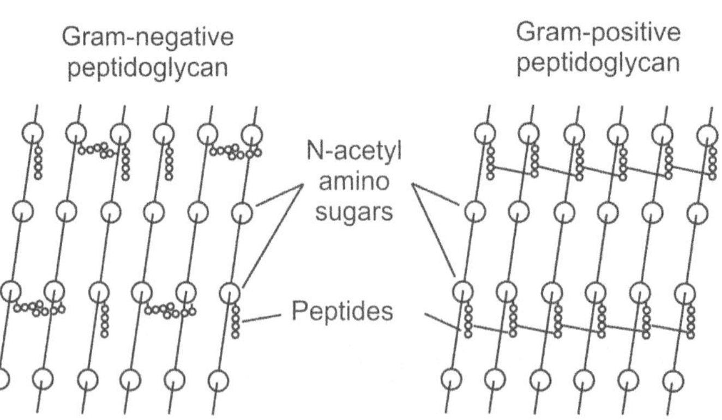

Figure 8.1 Diagrammatic representation of peptidoglycan structures with adjacent glycan strands cross-linked directly from the carboxyterminal D-alanine to the ε-amino group of an adjacent tetrapeptide or through a peptide cross bridge, N-acetylmuramic acid; N-acetylglucosamine.

Penicillins

Penicillins were first isolated from a common bread mold of the penicillium family. These are derived from a number of strains of *Pencillium notatum* and *Pseudononas chrysogenum*. Penicillin was discovered by Alexander Fleming in 1928 (He was preserving a culture of a pathogen and the plate became contaminated with an airborne fungus. The fungus not only grew but also produced a clear zone around its colony, indicating that the cells around it were being killed). Fleming recognized the significance of this discovery and tried to identify the contaminant. Unfortunately, he could not purify this compound because of its instability, but decade later two British scientists, Florey and Chain succeeded. In addition, they managed to produce the antibiotic on an industrial scale for widespread use. All three scientists shared the Nobel prize for this work, and rightly so - penicillin rapidly became the "wonder drug" which saved literally millions of lives during World War II. Pcnicillins arc the most widely used antibiotics. The basic nucleus of penicillin is 6-aminopenicillanic acid which consists of a thiazolidine ring (A) attached to a beta lactam ring (B).

Penicillins comprises of entire group of natural and semisynthetic penicillins and differ from one another in the R subsbtituent attached to 6-aminopenicillanic acid. Synthetic methods failed to replace the established fermentation processes as synthetic methods are providing fewer yields.

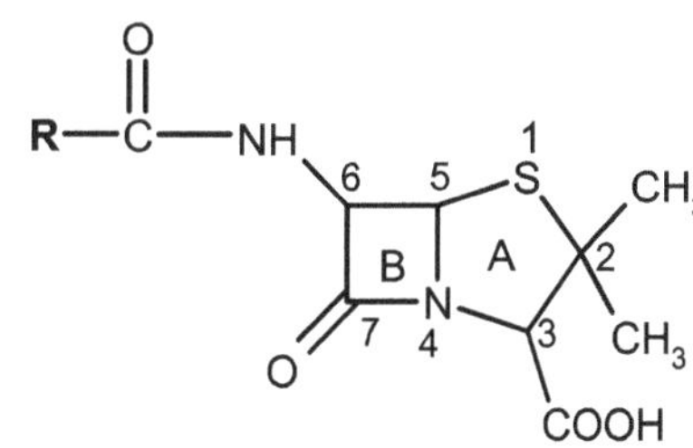

Classification

Penicillins are broadly classified basing on source of availability as:

1. **Natural penicillins :** Penicillin G, Penicillin V.
2. **Semi synthetic penicillins :** These semi synthetic penicillins can be further classified as:
   - (a) ***Broad spectrum penicillins*** **:** Ampicillin, amoxicillin etc.
   - (b) ***Penicillinase resistant parenteral penicillins*** **:** Methicillin, nafcillin etc.
   - (c) ***Penicillinase resistant oral penicillins*** **:** Oxacillin, cloxacillin, dicloxacillin etc.
   - (d) ***Penicillinase sensitive broad spectrum parenteral penicillins*** **:** Azlocillin, carbencillin, mezlocillin, ticarcillin etc.
   - (e) ***β-lactamase inhibitors*** **:** Clavulanic acid, sulbactam etc.

General characteristics

1. Penicillins are generally safe, having low toxicity, and can be used in pregnancy and during lactation.
2. Penicillins are poorly soluble, weak organic acids that are administered parenterally either as suspensions in water or oil, or as water-soluble salts. For example, sodium or potassium salts of penicillin G are highly water soluble and are absorbed rapidly from injection sites, whereas organic salts in microsuspension such as procaine penicillin G or benzathine penicillin G are gradually absorbed over 1-3 (or even more) days, respectively.

3. The trihydrate forms of the semisynthetic penicillins have greater aqueous solubility than the parent compounds and are usually preferred for both parenteral and oral use. They have low degree of direct toxicity and high incidence of allergic reactions. Penicillins are incompletely absorbed from the GIT when taken orally and possess short duration of action due to rapid excretion.

Structure-activity relationships (SAR)

Penicillins have been well studied and scientists were able to determine the following SAR. The following numbering is accordingly to USP nomenclature.

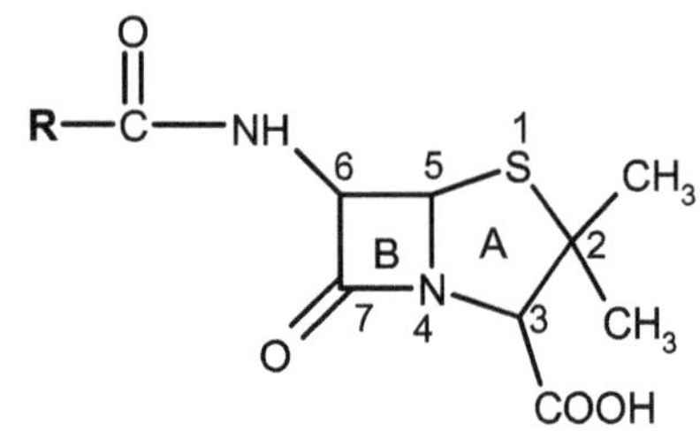

Basic structure of pencillins

1. Oxidation of the sulphur to a sulfone and sulfoxide will decrease the activity of penicillins which gives better acid stable activity. The methyl groups at position 2 are essential.
2. β-Lactam carbonyl and nitrogen are absolutely needed for activity.
3. The carbonyl on the β-lactam at position-7 is must.
4. The carboxylic acid of the thiazolidine at position-3 is required for activity. If it is changed to an alcohol or ester, activity is decreased.
5. Nitrogen at position-4 is must for antibacterial activity.
6. A group attached to the amide carbonyl (the R group) is the basis for change in activity of acid stability and susceptibility to resistance.
7. Sodium or potassium salts of penicillins are water soluble and readily absorbed when administered by injection or orally.
8. Procaine and benzathine penicillins have poor solubility in water and are used as depot forms.
9. The penicillin molecule contains three chiral carbon atoms (C-3(S), C-5(5R),C-6(6R)). Disruption of this spatial arrangement results in loss of anti bacterial activity.
10. SAR of the R group :
    (i) Addition of an electron withdrawing group near the amide carbonyl decreases the availability of the oxygen electrons for intra-molecular attack and allows for greater acid stability / oral availability. Example of penicillins that are acid stable are penicillin V and amoxicillin.
    (ii) A bulky group linked to carbonyl carbon of amide group will prevent the penicillin from entering the active site of β-lactamases but still allow them to enter the active sites of PBP's. Example of penicillins and β-lactamase resistant are nafcillin and methicillin.
    (iii) Addition of polar groups to the R group will allow the molecule to pass more easily through the gram-negative cell wall via porins and increase the spectrum of action. Example of penicillins with an extended spectrum of action include amoxicillin and dicloxacillin.

(iv) A "Urea-like" or polar and bulky R groups will add anti-pseudomonal activity to the penicillins. Example of anti-pseudomonal drugs are piperacillin and ticarcillin.

Mechanism of action

Penicillins were found to bind covalently to certain proteins in the bacterial membrane known as penicillin binding proteins (PBP's) and these appear to be involved in cell wall synthesis and the rigidity. They inhibit the synthesis of bacterial cell walls and prevent linkage of structural components to the cell. They are active against gram-positive and a few gram-negative organisms.

Stability

Most penicillins are strong monobasic acids with pK_a values in the range of 2.5 to 3.0. The free acids are unstable hence they are unsuitable for oral or parenteral administration. The alkali metal salts of penicillins are stable, soluble in water and readily absorbed orally as parenterally. Enzyme penicillinases (β-lactamases or acylases), alkalis and strong acids ($pH < 3$) degrade the penicillins basic nucleus and side chain to yield degradation products by following chemical reactions.

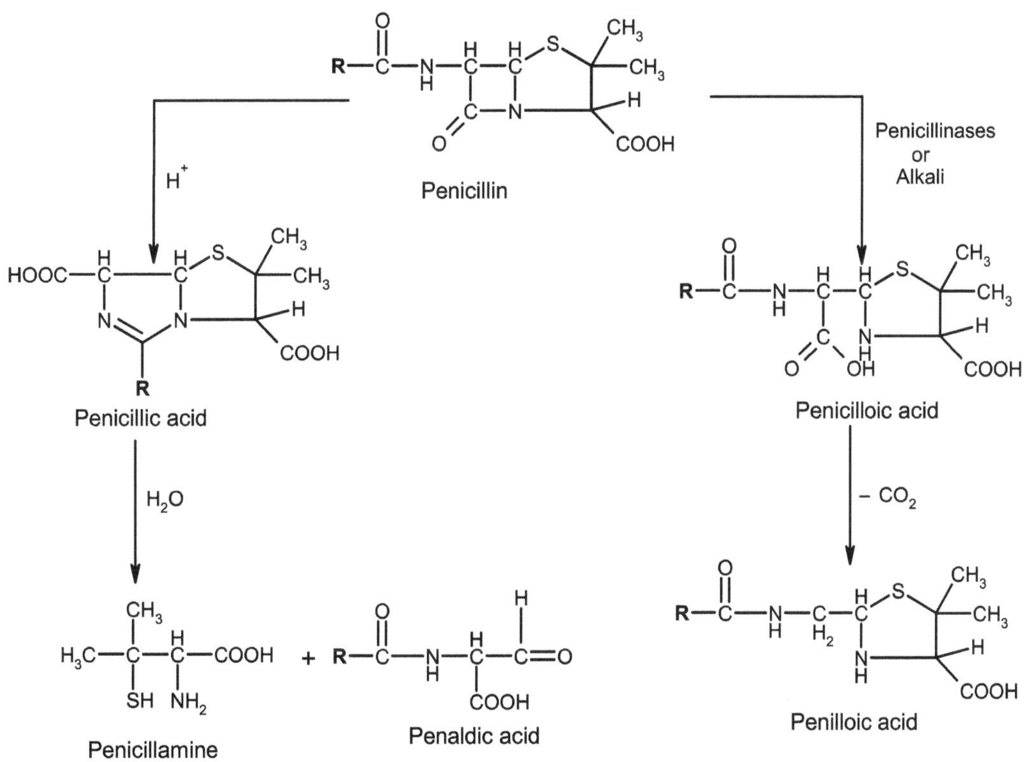

Figure 8.2 Instability of penicillins.

Penicillins contain a β-lactam nucleus that when cleaved by a β-lactamase enzyme (penicillinase) produces penicilloic acid derivatives that are inactive but which may act as the antigenic determinants for penicillin hypersensitivity.

Side effects

1. Most important side effects of penicillins are hyper sensitivity and anaphylaxis.
2. Penicillins are most common cause of allergies.
3. Cross-reactions among the penicillins.

Natural penicillins

The two natural penicillins obtained from culture filtrates of *Penicillium notatum* or the closely related species *Pseudomonas chrysogenum* are penicillin G and the more acid-resistant penicillin V. They are active only against gram-positive bacteria (which have a thick layer of peptidoglycan in the wall) and not against gram-negative species, including many serious pathogens like *Mycobacterium tuberculosis* (the cause of tuberculosis). Nevertheless, the natural penicillins were extremely valuable for treating wound pathogens such as *Staphylococcus* in Europe during wartime.

Penicillin G or benzyl penicillin: The first penicillin that was widely used is benzyl penicillin,or Penicillin G. Penicillin G possesses many of the qualities of an "ideal" antibiotic. It is relatively non-toxic to the host (or patient) and it is effective against a wide variety of organisms including fungi. It is obtained from fermentations of Penicillium chrysogenum mold and is classified as a narrow-spectrum drug effective against many gram-positive, some gram-negative organisms and some anaerobes. Benzyl penicillin is available as benzyl penicillin sodium or benzyl penicillin potassium.

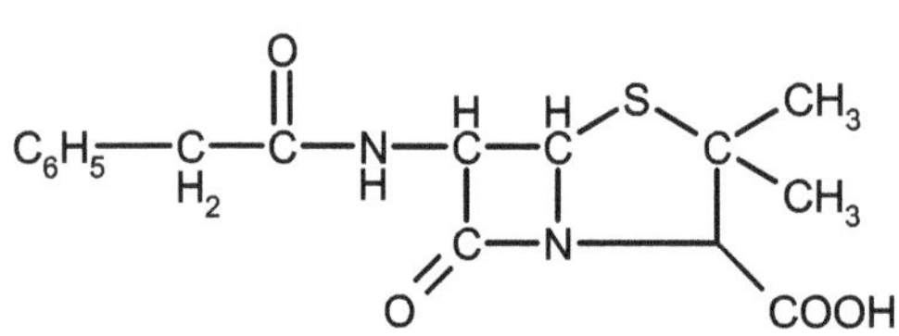

Penicillin G(Benzyl penicillin)

Penicillin G is a highly acidic drug, with a pK_a of 2.74. It is amorphous white powder. It is sparingly soluble in water and is soluble in ethanol, ether, ethyl acetate, benzene, chloroform and acetone. It is insoluble in petroleum ether. Benzyl penicillin sodium or potassium is freely soluble in water. One I.U. (International Unit) penicillin is equivalent to 0.00059 mg of benzyl penicillin. It is not acid-stable hence given (by injection) as parenteral. Penicillin G is short acting, but its salt forms, procaine and benzathine have extended duration of action because they can distribute into storage tissues to be released slowly.

Uses: Penicillin G is typically given by a parenteral route of administration because it is unstable to the hydrochloric acid of the stomach. Penicillin G is a bactericidal drug that is active against the *pneumococcus, Streptococcus, Gonococcus, Treponema, Anthrax, Clostridia*, penicillinase negative staphylococcus and against the actinomycosis fungus. Specific indications for benzyl penicillin include: Bacterial endocarditis, meningitis, aspiration pneumonia, lung abscess, community-acquired pneumonia, syphilis and septicaemia in children.

Penicillin V (phenoxymethyl penicillin)

Phenoxymethyl penicillin, commonly known as penicillin V, is the *orally-active* form of penicillin. It is also a narrow spectrum β-lactam antibiotic. It is obtained by adding 2-phenoxyethanol to *Penicillium notatum* on culture media.

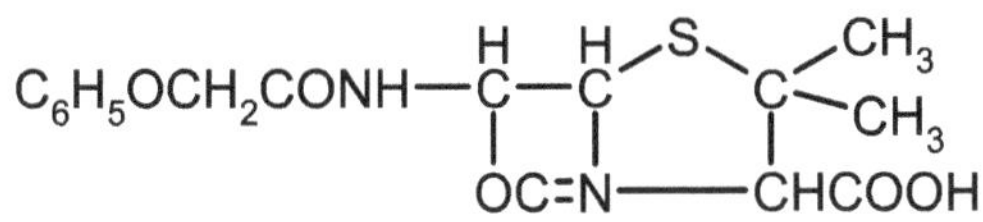

Peniclin V

It differs from penicillin G by being acid-stable and can be taken orally. It is effective against gram-positive cocci (*Streptococcus, Neisseria, Meningitis*), *Treponoma pallidum* (syphilis), *Burrelia burg dorferi* (lyme diseases), Some anaerobes (*Clostridium, Corynebacterium diphtheriae, Actinomyces, Bacillus anthracis* and *Listeria*). Specific indications for phenoxymethyl penicillin include: Infections caused by *Streptococcus pyogenes,* tonsilitis, pharyngitis, skin infections, prophylaxis of rheumatic fever, moderate-to-severe gingivitis (with metronidazole).

Benzathine benzylpenicillin, is slowly absorbed into the circulation, after intramuscular injection, and hydrolyzed to benzylpenicillin *in vivo*. It is the drug-of-choice when prolonged low concentrations of benzylpenicillin are required and appropriate, allowing prolonged antibiotic action over 2–4 weeks after a single IM dose.

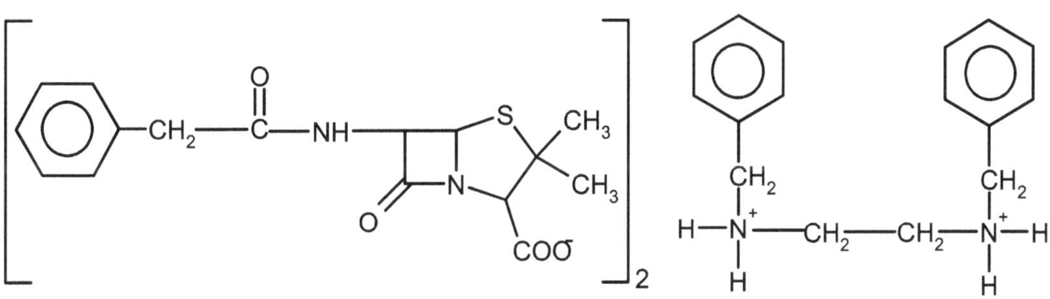

Benzathine penicillin

Semi-synthetic penicillins

Natural penicillins can be modified chemically by substitution of 6-amino group of 6-aminopenicillanic acid that confer new properties. The new acylated products produced are termed as semi-synthetic penicillins. These modern semi-synthetic penicillins such as ampicillin, carbenicillin and oxacillin have various specific properties such as:

- Resistance to stomach acids so that they can be taken orally,
- A degree of resistance to penicillinase (a penicillin-destroying enzyme produced by some bacteria),
- Extended range of activity against some gram-negative bacteria.

Ampicillin : Ampicillin is an amino penicillin and as such, is a broad-spectrum antibiotic and has been used extensively to treat bacterial infections since 1961. Ampicillin possesses

D-α-aminophenylacetamido side chain at position-6. It can sometimes results in allergic reactions that range in severity from a rash to potentially lethal anaphylaxis. Chemically, it is D-(-)-6-(2-amino-2-phenylacetamido)-3,3-dimethyl-7-oxo-4-thia-1-azabicyclo [3.2.0] heptane-2-carboxylic acid trihydrate.

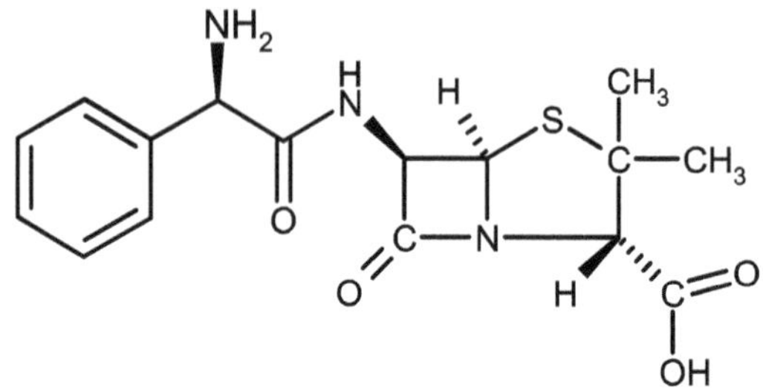

Ampicillin

Mechanism of action: Belonging to the group of beta-lactam antibiotics, ampicillin is able to penetrate gram-negative bacteria. It inhibits the third and final stage of bacterial cell wall synthesis, which ultimately leads to cell lysis.

Indications: It is more stable in stomach acids and therefore may be given orally; it is also more active against certain strains of bacteria. It is used regularly to treat common urinary-tract infections, some respiratory infections, and bacterial meningitis in children, although many strains of *Hemophilus influenzae* (the most common cause of bacterial meningitis) are now resistant to ampicillin, and it is commonly used along with other drugs. The potential side effects of ampicillin are similar to those of other penicillins – i.e., chiefly allergic reactions ranging from skin rashes and hives to life-threatening anaphylactic shock (very rare). People who are allergic to other drugs in this family are also likely to react to ampicillin. The incidence of skin rashes is higher with ampicillin than with other penicillins.

Amoxicillin: Amoxicillin is a moderate spectrum β-lactam antibiotic used to treat bacterial infections caused by susceptible microorganisms. It differs from ampicillin in p-hydroxyl functional group on benzene nucleus in side chain. It is usually the drug of choice within the class because it is better absorbed, following oral administration, than other β-lactam antibiotics. Amoxicillin is susceptible to degradation by β-lactamase producing bacteria, and so may be given with clavulanic acid to decrease its susceptibility.

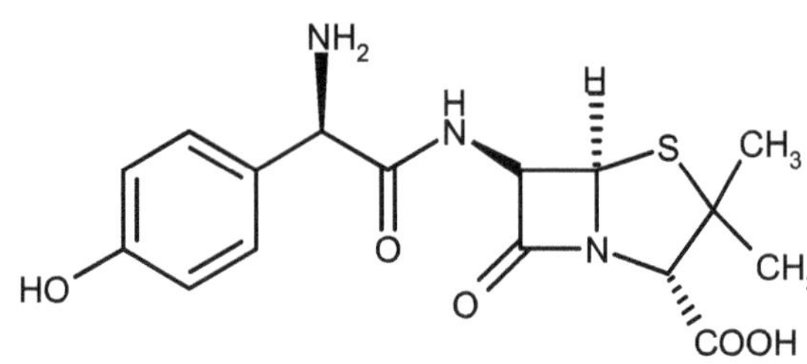

Amoxicillin

Mode of action : Amoxicillin acts by inhibiting the synthesis of bacterial cell walls. It inhibits cross-linkage between the linear peptidoglycan polymer chains that make up a major component of the cell wall of gram-positive bacteria.

Uses : Amoxicillin is a moderate-spectrum antibiotic active against a wide range of gram-positive (*Streptococcus* spp., *Diplococcus pneumoniae*, non β-lactamase-producing *Staphylococcus* spp., and *Streptococcus faecalis)*, and a limited range of gram-negative (*Haemophilus influenzae*, *Neisseria gonorrhoeae*, *Neisseria meningitis*, *Escherichia coli*, *Proteus mirabilis* and *Salmonella spp.)* organisms. Amoxicillin (in either trihydrate or sodium salt forms) may be combined with clavulanic acid (as potassium clavulanate), a β-lactamase inhibitor, to increase the spectrum of action against gram-negative organisms, and to overcome bacterial antibiotic resistance mediated through β-lactamase production.

Methicillin : Methicillin is a narrow spectrum β-lactam antibiotic which possess a 2, 6-dimethoxybenzamido group at 6-position. It is previously used to treat infections caused by susceptible gram-positive bacteria, particularly β-lactamase producing organisms such as *Staphylococcus aureus* but it is no longer clinically used. Its role in therapy has been largely replaced by flucloxacillin and dicloxacillin.

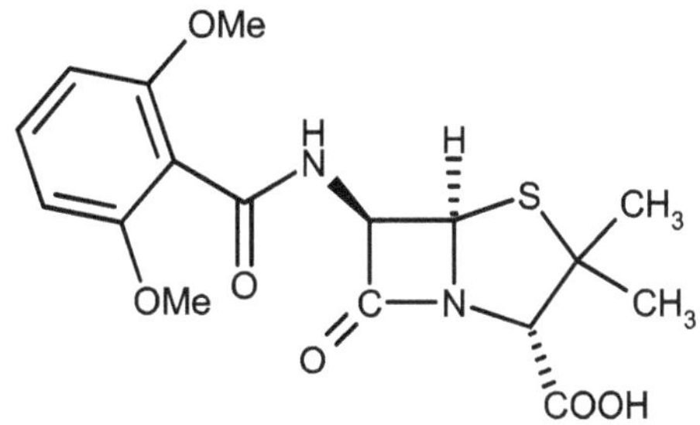

Methicillin

Methicillin is insensitive to β-lactamase (also known as penicillinase) enzymes secreted by many penicillin-resistant bacteria. The presence of the ortho-dimethoxyphenyl group directly attached to the side chain carbonyl group of the penicillin nucleus facilitates the β-lactamase resistance, since those enzymes are relatively intolerant of side chain steric hindrance. Thus it is able to bind to penicillin binding proteins (PBPs) and inhibit peptidoglycan cross-linking, but is not bound by or inactivated by β-lactamases.

Methicillin is not commonly used in clinical practice, but serves a purpose in the laboratory to determine antibiotic sensitivity in microbiological culture. Methicillin was previously used to treat infections caused by susceptible gram-positive bacteria. It is unstable in the presence of gastric acid, with a degradation half-life of 5 minutes at pH 2, so it must be administered by injection.

Nafcillin: Nafcillin is a semisynthetic β-lactam antibiotic derived from 6-amino-penicillanic acid. It is available as sodium salt in a parenteral dosage form. It has a molecular formula of $C_{21}H_{21}N_2NaO_5S \cdot H_2O$. Nafcillin is denoted chemically as: 4-Thia-1-azabicyclo [3.2.0] heptane-2- carboxylic acid, 6[[(2-ethoxy-1-naphthalenyl) carbonyl] amino]-3, 3-dimethyl-7-oxo-monosodium salt. It is available as white to yellowish white powder.

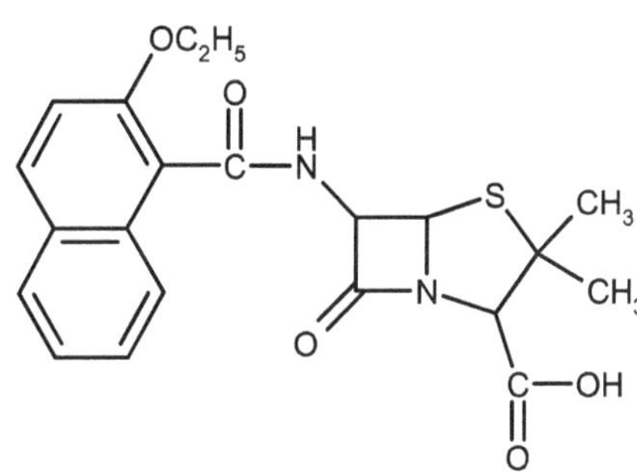

Nafcillin

Nafcillin can be given either orally or by injection. It is resistant to β-lactamase and is used to treat infections caused by gram-positive bacteria, particularly species of Staphylococci, that are resistant to other penicillins.

Penicillinase-resistant penicillins

Penicillinase-resistant penicillins are resistant to the β-lactamases as the name indicates. In these penicillins amide carbonyl group is attached with a bulky group which protects β-lactam ring from β-lactamases. These penicillinase-resistant penicillins have a more narrow spectrum of activity than the natural penicillins. Their antimicrobial efficacy is aimed directly against penicillinase-producing strains of gram positive cocci, particularly *Staphylococcal* species. They are sometimes called anti-staphylococcal penicillins. The penicillinase-resistant penicillins are inactive against *Rickettsia*, mycobacteria, fungi, *Mycoplasma* and viruses.

Cloxacillin, dicloxacillin, oxacillin and flucloxacillin have nearly identical spectrums of activity and can be considered therapeutically equivalent when comparing *in vitro* activity. These are white (or) almost white, crystalline compounds. They are hygroscopic and freely soluble in water and in methanol.

Cloxacillin : Cloxacillin is a semisynthetic penicillinase-resistant antibiotic. It is an isoxazolyl-penicillin antibiotic. Chemical designation is [2S (2α, 5α, 6β)]-3,3-dimethyl-6-[[3-(2-chlorophenyl)-5-methyl-4-isoxazolyl)carbonyl]amino]-7-oxo-4-thia-1-aza bicyclo [3.2.0] heptane-2-carboxylic acid, monosodium salt. It is available commercially as the monohydrate sodium salt which occurs as an odorless, bitter-tasting, white, crystalline powder. It is freely soluble in water and soluble in alcohol and has a pK_a of 2.7. One mg of cloxacillin sodium contains not less than 825 micrograms of cloxacillin. Cloxacillin sodium is resistant to acid inactivation in the gut, but is only partially absorbed. The bioavailability after oral administration in humans has been reported to range from 37-60% and if given with food both the rate and extent of absorption is decreased.

Cloxacillin benzathine occurs as white or almost white powder that is slightly soluble in water and alcohol. A 1% (10 mg/ml) suspension has a pH ranges from 3 - 6.5.

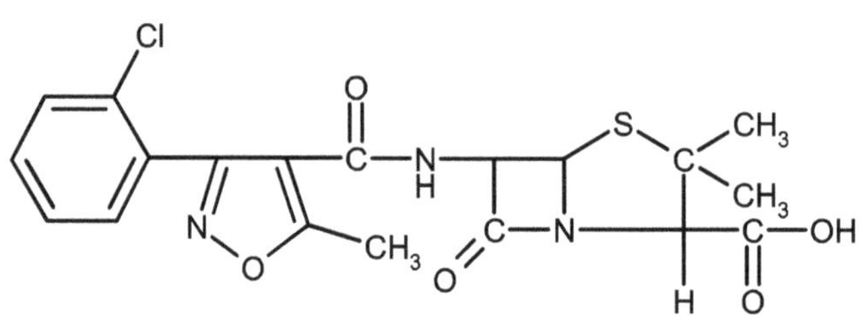

Cloxacillin

Cloxacillin is used against Staphylococci that produce β-lactamase.

- Mild to moderate infections caused by penicillinase-producing *Staphylococci*
- Upper respiratory tract infections
- Localized soft tissue/skin infections
- Lower respiratory tract infections
- Disseminated infections

Oxacillin : Oxacillin, derived from 6-aminopenicillanic acid, is a semisynthetic penicillinase-resistant penicillin against *Staphylococci* primarily. It is available as sodium salt. Chemically oxacillin sodium is [2S (2α, 5α, 6β)]-3,3-dimethyl-6-[[(5-methyl-3-phenyl-4-isoxazolyl) carbonyl] amino]-7-oxo-4-thia-1- azabicyclo [3.2.0]heptane-2-carboxylic acid, monosodium salt. Oxacillin sodium exists as white to off-white crystalline powder.

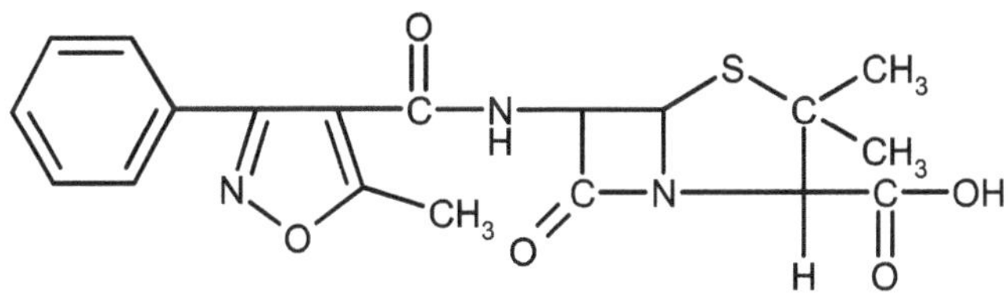

Oxacillin

Oxacillin is a β-lactam antibiotic used in the treatment of bacterial infections caused by susceptible, usually gram-positive organisms. The name "penicillin" can either refer to several variants of penicillin available, or to the group of antibiotics derived from the penicillins. Oxacillin has *in vitro* activity against gram-positive and gram-negative aerobic and anaerobic bacteria. The bactericidal activity of oxacillin results from the inhibition of cell wall synthesis and is mediated through oxacillin binding to penicillin binding proteins (PBPs). Oxacillin is stable against hydrolysis by a variety of β-lactamases, including penicillinases, and cephalosporinases and extended spectrum β-lactamases. It has been used particularly in the treatment of *Staphylococcus aureus* bacteria, and resistant strains are often called oxacillin-resistant *Staphylococcus aureus*. Oxacillin is more resistant to degradation on storage and is more likely to detect most heteroresistant strains.

Flucloxacillin : Flucloxacillin is a β-lactam penicillin antibiotic used in the treatment of bacterial infections caused by susceptible, usually Gram-positive organisms. Chemically it is 7-[3-(2-chloro-6-fluorophenyl)-5-methyloxazol-4-yl]carbonyl]amino]3,3-dimethyl-7-oxo-4-thia-1-azabicyclo [3,2,0] heptanecarboxylic acid. Flucloxacillin is stable against hydrolysis by a variety of β-lactamases, including penicillinases, and cephalosporinases and extended spectrum β-lactamases.

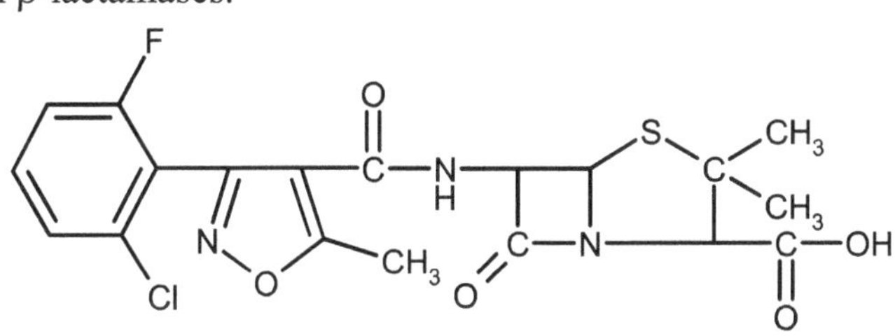

Flucloxacillin

Mechanism of Action: Flucloxacillin has *in vitro* activity against gram-positive and gram-negative aerobic and anaerobic bacteria. By binding to specific penicillin-binding proteins (PBPs) located inside the bacterial cell wall, flucloxacillin inhibits the third and last stage of bacterial cell wall synthesis. Cell lysis is then mediated by bacterial cell wall autolytic enzymes such as autolysins; it is possible that flucloxacillin interferes with an autolysin inhibitor.

Dicloxacillin : Dicloxacillin is a narrow spectrum β-lactam antibiotic. It is insensitive to β-lactamase (also known as penicillinase) enzymes secreted by many penicillin-resistant bacteria. The presence of the isoxazolyl group on the side chain of the penicillin nucleus facilitates the β-lactamase resistance, since they are relatively intolerant of side-chain steric hindrance. Dicloxacillin is more acid-stable than many other penicillins and can be given orally, in addition to parenteral routes. However, like methicillin, it is less potent than benzylpenicillin against non-β-lactamase producing gram-positive bacteria. It is commercially available as the sodium salt. Dicloxacillin has similar pharmacokinetics, antibacterial activity and indications to that of flucloxacillin and the two agents are considered interchangeable. It is believed that dicloxacillin have lower incidence of severe hepatic adverse effects than flucloxacillin, but a higher incidence of renal adverse effects.

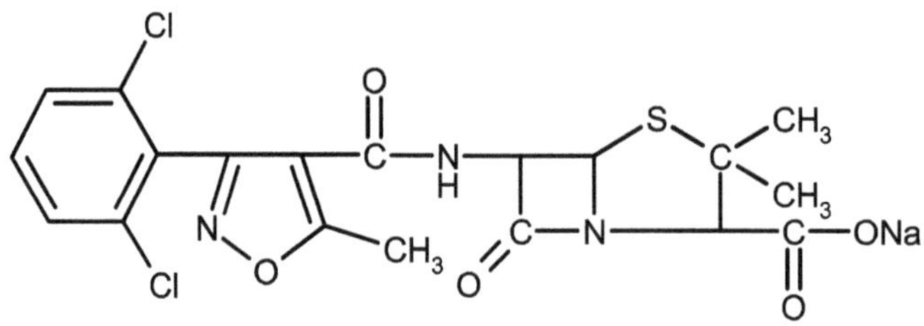

Dicloxacillin

Dicloxacillin exerts a bactericidal action against penicillin-susceptible microorganisms during the state of active multiplication. All penicillins inhibit the biosynthesis of the bacterial cell wall. By binding to specific penicillin-binding proteins (PBPs) located inside the bacterial cell wall, dicloxacillin inhibits the third and last stage of bacterial cell wall synthesis. Cell lysis is then mediated by bacterial cell wall autolytic enzymes such as autolysins; it is possible that dicloxacillin interferes with an autolysin inhibitor.

Indications: Dicloxacillin is indicated for the treatment of infections caused by susceptible bacteria. Specific approved indications include:

Staphylococcal skin infections and cellulitis including impetigo, otitis externa, folliculitis, boils, carbuncles, and mastitis.

- Pneumonia (adjunct)
- Osteomyelitis, septic arthritis
- Septicaemia
- Empirical treatment for endocarditis
- Surgical prophylaxis

Carbenicillin : Carbenicillin is a semisynthetic penicillin. Chemically it is 6-[(2-carboxy-2-phenyl-acetyl)amino]-3,3-dimethyl-7-oxo-4-thia-1-azabicyclo[3.2.0] heptane-2-carboxylic acid.

Carbenicillin is acid stable, and rapidly absorbed from the small intestine following oral administration. It provides substantial *in vitro* activity against a variety of both gram-positive and gram-negative microorganisms, the most important aspect of its profile is in its antipseudomonal and antiprotozoal activity. Because of the high urine levels obtained following administration, carbenicillin has demonstrated clinical efficacy in urinary

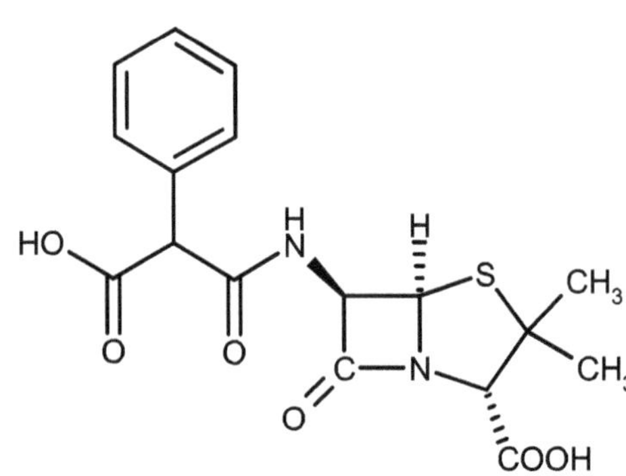

Carbenicillin

infections due to susceptible strains of *Escherichia coli*, *Proteus mirabilis*, *Proteus vulgaris*, *Morganella morganii*, *Pseudomonas* species, *Providencia rettgeri*, *Enterobacter* species, and *Enterococci* (*S. faecalis*).

Mechanism of Action: Free carbenicillin is the predominant pharmacologically active fraction of the salt. Carbenicillin exerts its antibacterial activity by interference with final cell wall synthesis of susceptible bacteria. It inactivates transpeptidase enzyme which prevents the formation of a cross-link of two linear peptidoglycan strands, inhibiting the third and last stage of bacterial cell wall synthesis.

Ticarcillin : Ticarcillin is an α-carboxypenicillin. It is derived from the basic penicillin nucleus, 6-amino-penicillanic acid. Chemically, ticarcillin disodium is *N* -(2-Carboxy-3,3-dimethyl -7-oxo-4-thia-1-azabicyclo[3.2.0] hept-6-yl)-3-thio-phenemalonamic acid disodium salt and may bc rcprcscnted as:

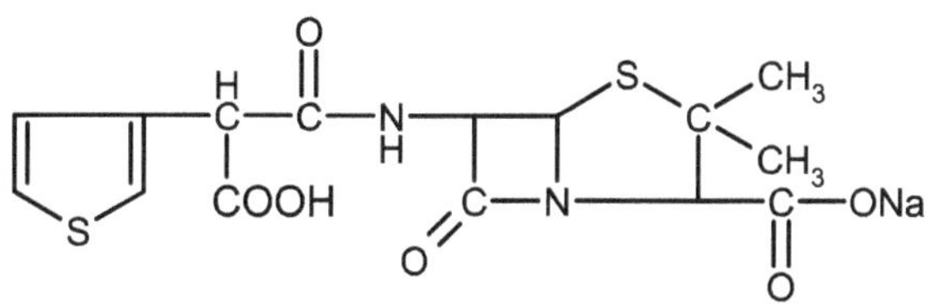

Ticarcillin

Ticarcillin disodium occurs as a white to pale yellow, hygroscopic powder or lyophilized cake with pK_a of 2.55 and 3.42. Ticarcillin is not appreciably absorbed after oral administration and must be given parenterally to achieve therapeutic serum levels. When given IM to humans, the drug is readily absorbed with peak levels occurring about 30-60 minutes after dosing. The reported bioavailability in the horse after IM administration is about 65 per cent.

Uses : Ticarcillin disodium is administered in combination with the β-lactamase inhibitor-clavulanate potassium (the potassium salt of clavulanic acid) by intravenous administration.

Azlocillin : Azlocillin is an acylampicillin antibiotic with an extended spectrum of activity and greater *invitro* potency than the carboxy penicillins. Azlocillin is similar to mezlocillin and piperacillin. It demonstrates antibacterial activity against a broad spectrum of bacteria, including *Pseudomonas aeruginosa* and in contrast to most cephalosporins exhibits activity against *enterococci*.

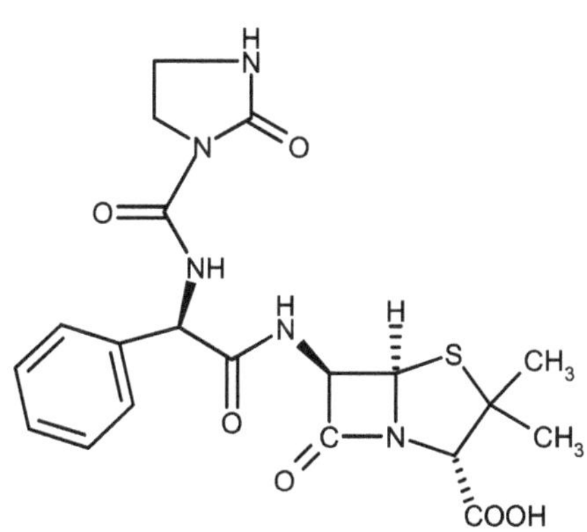

Azlocillin

Piperacillin : Piperacillin is an extended spectrum β-lactam antibiotic of the ureidopenicillin class. It is normally used together with the β-lactamase inhibitor tazobactam. The combination has activity against many gram-positive and gram-negative pathogens and anaerobes, including *Pseudomonas aeruginosa*. Piperacillin/tazobactam is administered intravenously. Its main uses are in intensive care medicine (pneumonia, peritonitis), some diabetes-related foot infections and empirical therapy in febrile neutropenia (e.g., after chemotherapy). It is administered by IV or IM injection.

β-Lactamase inhibitors

β-Lactamase inhibitors are proteins designed to inhibit or destroy the effectiveness of β-lactamase enzymes. Inhibitors generally have little antimicrobial properties themselves and so are combined with a β-lactam antibiotic. These inhibitors (clavulanic acid, sulbactam, tazobactam) function by binding to the β-lactamase enzymes more efficiently than the actual β-lactam antibiotic itself.

Clavulanic acid: Clavulanic acid is a β-lactamase inhibitor sometimes combined with penicillin group antibiotics to overcome certain types of antibiotic resistance. Specifically, it is used to overcome resistance in bacteria that secrete β-lactamase enzymes, which otherwise inactivate most penicillins. Most commonly, the potassium salt, potassium clavulanate is combined with amoxicillin or ticarcillin.

Clavulanic acid is produced by the fermentation of *Streptomyces clavuligerus*. It is a β-lactam structurally related to the penicillins and possesses the ability to inactivate a wide variety of β-lactamases by blocking the active sites of these enzymes. Chemically, clavulanate potassium is potassium (Z)-(2*R*,5*R*)-3-(2-hydroxyethylidene)-7-oxo-4-oxa- 1-azabicyclo [3.2.0] heptane-2-carboxylate and may be represented structurally as:

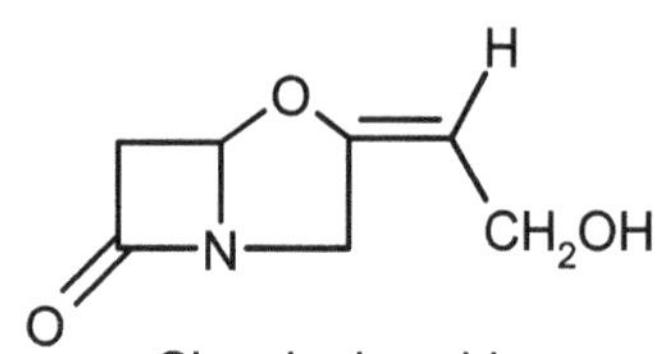

Clavulanic acid

Mechanism of action

Clavulanic acid has negligible intrinsic antimicrobial activity, despite sharing the β-lactam ring that is characteristic of β-lactam antibiotics. However, the similarity in chemical structure allows the molecule to act as a competitive inhibitor of β-lactamases secreted by certain bacteria to confer resistance to β-lactam antibiotics. This inhibition restores the antimicrobial activity of β-lactam antibiotics against β-lactamase secreting resistant bacteria.

Sulbactam

Sulbactam is a clinically useful injectable β-lactamase inhibitor sold by Pfizer. It is used in conjunction with a penicillin or cephalosporin to treat serious bacterial infections. Penicillins and cephalosporins are destroyed by a family of enzymes called β-lactamases, which hydrolyze the four-membered amide ring. Sulbactam inhibits these enzymes, allowing the drug to remain in circulation longer.

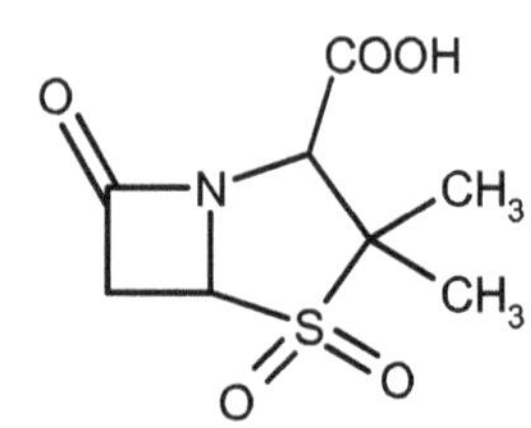

Sulbactam

9

CEPHALOSPORINS

Introduction

Cephalosporins are β-lactam antibiotics, which are obtained naturally from cephalosporium species or semisynthetically by chemical attachment of side chains to 7-aminocephalosporanic acid. The cephalosporin structure was first discovered in 1978. The cephalosporin ring structure is derived from 7-aminocephalosporanic acid (7-ACA), while the penicillins are derived from 6-aminopenicillanic acid (6-APA). Both structures contain the basic β-lactam ring but the cephalosporin structure allows for more Gram-negative activity than the penicillins and aminocillins. Modification of the 7-ACA side-chains resulted in the development of useful antibiotic agents, and the first agent cephalothin (cephalotin) was launched by Eli Lilly in 1964.

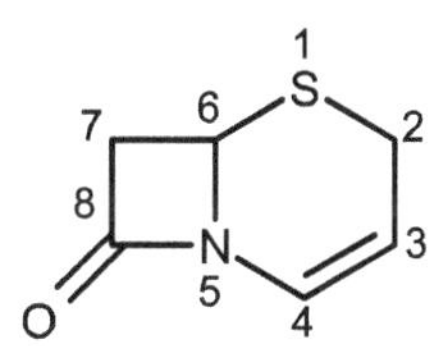

Cepham nucleus

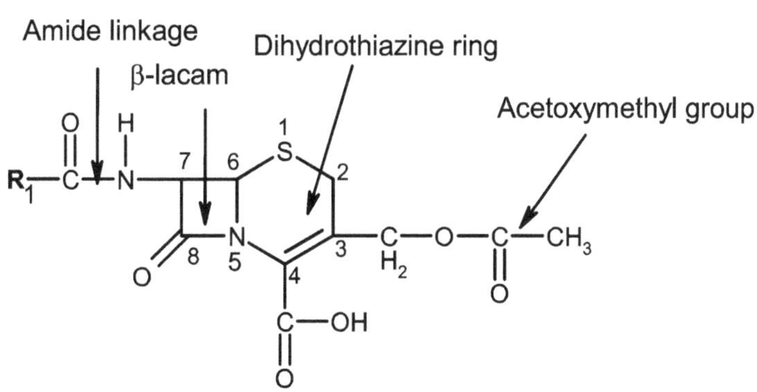

Cephalosporin nucleus

In 1948, Italian scientist Giuseppe Brotzu identified the first source of cephalosporins (*Cephalosporium acremonium*) in a sewage out fall off the Sardinian coast. Abraham and

Newton purified and established the structure of cephalosporin C (CPC). This molecule is the first of the cephalosporin antibiotic family. In CPC, the four-membered β-lactam ring is coupled to a six-membered dihydrothiazine ring to form the nucleus, 7- aminocephalosporanic acid (7-ACA), and a side chain, α-aminoadipic acid, is coupled via an amide bond to the nucleus. Cephalosporin C was shown to be active against a large number of pathogenic bacteria. However, its clinical use is hampered by a very low chemical stability.

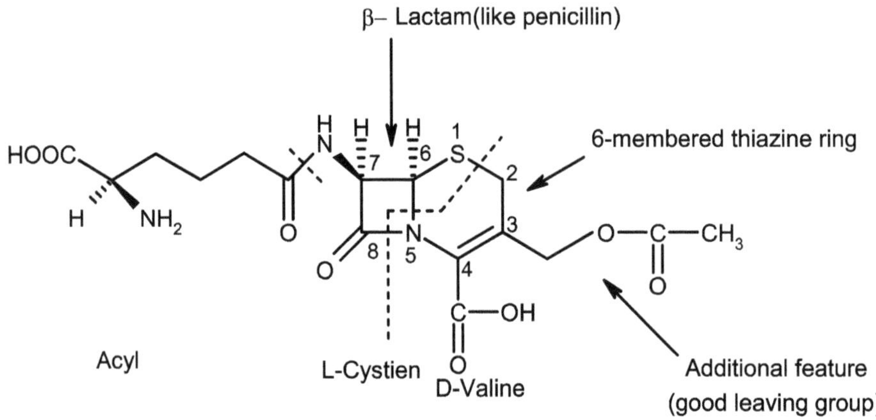

Cephalosporin C

Figure 9.1 Structure of cephalsporin C and the cell wall pentapeptide. The β-lactam ring of CPC is shown in bold. The structure closely resembles the two D-Alanine residues of the pentapeptide that is cross-linked in the bacterial cell wall. The bacterial transpeptidase enzyme cuts the amide bond between the two alanines (shown in bold), thereby removing one D-Alanine. Subsequently, it connects the rest of the pentapeptide to the lysine of a second pentapeptide via a pentaglycine. If the amide bond in the β-lactam ring of CPC is hydrolyzed, the dihydrothiazine ring remains attached and inhibits cross-linking and subsequent release of the enzyme.

Mode of action

Cephalosporins though possess similar to the penicillins in action have different chemical structures. They tend to be more stable than penicillins to many of the bacterial β-lactamases and have a broader spectrum of activity than penicillins. Their advantages over the penicillins are that they resist hydrolysis by the enzyme penicillinase that is secreted by a number of bacteria.

Cephalosporins have a bactericidal effect by inhibiting the synthesis of bacteria cell wall, resulting in cell lysis. Cell lysis occurs because the cell wall is deteriorated, causing the cell to be unprotected from the environment and subjective to burst under pressure. β-lactam antibiotics are structurally similar to D-alanyl-D-alanines(component of peptidoglycan), they are able to react chemically with penicillin-binding proteins [The final transpeptidation step in the synthesis of the peptidoglycan is facilitated by transpeptidases known as penicillin binding proteins (PBPs)] and inactivate them. Thus cephalosporins disrupt the synthesis of the peptidoglycan layer of bacterial cell walls (The peptidoglycan layer is important for cell wall structural integrity, especially in gram-positive organisms). Interfere with the bacteria's components and these antibiotics are not dangerous to the host cells.

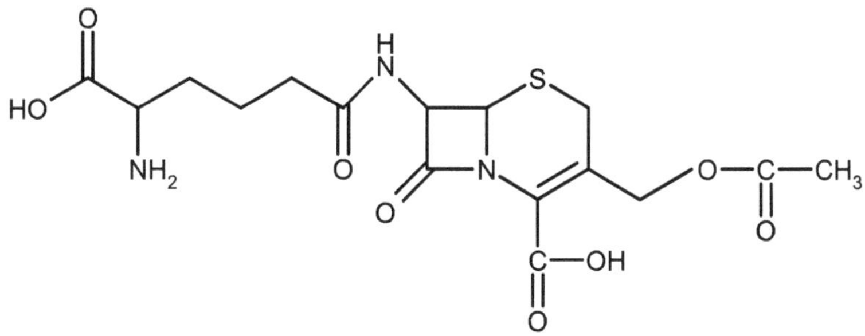

Cephalosporin C

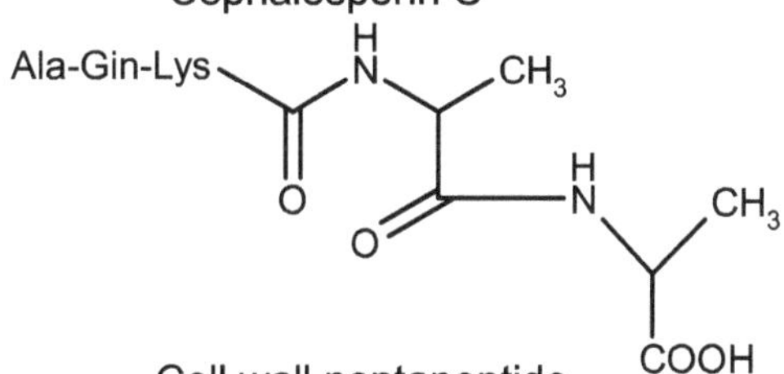

Cell wall pentapeptide

Stability of cephalosporins

The cephalosporin acylases are β-lactam acylases, highly specialized peptidases that are capable of cleaving the amide bond between a β-lactam nucleus and a side chain without damaging the β-lactam ring.

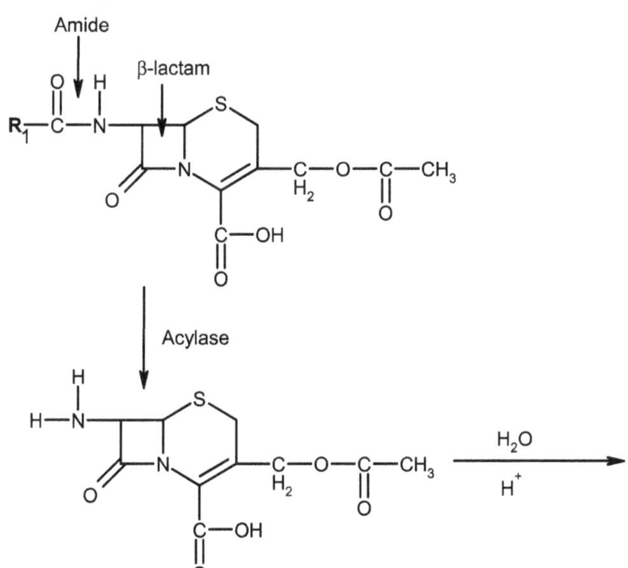

7-Aminocephalosporanic acid

Desacetyl-7-Aminocephalosporanic acid lactone

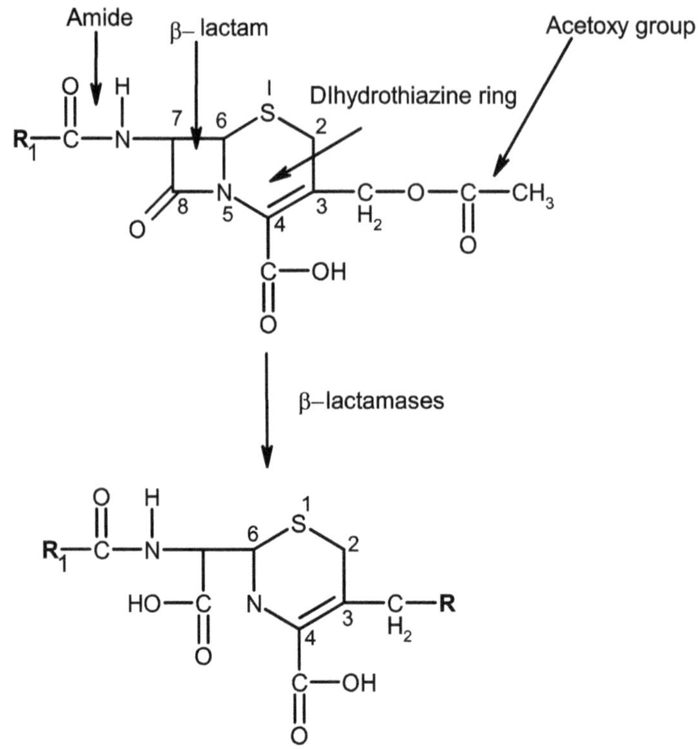

Cephalosporoic acid

Structure-activity relationships

1. In cephalosporins the β-lactam ring is bridged with a six member 1,3-dihydrothiazine ring. Intact β-lactam ring is required for PBP reactivity and antibacterial activity. The dihydrothiazine ring makes the β-lactam system of cephalosporin more stable to acids and penicillinase enzyme.

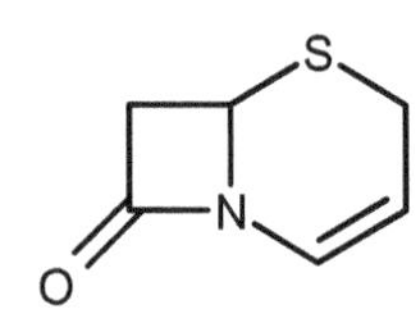

2. Natural cephalosporins biological activity is poor relative to penicillins, but the β-lactam ring is more stable to acid and to β-lactamases.
3. Semisynthetic cephalosporins have broad spectrum of activities. They are synthesized by adding different side chains at R_1 and R_2. The semisynthetic derivatives have increased acid stability, increased pharmacokinetic properties broad-spectrum activities, decreased allergic reactions and increased tolerance. E.g., Cephalotin, cefadroxyl, cefuroxime.
4. 3-CH_2OA_C in cephalosporin C provides another site for modification. The nature of subsbtituent at C-3 influences both pharmacokinetic and antibacterial activity. Replacement of 3-acetoxymethyl group with a group (H, CH_3, Cl, CH_2OCH_3, $CH{=}CHR^1$) yield cephalosporins with acid stable, metabolically stable, oral active derivatives.

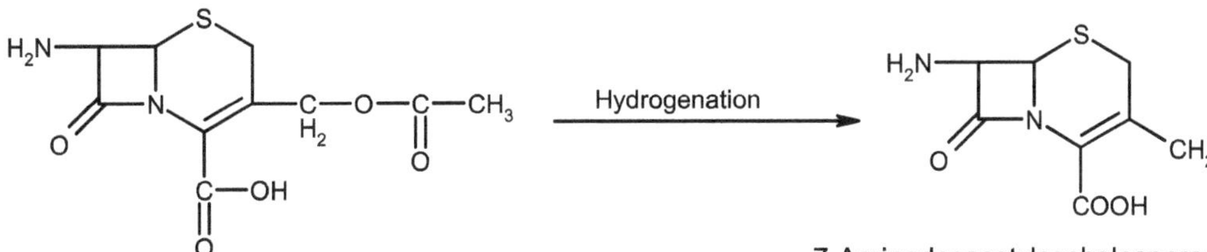

7-Aminocephalosporanic acid   7-Aminodesacetylcephalosporanic acid

(i) 3-Carbamoylcephalosporins are acid unstable but somewhat metabolically stable (more than cephalosporanic acids). They are minimally effective on spectrum of activity and not active orally.

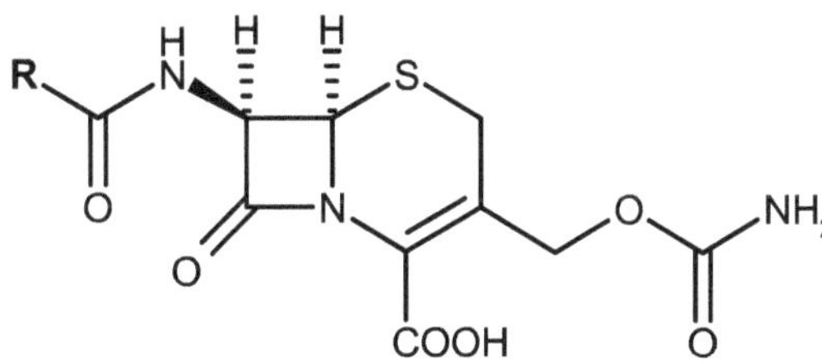

Introduction of thiothiadiazole at 3-position yield cephalosporins of acid unstable but metabolically stable and minimally active. They are not orally active.

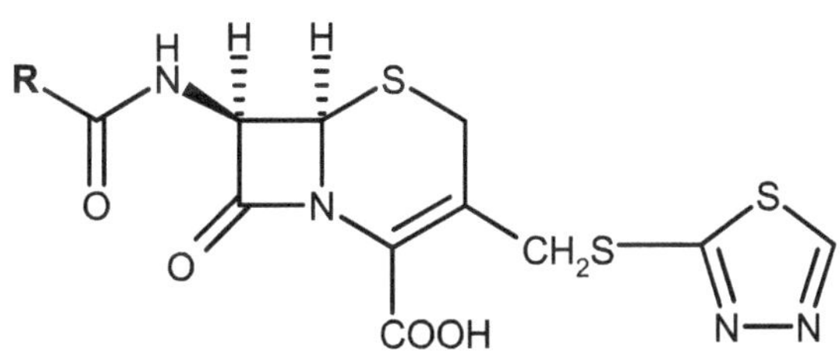

Introduction of N-methylthiotetrazole (NMTT) group or N-methylthiotetrazole-1-acetic acid or N-Methylthiotetrazole-1-methansulfonic acid at position-3 produces cephalosporin derivatives with minimal antibacterial effect.

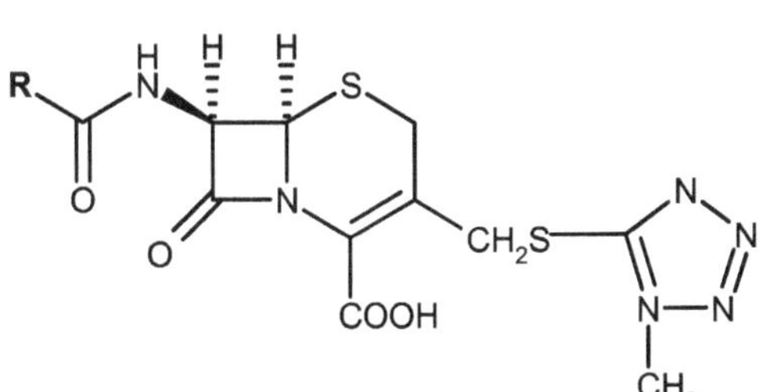

N-methylthiotetrazole

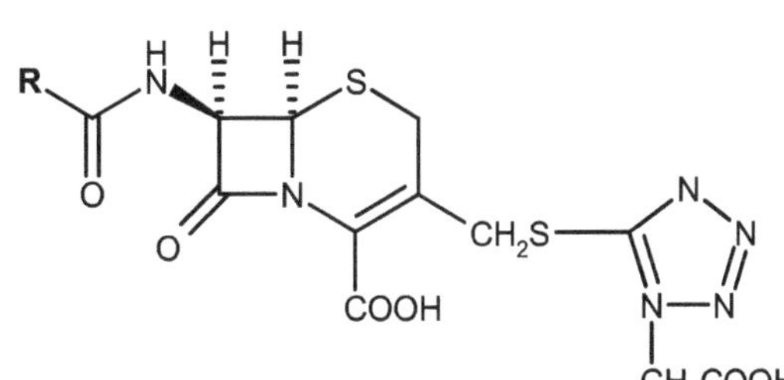

N-methylthiotetrazole-1-acetic acid

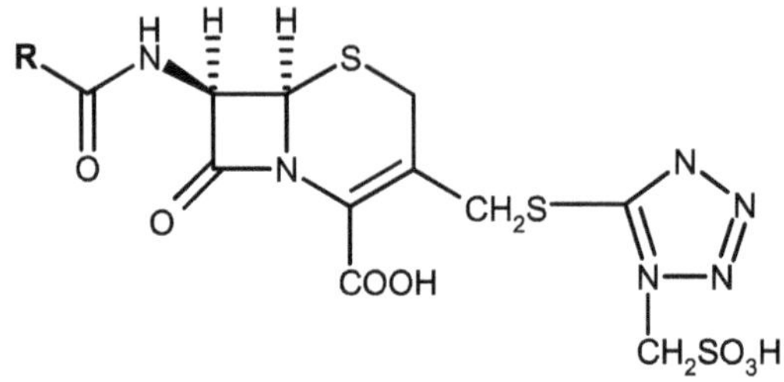

N-methylthiotetrazole-1-methansulphonic acid

(ii) Replacement of 3-acetoxymethyl group of 7-ACA by pyridine or imidazole moiety improves antibacterial activity against *Pseudomonas aeruginosa*. E.g., Cephaloridine, ceftazidine.

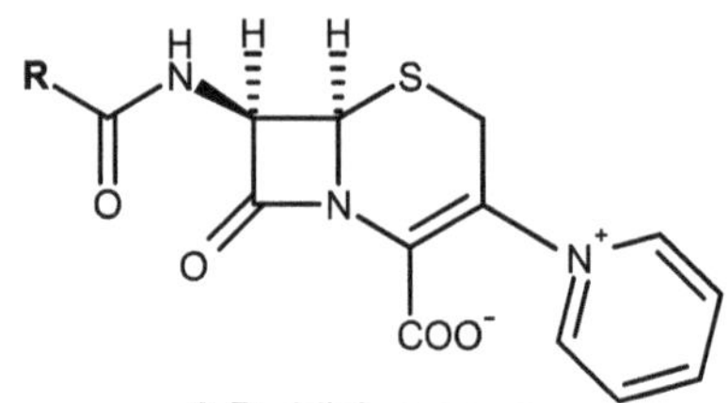

3-Pyridinium group

5. Changes in side chain at position 7 may cause changes in spectrum and β-lactamase resistance.

   (i) Acylation of 7-amino group increases antibacterial activity against Gram-positive organisms.

   (ii) Attachment of phenylglycyl substituent to nitrogen atom of C_7 increases the stability of lactam ring thus results in formation of orally active cephalosporins. E.g., Cefadroxyl, cephradine

   (iii) Substituents on aromatic phenyl ring increases Gram-positive activity due to increase in lipophilicity. E.g., Ceforanide

   (iv) Replacements of phenyl ring in side chain at position 7 with heterocycles such as thiophene or tetrazole or furan or pyridine or thiazole improves pharmacokinetic properties (ADME) and antimicrobial spectrum. They possess good β-lactamase stability and good PBP binding.

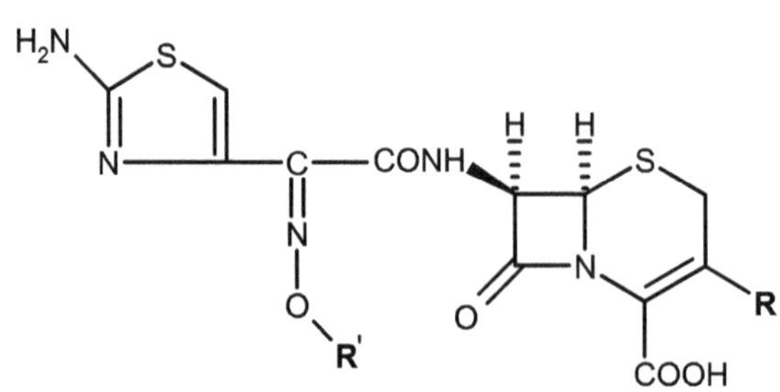

Aminothiazole alkoximines

(v) Presence of 1-methyl-5-thio tetrazole group leads to an extended spectrum of activity, higher potency and longer half-life. However 1-methyl-5-thio tetrazole group can cause bleeding due to hypoprothrombinaemia, as it will inhibit vitamin-K based enzymes that produce various clotting factors.

(vi) Addition of methoxy group at 7α-position leads to compounds that are very effective against β-lactamase producing bacteria.

6. Oxidation of sulphur of thiazole ring to sulphoxide or sulphone greatly diminishes antibacterial activity.
7. Double bond between C_3 and C_4 is essential for antibacterial activity. Carboxyl group at position 4 is also essential but can be esterified to get prodrugs which increases bioavailability of cephalosporins.

Classification

Cephalosporins are further classified basing on their antibacterial properties, generations and periods of their introduction. There are four generations of cephalosporins.

First generation drugs

These cephalosporins have activity against *Staphylococcus, Streptococcus, Proteus, Klebsiella*, and *Escherichia coli*. They show poor activity towards gram-negative organisms. E.g., Cephalothin, cephazolin, cephapirin, cephradine, cephalexin and cephadroxil etc.

Second generation drugs

The second generation cephalosporins have activity against *Staphylococcus, Streptococcus, Proteus, Klebsiella, Escherichia coli and Haemophilius influenzae.* E.g., Cefaclor, cefamandole, cefoxid, ceforanide and cefuroxime etc.

Third generation drugs

Third generation drugs are able to penetrate the central nervous system and have even greater activity on Gram negative organisms than the first and second generation drugs, but like the second generation may require testing to determine sensitivity. E.g., Cefotaxime, monolactam, cefoperazone, ceftazidime, ceftriaxone. The third generation drugs are even more resistant to β-lactamases than second generation cephalosporins.

Fourth generation drugs

Fourth generation cephalosporins are extended-spectrum agents with similar activity against gram-positive organisms as first-generation cephalosporins. They also have a greater resistance to beta-lactamases than the third generation cephalosporins. Many can cross blood brain barrier and are effective in meningitis. E.g., Cefclidine, cefepime, cefluprenam, cefozopran, cefpirome, cefquinome

First generation cephalosporins

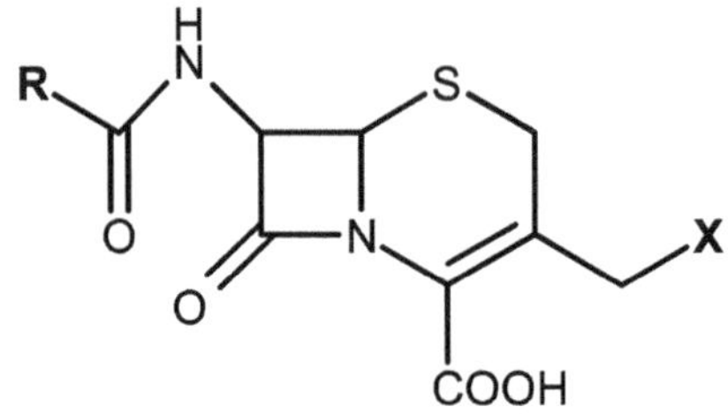

	R	X
Cephalothin (parenteral)	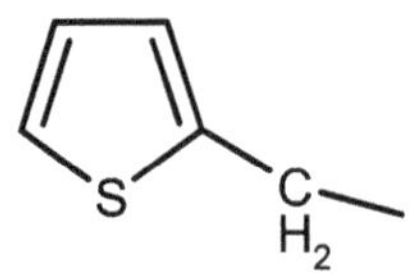	O–CO–CH_3
Cefazolin (parenteral)	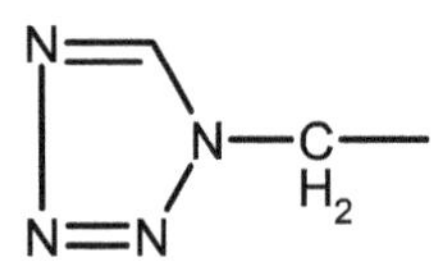	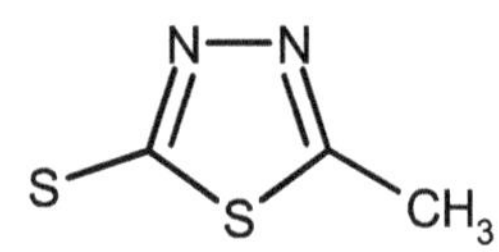
Cephalexin (oral)	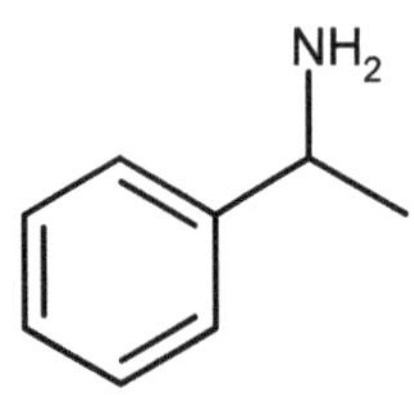	H

Cephalothin : Cephalothin was the first introduced cephalosporin, which is administered parenterally, as it is not absorbed by oral route. It is available as sodium salt and is effective against *Staphylococci.* However it has been replaced by other derivatives. It is synthesized by acylation of 7-ACA with 2-thienylacetylchloride.

3-[(acetoxy) methyl] – 8-oxo-7-[(2-thienylacetyl) amino] – 5-thia-1-azabicyclo [4.2.0] oct-2-ene-2-carboxylic acid

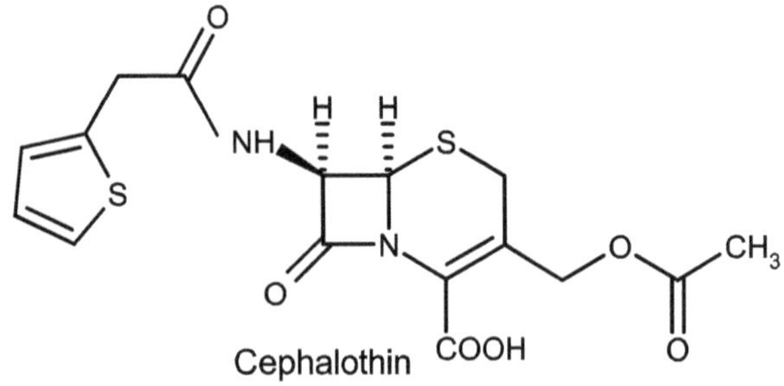

Cephalothin

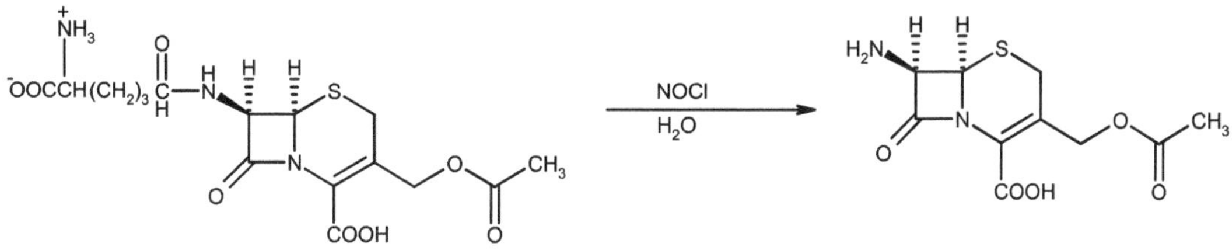

Cephalosporine C | 7-Aminocephalosporanic acid

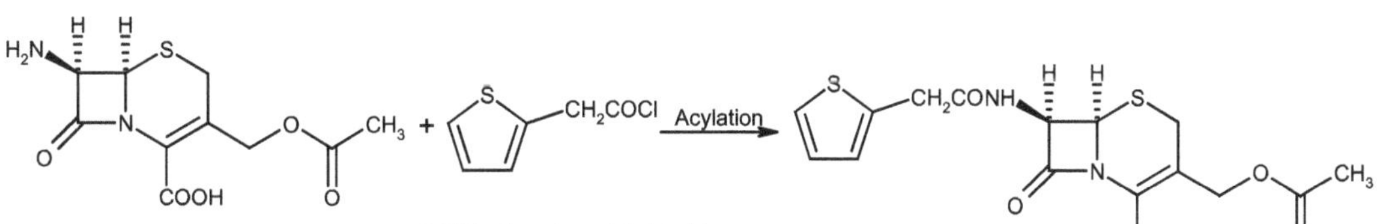

7-Aminocephalosporanic acid | 2-Thiophenyl acetyl chloride | Cephalothin

Cefadroxil : It is an orally active first generation broad-spectrum. It is a semisynthetic derivative of 7-anhydrodesacetylcephalosporanic acid. Chemically it is 7-{[2-amino-2-(4-hydroxyphenyl)-acetyl]amino}-3-methyl- 8-oxo-5-thia-1-azabicyclo [4.2. 0] oct-2-ene-2-carboxylic acid.

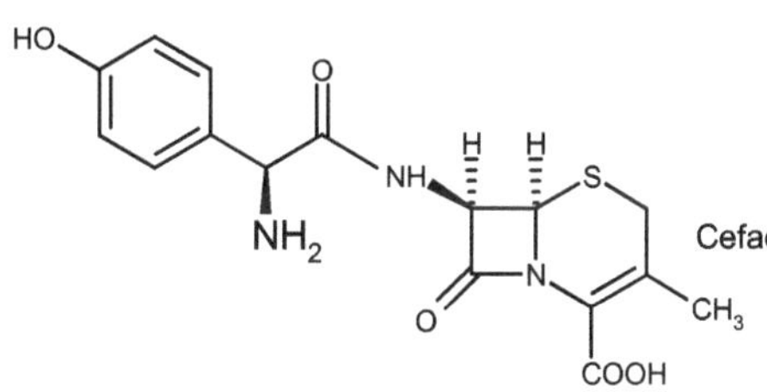

Cefadroxil

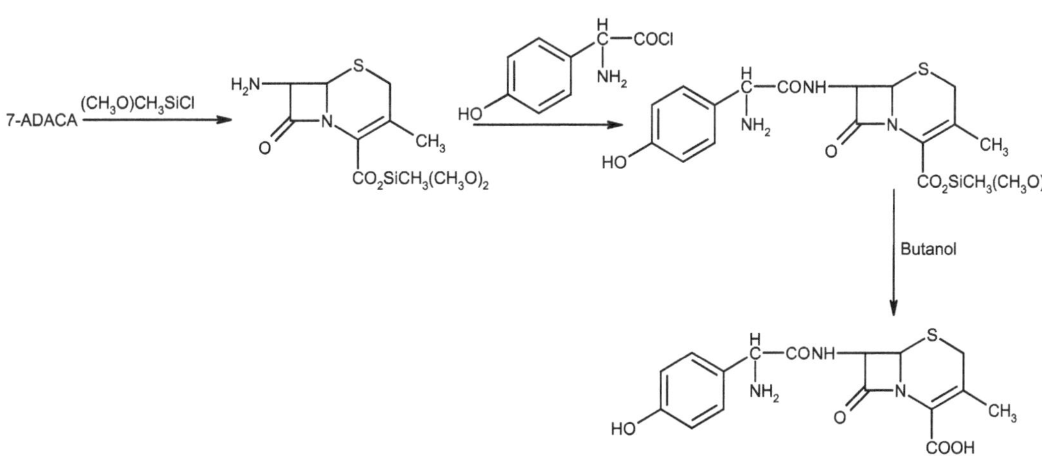

Cefadroxil

It occurs as white (or) almost white powder and is slightly soluble in water, very slightly soluble in alcohol.

***Uses*:** It is well absorbed orally and is effective against most gram-positive organisms. It, however, does not directly attack *mycoplasma*, but is useful in secondary infections such as skin, soft tissue and urinary tract. It is also used prophylactically in surgery to prevent infection.

Cephalexin: It is also orally active semisythetic cephalosporin antibiotic. Chemically cephalexin is 7-(2-amino-2-phenylacetyl) amino-3-methyl-8-oxo -5-thia-1-azabicyclo[4.2.0]oct-2-ene-2 carboxylic acid. It is an orally-administered agent with a similar antimicrobial spectrum to that of cephalothin. It crosses both placental and fetal serum and is not recommended during pregnancy. It does not enter cerebrospinal fluid (CSF). It does not show significant levels in breast milk, and may be given to lactating females. Cephalexin occurs as a white crystalline powder. It is sparingly soluble in water, practically insoluble in alcohol.

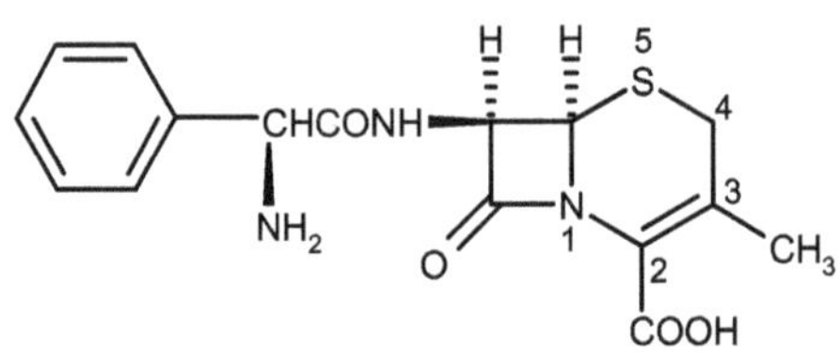

Cephalexin

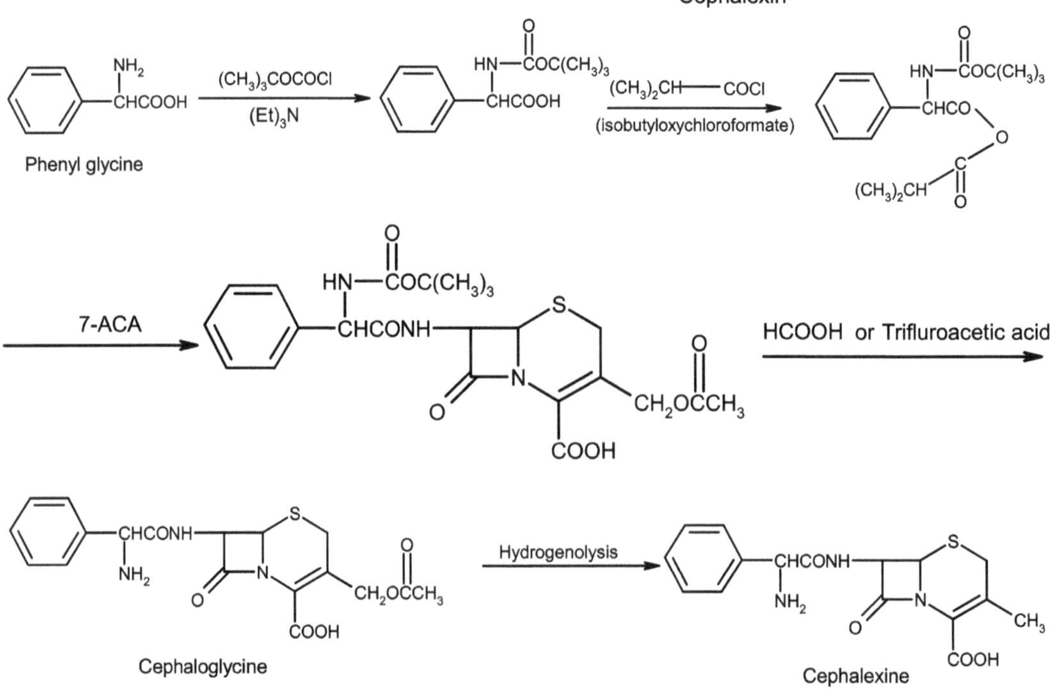

***Uses*:** It is effective against most gram-positive organisms such as β-Hemolytic streptococci, Staphylococus, Proteus, Escherichia coli, Klebsiella, Pasteurella and Salmonella. It has been used to treat deep skin (pyoderma), soft tissue, urinary tract infections (UTI) and as prophylactic following surgery to prevent infection.

Cefazolin: Cefazolin, is a first-generation antibiotic in the cephalosporin family. It is usually administrated either by intramuscular injection (injection into a large muscle) or an intravenous infusion (intravenous fluid into a vein). Cefazolin is mainly used to treat bacterial infections of the skin. It can also be used to treat moderately severe bacterial infections involving the lung, bone, joint, stomach, blood, heart valve, and urinary tract. It is effective only against infections caused by *Staphylococci* and *Streptococci* species of bacteria (These organisms are common on normal human skin).

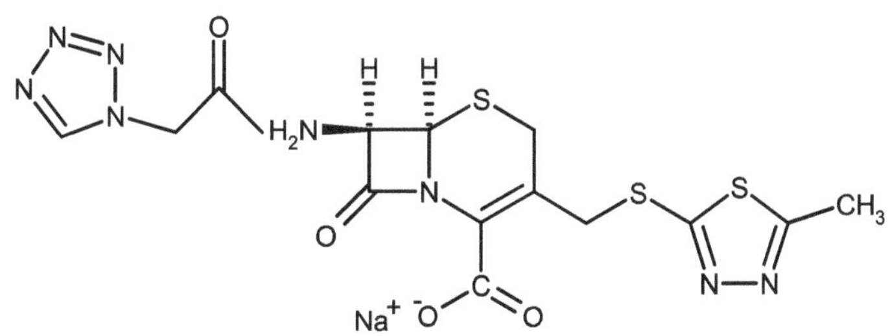

Cefazoline sodium

Cefradine : Cefradine is a first generation cephalosporin antibiotic. It has similar spectrum of activity to cephalexin. It is administered orally and parenterally.

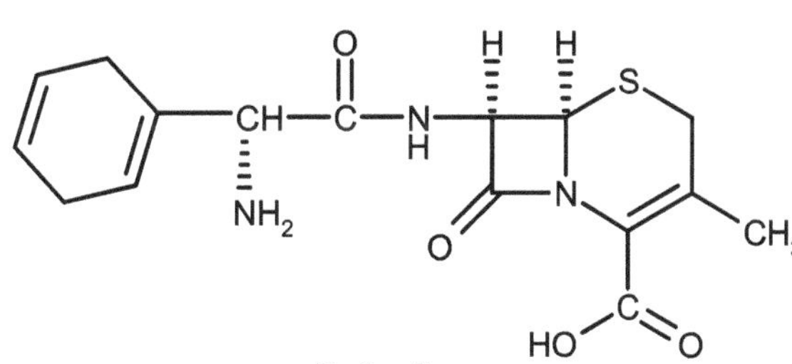

Cefradine

Second generation cephalosporins

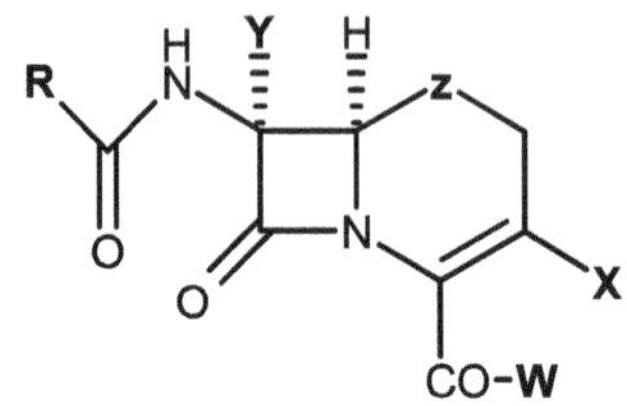

	R	W	X	Y	Z
Cefamandole (Parenteral)	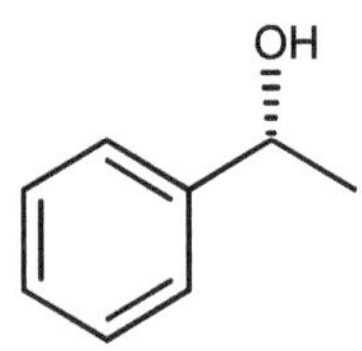	OH	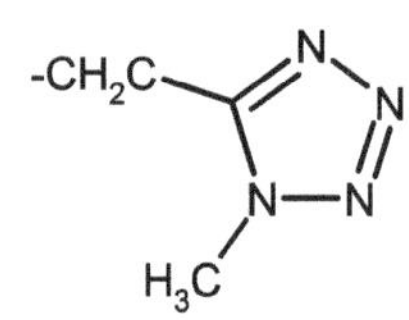	H	S
Cefoxitin (Parenteral)	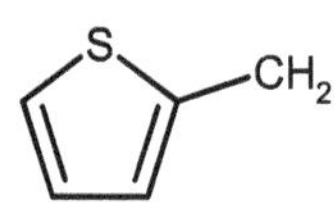	OH	CH_2OCONH_2	OMe	S
Cefaclor (Oral)	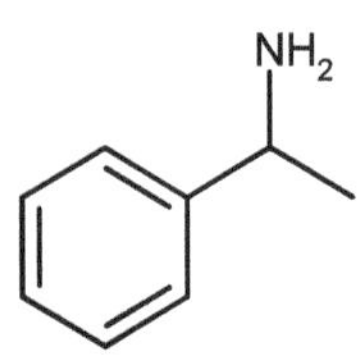	OH	Cl	H	S

Cefaclor: Cefaclor, also known as cefachlor, is a second generation cephalosporin antibiotic used to treat certain infections caused by bacteria such as pneumonia and ear, lung, skin, throat, and urinary tract infections. Chemically cefaclor is 7-[(2-amino-2-phenyl-acetyl)amino]-3-chloro-8-oxo-5-thia-1-azabicyclo[4.2.0]oct-2-ene-2-carboxylic acid.

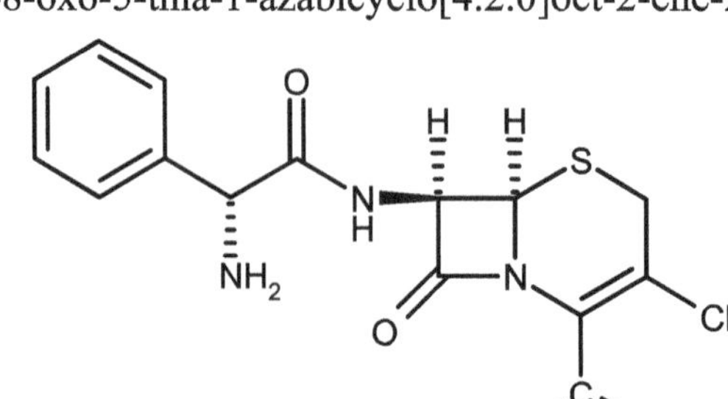

Cefaclor

It occurs as a white (or) slightly yellow powder, slightly soluble in water, practically insoluble in methanol and in methylene chloride.

Uses : It is used in the treatment of upper respiratory tract infections caused by Streptococcus pneumoniae and Haemophilius influenzae.

Cefamandole : It is a semisynthetic wide-spectrum cephalosporin with prolonged action, probably due to β-lactamase resistance. It is second generation cephalosporin. It is available as cefamandole nafate which rapidly hydrolyses to yield cefamandole. Chemically cephamandole is 5-thia-1-azabicyclo[4.2.0]oct-2-ene-2-carboxylic acid,–7-[[(2R)-(2-hydroxy)phenylacetyl]amino]-3-[[(1-methyl-1H-tetrazol-5-yl)thio]methyl]-8-oxo-monosodium salt, (6R,7R).

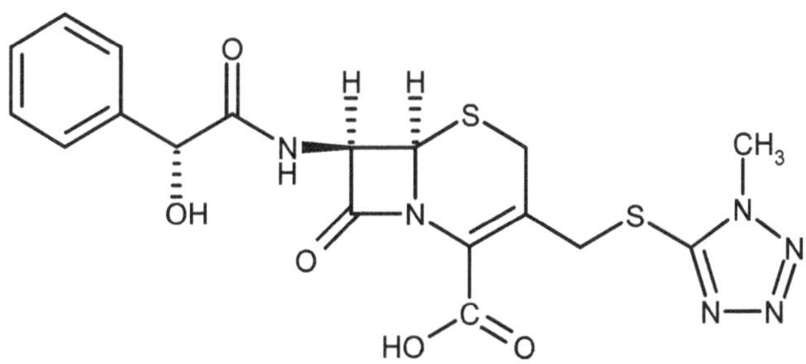

Cefamandole

It is available as white (or) almost white powder and is freely soluble in water, sparingly soluble in methanol.

Uses : It is used to treat :

(i) Lower respiratory tract infections, including pneumonia, caused by *Streptococcus pneumoniae, Haemophilius influenzae, Klebsiella* spp., *Staphylococcus aureus* (penicillinase- and non-penicillinase-producing), (β)-hemolytic streptococci, and *Pseudomonas mirabilis.*

(ii) Urinary tract infections caused by *Escherichia coli, Proteus* spp. (both indole-negative and indole-positive), *Enterobacter* spp., *Klebsiella* spp., group D streptococci (***Note:*** Most enterococci, e.g., *Enterococcus. faecalis,* are resistant), and *Staphylococcus epidermidis.*

(iii) Peritonitis caused by *Escherichia coli* and *Enterobacter* spp.

(iv) Septicemia caused by *Escherichia coli, Staphylococcus aureus* (penicillinase- and non-penicillinase-producing), *Streptococcus pneumoniae, Streptococcus pyogenes* (group A (beta)-hemolytic streptococci), *Haemophilius influenzae,* and *Klebsiella* spp.

(v) Skin and skin structure infections caused by *Staphylococcus aureus* (penicillinase and non-penicillinase producing), *Streptococcus pyogenes* (group A (β)-Hemolytic streptococci), *Haemophilius influenzae, Escherichia coli, Enterobacter* spp., and *Pseudomonas mirabilis.*

Cefoxitin : It is a semisynthetic antibiotic derived from cephamycin C; possessing high resistance to β-lactamase inactivation. It is available as cefoxitin sodium.

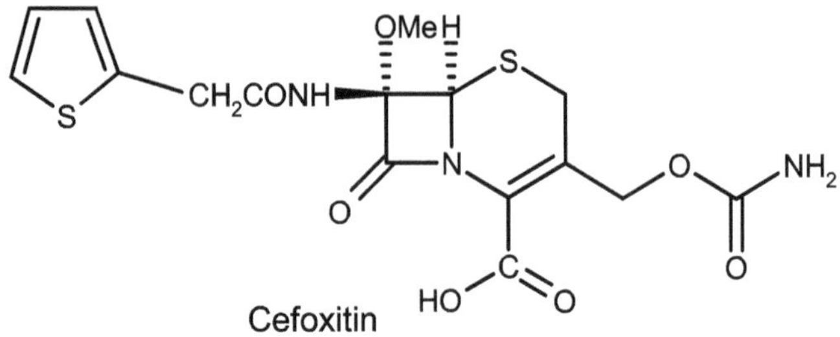

Cefoxitin

Cefoxitin sodium is available as white or almost white powder. It is hygroscopic and freely soluble in water. Cefoxitin sodium is administered parenterally by deep IM or IV injection or IV infusion.

Cefuroxime : Cefuroxime is a second generation cephalosporin antibiotic that has been widely available in the USA since 1977.

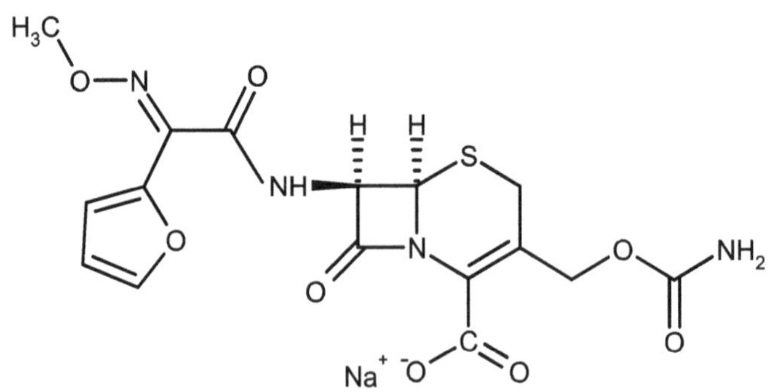

Cefuroxime sodium

Cefuroxime is available as cefuroxime sodium. Cefuroxime sodium is white or almost white powder and is freely soluble in water.

Uses : As a second-generation it is less susceptible to β-lactamase and so may have greater activity against *Haemophilus influenzae, Neisseria gonorrhoeae* and lyme disease.

Third generation cephalosporins

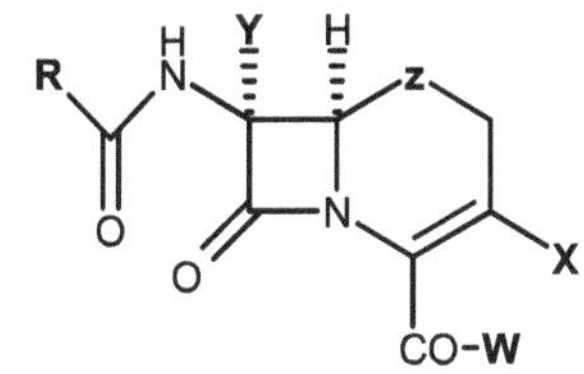

	R	W	X	Y	Z
Cefotaxime (parenteral)	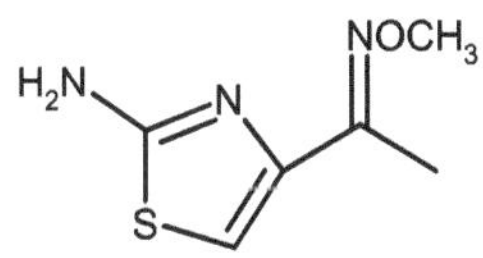	OH	CH_2OCOCH_3	H	S
Ceftazidime (parenteral)	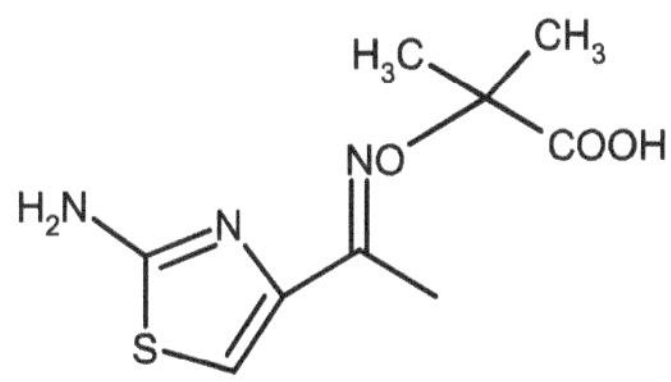	OH	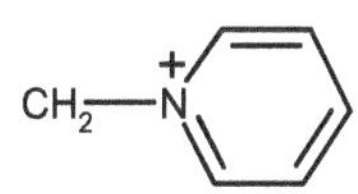	H	S
Cefixime (oral)	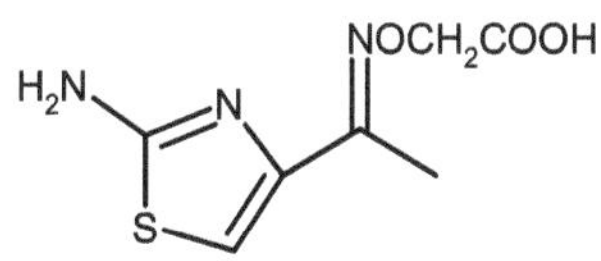	OH	$-CH_2{=}CH_2$	H	S

Cefotaxime : Cefotaxime is first third generation cephalosporin. It has broad spectrum of activity against gram-positive and gram-negative bacteria. In most cases, it is considered to be equivalent to ceftriaxone in terms of safety and efficacy. Chemically it is (6*R*,7*R*,*Z*)-3-(acetoxymethyl)-7-(2-(2-aminothiazol-4-yl)-2-(methoxy imino)acetamido)-8-oxo-5-thia-1-aza-bicyclo[4.2.0]oct-2-ene-2-carboxylic acid.

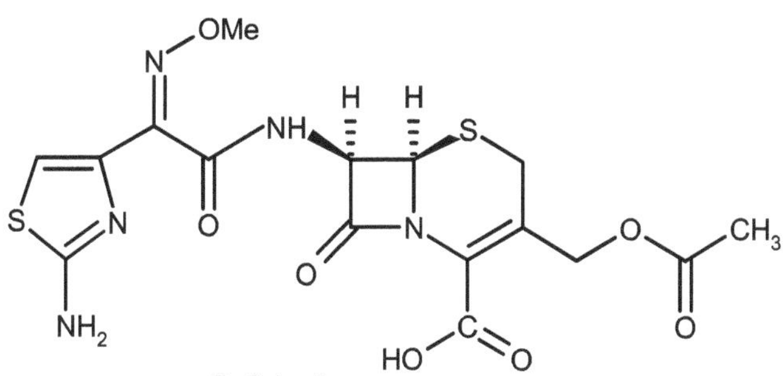

Cefotaxime

The *syn*-configuration of methoxyimino moiety confers stability to β-lactamase enzymes produced by many gram-negative bacteria.

Cefixime : Cefixime is an oral third generation cephalosporin antibiotic, it has an aminothiazole ring attached to an oximinoether containing side chain at C-7. It is used to treat gonorrhea. Cefixime is a white hygroscopic, powder. It is slightly soluble in water, soluble in methanol, sparingly soluble in ethanol, practically insoluble in ethyl acetate. It is well absorbed from suspension rather than from tablets.

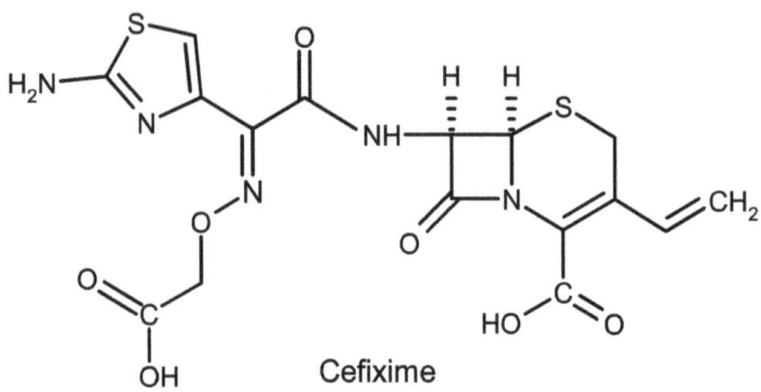

Cefixime

The vinyl group at 3-position of the cephem nucleus is responsible for the intestinal absorption of the intact molecule, primarily by a carrier-mediated transport mechanism. The aminothiazole ring and R-oximino group on the side-chain at 7-position are associated with an antibacterial activity similar to that of third generation cephalosporins.

Cefixime is highly stable in presence of β-lactamase enzymes. As a result, many organisms resistant to penicillins and some cephalosporins due to the presence of β-lactamases, may be susceptible to cefixime. The antibacterial effect of cefixime results from inhibition of mucopeptide synthesis in the bacterial cell wall.

Uses : First orally active broad spectrum cephalosporin. It is resistant to β-lactamases and has long life i.e., 4 hrs.

Cefoperazone : It is a broad spectrum third generation parenteral antipseudomonal cephalosporin containing an acylated side chain at C-7. It forms crystals from acetonitrile / water. It is stable at pH 4-7. It is slightly unstable in acid and highly unstable in alkaline solution. It is used as antibacterial agent against *Pseudomonas aeruginosa, Proteus species, Enterobacter* etc.

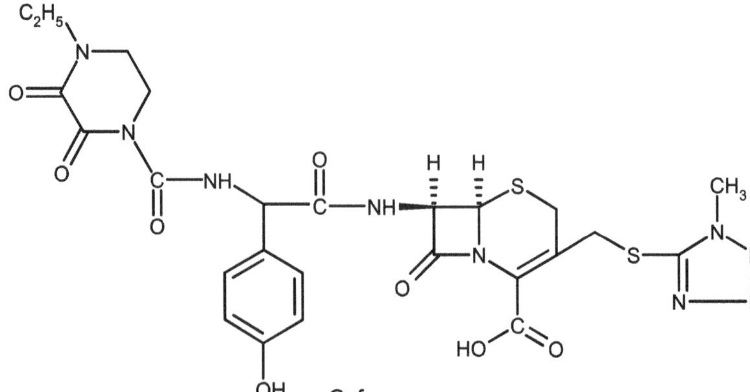

Cefoperazone

Ceftriaxone : Ceftriaxone is a third generation cephalosporin antibiotic. It possesses a 2,5-dihydro-6-hydroxy-2-methyl-5-oxo-1,2,4-triazin-3-yl-thioethyl moiety at C-3 in order to avoid some of the side effects of cephalosporins. Like other third-generation cephalosporins, it has broad spectrum of activity against gram-positive and gram negative bacteria. In most cases, it is considered to be equivalent to cefotaxime in terms of safety and efficacy. Ceftriaxone is a yellowish-orange crystalline powder which is readily soluble in water, sparingly soluble in methanol and very slightly soluble in ethanol. Chemically it is (6*R*,7*R*,*Z*)-7-(2-(2-aminothiazol-4-yl)-2-(methoxyimino)acetamido)-3-((6-hydroxy-2-methyl-5-oxo-2,5dihydro-1,2,4-triazin-3ylthio)methyl)-8-oxo-5-thia-1-aza-bicyclo[4.2.0]oct-2-ene-2-carboxylic acid.

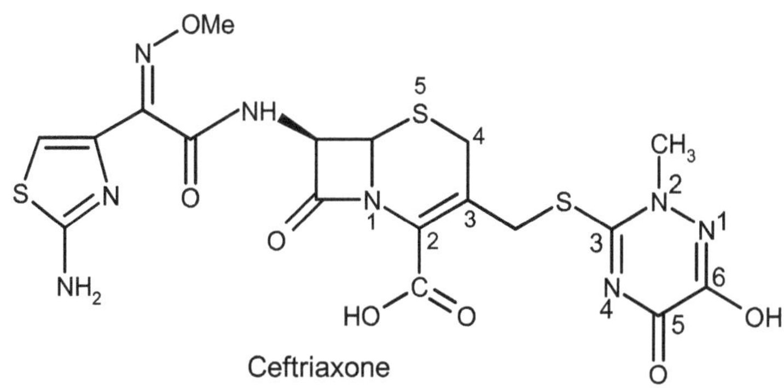

Ceftriaxone

The *syn*-configuration of methoxyimino moiety confers stability to β-lactamase enzymes produced by many gram-negative bacteria. Such stability to β-lactamases increases the activity of ceftriaxone against resistant gram-negative organisms. In place of the easily hydrolysed acetyl group of cefotaxime, ceftriaxone has a metabolically-stable thiotriazinedione moiety.

Ceftriaxone is often used (in combination with macrolide and/or aminoglycoside antibiotics) for the treatment of community-acquired pneumonia. It is also a choice drug for treatment of bacterial meningitis. In pediatrics, it is commonly used in febrile infants between 4 and 8 weeks of age who are admitted to the hospital to exclude sepsis. It has also been used in the treatment of lyme disease and gonorrhoea.

Cefpodoxime : Cefpodoxime is an oral third generation cephalosporin antibiotic. It is active against most gram-positive and gram-negative bacteria. Notable exceptions include *Pseudomonas aeruginosa*, *Enterococcus* and *Bacteroides fragilis*. It is commonly used to treat acute otitis media, pharyngitis, and sinusitis. It also finds use as oral continuation therapy when intravenous cephalosporins (such as ceftriaxone) are no longer necessary for continued treatment.

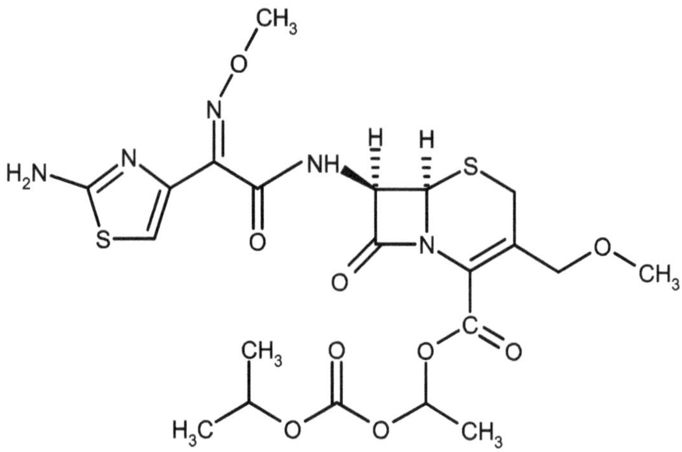

Cefpodoxime

Ceftazidime : Ceftazidime is a third generation cephalosporin antibiotic. Like other third generation cephalosporins, it has broad spectrum of activity against gram-positive and gram-negative bacteria. Unlike most third generation agents, it is active against *Pseudomonas aeruginosa*, however it has weaker activity against gram positive microorganisms. Chemically it is (6*R*,7*R*,*Z*)-7-(2-(2-aminothiazol-4-yl)-2-(2-carboxypropan-2-yloxyimino)acetamido)-8-oxo-3-(pyridinium-1-ylmethyl)-5-thia-1-aza-bicyclo[4.2.0]oct-2-ene-2-carboxylate.

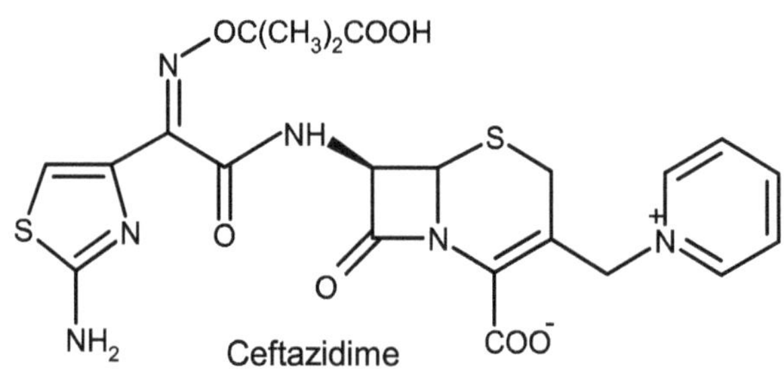

Ceftazidime

In addition to the *syn*-configuration of the imino side chain, compared to other third-generation cephalosporins, the more complex moiety (containing two methyl and a carboxylic acid group) confers extra stability to β-lactamase enzymes produced by many gram-negative bacteria. The extra stability to β-lactamases increases the activity of ceftazidime against gram-negative organisms including *Pseudomonas aeruginosa*. The charged pyridinum moiety increases water solubility.

Ceftazidime is usually reserved for the treatment of infections caused by *Pseudomonas aeruginosa*. It is also used to treat febrile neutropenia, in combination with other antibiotics.

Cefdinir : Cefdinir is a semi-synthetic antibiotic in the third generation of the cephalosporin family of antibiotics proven effective for common bacterial infections of the ear, sinus, throat, and skin. Cefdinir is administered orally. It is a broad-spectrum bactericide; it can be used to treat harmful bacteria including *Haemophilus influenzae, Moraxella catarrhalis, Esherichia coli, Klebsiella, and Proteus mirabilis, Staphylococcus aureus, Streptococcus pneumoniae and Streptococcus pyogenes*. It is not effective against Pseudomonas. Therapeutic uses of cefdinir include otitis media, soft-tissue infections, and respiratory tract infections. It was approved by the Food and Drug Administration (FDA) in December of 1997.

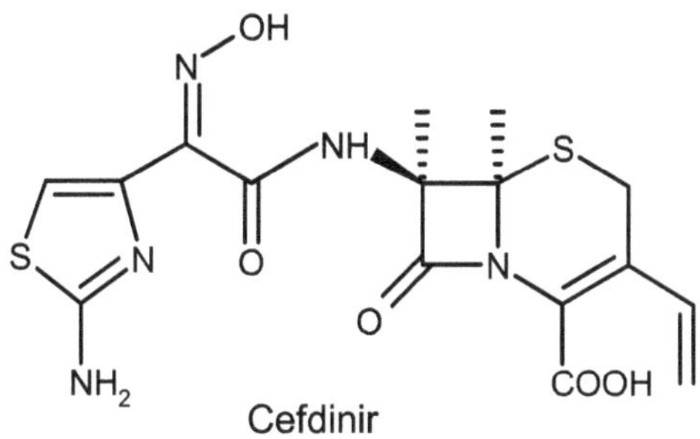

Cefdinir

Ceftibuten : Ceftibuten, a third generation oral cephalosporin, has excellent Gram-negative activity and possesses a high degree of β-lactamase stability. Current clinical trials indicate that ceftibuten (9 mg/kg/d in children and 400 mg/d in adults) is effective in the treatment of acute otitis media, streptococcal pharyngitis, acute exacerbations of chronic bronchitis, and urinary tract infections. In addition, ceftibuten's once-daily dosing may increase patient acceptance and tolerability.

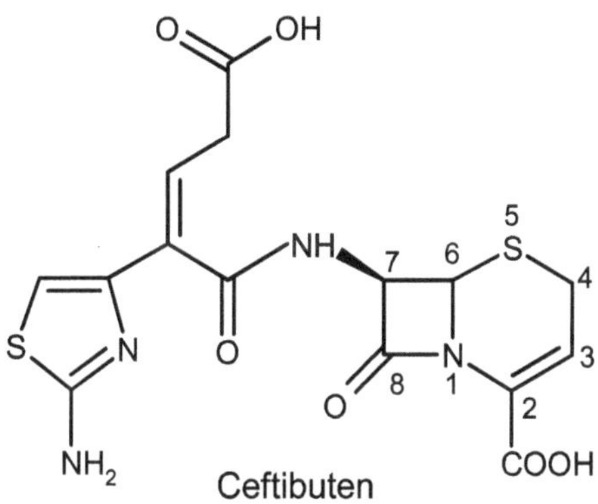

Ceftibuten

Cefepime : Cefepime is a fourth generation cephalosporin antibiotic developed in 1994. Cefepime has an extended spectrum of activity against gram-positive and gram-negative bacteria, with greater activity against both gram-negative and gram-positive organisms than third-generation agents. Cefepime hydrochloride was first marketed in 1994. The combination of the *syn*-configuration of the methoxyimino moiety and the aminothiazolyl moiety confers extra stability to β-lactamase enzymes produced by many bacteria. The *N*-methylpyrrolidine moiety increases penetration into gram-negative bacteria. These factors increase the activity of cefepime against resistant organisms including *Pseudomonas aeruginosa* and *Staphylococcus*. Chemically it is 7-(2-(2-aminothiazol-4-yl)-2-(methoxyimino)acetamido)-3-((1-methylpyrrolidinium-1-yl)methyl)-8-oxo-5-thia-1-aza-bicyclo[4.2.0]oct-2-ene-2 carboxylic acid.

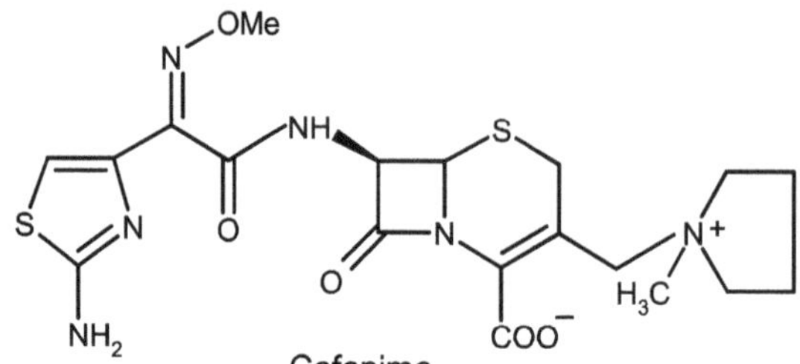

Cefepime

Carbapenems and monobactams

The β-lactam antibiotic thienamycin was isolated from the mold *Streptomyces cattlea*. It is a very interesting molecule, since it is an extremely potent antibiotic, and is also an effective inhibitor of β-lactamase. The sulphur atom is not part of the cyclic structure, but is exocyclic to the five membered ring. Thienamycin was never marketed, because in concentrated form the primary amine functionality attacks the β-lactam structure, thus inactivating the molecule. This problem was overcome by changing this amine to a less nucleophilic imino functionality, producing imipenem.

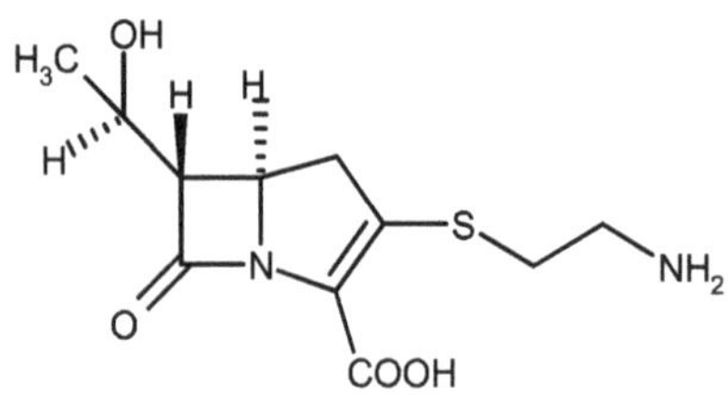

Thienamycin

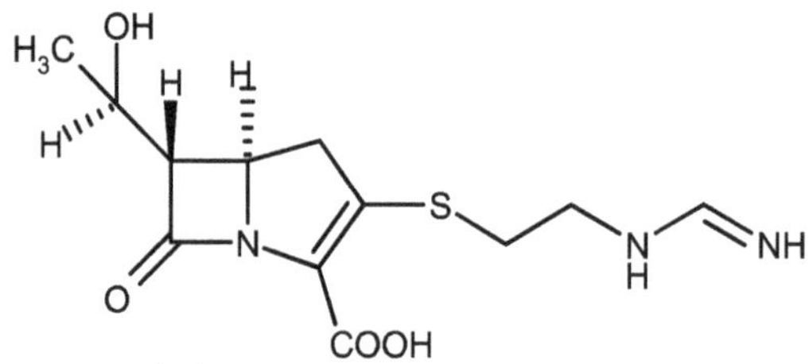

Imipenem

Imipenem penetrates bacterial porins well, and is stable to and inhibitory for many β-lactamases. It is not orally active, however imipenem can be used for urinary tract infections, but must be co-administered with cilastatin sodium, an inhibitor of renal dehydropeptidase 1, which attacks and inactivates imipenem.

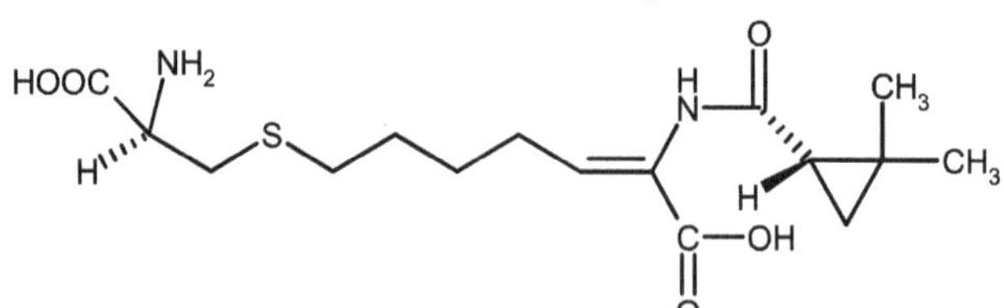

Cilastatin sodium

Fermentation of unusual microorganisms resulted in the isolation of certain monocyclic β-lactams called monobactams, of which aztreonam is the only important example. It is a totally synthetic parenteral antibiotic that is active almost entirely against gram-negative bacteria. Its mechanism is similar to the penicillins, and it has a particularly strong affinity for PBP-3.

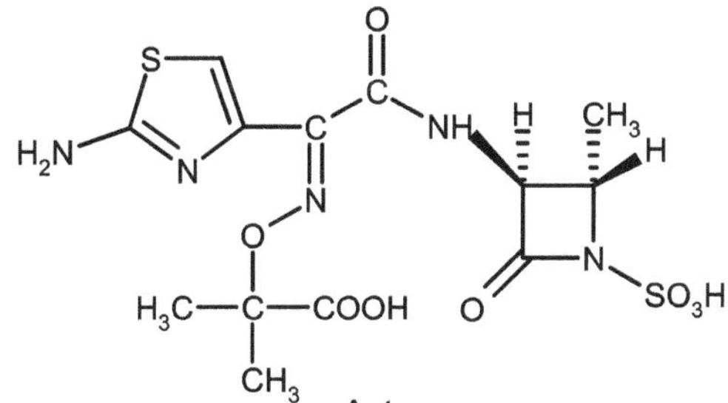

Aztreonam

10

AMINOGLYCOSIDES

Waksman introduced aminoglycosides by screening *streptomyces* species and these are the first agents effective against tuberculosis e.g., Streptomycin, gentamycin, amikacin, kanamycin. They are commercially produced by S*treptomyces* species: Streptomycin, neomycin, kanamycin, framycetin, and tobramycin and *Micromonospora* species: e.g., Gentamicin, sissomycin.

Aminoglycosides are a group of antibiotics which are effective against Gram-positive and Gram-negative organisms as well as *mycoplasma*. They show very potent activity against anaerobes (*Enterobacter, Esherichia coli, Klebsiella, Proteus, Serratia, Pseudomonas aeruginosa).*

Chemistry

Structurally aminoglycosides possess amino substituted sugars linked to aglycone (streptidine or 2-deoxystreptamine) by glycosidic linkages to form pseudo-oligo saccharides. Glycon may be an aminohexose sugar (or) a pentos sugar (like strepteomycinr, neomycin, paramomycin). Aglycone is 1,3-diaminoayclomexcin, or streptidine (streptomycin) or 2-deoxy streptamine [kanamycin, neomycin, gentamycin and tobramycin]. Aminoglycosides are basic in nature due to presence of several aminogrmps. They exist as cations in physiological pH. Generally aminoglycosides comprises of the following ring structures:

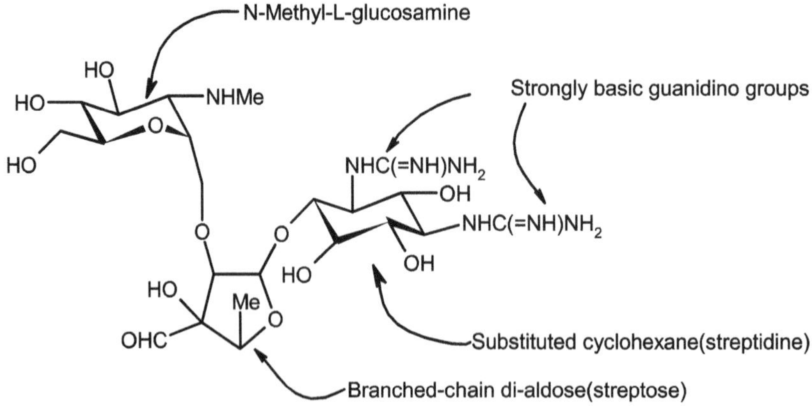

Streptomycin

Ring – I (Aminohexose sugar)

1. Ring-I is crucial for antibacterial activity and is the target for three different exzymatic mechanisms. Two attached hydroxyl groups are not essential for activity. All substitutions must be in equatorial position.
2. Acetylation of either 6' or 2' amino groups leads to severe decrease in potency. Methylation of 6' - carbon or 6'-amino group can lead to retention or improvement of potency.
3. Hydroxyl groups also play an important role in determining antibacterial activity. Replacement of hydroxyl group by hydrogen can lead to improved potency and spectrum of action, whilst other modifications result in considerable loss of potency. E.g., Replacement of 3' -hydroxyl group of kanamycin A by either methoxy or an amino group causes a loss of activity.

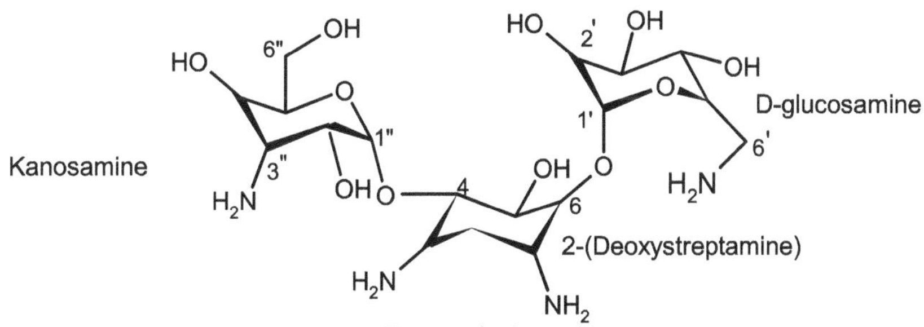

Kanamycin A

4. Unsaturation of ring 1 diminishes antibacterial activity whilst introduction of 4',5' - double bond to gentamycin gives a very potent compound.

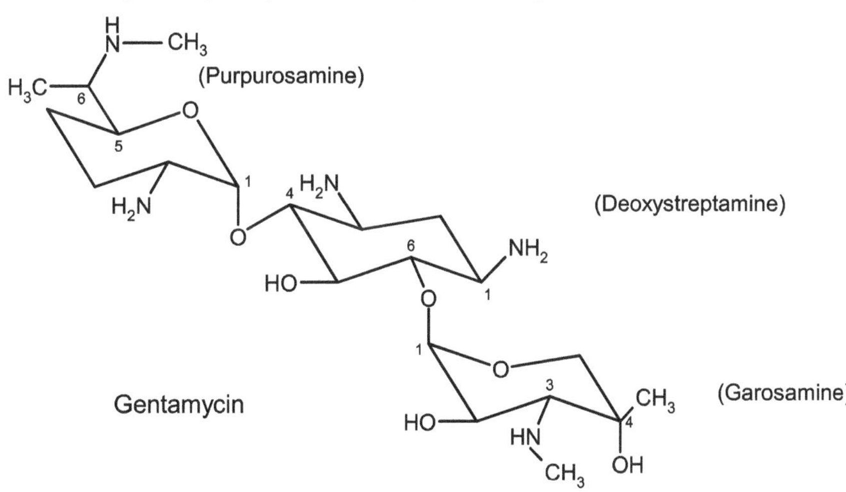

Gentamycin

Ring – II (Deoxystreptamine)

1. Acylation of 1-aminogroup of deoxystreptamine ring with 2-hydroxy-4-aminobutyric acid leads to improved antibacterial activity against pseudomonas.
2. S-Isomer of 2-hydroxy-4-aminobutyric acid derivative of kanamycin is more potent than R-isomer.

3. 2-Hydroxy-4-aminobutyric acid derivatives of gentamicin and tobramycin are also potent.

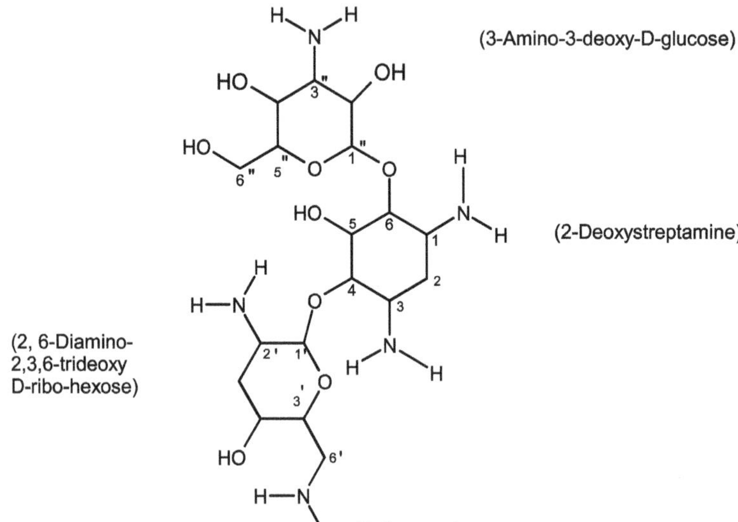

Tobramycin

Ring - III

1. Removal of 2-hydroxyl group or methylation of 2'-hydroxyl group decreases antibacterial activity. E.g., Gentamicin

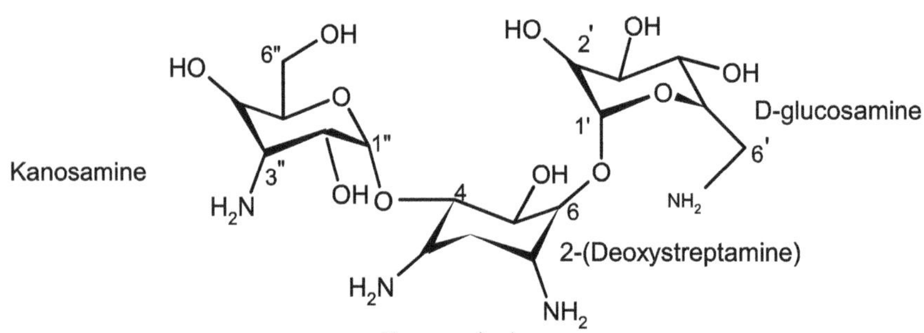

Kanamycin A

2. Replacement of 2'-hydroxyl group by amino group retains the antibacterial activity. E.g., Seldomycin

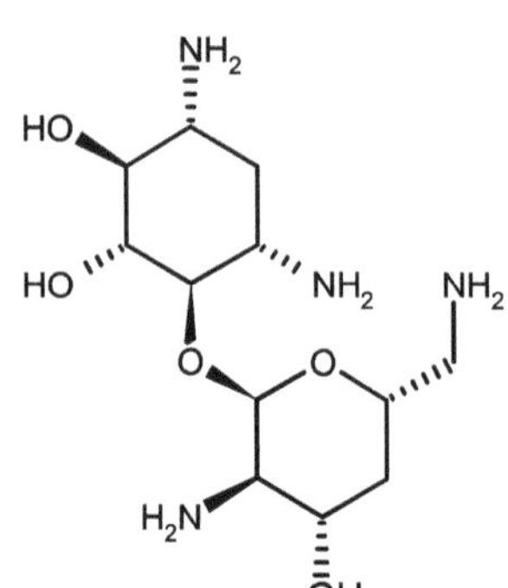

Seldomycin

3. 3′-Amino group may be 1° or 2° and 4'-hydroxyl group may be axial or equatorial or methylated
4. The Ring-III may have furanose arrangement, the 3''-hydroxyl group may be substituted. E.g., Neomycin

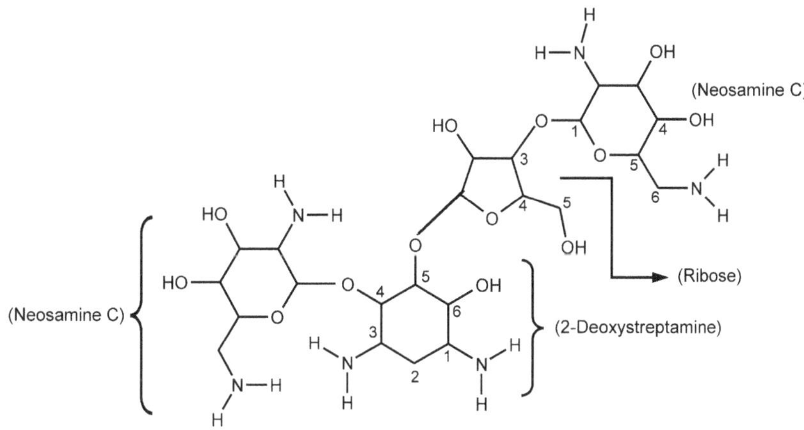

Neomycin

Ring - IV

Presence of fourth ring i.e., Ring-IV as in neomycin generally leads to increase in potency.

Mechanism of action

Aminoglycoside antibiotics exert their bactericidal activity and are mainly effective against gram-negative bacilli and some gram-positive organisms. Initially aminoglycosides bind to external lipopolysaccharides and diffuse into the cells in small amounts. They strongly bind to 30s subunits of the ribosome and interfere with protein synthesis by one of two mechanisms:

- They interfere with proper amino acid polymerization and elongation.
- Misreading the amino acid codons by t–RNA and impairing proof reading and thus incorporating incorrect amino acid and gives rise to nonsense proteins. These unnatural proteins are involved in upsetting bacterial membrane function.

Though aminoglycosides have broad antimicrobial spectra but their toxicity limits their clinical use to infection by gram-negative bacteria.

General characteristics

1. Aminoglycosides poly cations and are highly polar. They are water soluble at all pH.
2. They are basic and form salts with acids.
3. They are generally poorly absorbed after oral administration but completely absorbed by parenteral administration.
4. They are well distributed in body except central nervous system because as they cannot cross blood brain barrier but cross the placental barrier.

Streptomycin

Streptomycin is 5-(2,4-diguanidino-3,5,6-trihydroxy-cyclohexoxy)- 4-[4,5-dihydroxy-6-(hydroxymethyl)-3-methylamino-tetrahydropyran-2-yl] oxy-3 -hydroxy-2- methyl-tetrahydrofuran-3-carbaldehyde. Streptomycin is the first aminoglycoside antibiotic which was isolated from a strain of *Streptomyces griseus(1943)* in the laboratory of Solman Abraham Waksman at Rutgers University by Albert Schatz, (a graduate student in his laboratory). Waksman and his laboratory discovered several antibiotics, including actinomycin, clavacin, streptothricin, streptomycin, grisein, neomycin, fradicin, candicidin, candidin, and others. Two of these, streptomycin and neomycin, found extensive application in the treatment of numerous infectious diseases. Streptomycin was the first antibiotic that could be used to cure tuberculosis.

Structure

Streptomycin is a triacidic base. It possess two strongly basic guanidino groups and weakly basic methylamino group. Chemically it is 2,4-diguanidino-3,5,6-trihydroxycyclohexyl-5-deoxy-2-*O*-(2-deoxy-2-methylamino-α-l-glucopyranosyl)-3-C-formyl-α-L-lyxopentanofura noside. It possess three structural units: (a) Streptidine (b) Streptose (c) N-Methyl-L-glucosamine. The three units are connected together through glycosidic linkages (It is an aldo pentose sugar).

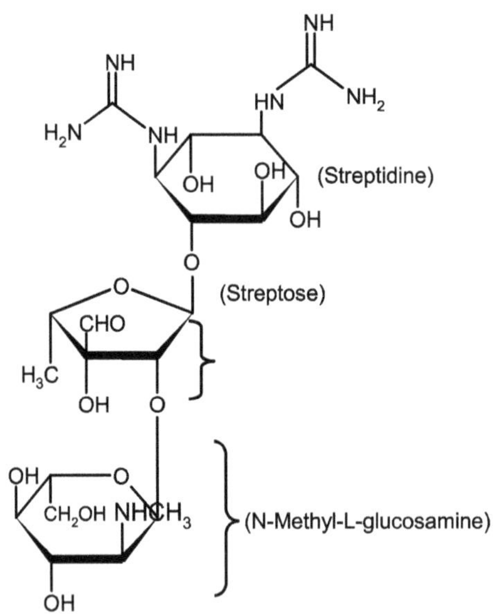

Structure activity relationship (SAR)

1. Reduction of aldehyde group of streptomycin to hydroxymethyl group retains antibacterial activity
2. Reduction of aldehyde group to a methyl derivative gives a compound which has only one-tenth of activity as streptomycin
3. Oxidation of aldehyde group to carboxylic acid results in poor activity

4. In N-methyl -L-glucosamine the nitrogen atom should be secondary amine as primary amine is weakly active and tertiary amine is inactive
5. Guanidino groups on streptidine ring are essential. Replacement of guanidino groups reduces antibacterial activity.

Properties

Streptomycin is a triacidic base. It occurs as white (or) yellowish white powder which is very soluble in water, very slightly soluble in alcohol, practically insoluble in acetone. Solutions of streptomycin are stable at pH between 4.5-7.0

Uses

Streptomycin is bacteriostatic (in low concentration) and bactericidal (in high concentration). It is effective against *Mycobacterium tuberculosis, Nocardia, Brucella, Actinobacillus mallei, Yersinia pestis, Francisella tularensis.* It is the drug of choice in tularemia and plague.

Dihydrostreptomycin sulfate

It is a semi-synthetic aminoglycoside antibiotic. It is a hydrogenated form of streptomycin; It is obtained by reduction of aldehyde group (-CHO) of streptomycin to primary alcohol (-CH_2OH). It occurs as a white to off-white crystalline powder. It is used against tuberculosis and tularemia and gram-negative organisms. Dihydrostreptomycin is more toxic than streptomycin hence it employed in veterinary practice.

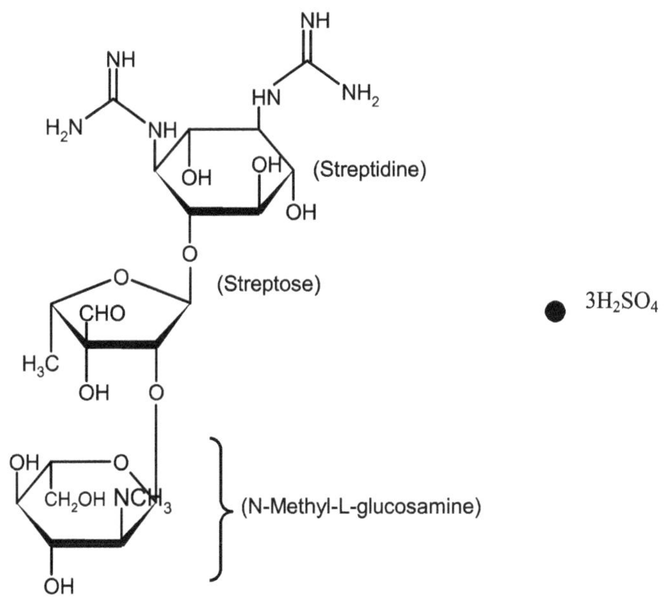

Neomycin

Neomycin was discovered in 1949 by the microbiologist Solman Waksman and his student Hubert Lechevalier. It is produced naturally by the bacterium *Streptomyces fradiae*. Neomycin is an aminoglycoside, which is used only for topical purpose because of its severe toxicity. It is a mixture of neomycin A, B and C. Neomycin is available as neomycin sulphate, which is administered parenterally because of poor absorption by oral route. It is widely used for the treatment of gastrointestinal infections, dermatological infections and acute peritonitis. It is combined with corticosteroids.

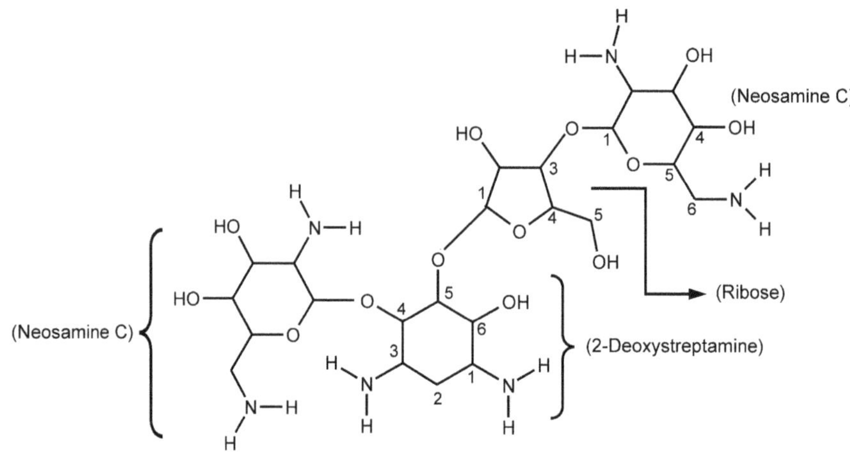

Kanamycin

Kanamycin is obtained from the soil bacterium *Steptomyces kanamycetius*. It consists of a major component (Kanamycin A) and two minor components (Kanamycin B and Kanamycin C). It is commercially available in pure Kanamycin A. The aglycone is 2-deoxystreptamine. Kanamycin differs from neomycin and streptomycin in having no ribose moiety hence it is less toxic. Chemically kanamycin A is 2-(aminomethyl)-6-[4,6-diamino-3-[4-amino-3,5-dihydroxy-6-(hydroxymethyl)tetrahydropyran-2-yl]oxy-2-hydroxy-cyclohexoxy]-tetrahydropyran-3,4,5-triol. Injections of kanamycin are painful hence local anaesthetics are employed.

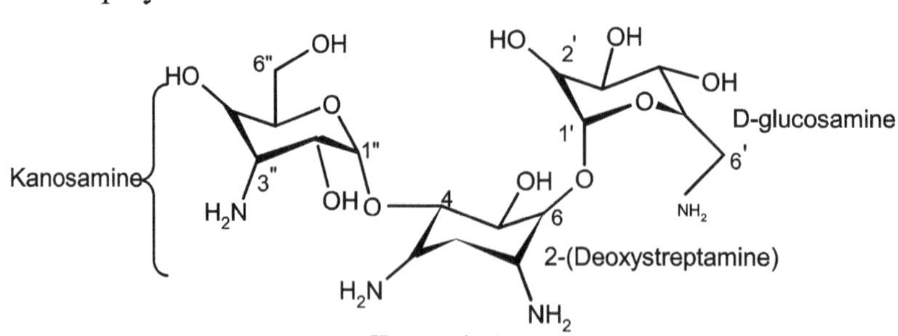

Kanamycin A

Properties: It is white crystalline powder which is freely soluble in water, practically insoluble in acetone; very slightly soluble in chloroform and in solvent ether.

Uses : Kanamycin works by affecting an unknown aspect of translocation, and by causing messenger RNA (mRNA) to be misread by the ribosome, causing a lethal level of translational errors. It is used parenterally against some gram-negative bacteria but *Pseudomonas aeruginosa*. It can also be used in combination with other drugs against certain *mycobacteria*. This antibiotic is used in crop genetic engineering as a selective marker.

Amikacin

Amikacin is a semisynthetic derivative of kanamycin A. It has the same spectrum of activity as gentamicin and tobramycin. Amikacin works by binding to the bacterial 30S ribosomal subunit, causing misreading of m – RNA and leaving the bacterium unable to synthesize proteins vital to its growth. Amikacin may be administered once or twice a day but must be given by intravenous or intramuscular route. Amikacin is synthesized from kanamycin A by acylation of 1-amino group with 1-N-L-(–)-amino-α-hydroxy butyric acid [L-AHBA].

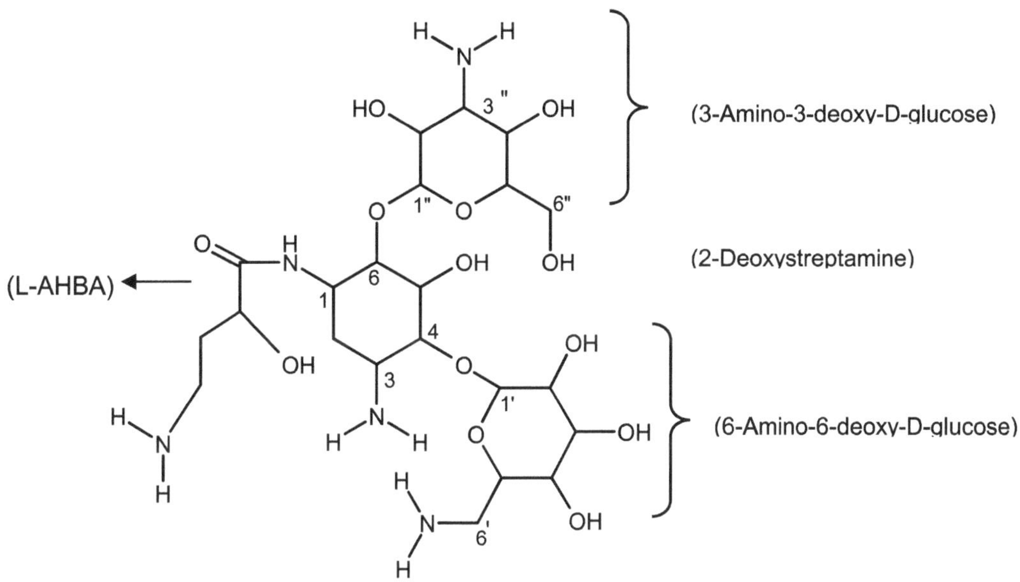

Amikacin

Properties

It is available as white powder, sparingly soluble in water, slightly soluble in methanol, practically insoluble in acetone and in alcohol. The drug is exclusively eliminated by glomerular filteration.

Uses

Amikacin is most often used for treating severe, hospital-acquired infections with multidrug resistant gram-negative bacteria such as *Pseudomonas aeruginosa, Acinetobacter*, and

Enterobacter. Amikacin may be combined with a β-lactam antibiotic to treat neutropenia and fever.

Gentamicin sulphate

Gentamycin is a aminoglycoside antibiotic, and can treat many different types of bacterial infections, particularly gram-negative infection. It is a mixture of several antibiotic components (C_1, C_2 and C_{1a}) obtained from *Microspora purpurea*.

Gentamicin works by binding to a site on the bacterial ribosome, causing the genetic code to be misread. Like all aminoglycosides, gentamicin does not pass the gastro-intestinal tract, so it can only be given intravenously, intramuscularly or topically. Gentamicin can cause deafness or a loss of equilibrioception.

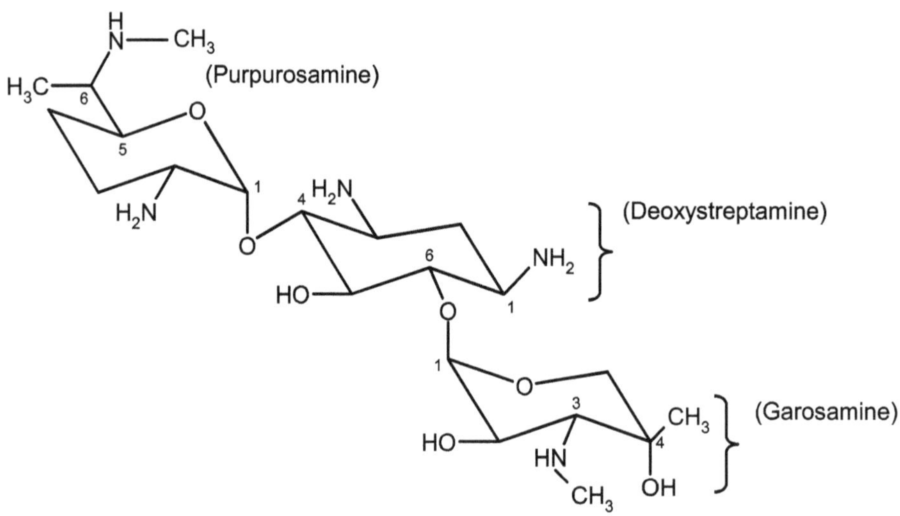

Structure

Chemically it is 2-[4,6-diamino-3- [3-amino-6-(1-methylaminoethyl) tetrahydropyran-2-yl]oxy-2-hydroxycyclohexoxy]-5-methyl-4-methylamino-oxane-tetrahy-dropyran-3,5-diol. The aglycone moiety in gentamycin is 2-deoxystreptamine. It occurs as white, hygroscopic powder and is freely soluble in water, practically insoluble in alcohol.

Uses

Gentamicin was one of the first antibiotics to have significant activity against *Pseudomonas aeruginosa* infections. It is frequently used in burns, skin infections, pneumonia and urinary tract infections (*Pseudomonas aeruginosa* is commonly encountered in burns, pneumonia and in urinary tract infections). It can be used in bone and joint infections caused by susceptible gram-negative organisms as well as to prevent fouling of contact lenses. Gentamicin should not be used with carbenicillin because of chemical incompatibility.

Tobramycin

It is obtained from *Streptomyces tenebrarius* which occurs as sulphate salt. Chemically it is 4-amino-2-[4,6-diamino-3-[3-amino-6-(aminomethyl)-5-hydroxy-tetrahydropyran-2-yl]oxy-2-hydroxy-cyclohexoxy]-6-(hydroxymethyl) tetrahydropyran-3,5-diol. Tobramycin sulphate is an aminoglycoside antibiotic used to treat various types of bacterial infections, particularly gram-negative infections. Tobramycin works by binding to a site on the bacterial ribosome, causing the genetic code to be misread. Tobramycin does not pass the gastro-intestinal tract, so for systemic use it can only be given intravenously or intramuscularly. It is white (or) almost white powder which is freely soluble in water, very slightly soluble in alcohol.

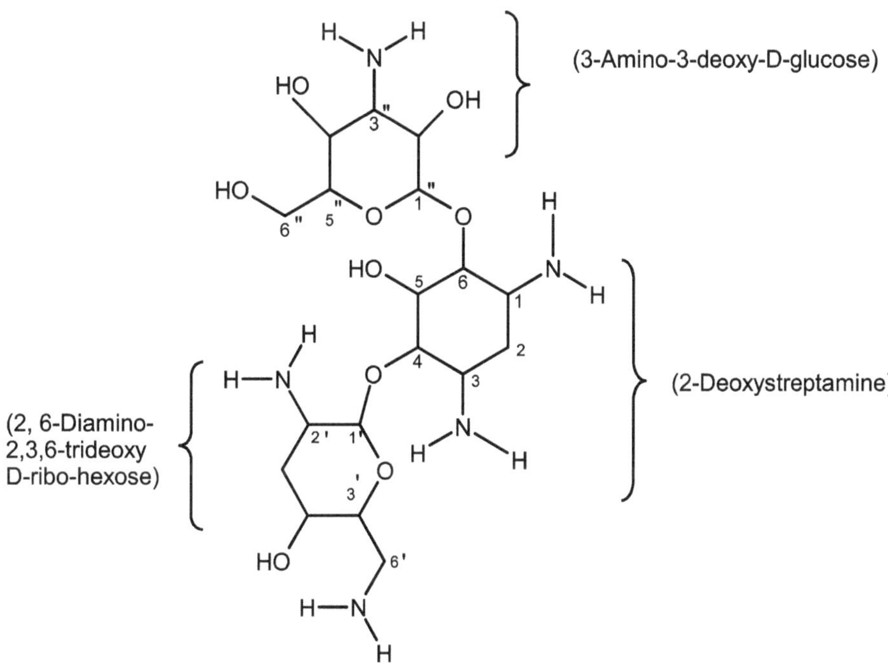

Uses

The antibacterial activity and pharmacokinetic properties of tobramycin are similar to gentamycin. It has superior activity against *Pseudomonas* species. It is used topically for eye infections. Like other aminoglycosides, tobramycin can cause deafness or a loss of equilibrioception in genetically susceptible individuals.

11

TETRACYCLINES

Introduction

Tetracyclines are introduced 50 years ago as broad spectrum antibiotics. They are closely congeneric derivatives of the polycyclic naphthacene. All tetracycline derivatives must possess fused tetracycline ring to exhibit antibacterial activity. Tetracyclines are biosynthesised from acetic acid or propionic acid units in microorganisms. Tetracyclines possess a wide spectrum of activity i.e., against gram-positive and gram-negative bacteria, chlamydias, rickettsias, mycoplasms, spirochaetes, some protozoa and mycobacteria. They are usually administered by oral route but most of them are administered by IV or IM injections.

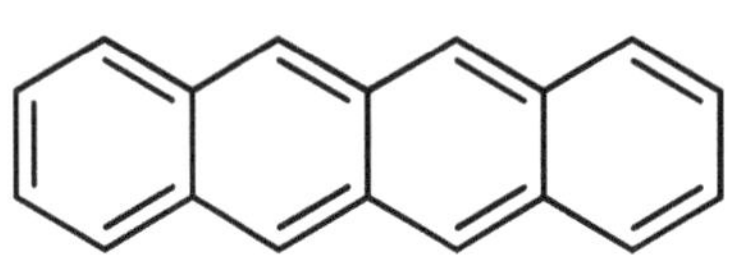

Naphthacene

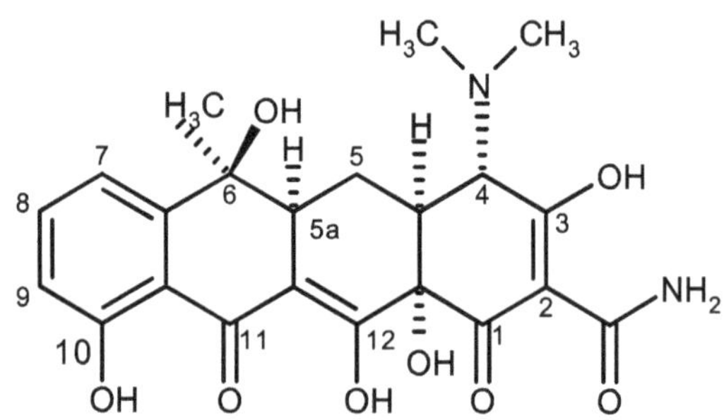

Tetracycline

Tetracyclines are amphoteric and possess three acid constants (pK_a) in aqueous solutions of tetracycline salts. The following groups are responsible for acidity constants:

pK_{a1} [2.8–3.3] = Conjugated trione system between C_1 to C_3

pK_{a2} [7.2–7.8] = Conjugated phenolic enone system between C_{10} to C_{12} through C_{11}

pK_{a3} [9.1–9.7] = Group present at C_4 i.e., dimethyl amino group. This group is responsible for formation of water soluble hydrochloride salts.

Structure activity relationships

1. The keto-enol tautomerism between C-2 and C-3 is very important for tetracyclines to show biological activity. Any modification in this system can be resulted in loss of activity.

2. The amide group is essential for activity. Substitutions at this amido group can result in hydrophilic compounds which can be taken orally.
3. Due to the presence of dimethylamino group at C-4 position tetracycline exists as zwitter ion, which enables it to distribute in body. Loss of activity is observed when dimethylamino group is removed. The epitetracyclines which are formed by structural modification at C-4 due to pH changes are less potent than the natural ones.
4. Substitution at 5th and 6th positions with hydroxyl groups produce water soluble derivatives which can be administered orally.
5. Eliminating 6-OH group causes an increase in lipophilicity and more stable to acids. Eg: Doxycycline, Minocycline. Methylenation at the C-6 position resulted in compounds having good antibacterial activity. Eg: Methacycline
6. Substitution of dimethylamino group at C-7 can result in increased antibacterial activity.
7. Electron withdrawing groups and electron donating groups equally potentiate the C-7 position.
8. Any modification at C-11, C-12, C-11a and C-12a positions result in loss of activity. A cis-type arrangement at A/B rings with β-hydroxyl group at C-12a is important for the activity of tetracyclines.
9. Any changes made to oxygen atoms at the C-11, C-12 reduces the biological activity.
10. Tetracyclines which are obtained by substitution of sulphur atom at C-6 position has shown very potent activity in comparison to minocycline.

Mechanism of action

Tetracyclines enter bacterial cells by either passive diffusion through pores or by an active transport (energy dependent process which requires ATP and magnesium ions). Inside the bacterial cells, they bind specifically to 30S ribosomes, thereby blocking binding of t-RNA to m-RNA ribosome complex, inhibiting protein synthesis.

Tetracyclines form chelate complexes with many metals including calcium, magnesium and iron. It has been suggested that they remove these divalent metallic cations from sites where they are required for enzyme activation.

Clinical uses of tetracyclines

Tetracyclines are clinically used in chronic bronchitis, atypical pneumonia, rickettsial infections, non-specific urethritis, lymphogranuloma venereum, trachoma, cholera, syphilis, anthrax, meningococcal carriers and amoebiasis.

Tetracycline

Tetracycline is commonly used antibiotic produced by *Streptomyces* species. Chemically it is 4-(dimethylamino)-1,4,4a,5,5a,6,11,12a-octahydro-3,6,10,12,12a-pentahydroxy-6-methyl-1,11-dioxo-2-naphthacenecarboxamide.

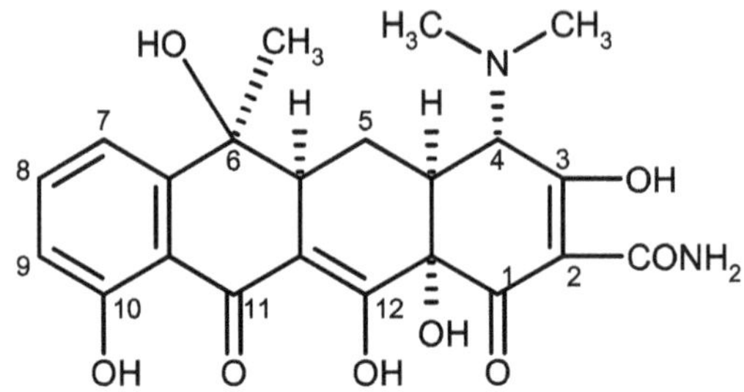

Tetracycline

Properties

Tetracycline hydrochloride is an yellow colored, crystalline, odorless, hygroscopic powder. It is amphoteric and darkens in moist air on exposure to sunlight. It is soluble in water, alkali hydroxides and carbonates but insoluble in acetone and ether.

Uses

It is used as antiamoebic, antibacterial and antirickettsial agent.

Chlortetracycline (Aureomycin or 7-Chlortetracycline)

It is a natural tetracycline obtained from the substrate of *Streptomyces aureofaciens*. Chemically chlortetracycline is 7-chloro-4-(dimethylamino)1,4,4a,5,5a,6,11,12a-octahydro-3,6,10,12,12a-pentahydroxy-6-methyl-1,11-dioxo-2-naphthacenecarboxamide.

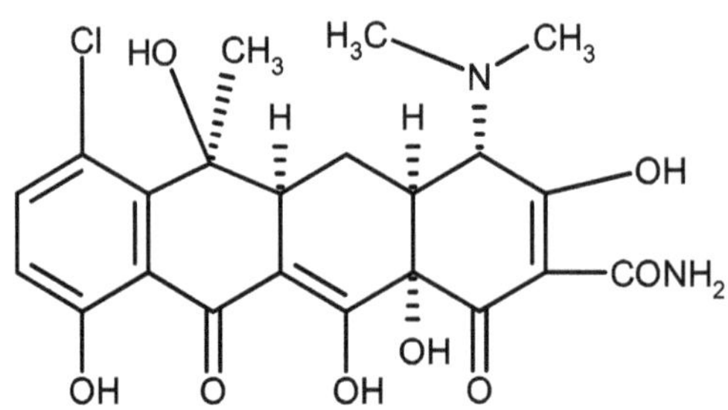

Chlortetracycline

Properties

Chlortetracycline is available as chlortetracycline hydrochloride. Chlortetracycline hydrochloride is a golden yellow crystals having a melting point of 168°C. It is soluble in water, very soluble in aqueous solvents and practically insoluble in ether.

Uses

It is used as antiamoebic and antibacterial agent.

Oxytetracycline

Oxytetracycline is a (4S,4aR,5S,5aR,6S 12aS)-4-(dimethylamino)-3,5,6,10,11,12a-hexahydroxy-6-methyl-1,12-dioxo-1,4,4a,5,5a,6,12,12a-octahy, rotetracene-2-carboxamide. Antibiotic substance isolated from the elaboration products of the *Actinomycetes, Streptomyces rimosus*; grown on a suitable medium.

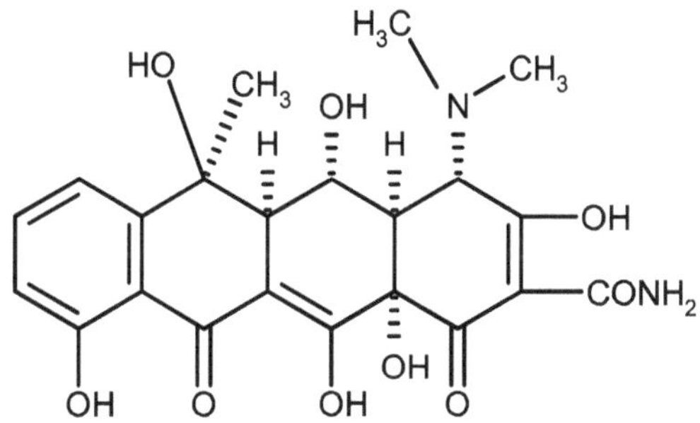

Oxytetracycline

Properties

Oxytetracycline occurs as yellow platelets, which are very soluble in water. These crystals show no loss in potency on heating for 4 days at 100°C.

Uses

To treat lethal yellowing in palm trees and used as an antibacterial agent.

Demeclocycline

Demeclocycline is obtained from the strains of *Streptomyces aureofaciens*. Chemically it is 7-chloro-4-(dimethylamino)1,4,4a,5a,6,11,12a-octahydro-3,6,10,12,12a-pentahydroxy-1,11-dioxo-2-naphthacenecarboxamide. Demeclocycline does not possess methyl group at 6th position as in chlortetracycline hence stability is improved against acid and alkali.

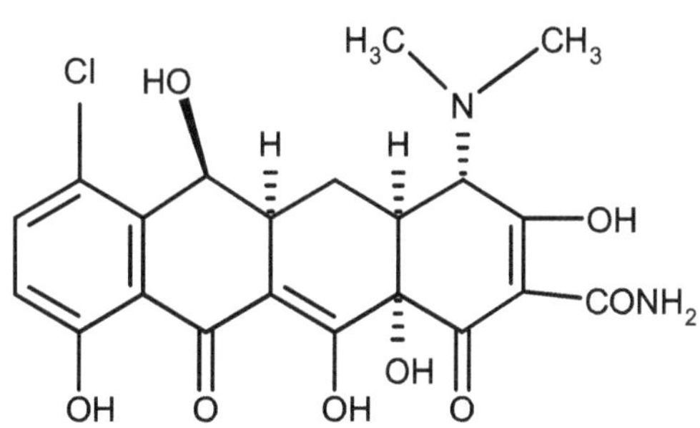

Demeclocycline

Properties

Demeclocycline HCl is yellow colored, melts at 175°C, odorless, crystalline compound.

Uses

It is used as an antibacterial agent.

Meclocycline

It is a semi-synthetic antibiotic derived from tetracycline. It is 7-chloro-6-deoxy-6-demethyl-6-methylene-5-oxytetracycline.

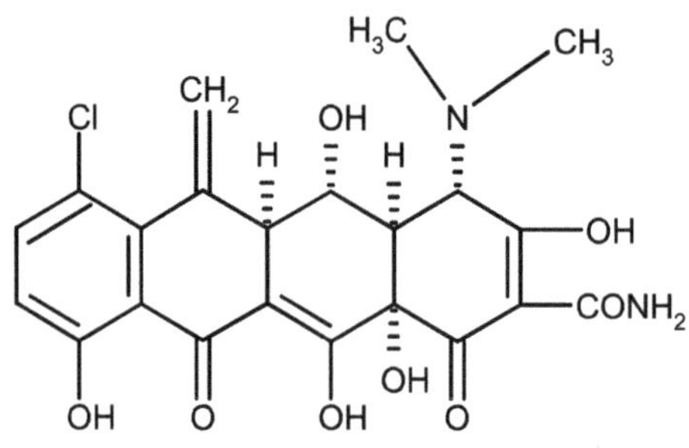

Meclocycline

Uses

It is available as 1% cream for external use as an antibacterial agent.

Doxycycline

Doxycycline is (4S,4aR,5S,5aR,6R,12aS)-4-(dimethylamino)-3,5,10,12,12a-pentahydroxy-6-methyl-1,11-dioxo-1,4,4a,5,5a,6,11,12a-octahydrotetracene-2-carboxamide. Doxycycline is a second generation tetracycline. It is a 6α-methylepimer and is three times more potent to its β-epimer like oxytetracycline. It is more stable in acids and bases due to absence of 6-hydroxy group.

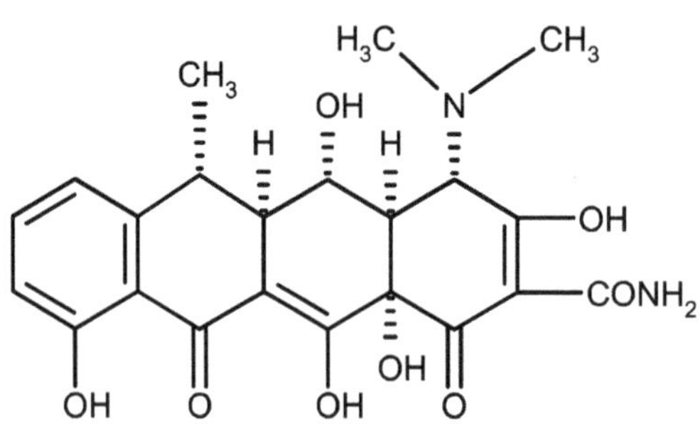

Doxycycline

Doxycyline is prepared by catalytic hydrogenation of methacycline.

Minocycline

Minocycline is 7-di-methylamino-6-demethyl-6-deoxytetracycline. Minocycline is a second generation antibiotic. It is the most potent currently used tetracycline. It is prepared by reductive methylation of 7-di-methylamino-6-demethyl-6-deoxytetracycline. It does not possess 6-hydroxyl group hence it is stable to acids.

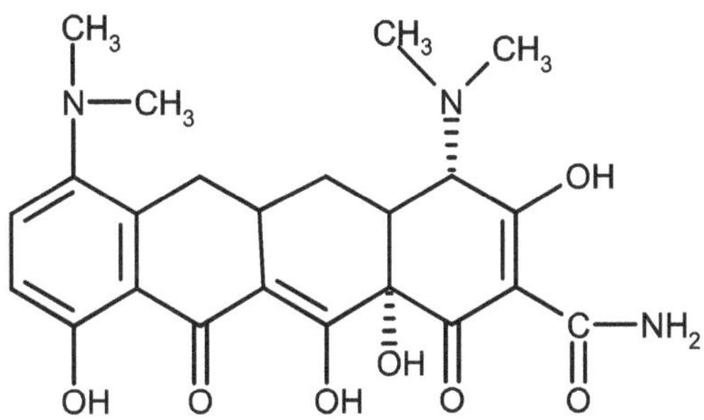

Minocycline

Minocycline is well absorbed by oral route and has long duration of action. It is used to treat staphylococcal and streprococcal infections such as chronic bronchitis, upper respiratory tract infections and urinary tract infections.

12

MACROLIDES

Macrolides are a group of antibiotics possessing a macrolide ring (a large lactone ring to which one or more deoxy sugars, usually cladinose and desosamine, are attached). The lactone ring can be 14, 15 or 16-membered. Macrolides belong to the polyketide (Polyketides are secondary metabolites from bacteria, fungi, plants, and animals. They are derived from polymerization of acetyl and propionyl subunits in a similar process to fatty acid synthesis) class of natural products.

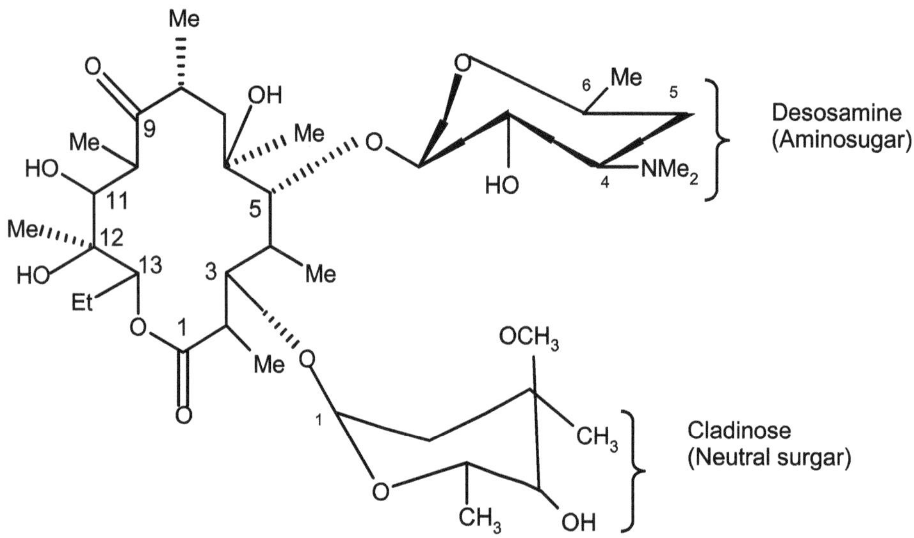

Macrolides are different from one another in their chemical substitutions on the structure of various carbon atoms and the amino and neutral sugars. Macrolides are products of actinomycetes (soil bacteria) (or) semi-synthetic derivatives of them. They are effective aganist gram-positive cocci such as *Streptococci*, *Staphylococci*, as well as *Mycobacterium*, *Mycoplasma*, *Chlamydia*, *Rickettsia* and some strains of gram-negative bacteria such as *Niessria* and *Haemophilus*.

Mechanism of action

The macrolide binding site is primarily of r-RNA. They inhibit bacterial protein synthesis by binding reversibly to 50S subunit of bacterial ribosome (50S subunit of ribosomes does not exist in human cells), thereby inhibiting translocation of peptidyl-t-RNA from A to P site. This action is mainly bacteriostatic, but can also be bactericidal in high concentrations. Macrolides tend to accumulate within leukocytes, and are therefore actually transported into the site of infection.

Erythromycin

In 1949, J. M. McGuire (Eli Lilly's research team), isolated erythromycin from the *Streptomyces erythreus* in soil samples. Erythromycin was formerly also called Ilotycin®. In 1981, Robert B. Woodward and a large team of researchers reported the first stereocontrolled asymmetric chemical synthesis of Erythromycin A.

Chemistry

Erythromycin is a macrolide antibiotic isolated from saccharopoly spora erythrea (streptomyces erythraeus). It has an antimicrobial spectrum similar to or slightly wider than that of penicillin, and is often used for people who have an allergy to penicillins. Structurally, this macrocyclic compound contains a 14-membered lactone ring with ten asymmetric centers and two sugars (L-cladinose and D-desoamine), making it a compound very difficult to produce via synthetic methods. Chemically erythromycin is 6-(4-dimethylamino-3-hydroxy-6-methyl-oxan-2-yl)oxy-14-ethyl-7,12,13-trihydroxy-4-(5-hydroxy -4-methoxy-4,6-dimethyl-oxan-2-yl)oxy-3,5,7,9,11,13-hexamethyl-1-oxacyclotetradecane-2, 10-dione.

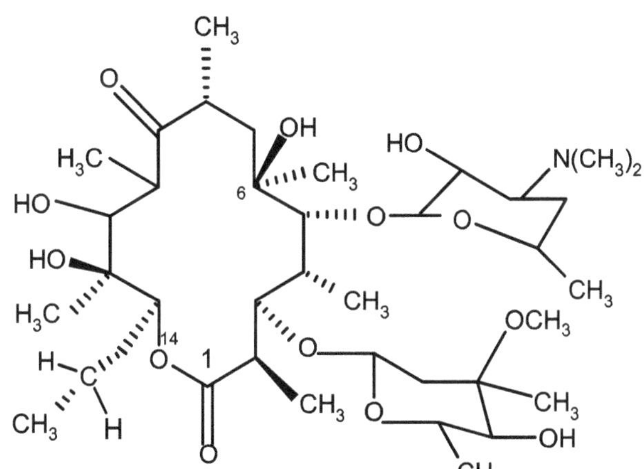

Erythromycin

Most of erythromycin is metabolised by demethylation in the liver. Its main elimination route is in the bile, and a small portion in the urine. Erythromycins half-life is 1.5 hours.

Mechanism of action

Erythromycin prevents bacteria from growing, by interfering with their protein synthesis. It binds to the 23S rRNA molecule in the 50S of the bacterial ribosome, blocking the exit of the growing peptide chain thus inhibiting the translocation of peptides.

Uses

- Particularly useful in respiratory infections.
- Treatment of pertussis.
- Prophylaxis in pencillin-sensitive patients, particularly in pregnant women.

Clarithromycin

Clarithromycin is *(3R,4S,5S,6R,7R,9R,11S,12R,13S,14S)* -6- {[2S,3R,4S,6R) -4-(dimethylamino)-3-hydroxy-6-methyloxan-2-y1]oxy}-14-ethyl-12,13-dihydroxy-4-{[(2*R*,4*S*,5*S*,6*S*)-5-hydroxy -4methoxy-4,6-dimethyloxan-2yl]oxy}-7 -methoxy-3,5,7,9,11,13-hexamethyl -1-oxacyclotetradecan-2-one The antibiotic clarithromycin was invented by scientists at the Japanese drug company Taisho Pharmaceutical in the 1970s as a result of their efforts to overcome the acid instability of erythromycin. It is 6-methyl ether of erythromycin which is a semisynthetic erythromycin obtained from erythromycin by simple methylation of 6-hydroxyl group in erythromycin. It occurs as water-insoluble white crystalline solid.

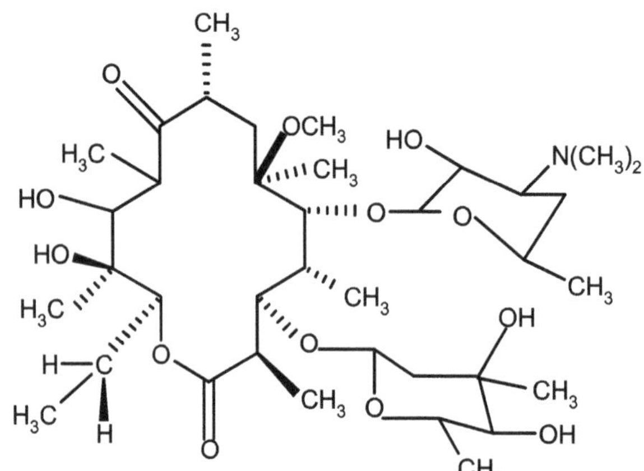

Clarithromycin

Clarithromycin exhibits greater potency than erythromycin against *Mycoplasma pneumoniae, Legionella, Chlamydia pneumoniae, Haemophilus influenzae,* and *Moraxella catarhalis*. It is also effective against *Borrelia burgdorferi, Mycobacterium avium* complex.

Azithromycin

Azithromycin is a (2*R*,3*S*,4*R*,5*R*,8*R*,10*R*,11*R*,12*S*,13*S*,14*R*)-2ethyl-3,4,10-trihydroxy-3,5,6,8,10,12,14-heptamethyl-15-oxo- 11-{[3,4,6-trideoxy-3- (dimethylamino)-β-D-*xylo*-]oxy}-1-oxa-6azacyclopentadec-13-yl 2,6- dideoxy3-*C*-methyl-3-*O*-methyl-α-L-*ribo*-hexopyranoside. Azithromycin is a nitrogen containing 15-membered lactone ring macrolides (Azalides). It is a semisynthetic derivative of erythromycin. It is primarily bacteriostatic, but can be bactericidal depending on the concentration given. It is acid stable than erythromycin because weakly basic tertiary amino group is introduced in place of 9-keto group of erythromycin.

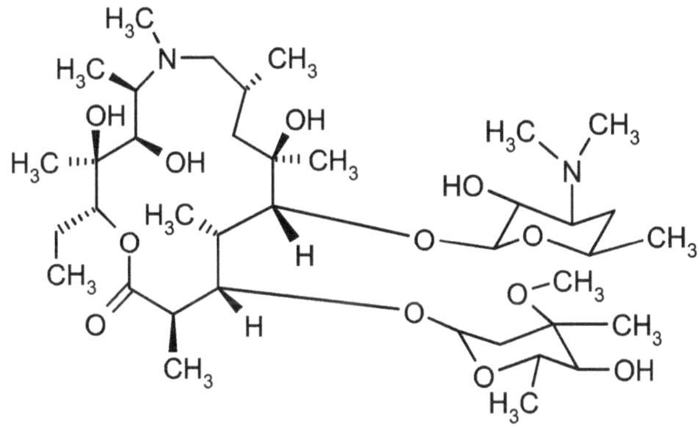

Azithromycin

It occurs as white (or) almost white powder, practically insoluble in water, freely soluble in ethanol and in methylene chloride.

Uses

Azithromycin has wide spectrum of activity (effective against *Halmophilus influenza, Chalamydia trachomatis, Micobacterium avium, Mycoplasma, Legionella, Moraxella, Camphylobacteria, Helicobacter pylori* etc) but it is effective against erythromycin resistant bacteria. It is more active against Gram-negative bacteria but less effective against gram-positive bacteria. It is widely prescribed for the treatment of respiratory tract infections because of its high efficacy and safety.

Roxithromycin

Roxithromycin is (3*R*,4*S*,5*S*,6*R*,7*R*,9*R*,11*S*,12*R*,13*S*,14*R*)-6-[(2S,3R4S,6R)-4-d-3-hydroxy-6-methyloxan-2-yl]oxy-14-ethyl-7,12,13-trihydroxy-4-[(2*R*,4*R*,5*S*,6*S*)-5-hydroxy-4-methoxy-4,6-dimethyloxan-2-yl]oxy-10-(2-methoxyethoxymethoxyimino)-3,5,7,9,11,13-hexamethyl-1-oxacyclotetradecan-2-one. Roxithromycin is a semi-synthetic macrolide antibiotic. It is a semi-synthetic 14-membered-ring macrolide antibiotic in which the erythronolide A lactone ring has been altered to prevent inactivation in the gastric milieu. It is derived from erythromycin, however, an N-oxime side chain is attached to the lactone ring. Roxithromycin is very similar in composition, chemical structure (semi-synthetic) and mechanism of action to erythromycin, azithromycin, or clarithromycin.

Roxithromycin is absorbed well into the gastro-intestinal tract, with few side effects, and actively responds to the presence of cryptosporidium, pneumocystis carinii (PCP), toxoplasma gondii, and Mycobacterium avium complex (MAC). The *in vitro* activity of roxithromycin is well documented and similar to that of other macrolide antibiotics.

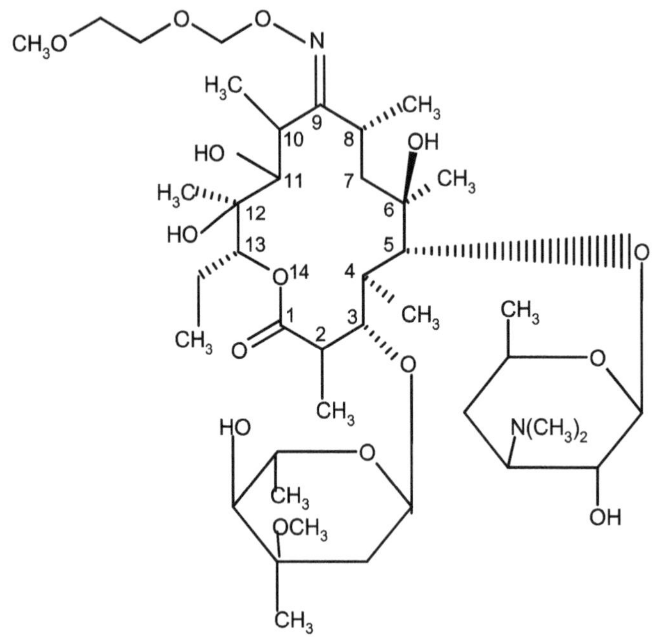

Roxithromycin

Mechanism of action

Roxithromycin act, by interfering with protein synthesis in bacteria. It binds to the subunit 50S of the bacterial ribosome, and thus inhibits the translocation of peptides. Roxithromycin has similar antimicrobial spectrum as erythromycin, but is more effective against certain gram-negative bacteria, especially *Legionella pneumophila*.

Uses: Roxithromycin is active against gram-positive bacteria like *Staphylococci*, *Streptococci*, *Listeria*, *Corynebacteria*; gram-negative bacteria such as *Gonococci*, *Haemophilus influenzae*, *Haemophilus ducreyi*, *Legionella*, *campylobacter*, and atypical pathogens like *Mycoplasma* and *Chlamydia*. It has been found useful in the treatment of upper and lower respiratory, otorhinolaryngological, skin, dental and genital infections. It is well tolerated by adults and children. Roxithromycin has less interactions than erythromycin as it has a lower affinity for cytochrome P450. It appears to interact with warfarin.

Dirithromycin

Dirithromycin is a prodrug, which is converted non-enzymatically during intestinal absorption into the microbiologically active moiety erythromycylamine. Chemically dirithromycin is 9-(4-dimethylamino-3-hydroxy-6-methyl-oxan-2-yl)oxy-3-ethyl-2,10dihydroxy-7-(5-hydroxy-4 meth -oxy-4,6-dimethyl-oxan-2-yl)oxy-152methoxyethoxymethyl)-2,6,8,10,12,17-hexamethyl-4,16 dioxa-14 azabicyclo[11.3.1] heptadecan-5-one Dirithromycin was more active *in vitro* against *Campylobacter jejuni* and *Borrelia burgdorferi* than erythromycin or clarithromycin, but in general demonstrated less activity than erythromycin, clarithromycin, azithromycin against a majority of microorganisms. Dirithromycin is used to treat many different types of bacterial infections, such as bronchitis, pneumonia, tonsillitis, and skin infections.

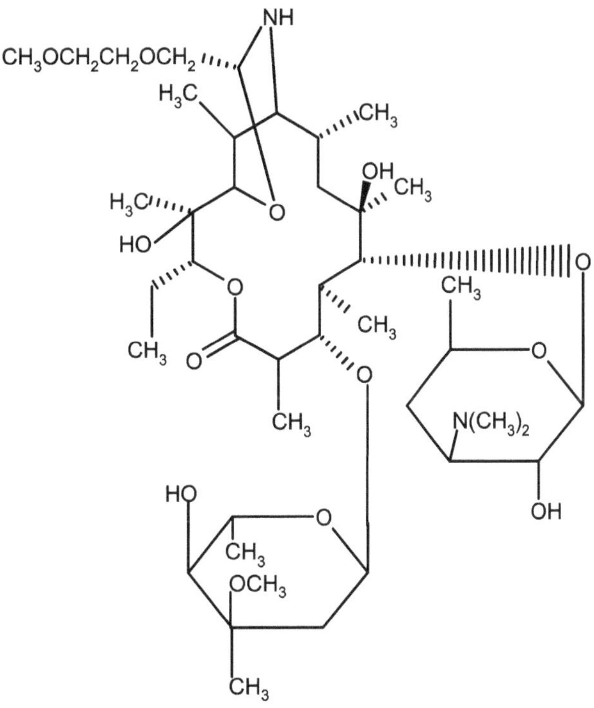

Dirithromycin

Erythromycylamine exerts its activity by binding to the 50S ribosomal subunits of susceptible microorganisms resulting in inhibition of protein synthesis. Dirithromycin/erythromycylamine has been shown to be active against most strains of the following microorganisms both *in vitro* and in clinical infections: *Staphylococcus aureus* (Methicillin susceptible strains only), *Streptococcus pneumoniae*, *Streptococcus pyogenes*, *Haemophilus influenzae*, *Legionella pneumophila*, *Moraxella catarrhalis*, and *Mycoplasma pneumoniae*.

Dirithromycin prevents bacteria from growing, by interfering with their protein synthesis. Dirithromycin binds to the 50S subunit of the 70S bacterial ribosome, and thus inhibits the translocation of peptides. Dirithromycin has over 10 times higher affinity to the subunit 50S than erythromycin. In addition, dirithromycin binds simultaneously into two domains of 23S RNA of the ribosomal subunit 50S, where older macrolides bind only in one. Dirithromycin can also inhibit the formation of ribosomal subunits 50S and 30S. Oral dirithromycin is rapidly absorbed, with an absolute bioavailability of approximately 10%. Dietary fat has little or no effect on the bioavailability of dirithromycin.

13

POLYPEPTIDE AND MISCELLANEOUS GROUP OF ANTIBIOTICS

Polypeptide antibiotics are composed of several aminoacid residues, which are linked through peptide linkages. Most of antibiotics are cyclic (except gramicidins) without sulphur bridges. Polypeptide antibiotics possesses D or L-amino acid units in addition to some unusual amino acid resides (α, β-diaminobutyric acid,α, β-diaminopropionic acid). *Eg:* Bacitracin, vancomycin, polymyxin, and gramicidin.

Antibiotics of the polypeptide class differ widely in their mechanism of action and antimicrobial properties. Eg: Bacitracin and Vancomycin interfere with bacterial cell wall synthesis and are effective only against gram-positive bacteria. Gramicidin and polymyxin interfere with cell membrane functions of bacteria.

Bacitracin

Bacitracin is (4*R*)-4-[2*S*)-2-({2-[(1*S*)-1-amino-2-methylbutyl]- 4,5-dihydro-1,3-thiazol-5-yl}fkormamido)-4-methylpentanamido]-4-{[(1*S*)-1-{[(3*S*,6*R*,9*S*,12*R*,15*S*,18*R*,21*S*)- 18-(3-aminopropyl)-12-benzyl-15-(butan-2-yl)-3-(carbomoylmethyl)- 6-(carboxymethyl)-9-(1*H*-imidazol-5-ylmethyl)-2,5,8,11,14,17,20- heptaoxo-1,4,7,10,13,16,19-heptaazacyclopentacosan-21-yl]carbamoyl}-2-methylbutyl]carbamoyl}butanoic acid. Bacitracin is obtained from *Bacillus subtilis*. It is a mixture of polypeptides. It is active at acidic pH (4 to 5) but inactive in alkaline pH and is also inactive with bivalent ions due to complexation. It is bactericidal against gram-positive bacteria. Bacitracin doesn't work well orally. However, it is very effective topically.

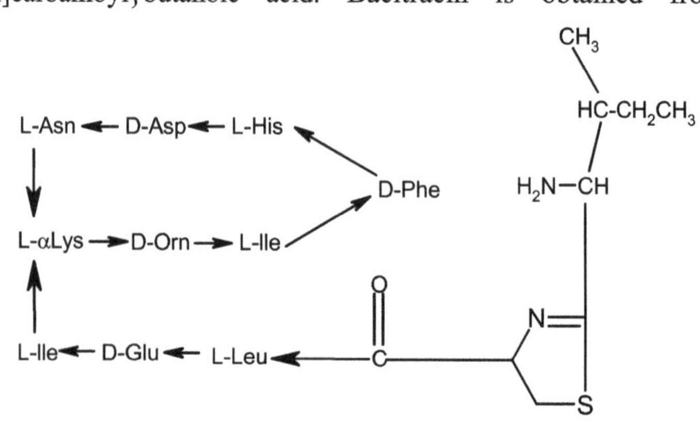

Mechanism of action

Bacitracin blocks dephosphorylation of the C_{55}-isoprenyl pyrophosphate, a molecule that carries the building blocks of the peptidoglycan bacterial cell wall outside of the inner membrane.

Uses

It is used for topical treatment of a variety of localized skin and eye infections. It is effective against gram-positive bacteria, including strains of *staphylococcus* that are resistant to penicillin is toxic to humans and is no longer used internally.

Gramicidin

Gramicidin is a heterogeneous mixture of polypeptide antibiotic compounds which are obtained from the soil bacterial species *Bacillus brevis*. It is bactericidal against gram-positive bacteria.

Gramicidin is available in a variety of topical preparations with other antibiotics (bacitracin, neomycin or polymyxin B) to treat local infections. Gramicidin acts as an ionophore in bacterial cell membranes to cause the loss of potassium ion from the cells.

Miscellaneous antibiotics

1. Spectinomycin

Spectinomycin is an aminocylitol antibiotic produced by a species of soil microorganism designated as *Streptomyces spectabilis*. It is effective against a number of Gram-negative bacteria. It is given by injection to treat gonorrhea. Side effects include itching, chills and red rash.

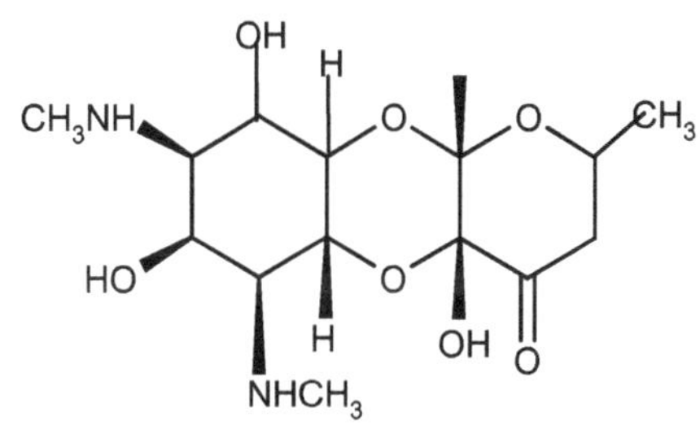

Spectinomycin

In vitro studies have shown spectinomycin to be active against most strains of *Neisseria gonorrhoeae* (minimum inhibitory concentration < 7.5 to 20 mcg/mL). Footprint studies indicate that spectinomycin exerts regional effects on ribosomal structure. Spectinomycin is an inhibitor of protein synthesis in the bacterial cell; the site of action is the 30S ribosomal subunit. It inhibits translocation of the peptidyl t-RNA from A site to the P site and is bacteriostatic in its action.

2. Lincomycins

Lincosamides are sulphur containing antibiotics obtained from *Streptomyces lincolnensis* useful for the treatment of infections caused by gram-positive bacteria such as *Streptococci, Staphylococci*, and *enterococci*. They have very limited use because of their serious side effects. Lincosamides bind to 50S ribosomal subunit, which block t-RNA binding, thereby inhibiting protein synthesis. They are widely different from erythromycin and other macrolide antibiotics in chemical structures but they have similar antimicrobial profiles and they act on the same site on bacterial ribosomes to suppress protein synthesis. *E.g :* Lincomycin, Clindamycin.

Lincomycin is the first lincosamide antibiotic obtained from the bacteria *Streptomyces lincolnensis*. However, because of its adverse effect and toxicity, it is rarely used for patients who are either allergic to penicillin or where bacteria has developed resistance. Lincomycin hydrochloride is methyl 6,8-dideoxy-6-(1-methyl-trans-4-propyl-L-2-pyrrolidine carboxamido)-1-thio-D-erythro-α-D-galacto-octopyranoside monohydro-chloride monohydrate. Lincomycin is composed of an amino acid portion, trans-N-methyl-4-N-propyl-L-proline, linked through an amide bond to an unusual sugar i.e., 6-amino-6, 8-dideoxy-1-thio-α-D-galacto pyranoside. The structural formula is represented below:

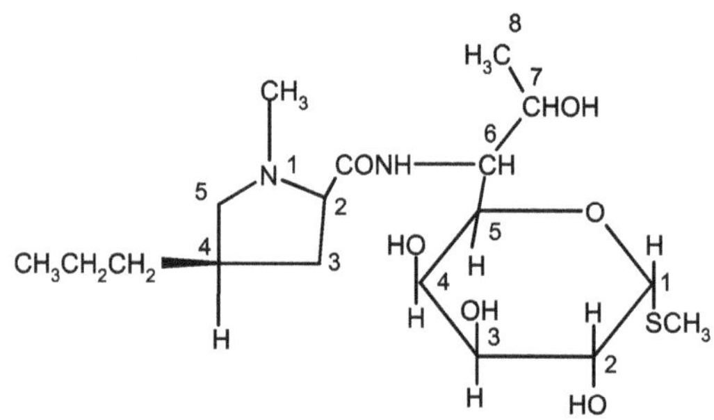

Lincomycin

Lincomycin hydrochloride is a white, crystalline powder and is odorless. Its solutions are acid and are dextrorotatory. Lincomycin hydrochloride is freely soluble in water dimethylformamide and slightly soluble in acetone. Lincomycin is effective against gram-positive cocci, *Haemophilus, Neisseria, Staphylococci, Pneumococcus, Corynebacteria* etc. it acts by inhibition of protein synthesis.

3. Clindamycin

Clindamycin is a semisynthetic antibiotic derived from lincomycin by 7(S)-chloro-substitution of the 7(*R*)-hydroxyl group of the lincomycin. Clindamycin is a chlorinated semisynthetic derivative of lincomycin but shows better absorption and antimicrobial activity than lincomycin. Chemically it is (2*S*,4*R*)-*N*-((1*R*)- 2-chloro-1-((3R,4R,5S,6R)-3,4,5-trihydroxy-6-(methylthio)-tetrahydro-2H-pyran-2yl)propyl)-1-methyl-4-propylpyrroli-dine-2-carboxamide. It is bactericidal against gram-positive cocci; *Staphylococci, Pneumococci, Corynebacteria*. It acts by inhibiting bacterial protein synthesis. It is recommended for the treatment of a wide variety of upper respiratory, skin and soft tissue infections caused by bacteria. Clindamycin can be administered orally or parenterally. Its half-life is 2 hours. In patients with hypersensitivity to penicillins, clindamycin may be used to treat susceptible aerobic infections as well. It is also used to treat bone infections caused by *Staphylococcus aureus*. Topical application of clindamycin phosphate can be used to treat severe acne. Clindamycin is now usually preferred to lincomycin as it is more active and has fewer side effects.

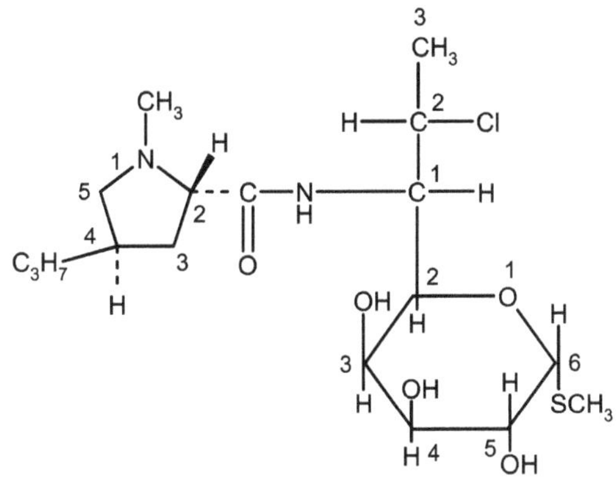

Clindamycin

4. Novobiocin

Novobiocin is a coumarin antibiotic used to treat *Staphylococcus epidermidis*. It is an aromatic ether compound acts by inhibiting DNA gyrase, an enzyme that mediates the supercoiling of DNA. DNA gyrase has no mammalian equivalent. Chemically it is N-[7-[[3-O-Aminocarbonyl-6-deoxy-5-C-methyl-4-O-methyl-β-L-lyxo-hexopyranosyl]oxy]-4-hydroxy-8-methyl-2-oxo-2H-1-benzopyran-3-yl]-4-hydroxy-3-(3-methyl-2-butenyl)benzamide.

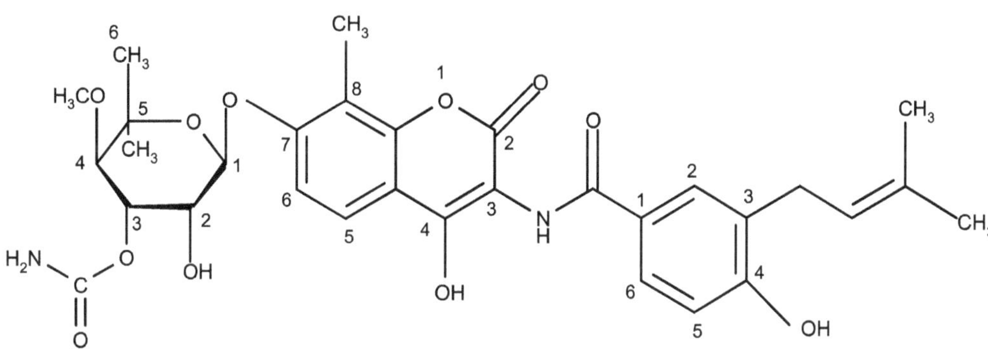

Novobiocin

5. Vancomycin

Vancomycin is (1*S*,2*R*,18*R*,19*R*,22*S*,25*R*,28*R*,40*S*)- 48- {[(2*S*,3*R*,4*S*,5*S*,6*R*)- 3-{[(2*S*,4*S*,5*S*,6*S*)-4-amino-5-hydroxy-4,6-dimethyloxan-2-yl]oxy}-4,5- dihydroxy-6-(hydroxymethyl)oxan-2-yl]oxy}-22-(carbomoylmethyl)-5,15-dichloro-2,18,32,35,37-pentahydroxy-19-[(2R)-4-methyl- 2- (methylamino)petanamido]-20,23,26,42,44-pentaoxo- 7,13- dioxa- 21,24,27,41,43- pentaazaoctacyclo $[26.14.2.2^{3.6}.2^{14.17}.1^{8,12}.1^{29,33}.0^{10,25}.0^{34,39}]$pentaconta-3,5,8(48),9,11,14,16,29(45), 30,32,34,36,38,46,49-pentadecaene- 40- carboxylic acid. Vancomycin is a glycopeptide bactericidal antibiotic obtained by growth of *Streptomyces orientalis*. It acts by inhibiting cell wall synthesis and is effective against gram-positive bacteria. Vancomycin relies heavily on a series of hydrogen bonds between the drug and the D-ala-D-ala side chains of the cell-wall peptidoglycan. It is mainly used to treat pseudomembraneous colitis and multiresistant staphylococcal infections.

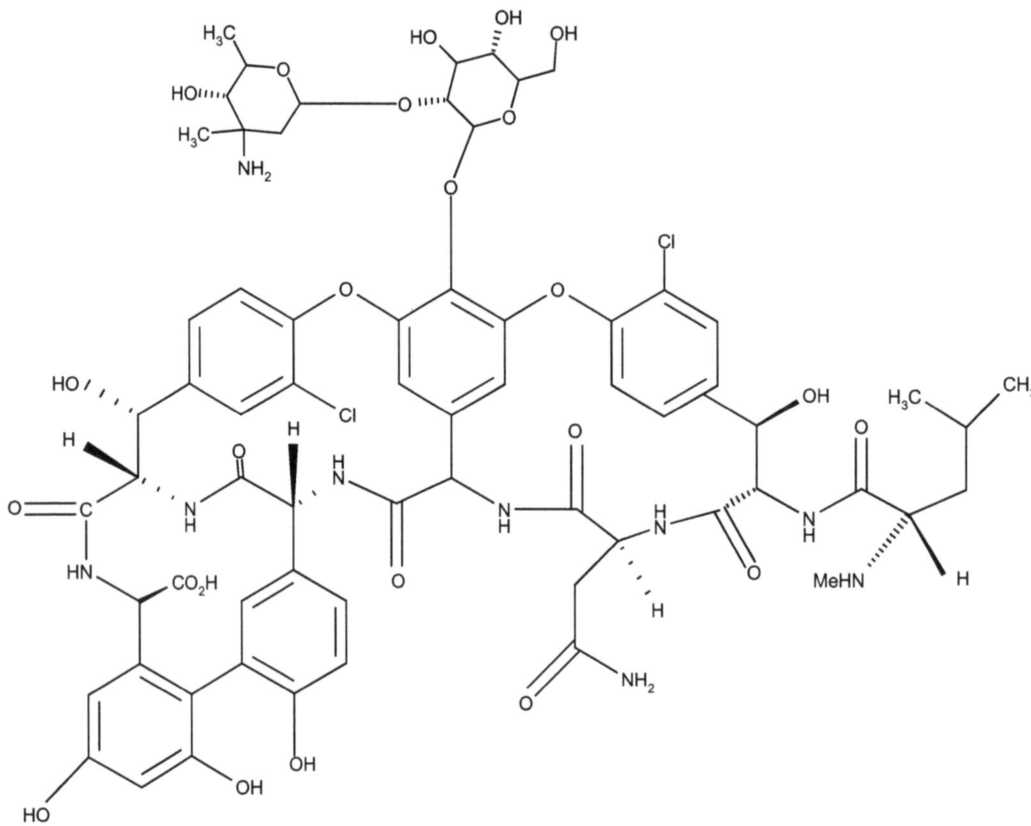

Vancomycin

Vancomycin consists of a complex cyclic peptide as aglycone. The aglycone is glycosidically linked to two sugar residues (Glucose and Vancosamine). It is decomposed in GIT hence it is administered by IV route.

6. Rifamycins

Rifamycins is (2S, 12Z, 14E, 16S, 17S, 18R,19R, 20R, 21S, 22R, 23S, 24E)-5,6,9,17,19-pentahydroxy-23-methoxy-2,4,12,16,18,20,22-heptamethyl-1,11-dioxo-1,2-dihydro-2,7-(epoxypentadecal[1,11,13]trienimino)naphtha[2,1-b]furan-21-yl acetate. Rifamycins are a group of antibiotics produced by *Streptomyces mediterranei*. They were first isolated in 1957 from a fermentation culture of *Streptomyces mediterranei* by Piero Sensi, with the

Israeli scientist Pinhas Margalith. Eventually around seven rifamycins were discovered, named Rifamycin A, B, C, D, E, S and SV. They possess a macrocyclic ring bridge across two nonadjacent positions of an aromatic nucleus. Rifamycins are active against gram positive organisms and some gram-negative organisms and *Mycobacterium tuberculosis* and *Mycobacterium leprae*. They are bactericidal, act by inhibiting nucleic acid synthesis.

E.g.: Rifampicin, rifamycin.

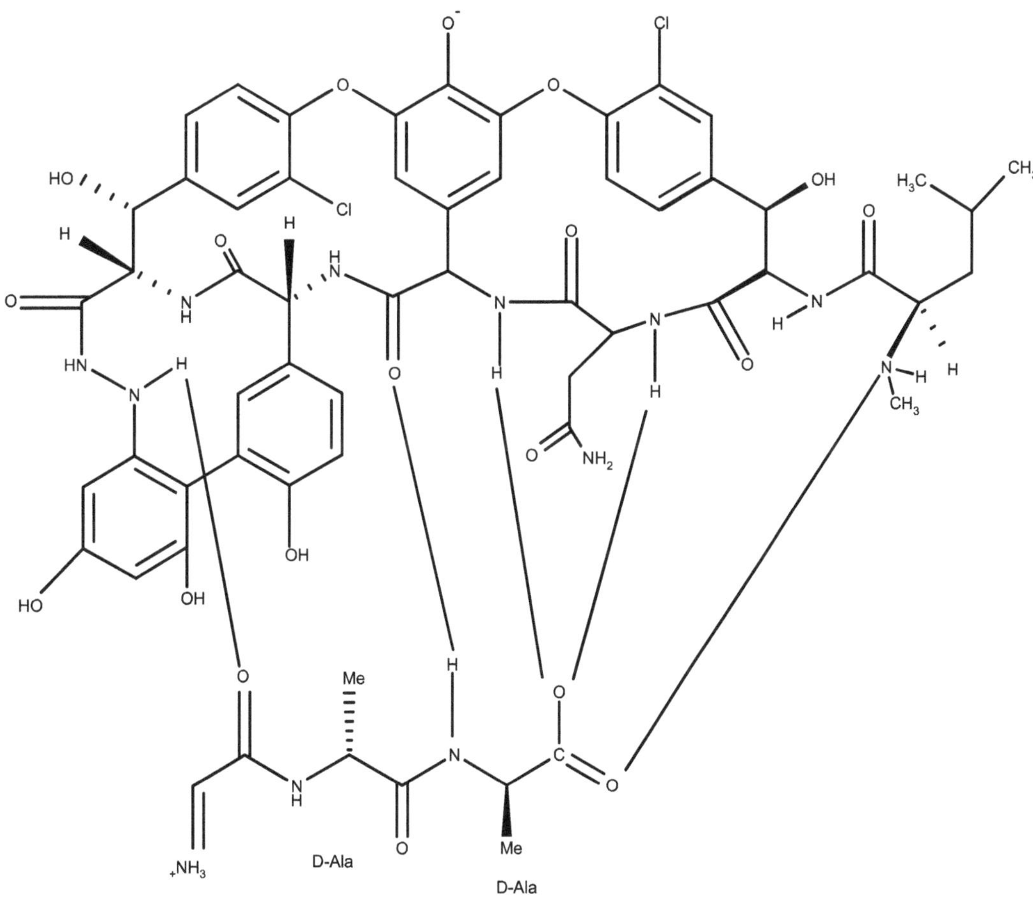

In vancomycin susceptible bacteria

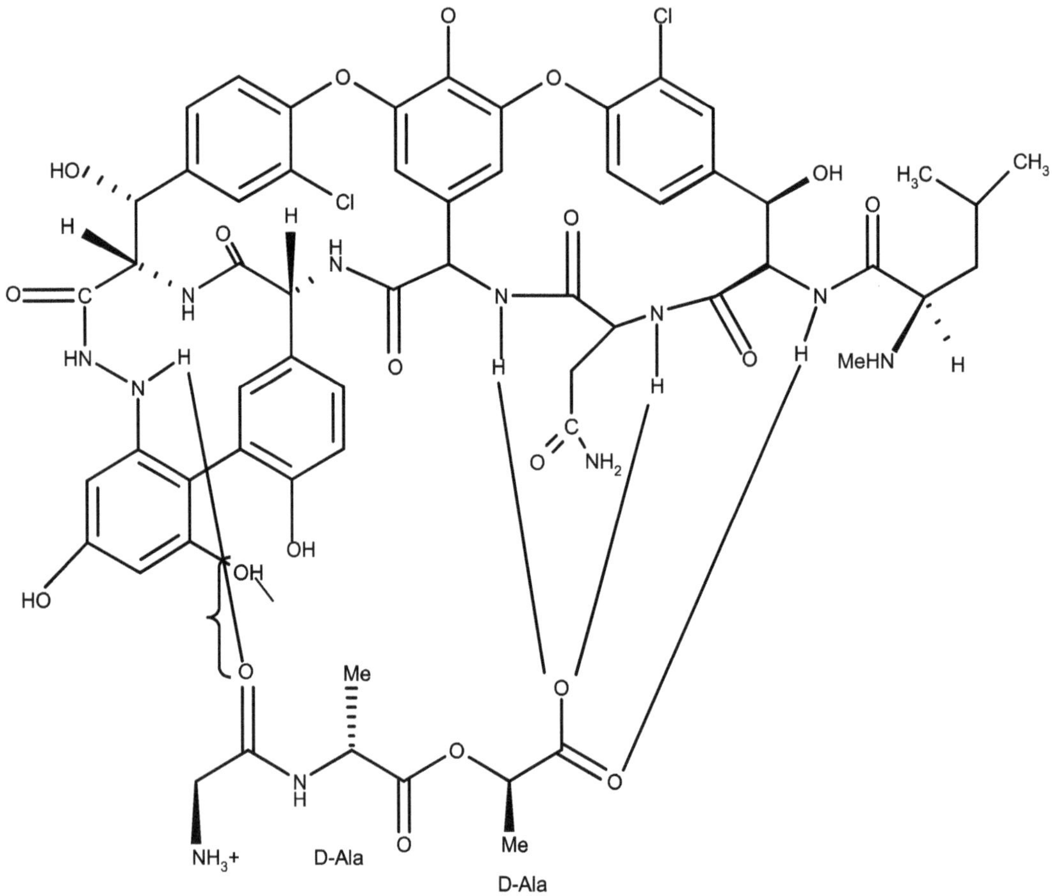

In vancomycin resistant bacteria

Rifamycin B

Rifamycin B is produced by fermentation, and its biosynthesis involves the assembly of a polypeptide by addition of acetate and propionate chain extension units to a unique starter unit, 3-amino-5-hydroxybenzoic acid (AHBA). Of the various rifamycins Rifamycin B was first introduced commercially. Lepetit introduced Rifampicin, an orally active rifamycin, around 1966. Rifabutin, a derivative of rifamycin S, was invented during 1975.

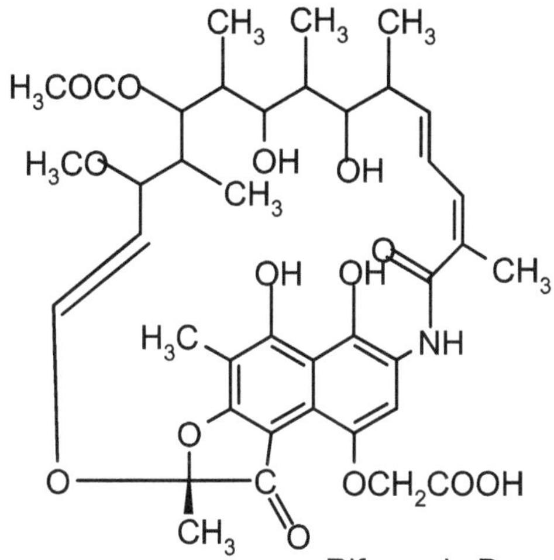

Rifamycin B

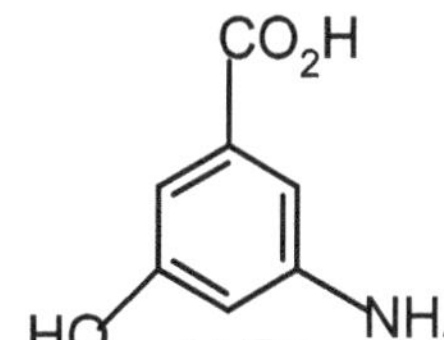

AHBA

Rifampicin or Rifampin

Rifampicin or rifampin is (*7S*,*9E*,*11S*,*12R*,*13S*,*14R*,*15R*,*16R*,*17S*,*18S*,*19E*,*21Z*)-2,15,17,27,29-pentahydroxy-11-methoxy-3,7,12,14,16,18,22-heptamethyl-26-{(E)-[(4- methylpiperazin-1-yl)imino]methyl}-6,23-dioxo-8,30-dioxa-24-azatetracyclo $[23.3.1.1^{4,7}.0^{5,28}]$triaconta-1(28),2,4,9,19,21,25(29),26-octaen-13-yl acetate. Rifampicin or rifampin is a bactericidal antibiotic of rifamycin group. Rifampin is a semisynthetic derivative of rifamycin B, an antibiotic produced by *Streptomyces mediterranei*.

Mechanism of action

Rifampicin affects mainly Gram-positive bacteria. Gram-negative bacteria are much less sensitive to Rifampicin (Gram-negative bacteria possess an outer membrane that is probably too great a barrier for the transport of Rifampicin into the cell). Rifampicin's bactericidal effect is caused by the inhibition of RNA synthesis in bacteria. The antibiotic interacts with RNA polymerase, thus inhibiting the synthesis of long RNA strands. Rifampicin's binding site lies on the β-subunit of the enzyme. The antibiotic, however, does not bind to the isolated subunit but only to the complete holo enzyme. Rifampicin does not interact with eukaryotic RNA polymerases. It is, however, active against RNA polymerases present in chloroplasts and mitochondria. This makes Rifampicin a toxic agent for plant and mammal cells. Resistance to Rifampicin can be built up rapidly and is based on a change in the bacterial RNA polymerases.

Rifampin is a red-brown crystalline powder very slightly soluble in water at neutral pH, freely soluble in chloroform, soluble in ethyl acetate and in methanol. The chemical name for rifampin is: 3-[[(4-Methyl-1-piperazinyl)imino]methyl]rifamycin or 5,6,9,17,19,21 hexahydroxy-23-methoxy-2,4,12,16,20,22-heptamethyl-8-[N-(4-methyl-1 piperazinyl)formi midoyl]-2,7-(epoxypentadeca[1,11,13]trienimino)naphtha [2,1-b] furan-1,11(2H)-dione 21-acetate.

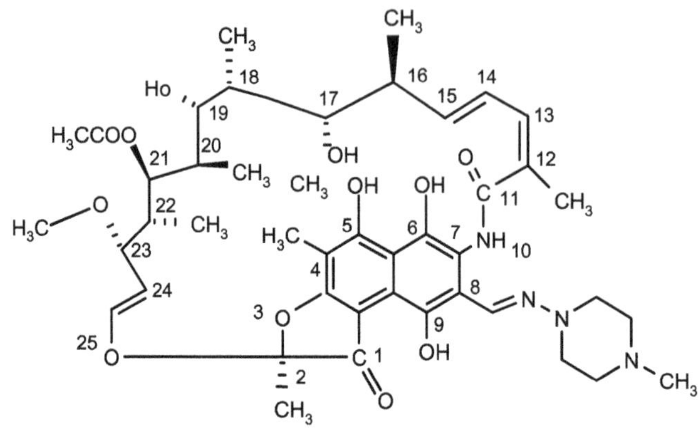

Rifampicin

Uses

It is typically used to treat *Mycobacterium* infections, including tuberculosis and leprosy and also has a role in the treatment of methicillin resistant *Staphylococcus aureus* (MRSA) in combination with fusidic acid. It is used in prophylactic therapy against *Neisseria meningititis* (meningococcal) infection. It is also used to treat *Listeria* species, *Neisseria gonorrhoeae*, *Haemophilus influenzae* and *Legionella pneumophila.*

Rifabutin

Scientists at the Italian drug company Achifar discovered rifabutin in 1975. Rifabutin is an antibiotic primarily used in the treatment of tuberculosis. It is a derivative of rifamycin S. Chemically it is 1',4-didehydro-1-deoxy-1,4-dihydro-5'-(2-methylpropyl)-1-oxorifamycin or (9 S , 12 E , 14 S , 15 R , 16 S , 17 R , 18 R , 19 R , 20 S , 21 S , 22 E , 24 Z)-6,16,18,20-tetrahydroxy-1'-isobutyl-14-methoxy-7,9,15,17,19,21,25-heptamethyl-spiro[9,4-(epoxypentadeca [1,11,13]trienimino)-2 H -furo[2',3':7,8]naphth[1,2- d]imidazole-2, 4'-piperidine]-5,10,26-(3 H ,9 H)-trione-16-acetate.

Rifabutin is a red-violet powder soluble in chloroform and methanol, sparingly soluble in ethanol, and very slightly soluble in water (0.19 mg/ml). Its log P value (between octanol and water) is 3.2. Its chemical structure is:

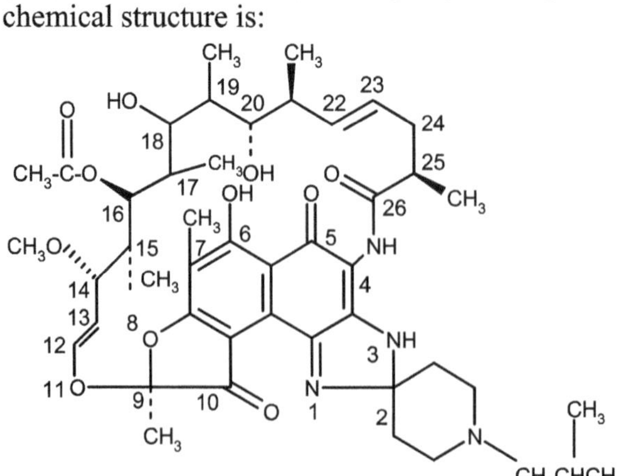

Rifabutin

Rifabutin is well absorbed when taken orally and is distributed widely in body tissues and fluids, including the CSF. It is metabolized in the liver and eliminated in bile and, to a much lesser extent, in urine, but dose adjustments are unnecessary with renal insufficiency. Rifabutin is readily absorbed from the gastrointestinal tract, with an absolute bioavailability averaging 20%.

Rifabutin inhibits DNA-dependent RNA polymerase activity in susceptible cells. Specifically, it interacts with bacterial RNA polymerase but does not inhibit the mammalian enzyme. It is bactericidal and has a very broad spectrum of activity against most Gram-positive and gram-negative organisms (including *Pseudomonas aeruginosa*) and specifically *Mycobacterium tuberculosis*. It is used in the treatment of *Mycobacterium avium* complex disease, a most commonly AIDS related bacterial infection.

Chloramphenicol

Chloramphenicol is 2,2-dichloro-N-[1,3-dihydroxy-1-(4-nitrophenyl)propan-2-yl]acetamide. Chloramphenicol was isolated from a soil sample from *Streptomyces venezuelae*. It contains a nitro benzene moiety and is considered as a derivative of dichloro acetic acid. It is prepared by the following steps:

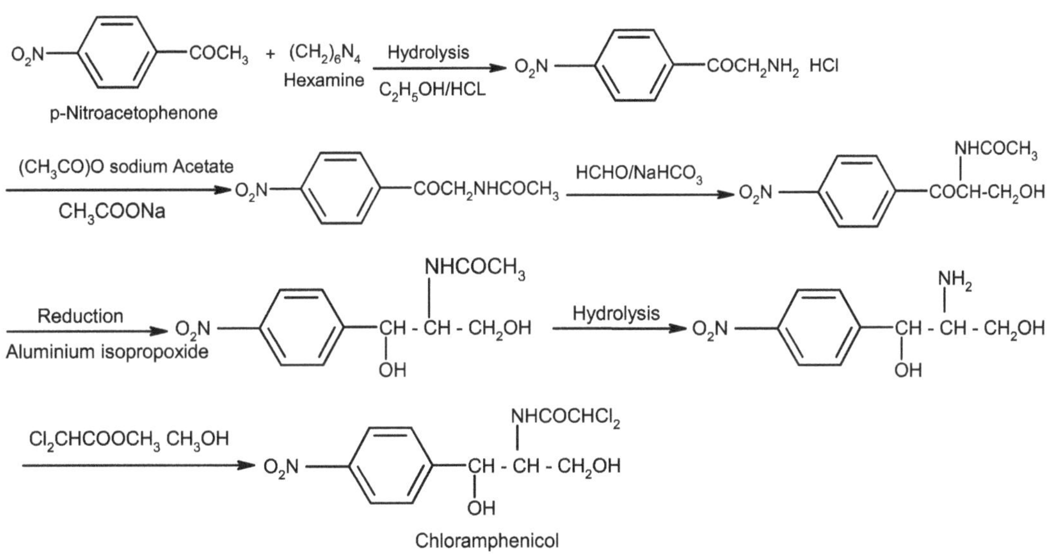

Chloramphenicol

SAR

1. Replacement (or) any modifications of the nitro group leads to reduction in activity.
2. Replacement of phenyl group with aryl groups shown similar activity but with alicyclic groups resulted in loss of activity.
3. The difluoro acetamide shown greater activity yet only shorter duration of time.

4. The primary alcohol group is essential for activity any alteration resulted in decrease in activity.
5. It has two chiral centers which can form four isomers, of which D(-) threoisomer is biologically active.

Mechanism of action

Chloramphenicol is bacteriostatic broad spectrum antibiotic. It binds to p-site of 50S ribosomal subunit of susceptible bacteria and prevents bacterial protein synthesis. It acts against both gram-positive and gram-negative organisms. It can cross the blood brain barrier and parental barrier.

Properties

It occurs as needles (or) elongated plates having a melting point of 157.5°C. It is very soluble in methanol, ethanol, butanol, ethyl acetate, acetone. Fairly soluble in ether. insoluble in benzene, petroleum ether and vegetable oils.

Uses

Chloramphenicol has a broad spectrum of activity against both aerobic and anaerobic gram-negative and gram-positive bacteria. But it is now infrequently used because of its toxicity (aplastic anaemia). It is used to treat serious infections due to organisms resistant to others antibiotics (or) when its penetration into the site of infection is clinically superior to other antibiotics. Those bacteria sensitive to this include *Clostridium*, *Chlamydia*, *Mycoplasma* and *Salmonella*.

14

URINARY ANTISEPTICS

The urinary tract consists of the kidneys, bladder, ureters and urethra. The kidneys produce urine by removing waste and water from the blood. The urine travels down the ureters and is stored in the bladder before being excreted through the urethra. Normal urine contains no bacteria, but germs may be introduced from the skin of the genital area. These bacteria can travel up the urethra into the bladder. When this happens, inflammation of the bladder can occur. Urinary tract infections (UTI's) are common, especially among women. Urinary tract infection is the second most common infection after respiratory tract infection. There are different types of UTI's. Most UTI's are restricted to the bladder and do not involve the kidneys. Bladder inflammations (cystitis) are usually very uncomfortable as they cause burning and stinging when passing urine. Kidney inflammation (pyelonephritis) is less common and more serious.

The agents of urinary tract infections

Majority of urinary tract infections are caused by *Escherichia coli*. Other organisms which cause urinary infections are *Staphylococcus faecalis*, *Staphylococcus aureus*, *Proteus mirabilis, Klebsiella pneumoniae, Pseudomonas aeruginosa*.

Signs and symptoms

- Pain or burning when urinating
- The need to urinate more often than usual
- A feeling of urgency when you urinate
- Blood or pus in the urine
- Cramps or pain in the lower abdomen
- Chills or fever (fever may be the only symptom in infants and children)
- Strong-smelling urine
- Pain during sexual intercourse

Drugs for urinary tract infections

Urinary tract infections are usually treated with the follwing classes of drugs:

I. Quinolones :

(i) Non-fluorinated quinolones: Nalidixic acid

(ii) Fluorinated quinolones: Ciprofloxacin, norfloxacin, enoxacin, gatifloxacin, pefloxacin, sparfloxacin, levofloxacin etc.

II. Antibiotics : Cephalosporins, ampicillin, carbenicillin, streptomycin

III. Sulphonamides : Sulphamethoxzole

IV. Pyrmidines : Trimethoprim

V. Miscellaneous drugs : Methenamine, nitrofurantoin

Quinolones

The discovery of nalidixic acid (1,8-naphthyridine) in 1960s began the steady advancement of the development of quinolones. They are generally used to treat urinary tract infections. The following fluoroquinolones are widely used as urinary antiseptics:

1. First generation: These molecules include norfloxacin, pefloxacin, ofloxacin and ciprofloxacin and showed increased gram-negative activity.
2. Second generation: Temafloxacin, sparfloxacin, grepafloxacin. These agents showed an increase in gram-positive activity.
3. Third generation: Clinifloxacin, trovafloxacin, moxifloxacin. These agents showed an increase in anaerobic activity.

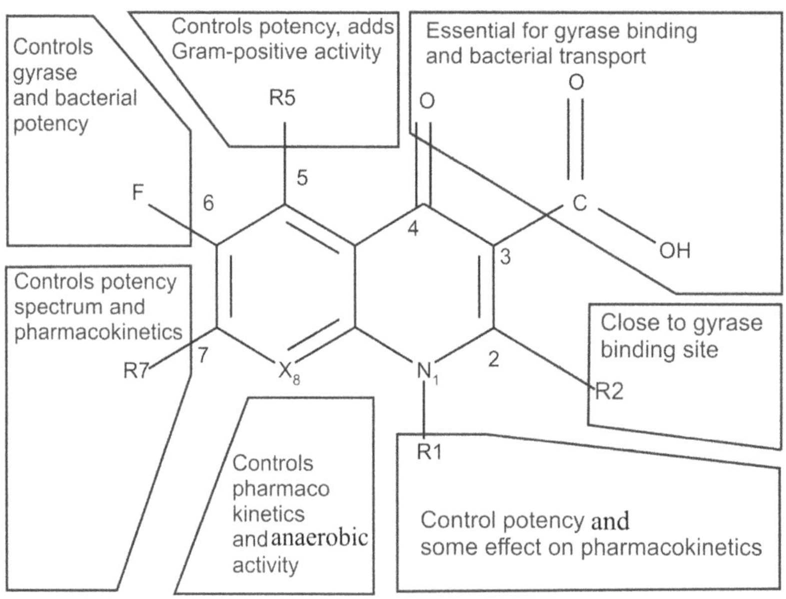

Figure14.1 Structure of quinolone and naphthyridone molecule. In molecules where X is a carbon atom, the molecule is a quinolone (cinoxacin, norfloxacin, ofloxacin, ciprofloxacin, temafloxacin, sparfloxacin, grepafloxacin, levofloxacin, clinafloxacin, moxifloxacin, gatifloxacin). Where X is a nitrogen atom, the molecule is a naphthyridone (nalidixic acid, enoxacin, tosufloxacin, trovafloxacin, gemifloxacin).

Mechanism of action

Two bacterial enzymes (DNA gyrase and topoisomerase IV) were identified as sites for antibacterial activity of quinolones. These enzymes are responsible for unwinding and supercoiling of DNA in bacteria prior to replication. They enter the cell by passive diffusion mechanism through water filled protein channels. They inhibit the replication of bacterial DNA by interfering with the action of DNA gyrase (Topoisomerase II) during bacterial DNA. Fluoro quinolones are active against-*Pseudomonas aeruginosa, rickettsias, plasmodium falciparum, Haemophilus, Neisseria, Mycoplasma, Chlamydia, Staphylococci* and a few of the *Streptococci.*

Nalidixic Acid

Nalidixic acid is a non-fluorinated quinolone derivative. It is primarily reserved for oral treatment of uncomplicated urinary tract infections caused by susceptible microorganisms such as *Escherichia coli.* It is active against gram-negative bacteria; uses for urinary tract infections (unpleasant side effects; poor pharmacokinetic profile; resistance developed quickly). Chemically it is 1-ethyl-1,4-dihydro-7-methyl-4-oxo-1,8-naphthyridine-3-carboxylic acid.

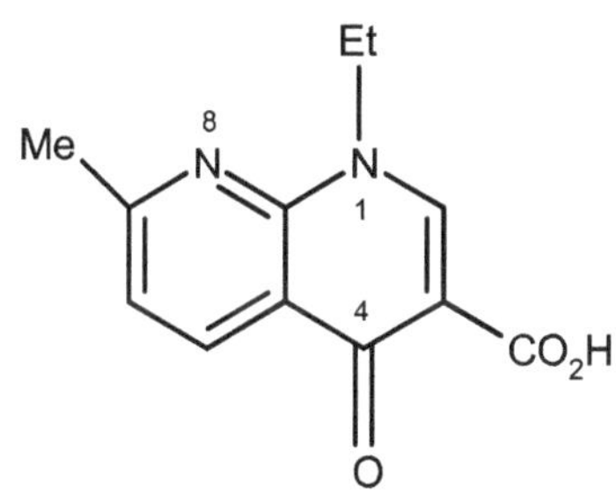

Nalidixic acid

Nalidixic acid is available as pale buff, crystalline powder having a melting point of 229°C. It is soluble in chloroform, toluene, methanol, ethanol, water and ether. It is synthesized by the following scheme:

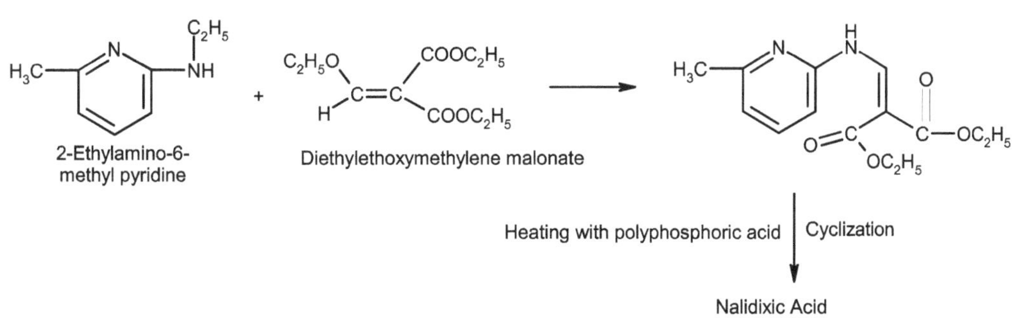

Nalidixic acid is primarily reserved for oral treatment of uncomplicated urinary tract infections caused by susceptible microorganisms such as *Escherichia coli, Enterobacter aerogenes, Klebsiella* species and *Proteus* species.

Norfloxacin

Chemically norfloxacin is 1-ethyl-6-fluoro-1,4-dihydro-4-oxo-7-(1-piperazinyl)-3-quinolinecarboxylic acid. It occurs as white to light yellow crystalline powder and it is soluble in water, methanol, ethanol and acetone. The solubility of norfloxacin in water is pH dependent, increasing sharply at pH < 5 or at pH > 10. It is photosensitive hence it should be protected from light. It is used to treat gonorrhea.

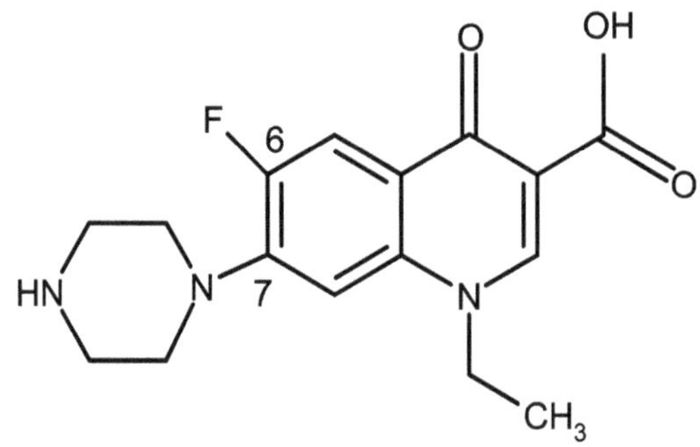

Norfloxacin

Ciprofloxacin

It is 1-cyclopropyl-6-fluoro-1,4-dihydro-4-oxo-7-(1-piperazinyl)-3-quinolinecarboxylic acid. It is light yellow crystalline powder having a melting point of 320°C. It is practically insoluble in water. Ciprofloxacin is available as ciprofloxacin HCl salt that is soluble in water. Ciprofloxacin is a potent drug with a broad spectrum of activity. It is effective against a wide variety of certain infections caused by bacteria, such as bone, joint, skin, ear, and urinary tract infections, pneumonia and other respiratory tract infections, gonorrhea, infectious diarrhea, typhoid fever, and inhalation anthrax.

It is synthesized by the following scheme:

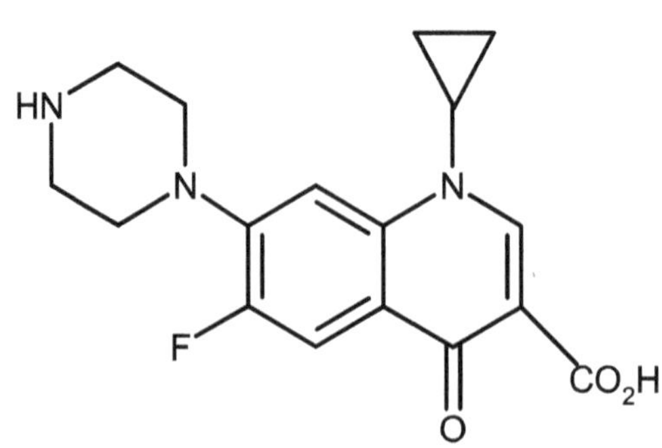

Ciproflozacin

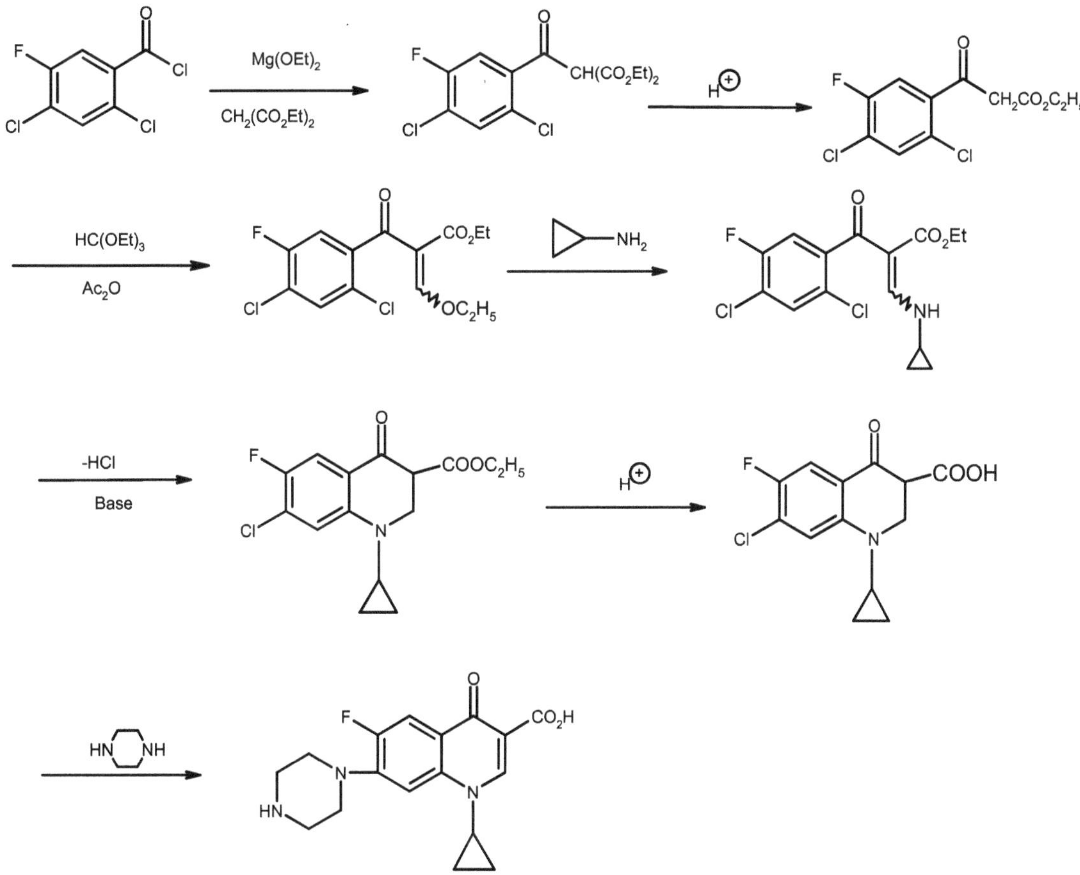

Ciprofloxacin

Enoxacin

Enoxacin is 1-ethyl-6-fluoro-1,4-dihydro-4-oxo-7-(1-piperazinyl)-1,8-naphthydrine-3-carboxylic acid. It is a 1,8-naphthydrine congener (isostere) of norfloxacin. Enoxacin occurs as crystals from ethanol having a melting point of 224°C.

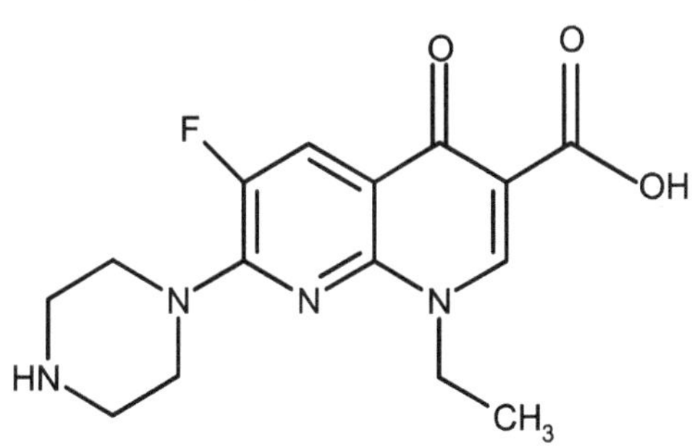

Enoxacin

Uses

It is used as an antibacterial in the treatment of urinary tract infections.

Ofloxacin

It is a quinolone derivative that has an oxazine ring bridged between 1 and 8 positions. It is a broad spectrum fluorinated quinolone. It is 9-fluoro-2,3-dihydro-3-methyl-10-(4-methyl-1-piperazinyl)-7-oxo-7H-pyrido[1,2,3-d,e]-1,4-benzoxazine-6-carboxylic acid. It is available as colorless needles having a melting point of 257°C. Ofloxacin is well absorbed from GIT.

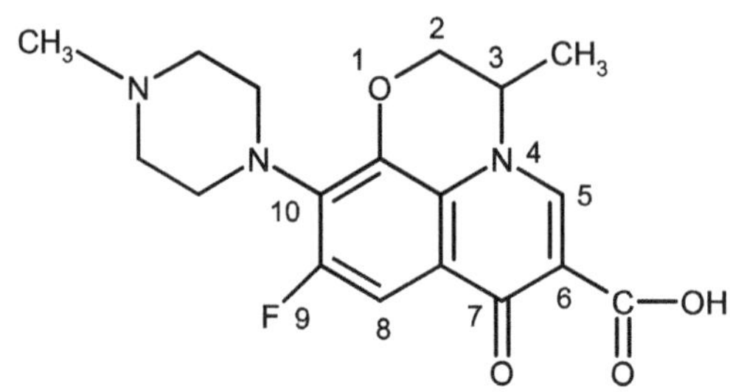

Ofloxacin

Uses

It works by inhibiting bacterial DNA-gyrase, which is involved in the production of genetic material (DNA). This therefore prevents the bacteria from reproducing and their growth is stopped. Ofloxacin is used to treat various bacterial infections such as bronchitis, pneumonia, chlamydia, gonorrhea, skin infections, urinary tract infections, and infections of the prostate. Ofloxacin is an alternative to ciprofloxacin used when there are contraindications to the use of ciprofloxacin itself. Penicillinase has no effect on the activity of ofloxacin. It is widely distributed to body fluids.

Enrofloxacin

Enrofloxacin is 1-cyclopropyl-7-(4-ethyl-1-piperazinyl)-6-fluoro-1,4-dihydro-4-oxo-3-quinolonecarboxylic acid. Enrofloxacin is a synthetic 6-fluoroquinolone used to treat a variety of infections, including skin infections, urinary tract infections, respiratory infections and wound infections caused by susceptible bacteria. Enrofloxacin is not effective for treating infections caused by viruses, parasites or molds. Its activity is concentration dependent. The mechanism of action is to inhibit bacterial DNA-gyrase, prevent DNA supercoiling and synthesis. It has activity against some gram-positive aerobes and a wide range of gram-negative bacilli and cocci, which include *Klebsiella*, *Pseudomonas*, *Salmonella*, and other organisms such as *Mycoplasma*, *Staphylococci* and *Chlamydia*.

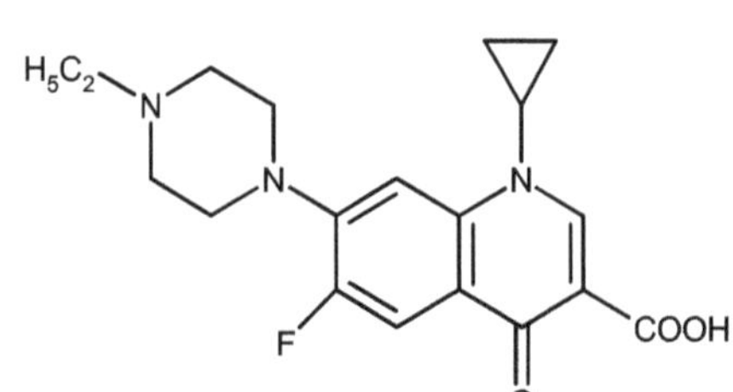

Enrofloxacin

Coplanar carbonyl groups (C = O) at positions 3 and 4 of the core structure are generally required for antimicrobial activity of the fluoroquinolones. They represent the binding site to the DNA gyrase complex. A fluorine atom, introduced at position 6, enhances the efficacy against gram-negatives and broadens the spectrum against gram-positive bacteria. The piperazine ring at position 7 further increases antimicrobial activity, especially against Pseudomonas organisms. The presence of a C_2H_5 group attached to the piperazine ring enhances tissue penetration and decreases central nervous system toxicity by reducing drug binding to GABA receptors in the brain. Due to the presence of carboxylic acid and one or more amine functional groups (basic), the molecule has amphoteric and zwitterionic properties. Thus, between pK_a of the acidic and basic functional groups, the substance is lipid soluble and able to penetrate tissues, pus and organic debris.

Enrofloxacin is a pale yellow, crystalline substance with a high degree of purity. In water at pH 7, it is slightly soluble. However, as it contains acidic and basic groups (betaine structure), it can readily be brought into solution when the pH values are either alkaline or acidic. Liquid formulations of baytril for parenteral administration contain freely soluble salts of enrofloxacin in an aqueous solution. Due to the high hydrolytic stability of the active ingredient, these solutions are very stable. The tablet formulations contain enrofloxacin in its original betaine form.

Gatifloxacin

Gatifloxacin is (±)-1-cyclopropyl-6-fluoro-1,4-dihydro-8-methoxy-7-(3-methyl-1-piperazinyl)-4-oxo-3-quinolinecarboxylic acid; It is a third generation quinolone antibiotic. This drug has been used to treat uncomplicated urinary tract infections, complicated urinary tract infections, pyelonephritis, sexually transmitted diseases, prostatitis, skin and tissue infections, urethral and cervical gonococcal infections, acute exacerbations of chronic bronchitis and community-acquired pneumonia. The antibacterial action of gatifloxacin results from inhibition of DNA gyrase and topoisomerase IV. DNA gyrase is an essential enzyme that is involved in the replication, transcription, and repair of bacterial DNA.

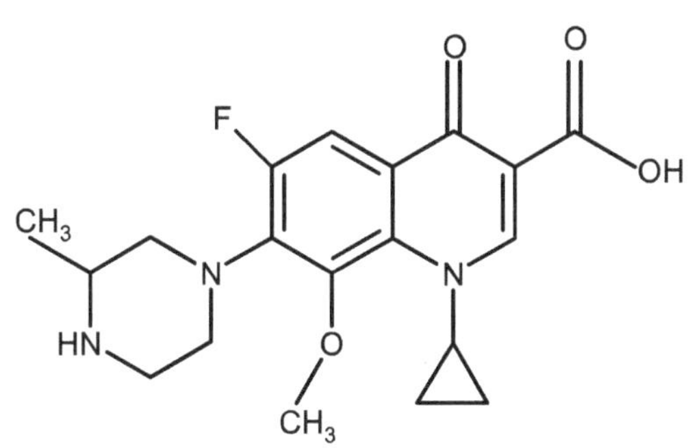

Gatifloxacin

Gatifloxacin pharmacokinetics are linear and time-independent at doses ranging from 200 to 800 mg administered over a period of up to 14 days. Steady-state concentrations are achieved by the third daily oral or intravenous dose of gatifloxacin.

Gemifloxacin

Gemifloxacin 7-[4Z)-3-(aminomethyl)- 4-methoxyimino-pyrrolidin-1-yl]- 1-cyclopropyl-6-fluoro-4-oxo- 1,8-naphthyridine-3-carboxylic acid. Gemifloxacin is a third generation quinolone antibiotic. Gemifloxacin (licensed from LG Chemical), currently in phase III trials worldwide, reported to have activity *against Streptococcus pneumoniae; Haemophilus influenzae; Moraxella catarrhalis* and *Acinetobacter*. It is used to treat uncomplicated urinary tract infections, complicated urinary tract infections, pyelonephritis, sexually transmitted diseases, prostatitis, skin and tissue infections, urethral and cervical gonococcal infections, acute exacerbations of chronic bronchitis and community-acquired pneumonia.

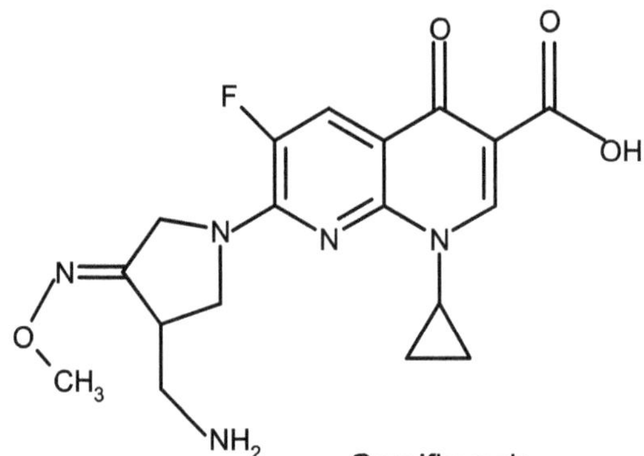

Gemifloxacin

Pefloxacin

Pefloxacin is 1-ethyl-6-fluro-7- (4-methylpiperazin-1-yl)- 4-oxo-quinoline-3-carboxylic acid. Pefloxacin is a third generation quinolone antibiotic. It is used to treat uncomplicated urinary tract infections, complicated urinary tract infections, pyelonephritis, sexually transmitted diseases, prostatitis, skin and tissue infections, urethral and cervical gonococcal infections, acute exacerbations of chronic bronchitis and community-acquired pneumonia.

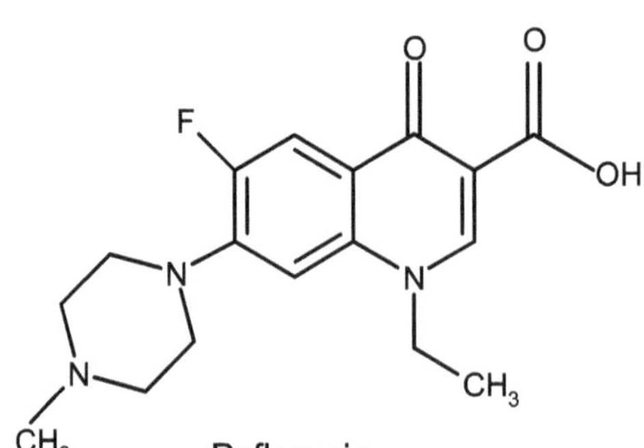

Pefloxacin

Sparfloxacin

Sparfloxacin is 5-amino-1-cyclopropyl-7-(*cis*-3,5-dimethyl-1-piperazinyl)-6,8-difluoro- 1,4-dihydro-4-oxo-3- quinoline carboxylic acid. It is a third generation quinolone antibiotic.

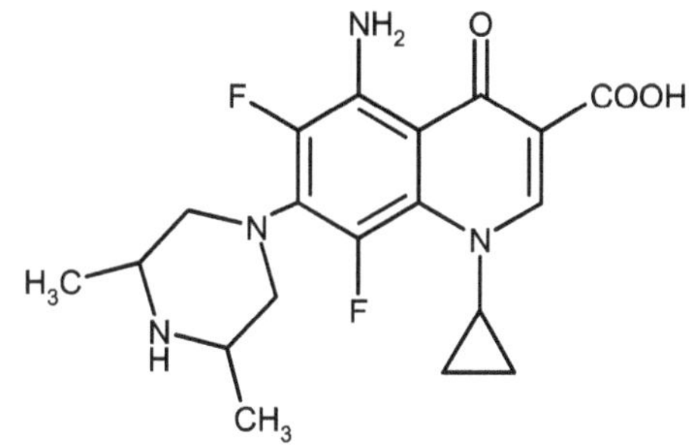

Spanflonacin

Grepafloxacin

Grepafloxacin is (*RS*)-1-cyclopropyl-6-fluro-5-methyl-7-(3-methylpinperazin-1yl]-4-oxo-quinoline-3-carboxylic acid. Grepafloxacin is a fourth generation quinolone antibiotics. It is used to treat the first, second and third-generation intra-abdominal infections, excluding complicated urinary tract infections, excluding pyelonephritis, nosocomial pneumonia, gynecologic and pelvic infections.

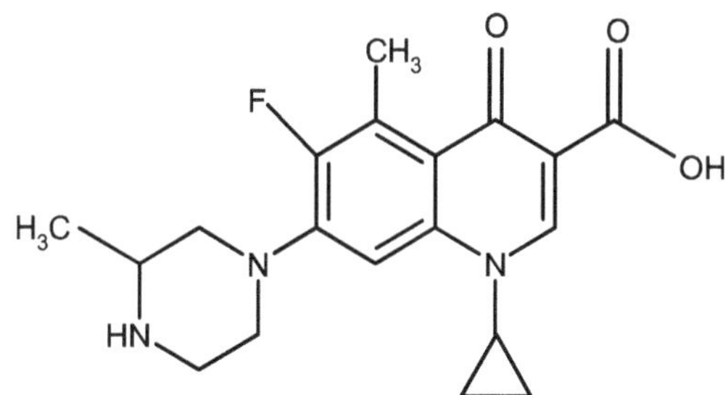

Grepafloxacin

Levofloxacin

Levofloxacin is (-)-(S)-9-fluoro-2 ,3-dihydro-3-methyl-10-(4-methyl-1-piperazinyl) -7-oxo-7H-pyrido[1,2,3-de]-1,4-benzoxazine-6-carboxylic acid; (-)-Ofloxacin; It is foruth generation quinolone antibiotics. Levofloxacin, the L- optical isomer (structurally a mirror image) of ofloxacin, has similar activity to ofloxacin in the laboratory and had similar efficacy to the macrolides against respiratory infection with *Chlamydophila pneumoniae*. It is used to treat first, second and third-generation intra- abdominal infections (excluding complicated urinary tract infections, excluding pyelonephritis), nosocomial pneumonia, gynecologic and pelvic infections.

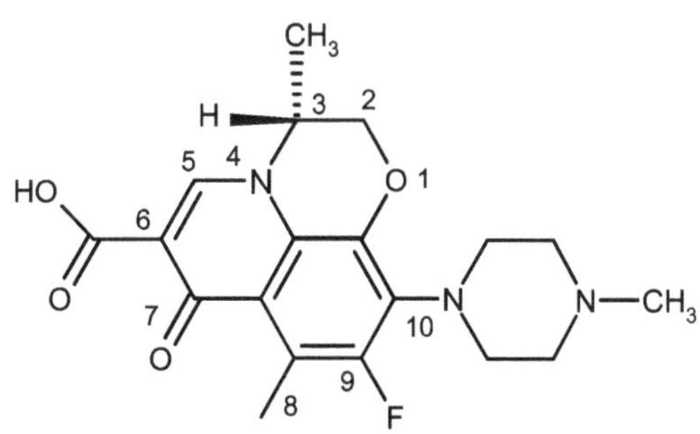

Levofloxacin

Moxifloxacin

Moxifloxacin is 1-cyclopropyl-7-[(S,S)-2,8-diazabicyclo[4.3.0]non-8-yl]-6-fluoro-8-methoxy-1,4-dihydro-4-oxo-3-quinoline carboxylic acid; It is fourth generation quinolone antibiotics. It is used to treat the first, second and third-generation intra- abdominal infections (excluding complicated urinary tract infections, excluding pyelonephritis), nosocomial pneumonia, gynecologic and pelvic infections.

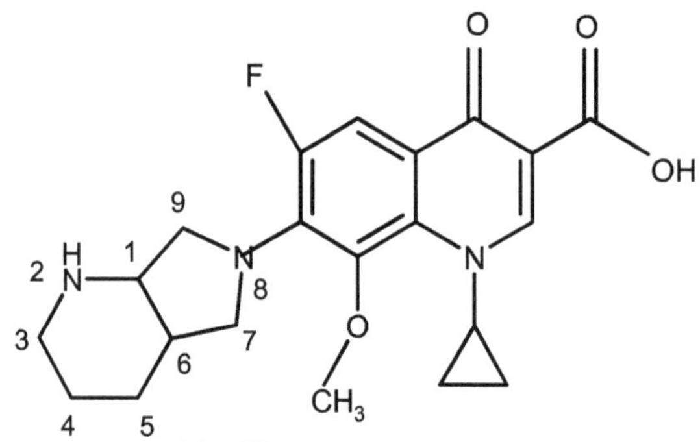

Moxifloxacin

SAR of Fluoroquinolones

1. The trisubstituted nitrogen atom at position 1 is essential to show activity.
2. The substitution of ethyl group at N-1 position showed an optimum activity but the substitution of cyclopropyl and diflurophenyl result in potent compounds.
3. Replacement of N-1 cyclo propyl with oxetane group showed increased activity against gram-positive.
4. Alterations of 3-carboxylic acid group produce compounds with decreased activity. Quinolones bind to DNA gyrase via the carboxy-group at C-3 in quinolone ring.
5. Replacement of 3-carboxylic acids with iso thiazole group produces most potent isothiazolo quinolone.
6. Presence of oxo group at position 4 is essential for activity.
7. Amino group substitution at position 5 gives active compounds.
8. Fluorine group at position 6 is essential for activity.
9. At position 7 piperazine and substituted piperazines give active compounds.
10. Replacement of 8-carbon atom with nitrogen atom resulted in active compounds.
11. Drugs that have 6-flouro, 7-piperazinyl groups show the most extended spectrum of activity including pseudomonas.

15

ANTI-TUBERCULAR DRUGS

Introduction

Tuberculosis (often called TB) is an infectious disease that usually attacks the lungs, but can also affect the central nervous system (meningitis), lymphatic system, circulatory system (Miliary tuberculosis), genitourinary system, bones and joints. Tuberculosis is one of the most deadly and major infectious diseases today, infecting two billion people, or approximately one-third (WHO TB) of the world's population. Tuberculosis spread from person to person through the air.

When people with TB in their lungs or throat cough, laugh, sneeze, sing, or even talk, the germs that cause TB may be spread into the air. If another person breathes in these germs there is a chance that they will become infected with tuberculosis.

Symptoms of TB

A person with TB disease may have any, all or none of the following symptoms:

- An unproductive cough
- Feeling tired all the time
- Weight loss and gradual loss of functions of vital organs
- Loss of appetite
- Fever
- Coughing up blood
- Night sweats, tachycardia, cyanosis and respiratory failure.

General Features

Mycobacterium tuberculosis is the organism that is the causative agent for tuberculosis (TB). There are other "atypical" mycobacteria such as *Mycobacterium kansasii* that may produce a similar clinical and pathologic appearance of disease. *Mycobacterium avium-intracellulare* (MAI) seen in immunocompromized hosts (particularly in persons with AIDS) is not primarily a pulmonary infection in terms of its organ distribution (mostly in organs of the mononuclear phagocyte system).

Mycobacterium tuberculosis is not classified as either gram-positive or gram-negative because it does not have the chemical characteristics of either, although the bacteria do contain peptidoglycan (murein) in their cell wall. If a gram stain is performed on *Mycobacterium tuberculosis*, it stains very weakly. *Mycobacterium* species, along with members of a related genus *Nocardia*, are classified as acid-fast bacteria due to their impermeability by certain dyes and stains.

The cell wall structure of *Mycobacterium tuberculosis* deserves special attention because it is unique among procaryotes and it is a major determinant of virulence for the bacterium. The cell wall complex contains peptidoglycan, but otherwise it is composed of complex lipids. Over 60% of the mycobacterial cell wall is lipid. The lipid fraction of mycobacterium cell wall consists of three major components.

Mycolic acids are unique α-branched lipids found in cell walls of *Mycobacterium* and *Corynebacterium.* They make up 50% of the dry weight of the mycobacterial cell envelope. Mycolic acids are strong hydrophobic molecules that form a lipid shell around the organism and affect permeability properties at the cell surface.

How does tuberculosis spread?

The Tuberculosis germ is carried on droplets in the air, and can enter the body through the airway. A person with active pulmonary tuberculosis can spread the disease by coughing or sneezing. The process of catching tuberculosis involves two stages: first, a person has to become infected; second, the infection has to progress to disease. To become infected, a person has to come in close contact with another person having active tuberculosis.

Tuberculosis Treatment

Administration of a single to treat tuberculosis drug often leads to the development of a bacterial resistant to that drug. Therefore effective regimens for the treatment of tuberculosis must contain multiple drugs to which the organisms are susceptible. If two or more drugs are used simultaneously, each helps to prevent the emergence of tubercle bacilli resistant to the others.

Classification

(a) Antitubercular drugs are classified on the basis of efficacy and safety as:

1. **First-Line drugs:** They have high-level efficacy and less toxicity.
   Eg : Isoniazid, rifampicin, pyrazinamide, ethambutol, streptomycin.
2. **Second-line drugs:** These are less tolerated and have higher toxicity.
   Eg : Ethionamide, para aminosalicylic acid, cycloserine, capreomycin, viomycin and thiacetazone.

(b) Antitubercular drugs are also classified on the basis of chemical moiety as:

(i)	Salicylic acid derivatives	:	Para aminosalicylic acid
(ii)	Pyridine derivatives	:	Ethionamide, isonicotinic acid hydrazide
(iii)	Pyrazine derivatives	:	Pyrazinamide
(iv)	Ethylenediaminobutanol derivatives	:	Ethambutol
(v)	Antibiotics	:	Streptomycin, cycloserine, capreomycin, rifampin, kanamycin
(vi)	Miscellaneous	:	(a) Mefloxacin, ciprofloxacin, sparfloxacin, ofloxacin, (b) Clarithromycin, azithromycin

First-Line Drugs
Isoniazid

Synthesis

Isoniazid is isonicotinohydrazide. Isoniazid (isonicotinic acid hydrazide, INH) first synthesized in 1952. It is a first-line synthetic anti-tubercular drug. INH is completely absorbed on oral administration. It is metabolized in the liver largely by acetylation and is excreted in urine.

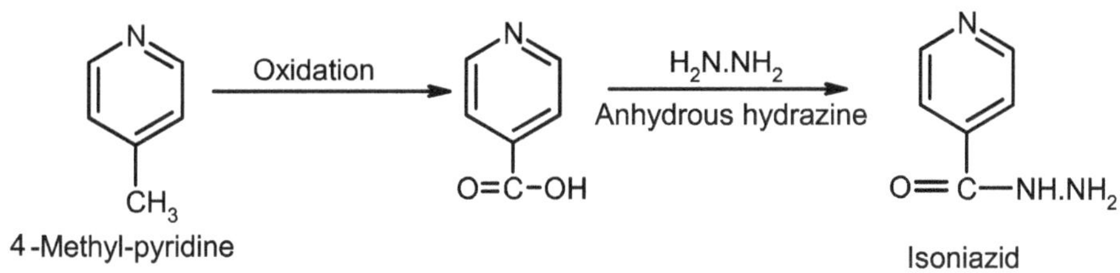

SAR

(a) The N-1 nitrogen in hydrazine side chain should be unsubstituted.

(b) N-2 nitrogen can be substituted with alkyl groups to get active compounds.

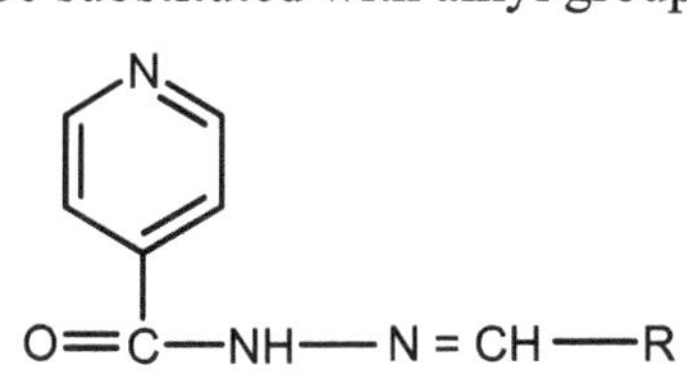

Isoniazid hydrazones

(c) Isonicotinic acid hydrazones are active but they are decomposed to INH in gastric acid pH medium.

Mechanism of action

INH is a prodrug and is activated by oxidation to isonicotinaldehyde, isonicotinic acid and isonicotinamide. The enzyme complex (catalase peroxidase) responsible for oxidation is present in mycobacterium.

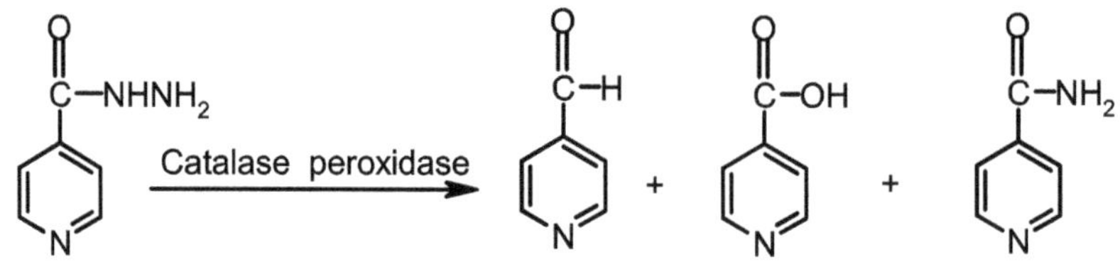

The reactive species generated attack critical enzyme required for mycolic acid synthesis in mycobacterium. The mycolic acids are important constituents of bacterial cell wall.

Properties

These are crystals from alcohol having a melting point of 171°C. It is soluble in water, alcohol, boiling alcohol and chloroform, practically insoluble in ether and benzene.

Uses

(a) Treatment of tuberculosis; usually two or three agents together or alone for prophylaxis of tuberculosis,

(b) Pyridoxine (vitamin B6) is given together with the isoniazid to correct the toxic reactions of INH.

Rifampin

Rifamycins are a group of structurally related complex macrocyclic antibiotics, which are produced by *Streptomyces mediterranei.* Rifampin is a semisynthetic derivative of one of these molecules (rifamycin B). Rifampin is a zwitter ion and is soluble in water at an acidic pH. Oral administration of rifampin produces peak plasma concentration in 2 to 4 hours.

Rifampin is effective against gram-positive bacteria such as *Staphylococcus aureus, Hemophilus influenzae and Neisseria meningitis* and gram-negative bacteria such as *echerichia coli, Proteus, Klebsiella* and *Pseudomonas,* as well as *Mycobacterium*, especially *Mycobacterium tuberculosis, Mycobacterium. kansasii and Mycobacterium fortuitum.*

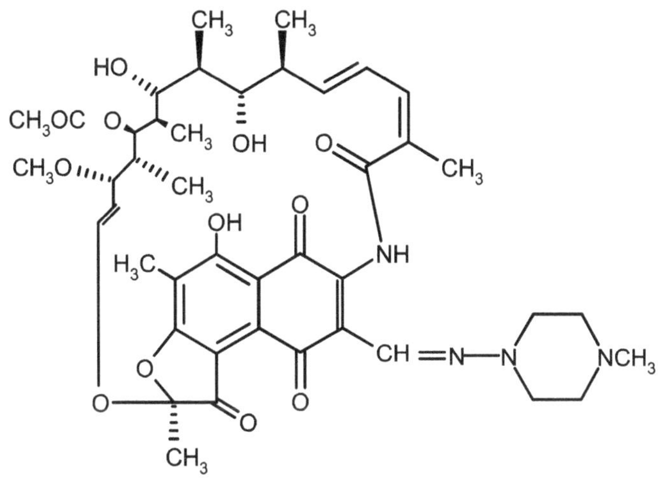

SAR

(a) Intact macrocyclic molecule is required for antimycobacterial activity.

(b) Double bonds in macrocyclic nucleus should not be reduced,

(c) Free hydroxyl groups should be present at C-1, C-8, C-21 and C-23 for good binding to DDRP DNA – dependent RNA polymerase.

Mechanism of action

- Rifampin is bactericidal at 0.005-0.2 μ g/ml vs. *Mycobacterium tuberculosis.*
- Rifamycins inhibit bacillary DNA-dependent RNA polymerase (DDRP) by binding strongly to its β-subunits and there by inhibiting the RNA synthesis. Rifampin is rapidly metabolized by deacetylation to active metabolite.

Uses

(a) In treatment of tuberculosis, together with isoniazid and others.

(b) For prophylaxis in people exposed to meningococcemia or *Haemophilus influenzae* type B meningitis.

(c) In cases of endocarditis or osteomyelitis resistant to other antibiotics.

(d) In leprosy.

Ethambutol

Ethambutol is (+)-2,2'-(ethylenediamino)-di-1-butanol. It has no effect on organisms other than mycobacteria. It is a stereospecific compound. The dextroisomer is 16 times more active than meso compound.

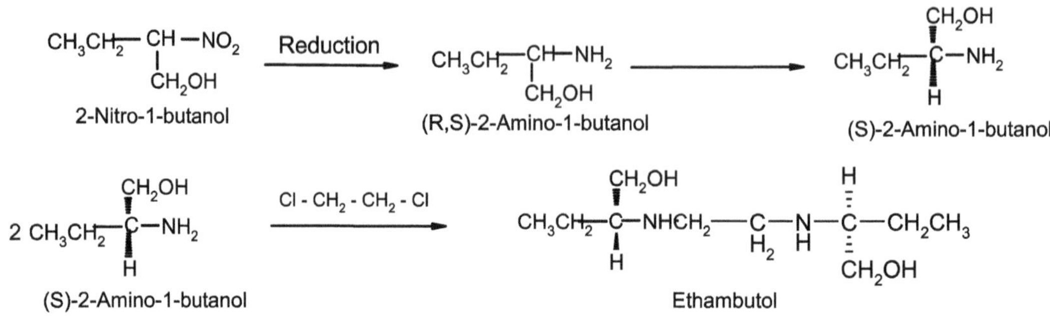

Properties

It has a melting point of 88.8°C. It is soluble in chloroform, methylene chloride, less soluble in benzene, sparingly soluble in water. It is rapidly absorbed by oral route.

Mechanism of action

- It is only active against Mycobacteria. Exact mechanism is not known. It appears to inhibit the mycobacterial cell wall synthesis.
- It inhibits arabinosyl transferase enzyme which is responsible to form outer envelope to cell wall (outer envelop consists of arabinofuranose and galactose units).
- Ethambutol is used in treatment of tuberculosis together with other drugs.

Streptomycin

Streptomycin is 5-(2,4-diguanidino-3,5,6-trihydroxy-cyclohexoxy) -4-[4,5-dihydroxy-6-(hydroxymethyl)-3-methylamino-tetrahydropyran-2-yl] oxy-3-hydroxy-2-methyl-tetrahydrofuran - 3-carbaldehyde. Streptomycin is an amino glycoside antibiotic. The chemistry, mechanism of action is discussed under amino glycoside antibiotics in **Chapter 10.**

Pyrazinamide (Pyrazinecarboxamide)

Pyrazinamide is pyrazine-2-carboxamide. It is synthesized from quinoxaline by oxidation

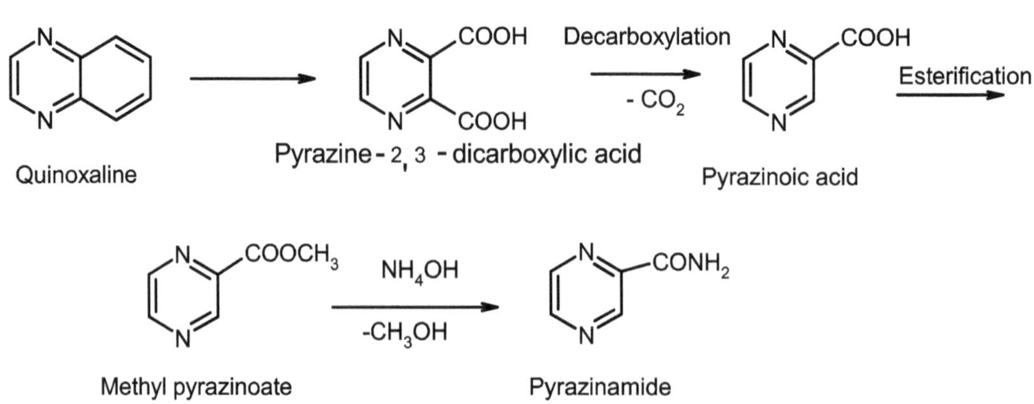

SAR

1. Pyrazinamide is a bioisostere of nicotinamide
2. Pyrazine nucleus should be unsubstituted
3. Pyrazine nucleus should not be replaced by other heterocyclic moieties.

Properties

Pyrazinamide is white crystalline powder. It is sparingly soluble in water.

Mechanism of action

- It is synthesized in 1952. Pyrazinamide (PZA) is the pyrazine analogue of nicotinamide.
- Pyrazinamide is readily absorbed after oral administration.
- Pyrazinamide is a prodrug and is hydrolyzed to active form pyrazinoic acid, intracellularly by pyrazinamidase (mycobacterial enzyme).
- Pyrazinoic acid is highly active. it might function as an antimetabolite of nicotinamide and interfere with the synthesis of NAD.
- Pyrazinamide may be bacteriostatic or bactericidal depending upon concentration.
- Pyrazinamide has potential hepatotoxicity.

Second-line drugs

p-Amino salicylic acid(PAS)

PAS is 4-amino-2-hydroxy-benzoic acid. PAS was first proposed in 1964 by Lehmann to treat tuberculosis. It is synthesized from nitrobenzene by the following chemical reactions:

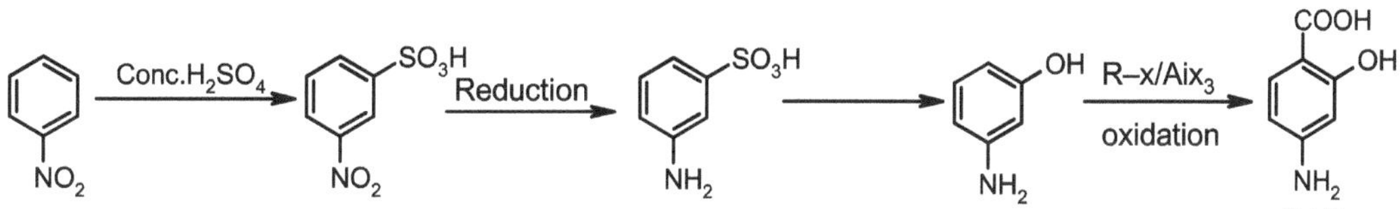

PAS

Properties

PAS exists as minute crystals having a melting point of 157°C. It is slightly soluble in ether, practically insoluble in benzene. It is soluble in dilute nitric acid, dilute sodium hydroxide. The aqueous solution of PAS has a pH of $\simeq$ 3.2.

Mechanism of action

PAS act as an antimetabolite and interfere with the incorporation of PABA into folic acid.

Uses

PAS is administered orally in the form of sodium salt. PAS is bacteriostatic against *Mycobacterium tuberculosis.* It is administered with INH to reduce acetylation of INH thus increases plasma levels of INH.

Ethionamide

It is a pyridine analogue used to treat tuberculosis. Chemically ethionamide is 2-ethylpyridine-4-carbothioamide.

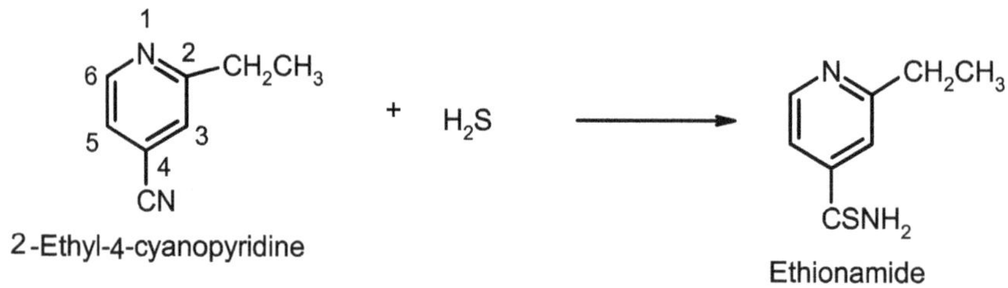

Properties

Ethionamide exists as minute yellow crystals having a melting point of 164°C. It is very sparingly soluble in water, ether, sparingly soluble in methanol, ethanol and propylene glycol. It is soluble in hot acetone, dichloroethane and freely soluble in pyridine.

Mechanism of action

Ethionamide is a prodrug which is oxidized to active acylating agent (ethionamide sulphoxide) by catalase peroxidase (by oxidation). The ethionamide sulphoxide inactivates reductase enzyme, which is responsible for synthesis of NAD^+ from NADH.

Uses

It is used in the treatment of tuberculosis in combination with other antitubercular drugs.

Antibiotics

Cycloserine

It is an antitubercular antibiotic obtained from *Streptomyces orchidaceus in 1955.*

Structure

Cycloserine is a chemical analogue of D-alanine and possess a chiral center with R-configuration. It is D-(+)-4-amino-3-isoxazolidinone.

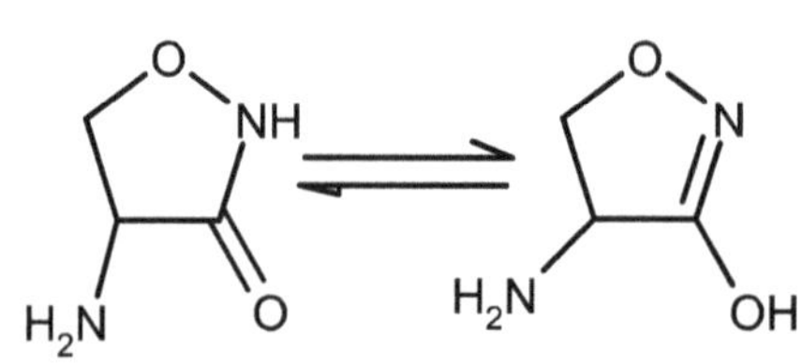

Mechanism of action

Cycloserine acts by inhibiting the enzyme alanine racemase, D-alanine ligase and thereby interferes with the incorporation of D-alanine into the mucopeptides of the bacterial cell wall (D-alanine is the important constitutent of mycobacterial cell wall).

Properties

Cycloserine available as colorless crystals which decompose at 155°C. It is soluble in water slightly soluble in methanol, propylene glycol.

Uses

It is used as tuberculostatic drug.

Capreomycin

Capreomycin is (3S)-3,6-diamino-N-[[2S,5S,8E,11S,15S)-15-amino-11-[(4R)-2-amino-3,4,5,6-tetrahydropyrimidin-4-yl]-8-[(carbamoylamino)methylidene]-2-(hydroxymethyl)-3,6,9,12,16-pentaoxo-1,4,7,10,13- pentazacyclohexadec-5-yl]methyl]hexanamide; (3S)-3,6-diamino-N-[[(2*S*,5*S*,8*E*,11*S*,15*S*)-15-amino-11-[(4*R*)-2-amino-3,4,5,6- tetrahydropyrimidin-4-yl]-8-[(carbamoylamino)methylidene]-2-methyl-3,6,9,12,16-pentaoxo-1,4,7,10,13-pentazacyclohexadec-5-yl] methyl]hexanamide. Capreomycin is cyclic peptide antibiotic similar to viomycin produced by *Streptomyces capreolus*. Capreomycin resembles in structure to viomycin. It is a second line anti-tubercular drug used in combination with other drugs. It is a highly toxic drug (damage to eighth cranial nerve and renal damage).

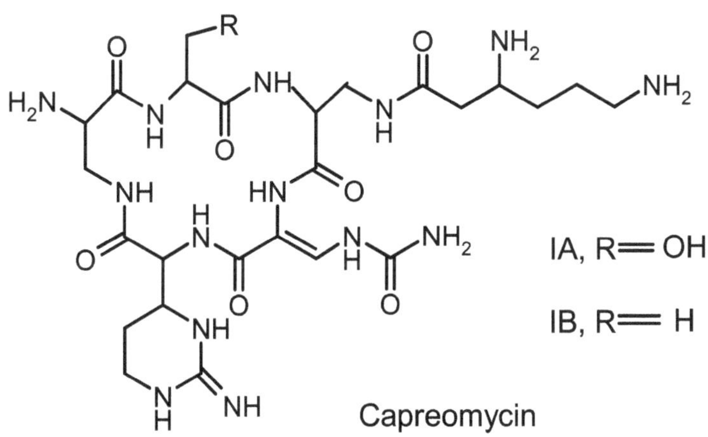

IA, R═OH

IB, R═H

Capreomycin

Capreomycin is a white solid which is soluble in water. Practically insoluble in most organic solvents.

Drugs for the treatment of *Mycobacterium avium* complex (MAC)

Mycobacterial infections caused by organisms like *Mycobacterium avium, Mycobacterium intracellulare, Mycobacterium kansasii, Mycobacterium murinum, Mycobacterium serofulaceum* are commonly termed as *Mycobacterium avium* complex (MAC). MAC is limited to infection of lungs in non-HIV infected individuals (healthy persons). MAC is resistant to many of the commonly used antitubercular drugs. The following drugs are used to treat MAC:

1. MAC infection is common in AIDS patient where it is a disseminated disease. In patients without AIDS, it is usually restricted to the lungs.
2. Like tuberculosis, the use of one drug increases resistance and so the regiments are 2, 3 or 4 drugs.
3. The basic regimen is ethambutol with either clarithromycin or azithromycin.
4. Prophylaxis with rifabutin for life is recommended for AIDS patients with CD4 count less than 100 cells/mm^3.

Rifabutin

Rifabutin is similar to rifampicin in structure and mechanism of action. However it is less effective against *Mycobacterium tuberculosis* and more effective against MAC. It is used in combination with clarithromycin and ethambutol for MAC infection.

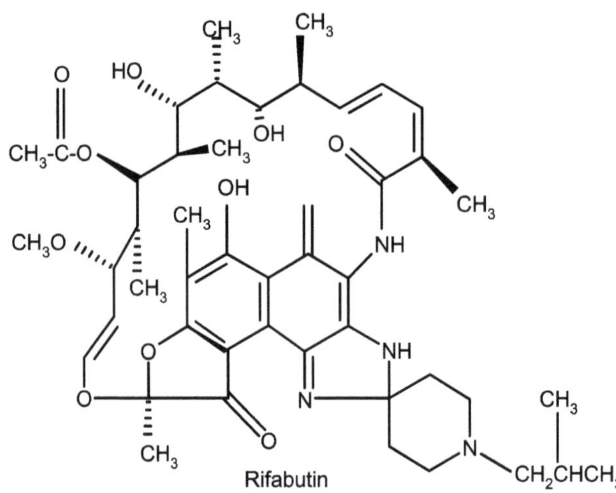

Rifabutin

Fluroquinolone derivatives

Fluroquinolones (ciprofloxacin, ofloxacin, lomefloxacin) are effective against MAC complex and *Mycobacterium tuberculosis*.

Precise mechanism of action is unknown, but the drug is bactericidal and appears to bind preferentially to mycobacterial DNA. Typical MACs are 0.1-1 µg/ml.

It also appears to have anti-inflammatory properties which is useful in controlling some MAC infections.

16

ANTILEPROTIC DRUGS

The drugs used in the treatment of leprosy are known as antileprotic drugs.

Leprosy

- Leprosy is an infectious disease caused by a bacillus, *Mycobacterium leprae.*
- *Mycobacterium leprae* multiplies very slowly; the incubation period for the disease is about five years.
- Leprosy is not highly infectious, it is transmitted via droplets, from the nose and mouth, during close and frequent contact with those infected who are not on treatment with multidrug therapy.
- Most people have natural immunity to leprosy and only a few people develop the disease.
- Leprosy mainly affects the skin and peripheral nerves.
- If detected early and treated, leprosy will not lead to disabilities.

Signs of leprosy

A leprosy patient is someone who has a skin patch or patches with a definite loss of sensation and who has not completed a full course of treatment with multidrug therapy.

Leprosy patches

- Can be pale or reddish or copper-colored
- Can be flat or raised
- Do not itch
- Usually do not hurt
- Lack sensations to heat, touch, or pain
- Can appear anywhere.

Other signs of leprosy include

Reddish or skin-colored nodules or smooth, shiny diffuse thickening of the skin on the face, ears and hands with no loss of sensation.

Diagnosis of leprosy

- Leprosy can be easily diagnosed on clinical signs alone. The main diagnostic sign is loss of feeling in the affected skin and is unique to the disease. The diagnosis can be made by gently touching the affected areas with a pointed object like a pen. Comparison can then be made with the sensation in normal skin. As the diagnosis is so simple, it can be made by paramedical staff with minimal training.
- Leprosy is classified into paucibacillary or multi bacillary leprosy based on the number of skin patches in order to choose the right treatment regimen. Paucibacillary cases have 1-5 skin patches; multibacillary cases more than five.

Classification

1. Sulphones	:	Dapsone, solapsone
2. Thiosemi carbazones	:	Amithiazone
3. Phenazines	:	Clofazimine
4. Antibiotics	:	Rifampicin
5. Natural oils	:	Chaulmoogra oil, hydnocarpus oil.

Drugs for the treatment of leprosy

Sulphones

1. Most widely used sulphone is dapsone (DDS).
2. Dapsone is bacteriostatic for *Mycobacterium leprae* and is given orally.
3. Sulphones were first used in the treatment of leprosy in 1941.

Structural characteristics

Several dapsone were synthesized to increase its antileprotic activity.

1. Replacement of one of the benzene rings with isosteric thiazolsulphone decreases antileprotic activity.
2. Substitution on aromatic ring of DDS reduces antileprotic activity.

Mechanism of action

Dapsone (4,4-diaminodiphenylsulphone) is a sulphone that is bactericidal as well as bacteriostatic against *Mycobacterium* leprae, the causative agent of leprosy. Dapsone appears to inhibit PABA biosynthesis or the incorporation of PABA into folate (similar to sulphonamides). Bacteria synthesize folic acid but host cells do not. DDS and clofazimine have significant anti-inflammatory actions.

Synthesis of dapsone

Following series of reactions

1. Two moles of 4-chloronitrobenzene is condensed with sodium sulphide to get di-(4-nitrophenyl) sulphide.
2. The above obtained di-(4-nitrophenyl) sulphide is oxidized with chromic acid to dinitrosulphone which on reduction yield dapsone.

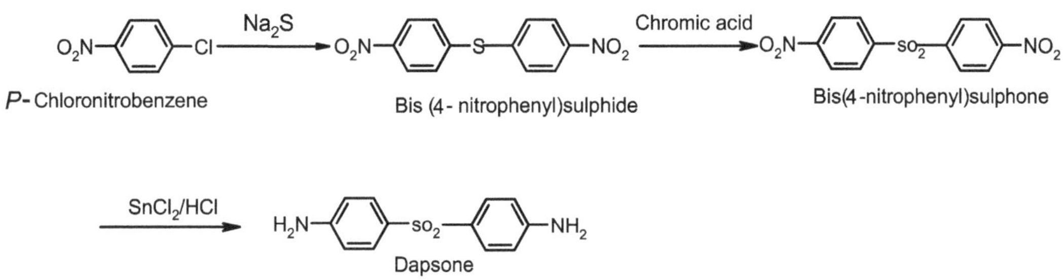

Clofazimine

Clofazimine is a *N*,5-bis(4-chlorophenyl)-3-(propan-2-ylimino)-3,5-dihydrophenazin-2-amine. Clofazimine is a phenazine derivative, which is a dye useful in the treatment of leprosy.

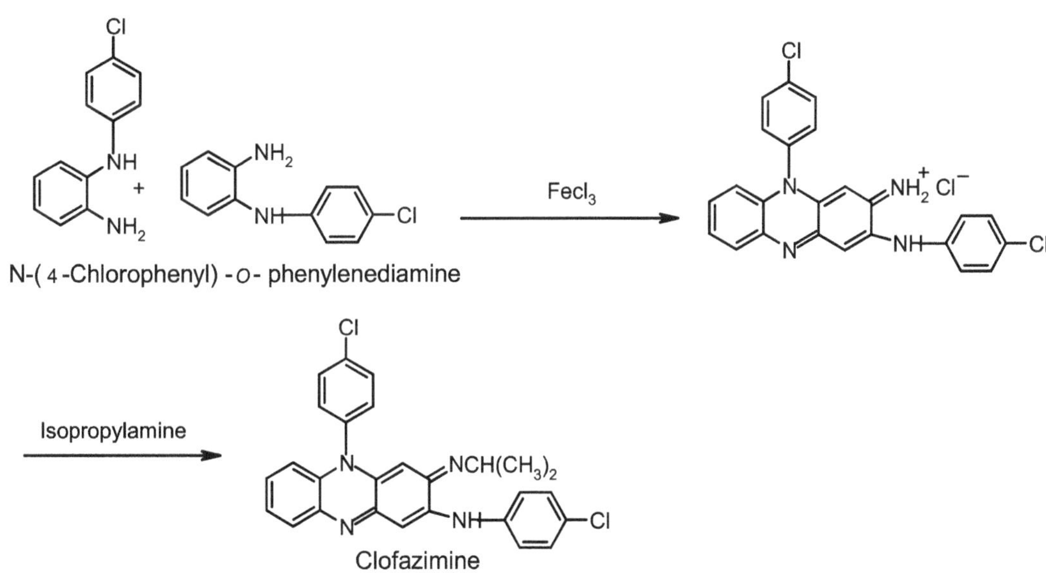

Properties

A reddish brown fine powder; odorless, exhibits polymorphism practically insoluble in water, soluble in chloroform, slightly soluble in ethanol (96%), very slightly soluble in ether.

SAR

1. Imino group at second position is essential for antileprotic activity.
2. Antileprotic activity of clofazimine increases by the substitution at amino group with alkyl or cycloalkyl groups.

Mechanism of action

Clofazimine possess direct antimycobacterial and immunosuppressive properties. It increases prostaglandin synthesis which releases antimicrobial oxidants from neutrophils. The released antimicrobial oxidants (super oxide anion) possess antileprotic effect.

Uses

It is highly useful in the treatment of leprosy in combination with dapsone and rifampicin.

17

ANTIMALARIALS

Introduction

Malaria is the major parasitic infection in many tropical and subtropical regions, leading to more than one million deaths (principally young African children) out of 400 million cases each year (WHO world health report 2000). More than half of the world's population lives in areas where they remain at risk of malaria infection. During last years, the situation has worsened in many ways, mainly due to malarial parasites becoming increasingly resistant to several antimalarial drugs.

In human beings *Plasmodium malariae, Plasmodium ovale, Plasmodium falciparum* and *Plasmodium vivax* cause malaria. All species of plasmodium have two hosts, a vertebrate and a mosquito. These plasmodia are found in female anopheles mosquito, which is a primary host of protozoa. They are transmitted to human beings by the bite of female anopheles mosquito. The salivary glands of the infected mosquito contain a large number of sporozoites and enter into blood stream of host. These sporozoites get attached to the parenchymal cells of liver where they grow and sporulate (pre-erythrocytic stage). After the pre-erythrocytic stage (seven days to several months) merozoites are released into the blood stream from liver cells. Merozoites then invade erythrocytes and undergo further multiplication (tropozoites). When the infected erythrocytes rupture and release merozoites the patient gets fever and chill. Again during the mosquito bite of an infected person, these merozoites (female and male gametocytes) enter mosquito, from the peripheral blood. In the gut of the mosquito the female gametocytes fertilizes to zygote to form oocyst, which ultimately gives rise to sporozoites. These sporozoites eventually reach the salivary glands of the mosquito and enter another human host with the mosquito's bite.

The figure shows various stages of the life cycle of Plasmodium species and the differences in sensitivity to drugs of the blood and liver forms of the parasite. *Plasmodium falciparum* is highly pathogenic because it affects all erythrocytes. Falciparum infections are potentially lethal. *Plasmodium vivax* and *Plasmodium malariae*, which affect fewer red cells are not usually lethal.

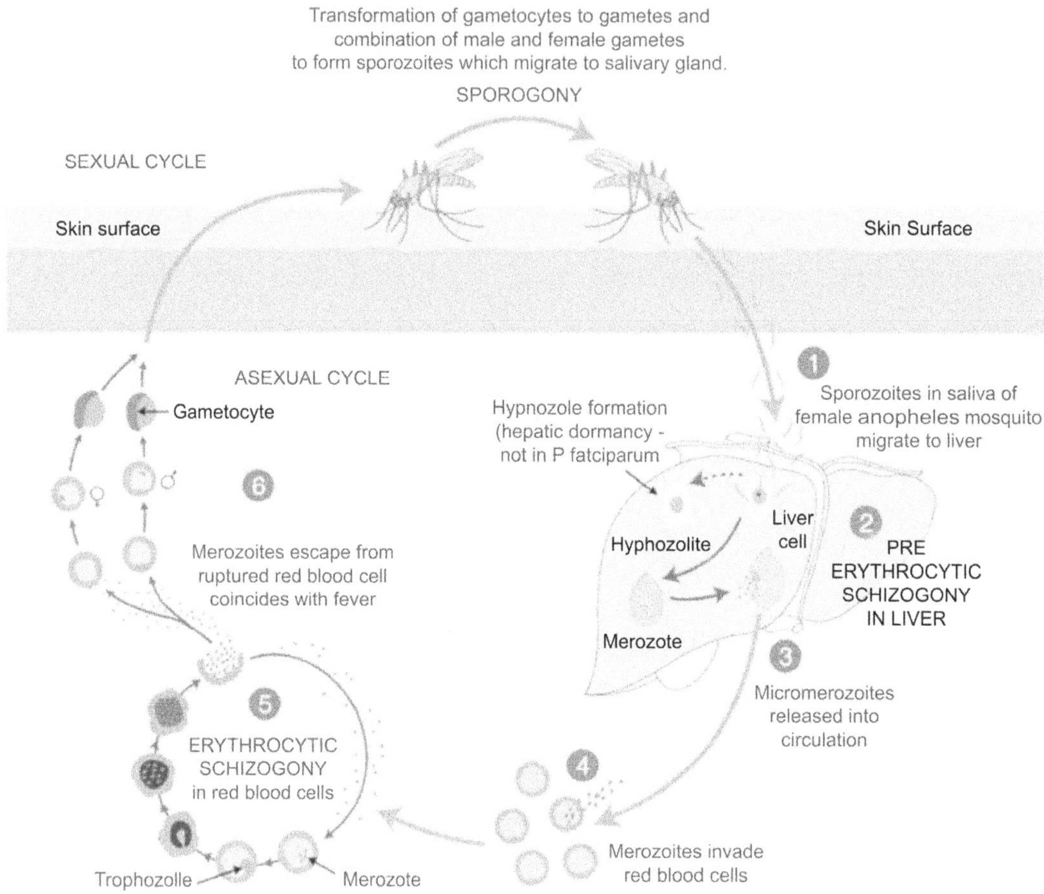

Figure 17.1 Life cycle of malarial parasite.

Classification of antimalarial drugs

The antimalarial drugs are classified basing on their chemical moiety:

1. Cinchona alkaloids – E.g., Quinine, cinchonine
2. 4-Amino quinoline – E.g., Chloroquine, amodiaquine
3. 8-Amino quinoline – E.g., Primaquine, pamaquine
4. 9-Amino acridines – E.g., Quinacrine, acridine
5. 2,4-Diamino pyrimidines – E.g., Pyrimethamine, trimethoprim
6. Biguanides – E.g., Proguanil, chlorguanil,
7. Sulphonamides – E.g., Sulphadoxine, sulphamethoxazole,
8. Newer drugs – E.g., Halofantrine, artemisinin, atovaquone.

Structural activity relationship of quinoline anti-malarials

1. Most of the antimalarial agents possess a quinoline ring system.
   E.g : Quinine, chloroquine, mefloquine, primaquine.

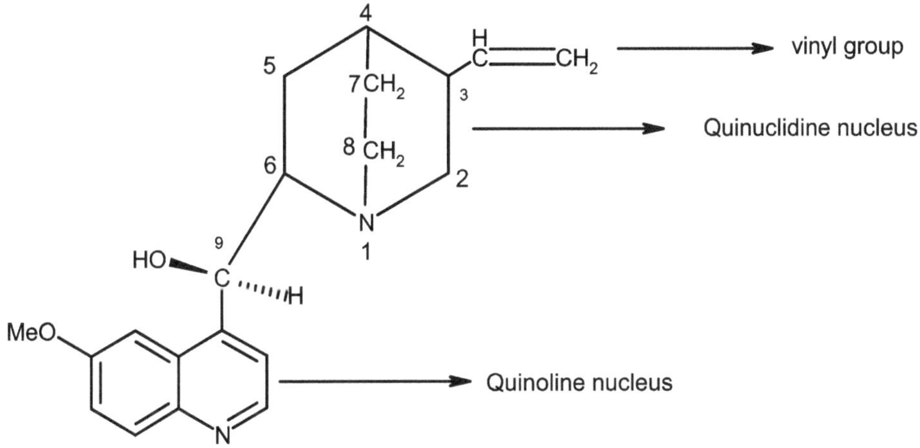

2. A chlorine group at C-7 provides maximum therapeutic activity in addition to maximum toxicity.

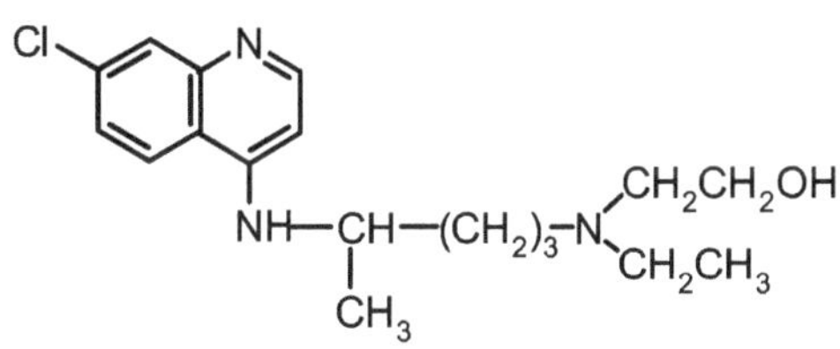

Hydroxychloroquine

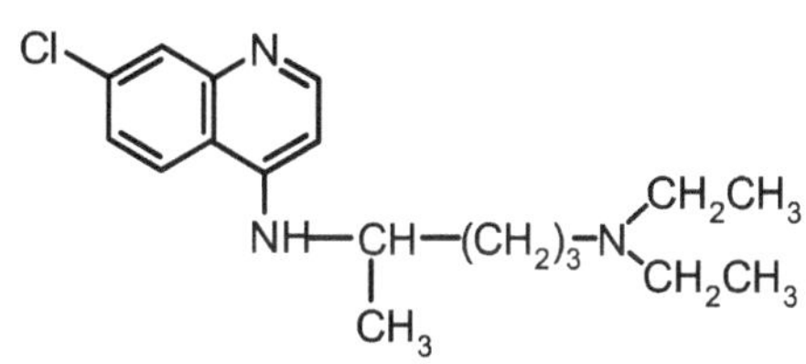

Chloroquine

3. Introduction of methoxy group at 2 (or) 4 (or) 6 position of quinoline yields more active compounds.

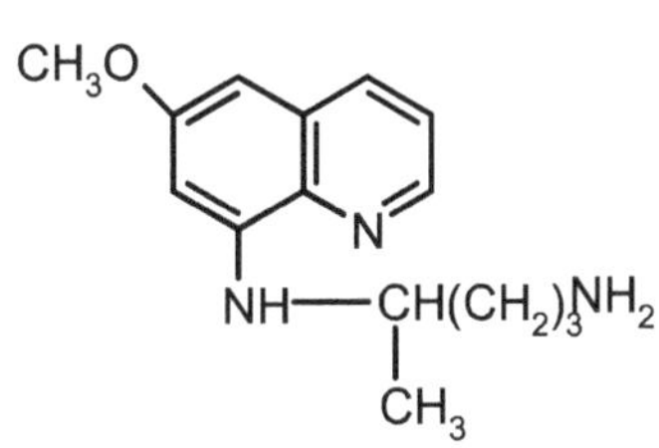

Primaquine

4. Introduction of dialkylaminoalkylamino side chains improves the antimalarial activity.

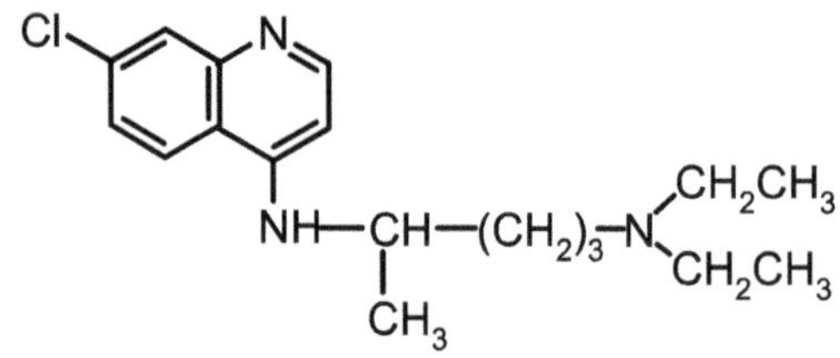

Chloroquine

5. 4-Aminoquinolines are not effective against exoerythrocytic parasites.

1. Cinchona alkaloids

Quinine

Quinine is the first antimalarial drug. It has been used in malaria treatment for more than 300 years. Quinine is the principle alkaloid obtained from cinchona bark. Quinine is (R)-(6-methoxyquinolin-4-yl)((1R,2S,4R,5S)-5-vinylquinuclidin-2-yl)methanol. It possess the following chemical features:

(a) A 6-methoxy quinoline nucleus

(b) A 3-vinyl quinuclidine moiety

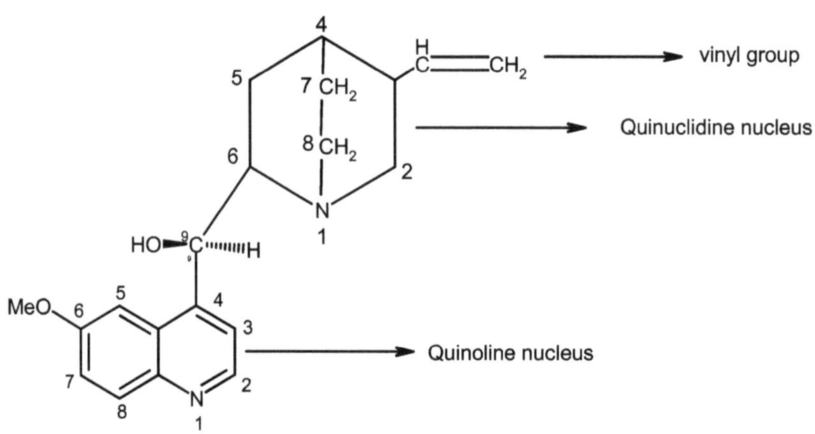

(c) Two asymmetric (8 and 9) carbon atoms.

Mechanism of action

Quinine is blood schizonticidal, effective against erythrocytic forms of all species of plasmodium. It acts by inhibiting parasites's haem polymerase. It is used to treat *Plasmodium falciparum* malaria either alone or with pyrimethamine (a sulphonamide) or with a tetracycline.

Uses

Quinine is used for the treatment of malaria and associated febrile states, leg cramps caused by vascular spasm, internal hemorrhoids, varicose veins and pleural cavities after thoracoplasty.

Cinchonine

Cinchonine is a (S)-(5-ethenyl-1-azabicyclo[2.2.2]octan-2-yl)-quinolin-4-ylmethanol hydrate hydrochloride. Cinchonine along with quinine isolated from the bark of various species of cinchona. It possess the following chemical structure:

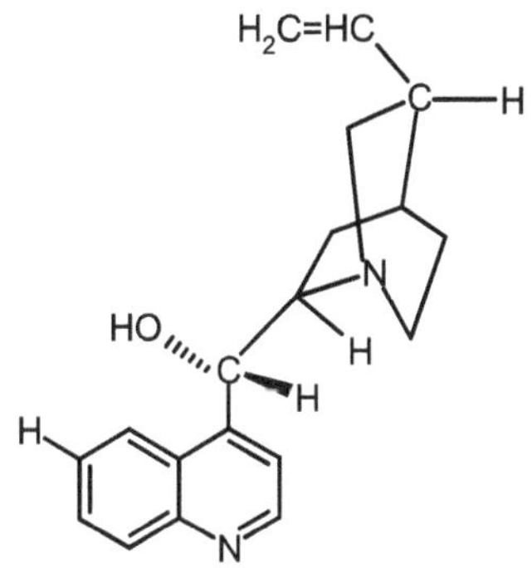

Uses

Cinchonine is used as an antipyretic and fitter stomachic.

2. 4-Aminoquinoline analogue

Chloroquine (4-aminoquinoline analogue)

Chloroquine possess quinoline moiety with a substituent at position-4 of quinoline nucleus. It also possess an asymmetric carbon in side chain. Chloroquine is 7-chloro-4-[(4-diethyl amino)-1-methyl butylamino]quinoline.

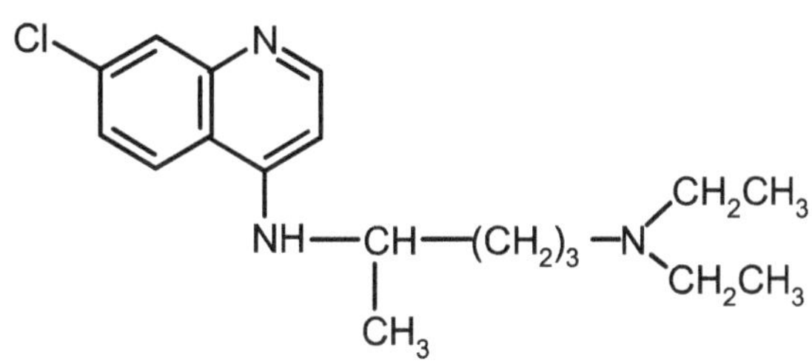

Chloroquine

Chloroquine is prepared by condensing 4,7-dichloroquinoline with 4-amino-1-diethylamino pentane in phenol.

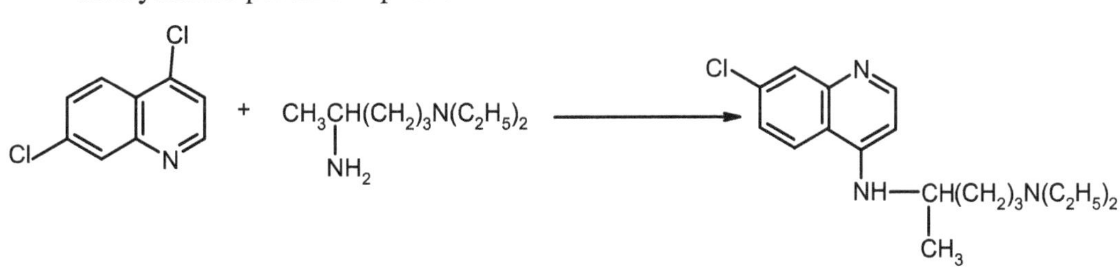

Chloroquine

Mechanism of action

1. Chloroquine act by preventing DNA and RNA synthesis in protozoa.
2. The complex formed by the interaction of chloroquine and ferriprotoporphyrin IX (formed from hemoglobin of decomposed erythrocytes) damage the membrane of parasite.

Properties

1. Chloroquine is colorless, odorless, bitter taste crystalline powder.
2. Chloroquine decolorizes on exposure to light.
3. It melts at 215°C.
4. It is slightly soluble in water, soluble in dilute acids, chloroform and ether.
5. Chloroquine is available as HCl or phosphate salt.

Uses

1. Chloroquine is used as therapeutic agent in the treatment of erythrocytic falciparum malaria.
2. It is also effective against asexual forms of *Plasmodium vivax* and *Plasmodium falciparum.*
3. It is also used in the treatment of extra intestinal amoebiasis.
4. Chloroquine also has anti-inflammatory action.

Hydroxychloroquine

Hydroxychloroquine is a 4- amino quinoline derivative. It possesses a hydroxy group on one of the ethyl groups in side chain at position 4 of quinoline nucleus. Chemically it is 2-({4-[(7-chloroquinolin-4-yl)amino]pentyl}(ethyl)amino)ethan-1-ol

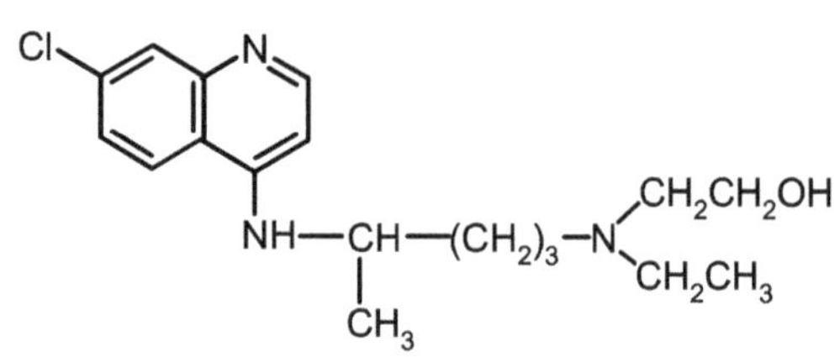

Hydroxychloroquine

Hydroxychloroquine can treat malarial infections caused by susceptible strains of *Plasmodium falciparum, Plasmodium vivax, Plasmodium malariae.* It is also used to treat acute or chronic rheumatoid arthritis and chronic discoid and systemic erythematosus.

Amodiaquine

Amodiaquine is a 4-amino quinoline derivative. Chemically it is 7-chloro-4-(3-diethylaminomethyl -4-hydroxyphenylamino) quinoline.

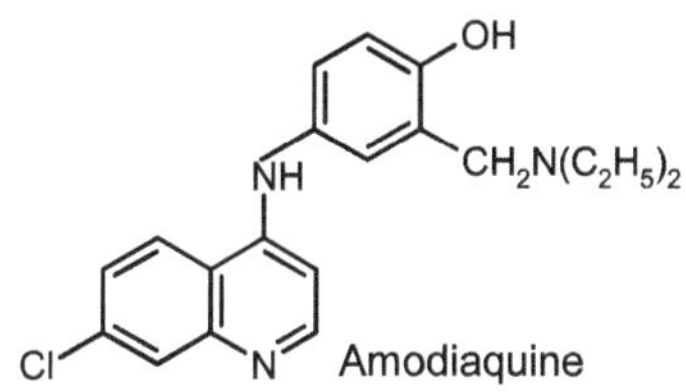

Amodiaquine

Amodiaquine is prepared by following chemical reaction:

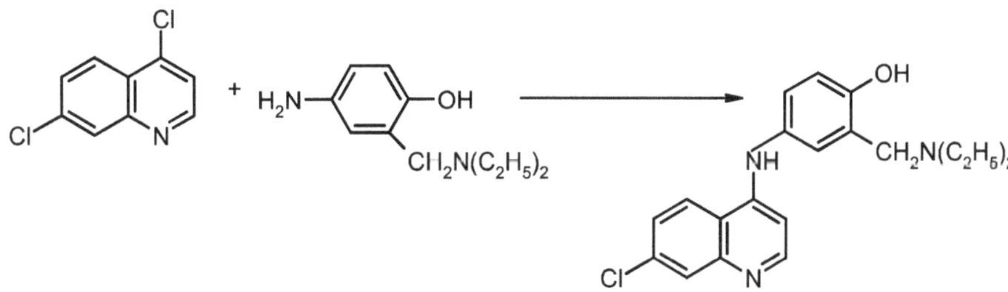

Amodiaquine

Properties

It occurs as colorless crystals from absolute ethanol having a melting point of 208°C. It is soluble in water, sparingly soluble in alcohol; very slightly soluble in benzene, chloroform, and ether.

Uses

It is used as an antimalarial drug. Amodiaquine is highly toxic due to hydroquinone (phenol) amine system, which readily oxidizes to quinone-imine (toxic metabolite).

Mefloquine

Mefloquine is [(R*,S*)-2,8-bis(trifluoromethyl)quinolin-4-yl]-(2-piperidyl)methano. It is structurally similar to chloroquine and primaquine. Mefloquine is used to treat chloroquine resistant *falciparum* malaria and *vivax* malaria. It is ineffective against hepatic forms of parasites hence it should be used with primaquine to treat *P.vivax* malaria. Mefloquine is useful in treating chloroquine resistant *Plasmodium falciparum malaria* and *Plasmodium vivax* malaria.

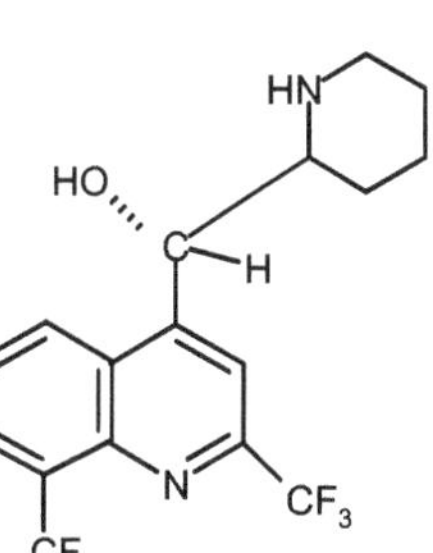

Mefloquine

Structurally mefloquine is different from other 4-aminoquinoline derivatives. It possess two trifluoromethyl groups (2 and 8 positions of quinoline) and no electronegative group either at 6 or 7 positions.

3. 8-Aminoquinolines analogue

8-Aminoquinolines possess a side chain at C-8 in quinoline nucleus. They possess a methoxy group at sixth position like natural antimalarials. The side chain is dialkylaminoalkylamine as in case of 4-aminoquinolines. They act against pre-and exo-erythrocytic forms of plasmodia. Eg: Primaquine, pamaquine and pentaquine.

Primaquine (8-Aminoquinoline analogue)

It is an 8-aminoquinoline derivative introduced in 1826. Currently primaquine is not in use because of its toxicity.

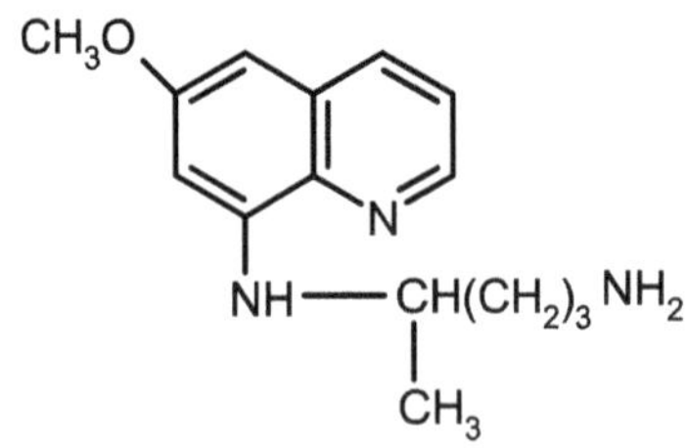

Primaquine

It is synthesized by condensing 6-methoxy-8-aminoquinoline with 2-chloropentylamine. The required 6-methoxy-8-amino- quinoline is synthesized from 4-amino-3-nitroanisole by Skraup's method:

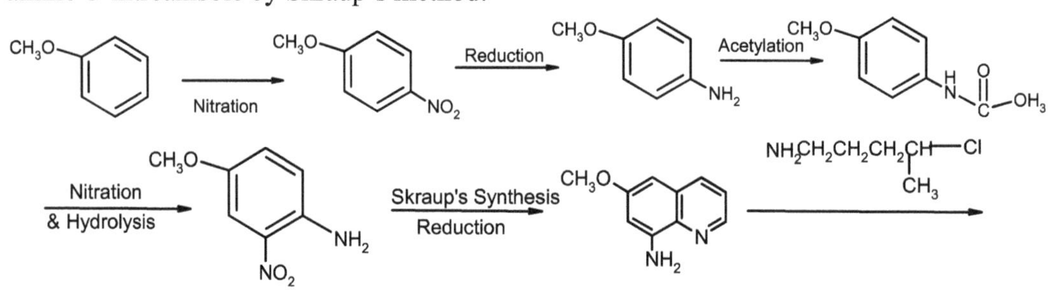

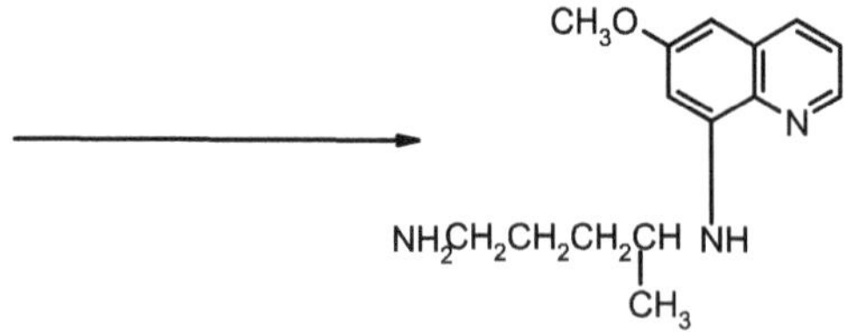

Primaquine

Mechanism of action

Exact mechanism of action is unknown. It is schizonticidal against pre-erythrocytic and exo-erythrocytic forms of *Plasmodium falciparum* and *Plasmodium vivax*. Primaquine is believed to act by cleaving parasitic mitochondria, thus cell division is inhibited.

Properties

1. Primaquine is viscous liquid but primaquine phosphate is orange-red colored, odorless, bitter taste crystalline powder.
2. It is insoluble in water but its phosphate salt is soluble in water.

Uses

1. It is very important for the radical cure of relapsing *plasmodium vivax* malaria.
2. It is used to treat toxoplasmosis.
3. Primaquine is also gametocidal for all four Plasmodia species.

Pamaquine

Pamaquine *N,N*-diethyl-*N'*-(6-methoxyquinolin-8-yl)pentane-1,4-diamine. Pamaquine is another 8-aminoquinoline derivative possessing the following structure:

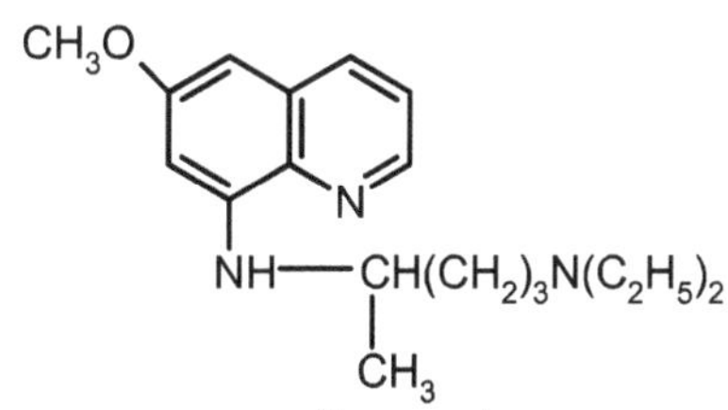

Pamaquine

It is prepared by following chemical reaction:

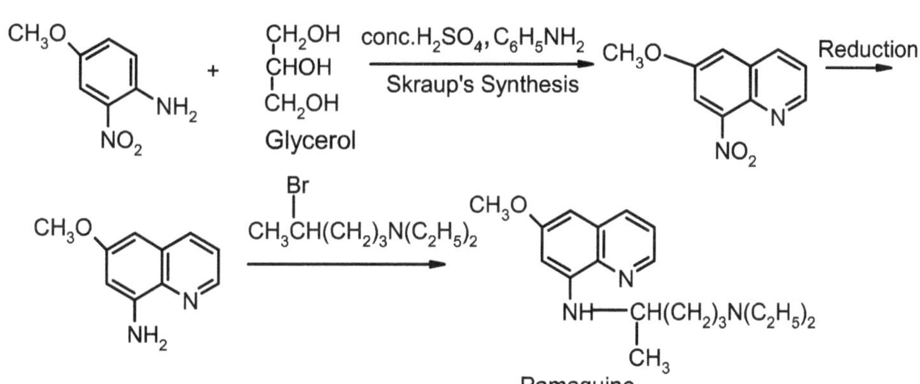

4. 2,4-Diaminopyrimidine analogue

Pyrimethamine (2,4-diaminopyrimidine analogue)

Pyrimethamine is a fully substituted pyrimidine. Chemically it is 2,4-diamino-5-(4-chlorophenyl)-6-ethyl pyrimidine.

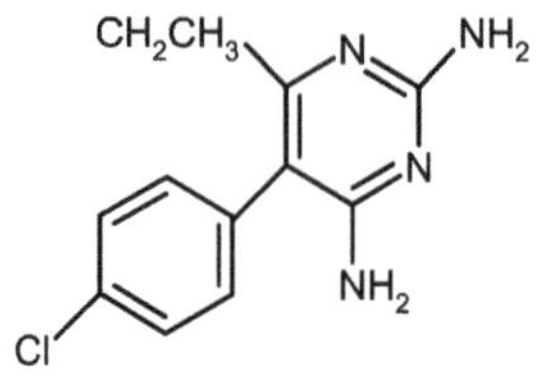

Pyrimethamine

Pyrimethamine is prepared by condensing p-chlorophenylacetonitrile with ethylpropionate in presence of sodium ethoxide to get cyanoketone:

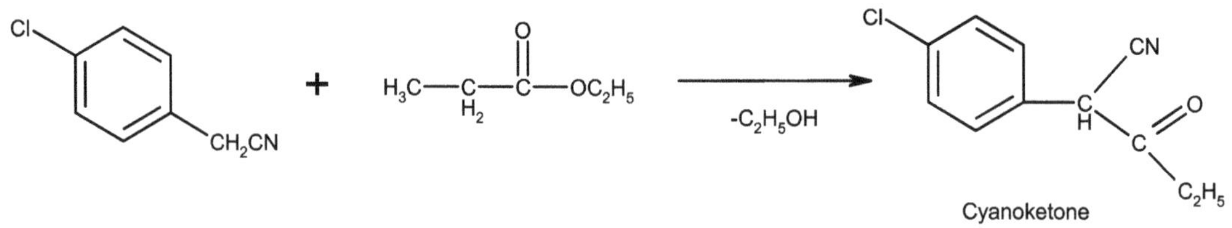

The above obtained cyanoketone on treatment with diazomethane yield methyl ether of cyanoketone which on condensation with guanidine produce pyrimethamine

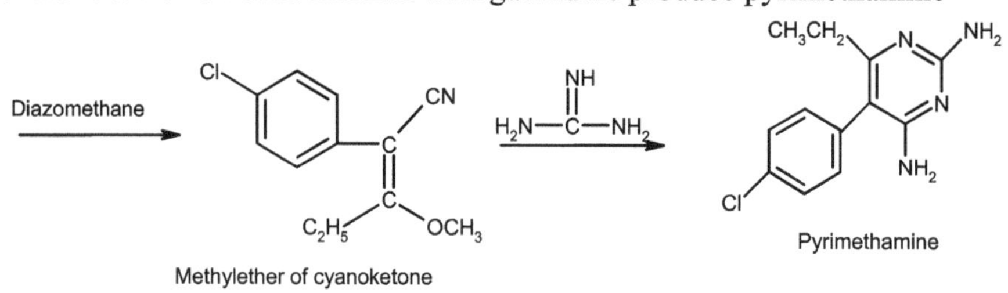

Properties

1. Pyrimethamine is colorless, odorless, slightly bitter taste crystalline powder.
2. It is insoluble in water but soluble in alcohol and chloroform.
3. It melts at 242°C.

Mechanism of action

1. Pyrimethamine is an antifolate agent.
2. It inhibits the biosynthesis of DNA by inhibiting the conversion of dihydrofolic acid to tetrahydrofolic acid (THF). The THF is required for many *fundamental* reactions like biosynthesis of pyrimidine bases.
3. Pyrimethamine is similar in structure to trimethoprim.

Uses

1. Pyrimethamine is also effective against *Plasmodium falciparum.*
2. Pyrimethamine (25 mg) in combination with sulphonamide (500 mg of sulphodoxine) is schizonticidal and is effective for treatment of *Plasmodium falciparum.* Sulphonamides block the incorporation of PABA to form dihydropteroic acid, which converts to dihydrofolic acid.

Trimethoprim (2,4 Diamino pyrimidine)

Trimethoprim is an antibacterial agent. It is 2,4-diamino-5-(3,4,5-trimethoxybenzyl) pyrimidine.

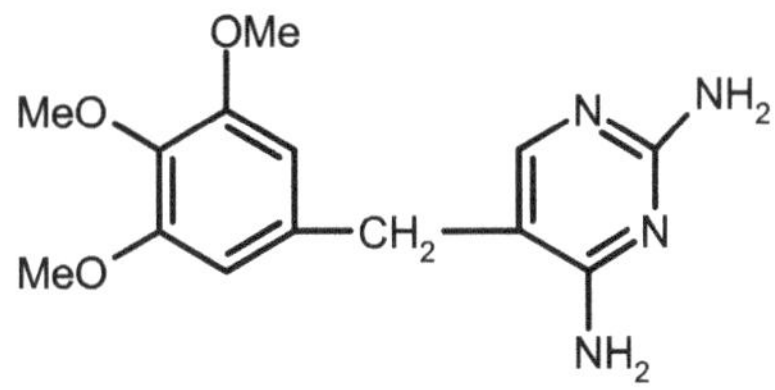

Trimethoprim is synthesized by the following steps:

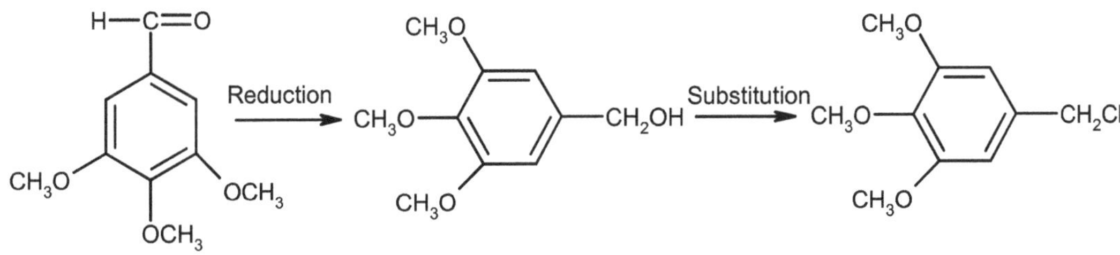

3,4,5-Trimethoxybenzaldehyde

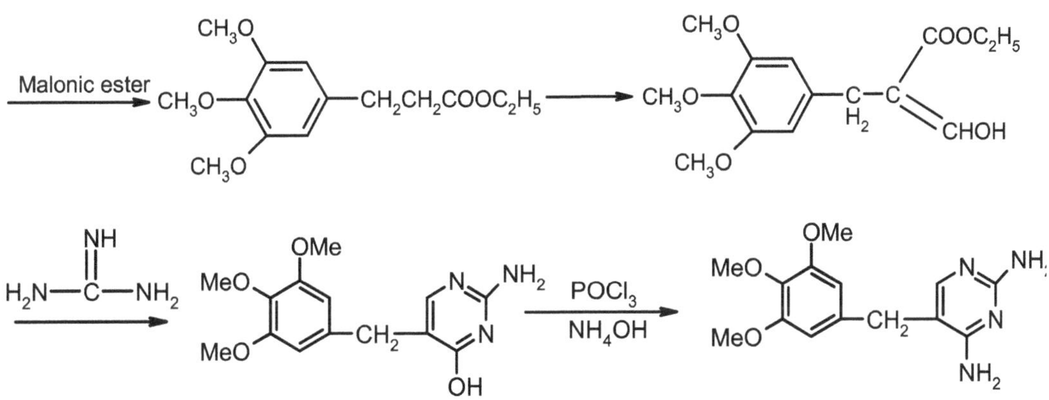

Trimethoprim

Mechanism of action

Same as pyrimethamine but for bacteria but not for protozoa.

Properties

1. Trimethoprim is a cream-colored, odorless, bitter taste crystalline powder.
2. It is very slightly soluble in water but soluble in absolute alcohol and chloroform.
3. It melts at 199°C.

Uses

1. It is used as an antimalarial drug (mostly against *Plasmodium falciparum*).
2. It is also used as an antibacterial agent.

5. 9-Amino acridines

Quinacrine

Quinacrine is 6-chloro-9-[[4-(diethyl amino)-1-methylbutyl]amino]-2-methoxy acridine. Compounds containing a quinoline nucleus with an additional benzene ring (an acridine ring) show antimalarial activity. Among various acridine derivatives quinacrine is a potent antimalarial with less toxicity. It also possesses chlorine atom, methoxyl group and an aminoalkylamino side chain.

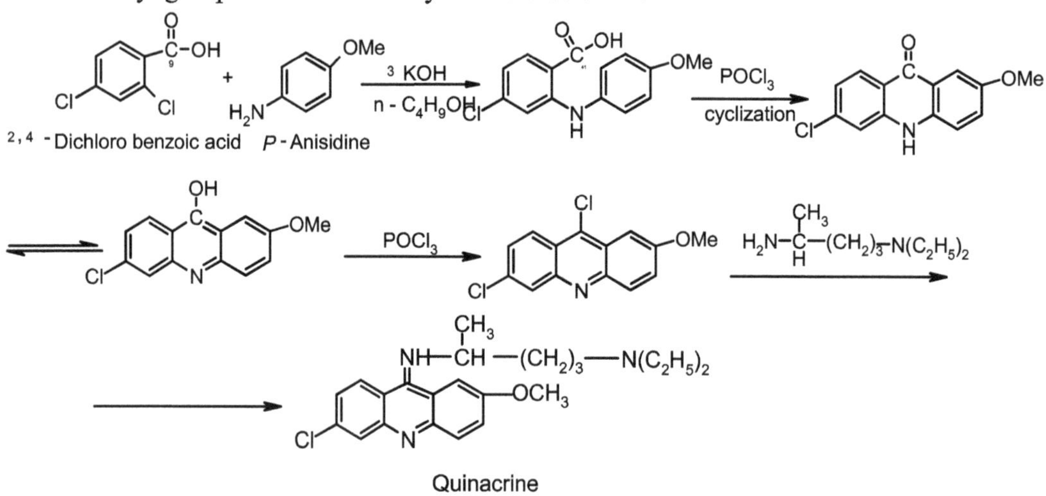

Uses

1. Quinacrine inhibits the erythrocytic stage of malarial parasite.
2. This also cures falciparum malaria.
3. Quinacrine is more effective and less toxic than quinine but it is more toxic and less effective than chloroquine.
4. Quinacrine is also used in the treatment of guinea-worm, amoebiasis, giardiasis, tapeworm and pinworm infestations.
5. It also possess anticonvulsant activity.

Biguanides

Biguanides are produced by condensation of two guanidine moieties:

E.g., Proguanil

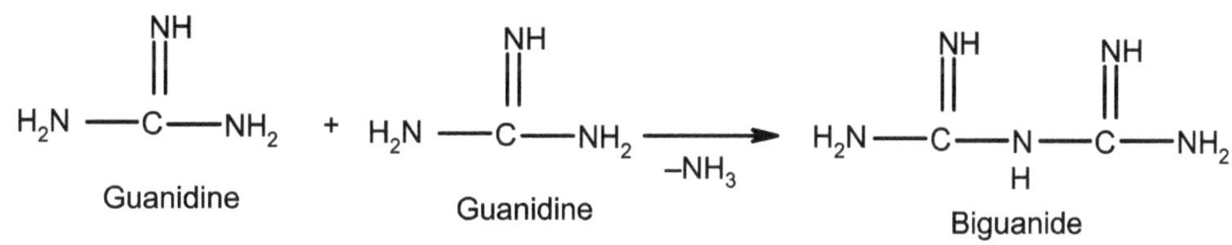

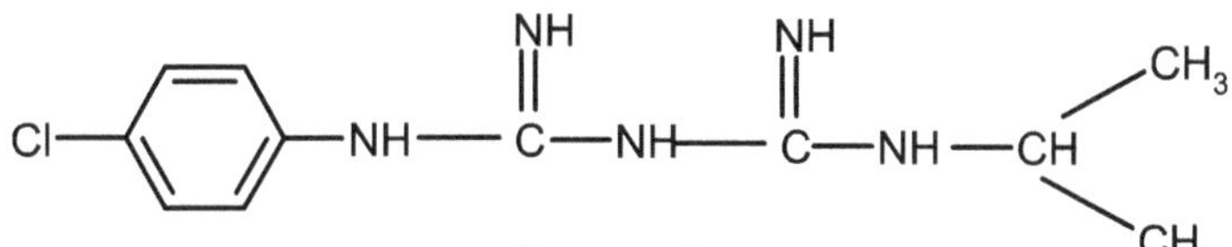
Proguanil

SAR

1. Presence of N-aryl group is essential for antimalarial activity.
2. Introduction of two halogen atoms at third and fourth positions of benzene ring yields potent anti malarial drugs.
3. Presence of alkyl groups on N1, N2 or N4 positions decreases activity.

Proguanil HCl (Chlorguanide)

In 1945 proguanil is developed. Chemically it is 1-(-4-chlorophenyl)-5-isopropylbiguanide. It is synthesized by the following steps from 4-chloroaniline.

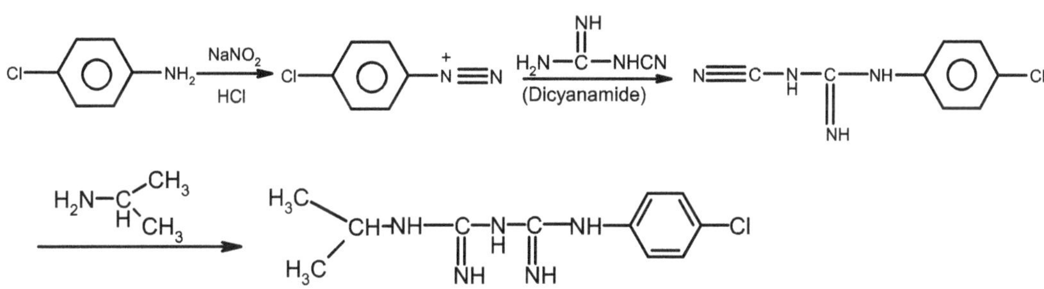

proguanil

Properties

1. Proguanil is a colorless, odorless, bitter taste crystalline powder.
2. Slightly soluble in water, sparingly soluble in alcohol. Practically insoluble in methylene chloride.

Uses

1. Proguanil is used as an antimalarial drug.
2. It is effective against pre-erythrocytic stage of malarial parasite.
3. Proguanil is a prodrug, which is metabolized to cycloguanil by CYP2C19 (hepatic enzyme). Cycloguanil inhibit dihydrofolate reductase enzyme thus protein synthesis is prevented.

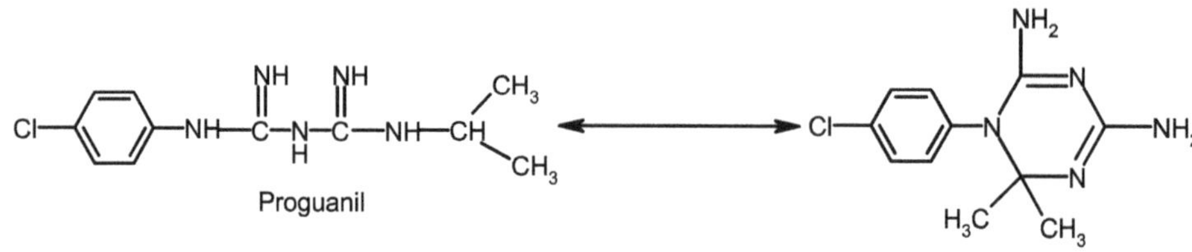

Proguanil

Cycloguanil(Active)

4. Proguanil is administered orally with atovaquone in 2.5:1 ratio (in milligrams). The combination drugs have antimalarial activity by two different mechanisms (atovaquone is a selective inhibitor of Plasmodium mitochondrial electron transport system). The combination is good effective against both erythrocytic and exoerythrocytic plasmodium. Atovaquone is also active against *Pneumocystis carinii* (fungus) which is chemically 2-[trans-4-(4-chlorophenyl)cyclohexyl]-3-hydroxy-1,4-naphthoquinone.

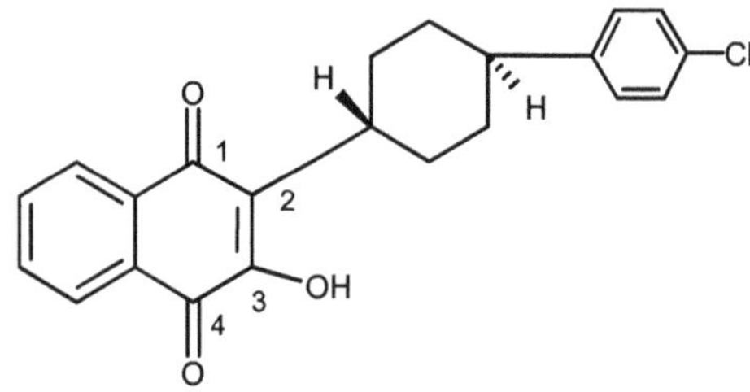

Atovaquone

6. Newer drugs

Halofantrine

Halofantrine is a trifluoromethyl substituted phenanthrene derivative. Chemically it is 3-dibutylamino-1-[1,3-dichloro-6-(trifluromethyl) phenanthren-9-yl]-propan-1-ol

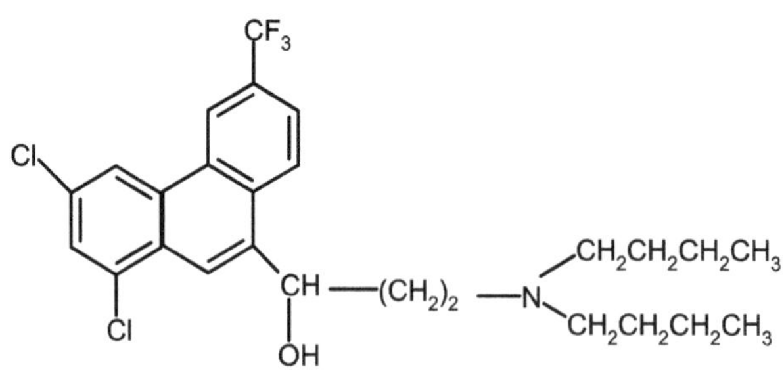

Properties

Practically insoluble in water, freely soluble in methanol, sparingly soluble in alcohol which is white (or) almost white powder.

Uses

It is a newer antimalarial agent, which is schizonticidal and has no effect on sporozoite, gametocyte or hepatic stages. It is used to treat mild to moderate malaria caused by *Plasmodium falciparum or Plasmodium vivax.*

Artemisinin

Artemisinin is the antimalarial principle isolated from *Artemisia annua*, a plant used in traditional Chinese medicine. It is a sesquiterpene lactone with a peroxide bridge linkage, responsible for antimalarial activity. When this group is lacking, compound (desoxoartemisinin) is inactive. Chemically it is (3R, 5a*S*,6*R*,8a*S*,9R,12*S*,12a*R*)-octahydro-3,6,9-trimethyl-3,12-epoxy-12H-pyrano[4,3-*j*]-1,2-benzodioxepin-10(3H)-one.

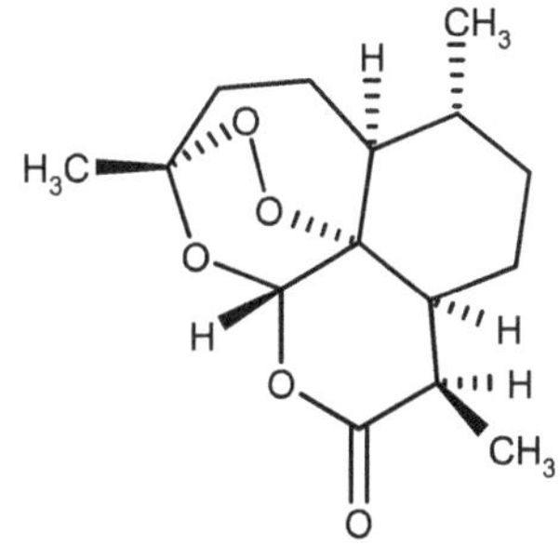

artemisinin

Mechanism of action of artemisinin

It acts by oxidative mechanism. At the molecular level it is possible that the o-o bond of the peroxide bridge is broken due to an electron transfer with the generation of an oxygen centered radical. This radical species could be responsible for the disruption of the membranes of plasmodium

Uses

Artemisinin derivatives are very efficient against malaria, especially against chloroquine-resistant strains of *Plasmodium falciparum.* Only low resistance of parasites to artemisinin derivatives has been observed so far.

18

ANTI-PROTOZOAL DRUGS

Drugs used to treat infections of *Entamoeba histolytica, Trichomonas vaginalis, Giardia lamblia, Leishmania, Trypanosoma, Toxoplasma gondii, Pneumocystis carinii, Enterocytozoon beeneusi, Balantidium coli, Plasmodia* are known as anti-protozoal drugs. Drugs act against *Plasmodia* (antimalarials) are discussed in **Antimalarials Chapter 17,** however drugs against *Amoeba, Trichomonas, Giardia, Leishmania* and *Trypanosoma* are discussed here.

Antiamoebic drugs

These are the drugs used to treat infection (amoebiasis) caused by *Entamoeba histolytica*. Amoebiasis has a worldwide distribution. Poor environmental sanitation and low socio-economic status are important factors in the spread of disease. It spreads by faecal contamination of food and water. *Entamoeba histolytica* has a two stage life cycle i.e., (a) vegetative (the trophozoite) stage and (b) the cystic stage. In cystic stage the organism can live for long periods both outside the body and within the human intestine. The infective cysts contain four nuclei which divide to form 8 nuclei. The cyst hatches in intestine and liberates 8 trophozoites. Trophozoites form amoebae which pass on to the colon. Some of amoebae enter the portal circulation and reach the liver and cause hepatitis and amoebic abscess.

Classification of antiamoebic drugs

1. Antiamoebic drugs are classified according to their site of action as follows:
   - (i) **Luminal amoebicides:** These are active against intestinal forms of amoebae.
     E.g : Diloxanide furoate, iodoquinol, tetracyclines, paromomycin.
   - (ii) **Tissue amoebicides :** These drugs primarily act in the bowel wall, liver and other extraintestinal tissues.
     E.g : Chloroquine, emetine, dehydroemetine.
   - (iii) **Mixed amoebicides:**
     E.g : Metronidazole.

2. Antiamoebic drugs are also classified on the basis of chemical structures as :

(i) **Alkaloids :** Emetine, dehydroemetine, emetine bismuth iodide.

(ii) **Halogenated hydroxy quinolines :** Diiodohydroxy quinoline, chloroquine.

(iii) **Nitroimidazoles :** Metronidazole, tinidazole, secnidazole, ornidazole.

(iv) **Organic arsenicals :** Acetorsol, carbarsone, glycobiarsol.

(v) **Antibiotics :** Oxytetracycline, bacitracin, paromomycin.

(vi) **Miscellaneous :** Diloxanide furoate.

Alkaloids

Emetine

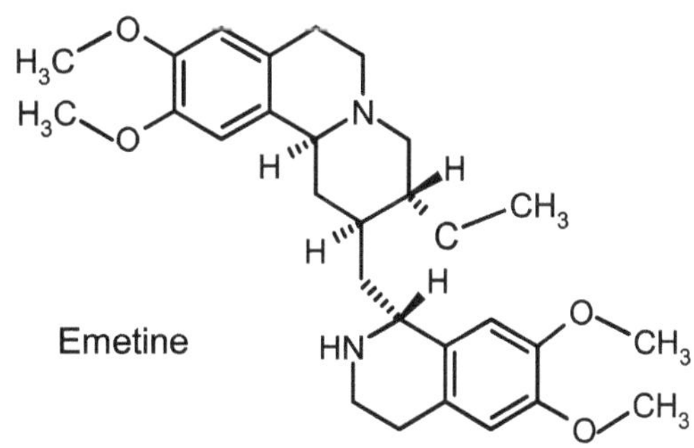

Emetine

Emetine is an alkaloid obtained from the dried roots of *Cephaelis ipecacuanha*. It is the most useful and potent of amoebicidal drugs. Emetine has direct lethal action on *Entamoeba histolytica*. Emetine in therapeutic doses acts against trophozoites. At higher doses it may be active against cysts. It inhibits protein synthesis by interfering with attachment of t-RNA to ribosomes. Chemically it is (2*S*,3*R*,11b*S*)-2-{[(1*R*)-6,7-Dimethoxy-1,2,3,4-tetrahydro-isoquinolin-1-yl]}-3-ethyl-9,10-dimethoxy-2,3,4,6,7,11b-hexahydro-1*H*-pyrido [2,1-a]isoquinoline

It is administered as intramuscular or subcutaneous injection and rarely orally as enteric-coated capsule. Emetine bismuth iodide is given orally. Emetine is a toxic drug even in therapeutic doses hence it is seldom used today. It is useful in the treatment of amoebic abscess of the liver. It is not effective on cystic forms of *E. histolytica*.

Dehydroemetine

Several molecular modifications emetine have been carried out of these, dehydroemetine has been studied extensively in animals and man. It retains the amoebicidal property of emetine but is less toxic. Chemically it is (11b*S*)-2-[[(1*R*)-6,7-dimethoxy-1,2,3,4-tetrahydroisoquinolin-1-b-yl]methyl]-3-ethyl-9,10-dimethoxy-4,6,7,11b-tetrahydro-1*H*-pyrido[2,1-a]isoquinoline

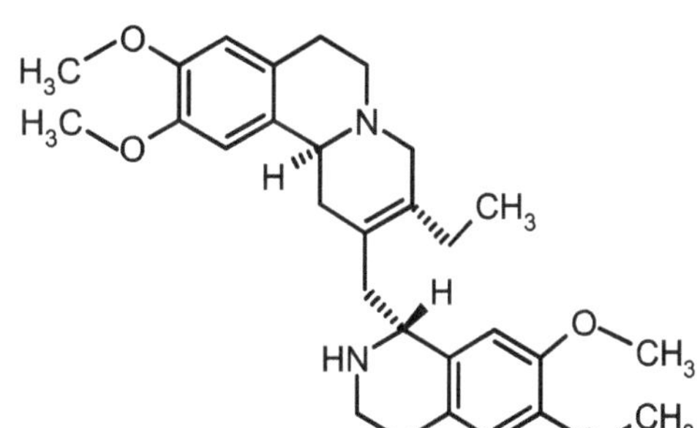

Dehydroemetine

Halogenated hydroxyquinolines

The currently used drugs of this group are chloroquine and iodoquinol.

Mechanism of action

They exert direct amoebicidal action against trophozoites and cysts of *Entamoeba histolytica* in intestines. The antiamoebic effects appear to be exerted by chelation of ferrous iron necessary for amoebal growth.

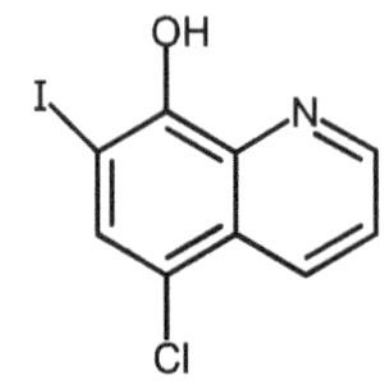

Iodochlorohydroxy quinoline

Iodochlorohydroxy quinoline is more effective in amoebic dysentery. It also produces antifungal effects and is useful to treat *Trichomonas vaginalis* in women.

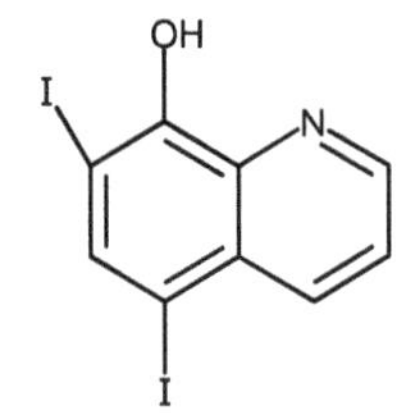

Diiodohydroxyquinoline

Diiodohydroxyquinoline is effective against both motile and cystic forms but ineffective against extra intestinal amoebiasis because it is not absorbed by oral route. Diiodohydroxyquinoline is synthesized by direct iodination of 8-hydroxy quinoline with iodine monochloride or potassium iodate.

Iodochlorohydroxyquinoline (quiniodochlor or clioquinol) is prepared from 5-chloro-8-hydroxyquinoline by iodination using KI and hypochlorite. (activating hydroxy group at 8th position in quinoline directs iodine into ortho position of homocyclic ring).

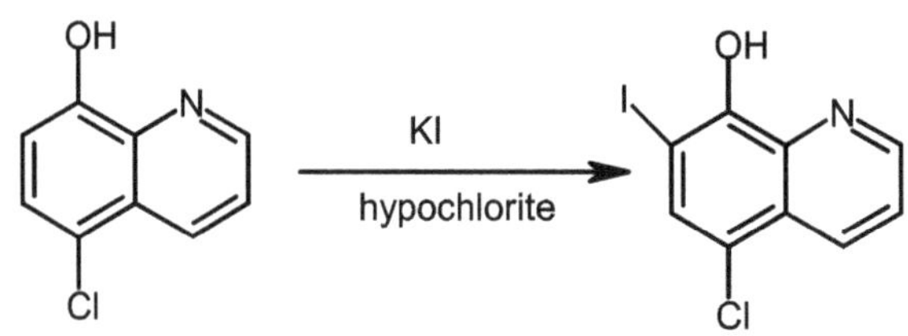

5-chloro-8-hydroxyquinoline   Iodochlorohydroxyquinoline

Quinoline derivatives on prolonged use have recently been reported to produce a serious complication called SMON (sub-acute myeloptic neuropathy: decreased sensations in limbs, muscular weakness, abdominal pain, decrease in vision).

5-Nitroimidazoles

5-Nitroimidazoles have both antiprotozoal and antibacterial activities. Nitroimidazoles act against trichomonads and amebae are metronidazole, tinidazole, nimorazole, flunidazole, and ronidazole. Metronidazole and nimorazole are effective in the treatment of giardiasis, while dimetridazole, ipronidazole, and ronidazole control histomoniasis in poultry. Several nitroimidazoles have activity against trypanosomes. Metronidazole, ornidazole, and other nitroimidazoles are active against anaerobic bacteria. Metronidazole is the compound that has been the most studied and is discussed as the prototype of the group.

Metronidazole

Metronidazole 2-methyl-5-nitroimidazole-1-ethanol. Metronidazole a member of a subgroup of nitrofurans called nitroimidazoles.

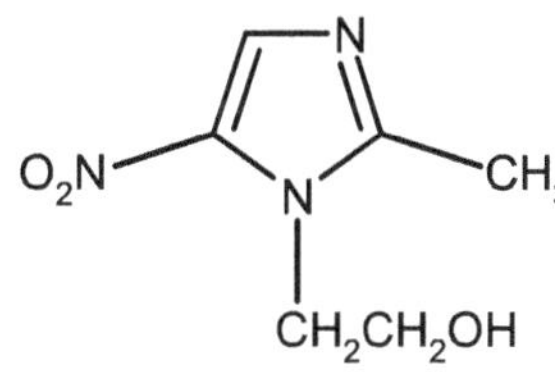

Metronidazole

It is prepared from 2-methylimidazole by following chemical reactions:

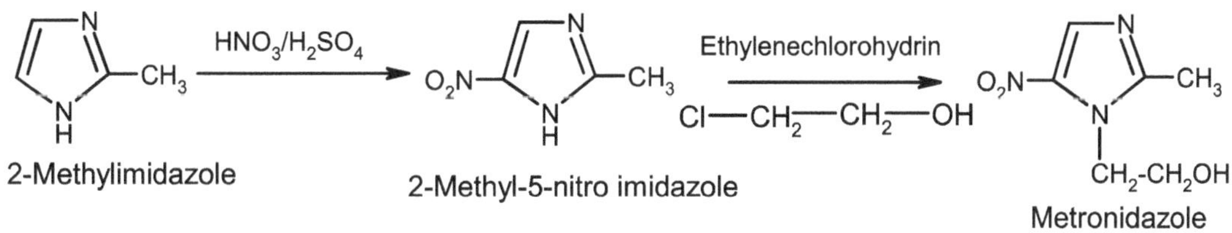

Mechanism of action

Metronidazole is bactericidal at higher concentrations. The precise mode of action is unclear, but it seems that after the drug enters a susceptible organism it is first reduced and then binds to DNA, causing loss of the helical structure, strand breakage, and impairment of DNA function.

Additionally, metronidazole is related to that of nitrofurans involving the reduction of the nitro group coupled with the formation of free radicals like hydroxyl which cause damage to the bacterial DNA.

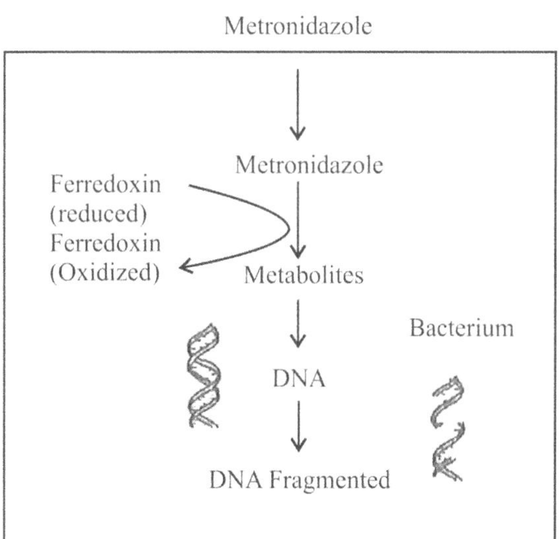

Figure 18.1 Mechanism of action of metronidazole.

Clinical Use

The principal clinical indications for metronidazole include the treatment of specific protozoal infections (amebiasis, trichomoniasis, giardiasis, and balantidiasis) and anaerobic bacterial infections such as those that may be seen in abdominal abscesses, peritonitis, empyema, genital tract infections, periodontitis, otitis media, osteitis, arthritis, and meningitis, and in necrotic tissue. Metronidazole has been successfully used to prevent infection after colonic surgery. Nitroimidazoles also act as radiosensitizers, and metronidazole has been used as an adjunct to the radiotherapy of solid tumors.

Metabolism

Metronidazole is metabolized by the cytochrome P_{450} system. The methyl group is oxidized to a hydroxymethyl ($-CH_2OH$) group which is an active metabolite. Additionally, the ethanol side chain is oxidized to an acid group ($-CH_2COOH$) which is also an active metabolite. A minor metabolite involving the splitting of the metronidazole ring results in a carcinogenic species in rats.

Tinidazole

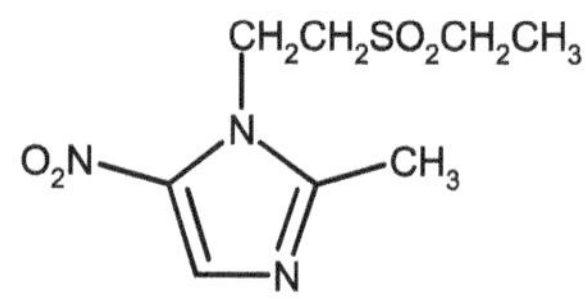

Tinidazole

Tinidazole, a second-generation synthetic 1-(2-ethylsulfonylethyl)2-methyl-5-nitro-imidazole with selective antimicrobial activity against anaerobic bacteria and protozoa. It is a structural analogue of metronidazole with sulphonyl side chain. The drug has activity against many species of infectious protozoa, including those which sexually transmitted and water borne. It was designed to be effective in the short term, with treatment usually ranging from just a single dose to as long as 3 days.

Mechanism of action

While the precise mechanism of action of tinidazole is unknown, cell extracts from *Trichomonas* have been shown to reduce the molecules nitro group, producing cytotoxic free radicals. The mechanism of action against *Giardia* and *Entamoeba* species is unknown but activity has been confirmed both *invitro* and *invivo*. It has been used to treat the following protozoal infections: Trichomooniasis caused by *Trichomonas vaginalis* in both male and female patients, Giardiasis caused by *Giardia duodenalis/Giardia lamblia*, Amebiasis and amebic liver abscess caused by *Entamoeba histolytica*.

Ornidazole

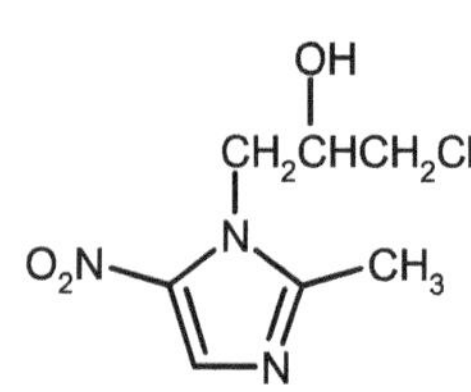

Ornidazole

Ornidazole is a synthetic nitroimidazole derivative used in the treatment of infections caused by anaerobic bacteria and protozoa. Chemically it is 1-(3-chloro-2-hydroxypropyl)-2-methyl-5-nitroimidazole. It is prepared by condensing 2-methylimidazole with epichlorhydrin in acidic conditions.

Nimorazole

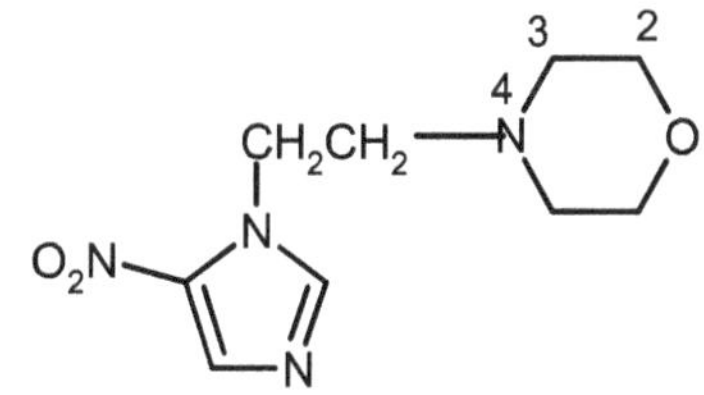

Nimorazole is 4-[2-(5-nitro-1*H*-imidozol-1-yl) ethyl] morpholine. It is an antitrichomonal agent which is effective either topically or orally and whose urinary metabolites are also trichomonicidal.

Organic arsenicals

Organic arsenicals have been used for chemotherapy of amoebiasis and trypanosomiasis. However they have been replaced by less toxic drugs. E.g: Carbarsone, acetarsol. carbarsone and acetarsol are pentavalent organic compounds. Pentavalent arsenic compounds such as carbarsone and acetarsone have been used in the treatment of amebiasis for many years. More recently, Anderson showed that the trivalent arsenic compounds–carbarsone oxide and its thioglycolic acid and thiosalicylic acid derivatives were active in human and monkey amebiasis.

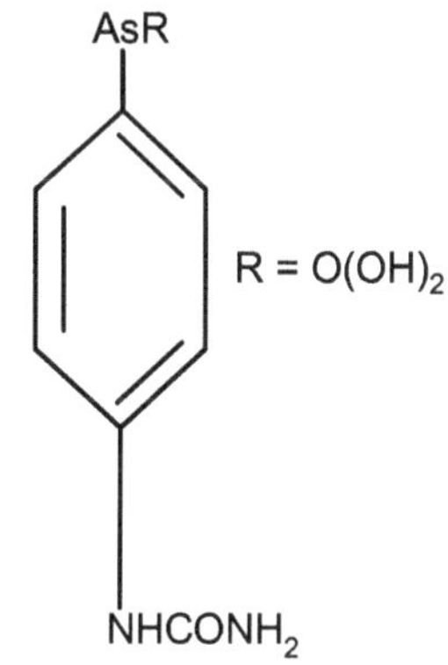

Carbarsone

Carbarsone is used in *Trichomonas vaginalis* and *Balantidium* dysentry.

Acetarsol is used in local treatment of *Trichomonas vaginalis*. It is less effective than carbarsone. Chemically acetarsol is 3-acetamido-4-hydroxy phenyl arsonic acid may be used concurrently, or sequentially, with other agents such as the nitroimidazoles in the treatment of invasive or extraintestinal forms of amoebiasis.

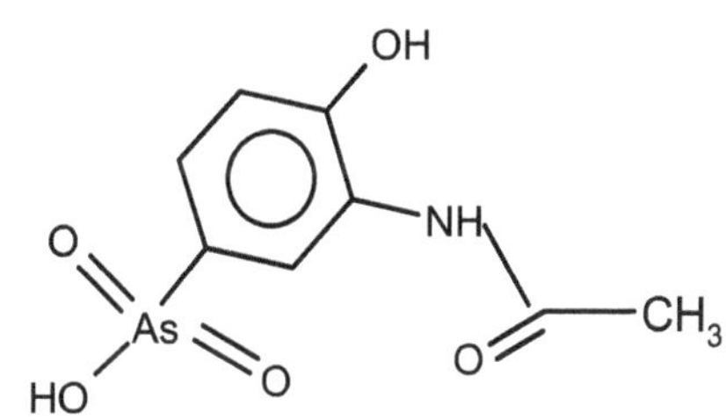

Acetarsol

Diloxanide furoate

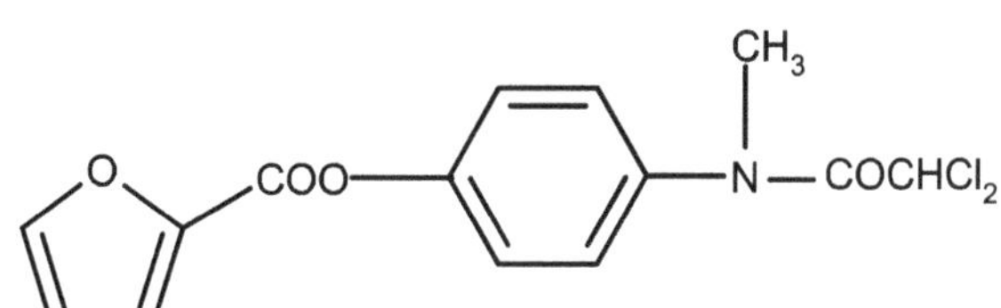

Diloxanide furoate

Diloxanide furoate is an aromatic ester of 2-furoic acid. Chemically it is 4-(N-methyl -2,2-dichloro acetancido phenyl-2-furoate. It is synthesized from 4-aminophenol.

It is Luminal amebicide. The mechanism of action of diloxanide is unknown. This agent destroys the trophozoites of *Entamoeba histolytica* that eventually form into cysts. The cysts are then excreted by persons infected with asymptomatic amebiasis. Diloxanide furoate is slowly absorbed from the gastrointestinal tract and can therefore provide an adequate concentration of the medication in the intestinal lumen for a long period of time. However, the parent compound, diloxanide, is rapidly absorbed and has a bioavailability of approximately 90%.

Diloxanide furoate is largely hydrolyzed into diloxanide and furoic acid in the intestinal lumen before being absorbed. The absorbed diloxanide is extensively conjugated with glucuronic acid, this conjugate is inactive. 99% of diloxanide occurs as glucuronide and 1% as free diloxanide in the systemic circulation.

Diloxanide is used alone as a primary agent in the treatment of asymptomatic (cystpassers) intestinal amebiasis caused by *Entamoeba histolytica*. This medication may also be used concurrently, or sequentially, with other agents such as the nitroimidazoles in the treatment of invasive or extra intestinal forms of amebiasis.

Antigiardial drugs

Giardiasis is caused by *Giardia lamblia*, a one-celled, microscopic parasite that lives in the intestines of people and animals. This protozoan was initially named *Cercomonas intestinalis* by Lambl in 1859 and renamed *Giardia lamblia* by Stiles in 1915, in honor of Professor A. Giard of Paris and Dr. F. Lambl of Prague. However, many consider the name, *Giardia intestinalis*, to be the correct name for this protozoan. The International Commission on Zoological Nomenclature is reviewing this issue.

How do people get giardiasis?

People get giardiasis by swallowing *Giardia* cysts, the infectious stage of the parasite. People can get giardiasis by:

- Putting anything into the mouth that has touched the stool of a person or animal with giardiasis
- Swallowing water (such as from a swimming pool, lake, river, pond, or stream) contaminated with sewage or stool from *Giardia*-infected people or animals.
- Eating uncooked or undercooked food contaminated with *Giardia* cysts
- Touching and bringing to the mouth cysts picked up from surfaces (such as toys, bathroom fixtures, changing tables, diaper pails) contaminated with stool from an infected person

Cysts are resistant forms and are responsible for transmission of giardiasis. Both cysts and trophozoites can be found in the feces. Infection occurs by the contaminated water, food, or by the fecal-oral route. In small intestine, excystation releases trophozoites (each cyst produces two trophozoites). Trophozoites multiply by longitudinal binary fission, remaining in the lumen of the proximal small bowel where they can be free or attached to the mucosa by a ventral sucking disk.

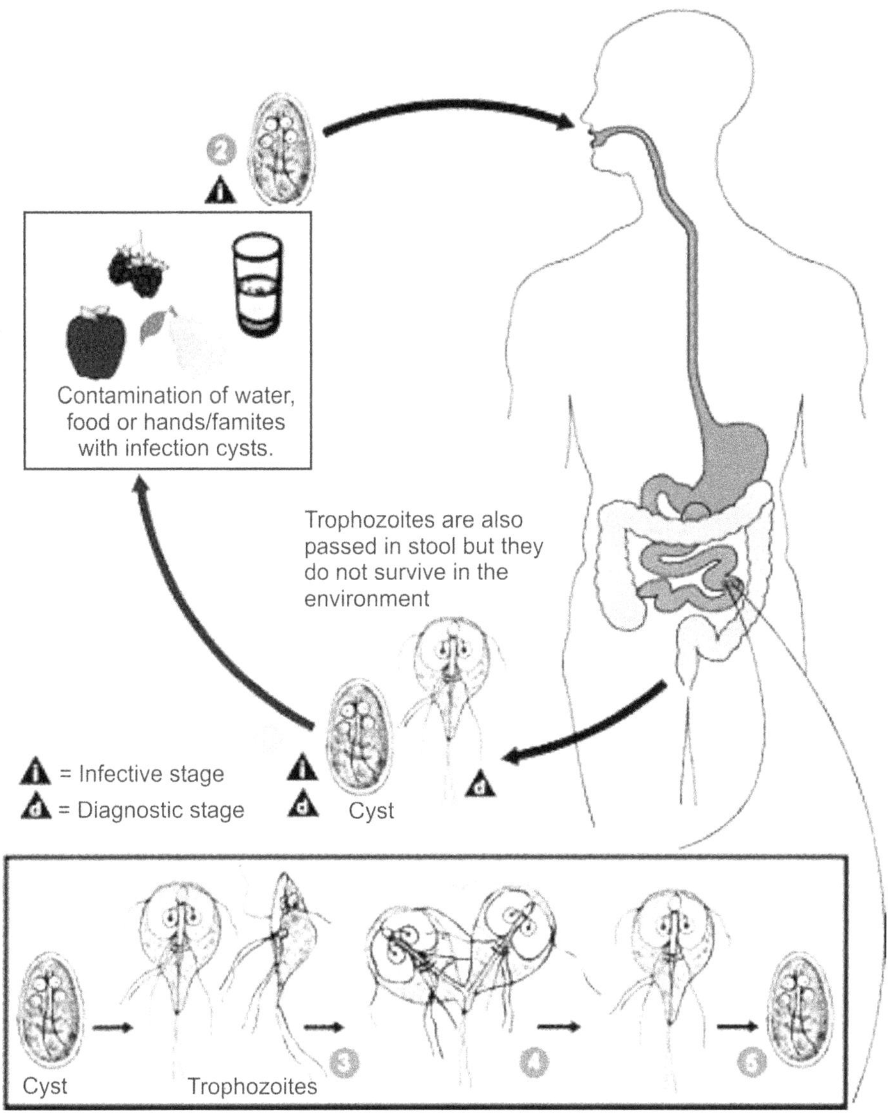

Figure 18.2 Life history of *Giardia lamblia.*

The signs and symptoms of giardiasis are similar to those of other intestinal illnesses:

- Diarrhea
- Abdominal cramps
- Nausea

These symptoms can lead to weight loss and dehydration (loss of fluids). However, not all infected persons have symptoms. Giardiasis is diagnosed by examining a stool sample under a microscope to look for *Giardia* cysts. Because a stool sample might contain only a few cysts, and they can be easy to miss, diagnosis sometimes requires several tests over several days.

Treatment of this debilitating disease is usually accomplished using one of several drugs.

Metronidazole is the treatment of choice but benzimidazoles are now being used more frequently. Other treatments include quinacrine, paromomycin and furozolidone. Even through these drugs are all used to treat the same disease, their modes of action differ in all cases. However, resistance is increasing and new alternatives are being sought. New wave antigardials all appear to have their roots in natural herbal remedies.

1. Metronidazole: Discussed under antiamoebics
2. Mepacrine: Discussed under antimalarials
3. Quiniodochlor: Discussed under antiamoebics
4. Furazolidone

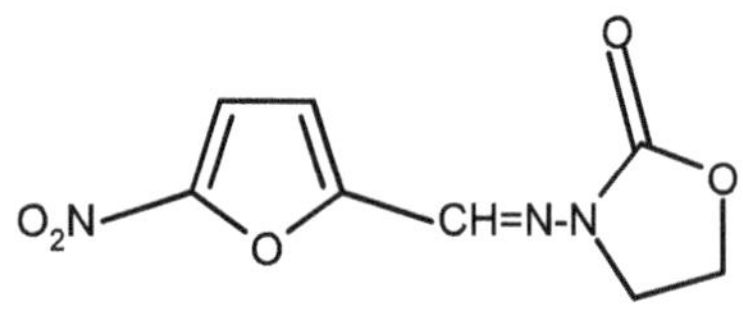

Furazolidone

Furazolidone is a synthetic nitro furan derivative that is an antibacterial and antiprotozoal agent.

It occurs as a yellow odorless crystalline powder with a bitter after taste. The drug is practically insoluble in water, alcohol and is decomposed by alkali. The drug should be protected by light because it darkens on exposure to strong light and thus should be stored in light resistant containers. Following oral administration, FZD is poorly absorbed and is inactivated in the intestine. About 5% of an oral dose of FZD is excreted in the urine as unchanged drug and metabolites, which may tint the urine brown.

Furazolidone is active against the protozoan *Giardia lamblia (Giardia intestinalis)* and against a range of bacteria *in vitro* including *staphylococci, enterococci*, *Escherichia coli, Salmonella* spp., *Shigella* spp., and *Vibrio cholerae.* It is bactericidal and appears to act by interfering with bacterial enzyme systems. It is used in the treatment of giardiasis, trichomoniasis, cholera and other vibrio infections. It has been suggested for other bacterial gastrointestinal infections but antibacterial therapy with furazolidone is regarded as unnecessary in mild and self-limiting gastro-enteritis. However, it has been reported to possess anti-helicobacter activity and to have some ulcer-healing properties

Mechanism of action

Furazolidone is bactericidal due to its interference with several bacterial enzyme systems, possibly including prevention of acetylation of coenzyme A. It also acts as a monoamine oxidase (MAO) inhibitor.

Synthesis of furazolidone

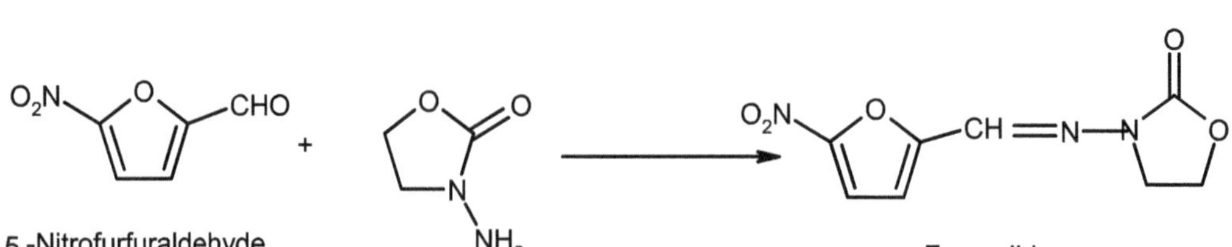

5 -Nitrofurfuraldehyde

Furazolidone

Trichomonacides

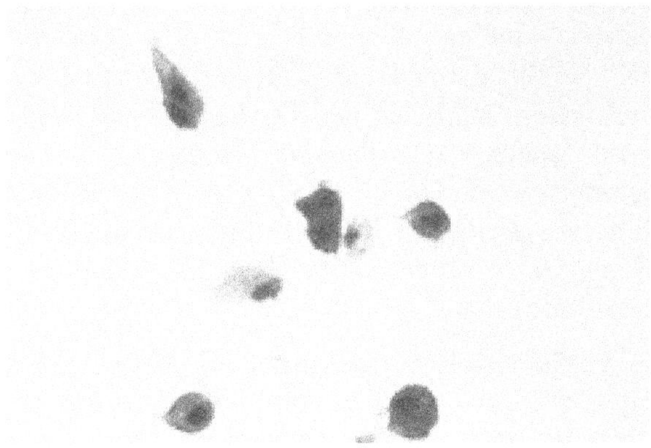

Figure 18.3 *Trichomonas vaginalis*

Trichomoniasis, sometimes referred to as "trich" or the ping pong disease, is a common sexually transmitted disease. It is caused by a single celled protozoan parasite *Trichomonas vaginalis*. Trichomoniasis is primarily an infection of the genitourinary tract; the urethra is the most common site of infection in men, and the vagina is the most common site of infection in women. Trichomoniasis, like many other sexually transmitted diseases, often occurs without any symptoms. Men almost never have symptoms, while 20% of women are asymptomatic. When women have symptoms, they usually appear within 5 to 28 days of exposure. The symptoms in women include a heavy, yellow-green or gray vaginal discharge, discomfort during intercourse, vaginal odor, and painful urination. Irritation and itching of the female genital area, and on rare occasions, lower abdominal pain also can be present. In about two-thirds of infected females, there is edema, inflammation, cell hypertrophy and metaplasia. The symptoms in men, if present, include a thin, whitish discharge from the penis and painful or difficult urination.

Trichomoniasis can usually be cured with the prescription drug, metronidazole, given by mouth in a single dose which is already discussed under antiamoebics.

Nimorazole

Nimorazole is 4-[2-(5-nitro-11*H*-imidazol-1-yl)ethyl]morpholine. It is an antitrichomonal agent which is effective either topically or orally and whose urinary metabolites are also trichomonicidal.

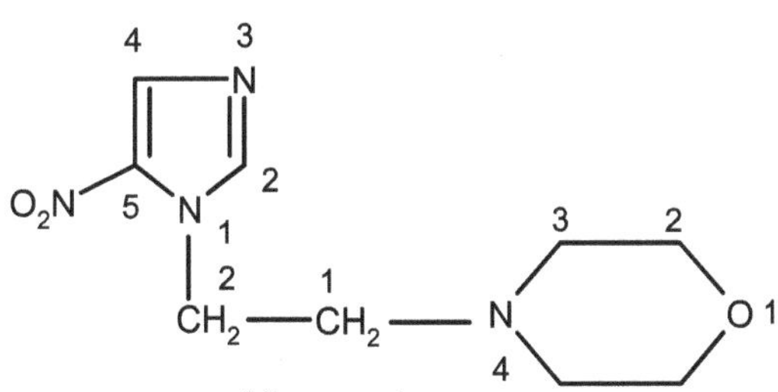

Nimorazole

Leishmanicides

Leishmaniasis is a disease caused by parasites that belong to the genus *Leishmania* and is transmitted by the bite of certain species of sandfly, including flies in the genus *Lutzomyia* in the new world and phlebotomus in the old world. Synonyms for leishmaniasis include kala azar, black fever, sandfly disease, dum-dum fever and espundia. Most forms of the disease are transmittable only from animals (zoonosis), but some can be spread between humans. Human infection is caused by about 21 of 30 species that infect mammals. These include the *Leishmania donovani* complex with three species (*Leishmania donovani, Leishmania infantum*, and *Leishmania chagasi*); the *Leishmania mexicana* complex with 3 main species (*Leishmania mexicana, Leishmania amazonensis*, and *Leishmania venezuelensis*); *Leishmania tropica; Leishmania major; Leishmania aethiopica*; and the subgenus *Viannia* with four main species (*Leishmania (Vianna) braziliensis, Leishmania (Viannia) guyanensis, Leishmania (Viannia) panamensis*, and *Leishmania (Viannia) peruviana*).

Leishmaniasis is transmitted by the bite of female phlebotomine sandflies. The sandflies inject the infective stage, promastigotes, during blood meals (1). Promastigotes that reach the puncture wound are phagocytized by macrophages (2) and transform into amastigotes (3). Amastigotes multiply in infected cells and affect different tissues, (4). This originates the clinical manifestations of leishmaniasis. Sandflies become infected during blood meals on an infected host when they ingest macrophages infected with amastigotes (5, 6). In the sandfly's midgut, the parasites differentiate into promastigotes (7), which multiply and migrate to the proboscis (8).

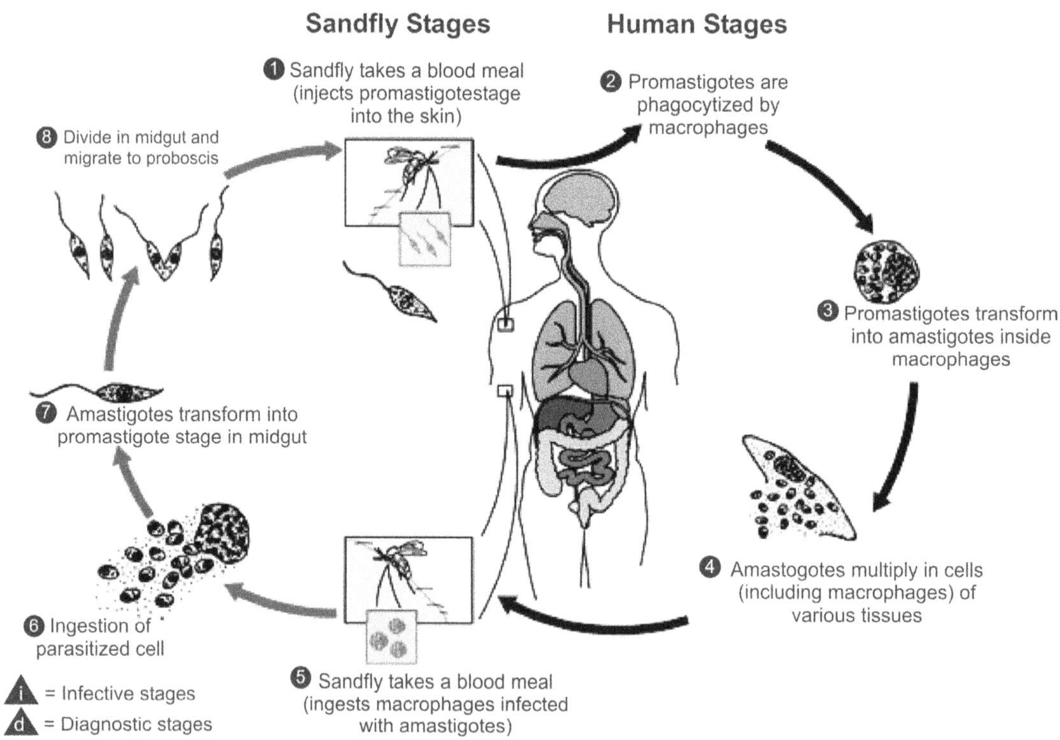

Figure 18.4 Life history of Leishmania parasites.

Signs and symptoms

The symptoms of leishmaniasis are skin sores which erupt weeks to months after the person affected is bitten by sand flies. Other consequences, which can become manifest anywhere from a few months to years after infection, include fever, damage to the spleen and liver, and anaemia.

There are four main forms of leishmaniasis:

- Visceral leishmaniasis - the most serious form and potentially fatal if untreated.
- Cutaneous leishmaniasis - the most common form which causes numerous sores on the body, which heal within a few months leaving unpleasant looking scars.
- Diffuse cutaneous leishmaniasis - this form produces widespread skin lesions which resemble leprosy and is particularly difficult to treat.
- Mucocutaneous leishmaniasis - commences with skin ulcers which spread causing tissue damage to (particularly) nose and mouth

The following Drugs are employed to treat leishmaniasis :

1. **Sodium stibogluconate**: Sodium stibogluconate it is a 2,2:2'4'-O-(oxydistibylidyne)bis[D-gluconic acid]. a pentavalent antimony derivative produced by the reaction of stibonic and gluconic acids, is the drug of choice for the treatment of leishmaniasis. It has been reported to be a complex mixture rather than a single compound.

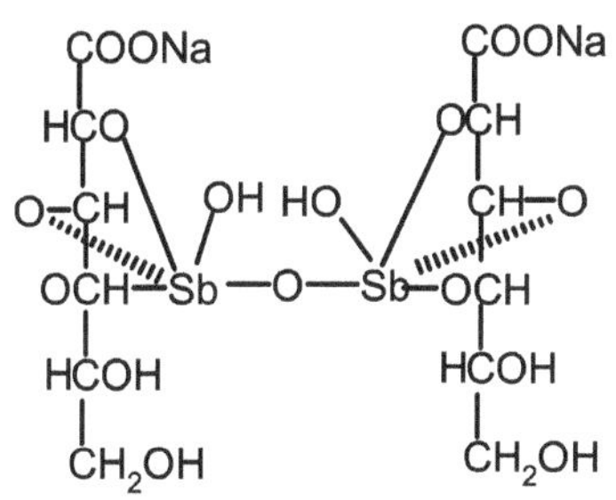

Sodium stibogluconate

2. **Meglumine antimonate (Glucantime; Merial):** Meglumine antimonate (Glucantime), a drug of choice for the treatment of leishmaniasis, is produced by the reaction of pentavalent antimony with *N*-methyl-D-glucamine, (a carbohydrate derivative).

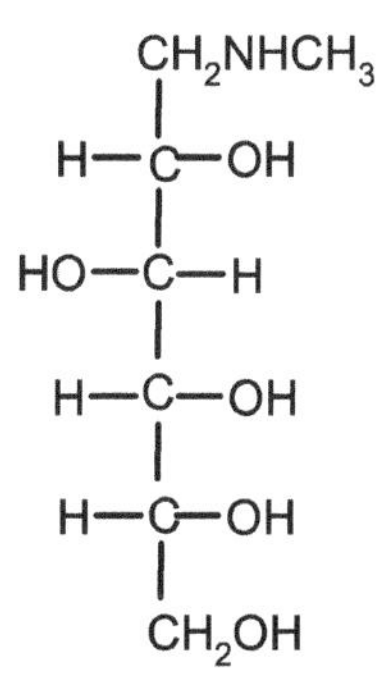

Meglumine

Meglumine antimonate blocks parasite metabolism by inhibition of parasite enzymes. It is administered by subcuticular injection.

3. **Pentamidine** isethionate is an antiparasitical/antiprotozoal drug primarily given for prevention and treatment of *Pneumocystis jiroveci pneumonia*, also formerly known as *Pneunocystis carinii pneumonia* (PCP), a type of pneumonia often seen in patients with HIV infection. Pentamidine has good clinical activity against the parasites causing Leishmaniasis. The exact nature of its antiprotozoal action is unknown. The drug has also activity against candida albicans in clinically relevant concentrations.

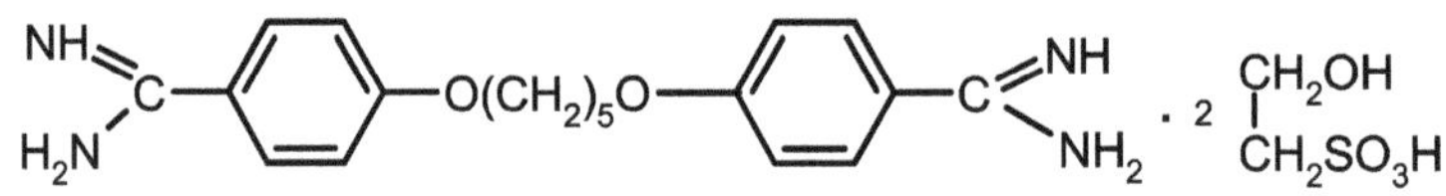

Pentamidine

4. **Allopurinol** is a white, powdery drug used to treat gout. Allopurinol is known chemically as 1, 5-dihydro-4H-pyrazolo [3,4-*d*]pyrimidin-4-one. Allopurinol is an analog of the natural purines in the body, and is quickly metabozied to oxipurinol which is also a xanthine oxidase inhibitor.

   It is a xanthine oxidase inhibitor which is administered orally and intravenously. It is a white amorphous mass. It has the structural formula below.

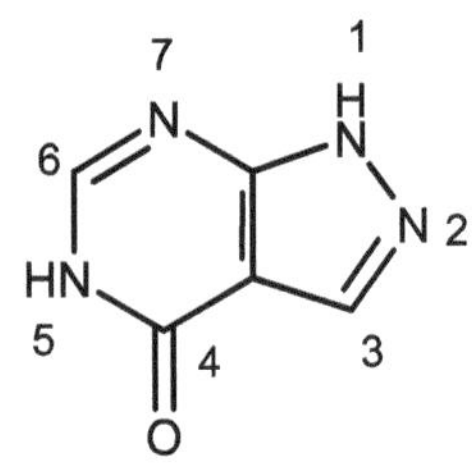

Allopurinol

It is an isomer of hypoxanthine and inhibits the production of uric acid, the metabolite responsible for gout, by inhibiting the enzyme xanthine oxidase. Allopurinol can also be given with some cancer treatments (E.g., CHOP) that increase uric acid (tumor lysis syndrome), as well as for kidney stones. These treatments result in large numbers of cells being disposed off by the body, which releases uric acid as part of the breakdown of DNA.

19

ANTHELMINTICS

Helminthiasis is a disease in which a part of the body is infested with worms such as pinworm, roundworm or tapeworm. Typically, the worms reside in the gastrointestinal tract but may also burrow into the liver and other organs. Worms may also be called helminths, especially the Nematoda (roundworms) and Cestoda (tapeworms).

Anthelmintics are group of drugs that are selectively toxic to parasites. These drugs act by either inhibiting the metabolic process vital to the parasite, or by causing the parasite to be exposed to a higher concentration of drug than the host cells. They can accomplish during the treatment by: interfering with the integrity of parasite cells, inhibiting neuromuscular transmission and coordination, or by interfering with the mechanisms which protect against host immunity that ultimately lead to the starvation, neuromuscular paralysis, death and expulsion of the parasite.

Anthelmintics can be administered by drench, paste, orally, or by injection. The drugs are absorbed into the blood stream and widely diffused. They are metabolized in liver and excreted in feces and urine.

Albendazole

Albendazole is an orally administered broad-spectrum anthelmintic. Chemically it is methyl 5-(propylthio)-2-benzimidazolecarbamate. Its molecular formula is $C_{12}H_{15}N_3O_2$ S and has the following chemical structure:

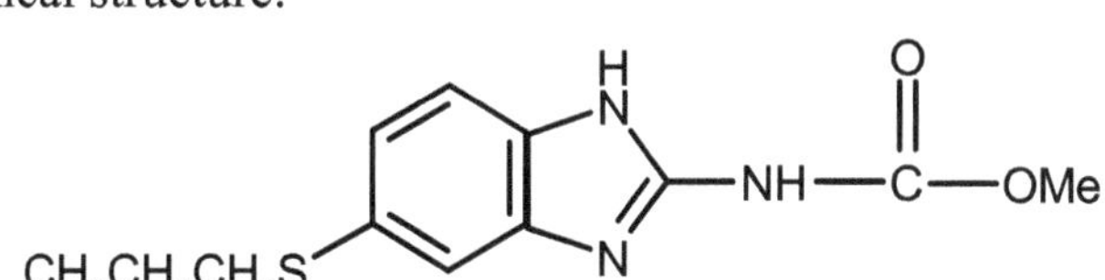

Albendazole

Albendazole is synthesized by the following steps:

1. 2-Nitro-4-mercaptoacetanilide is etherified with n-propylbromide to yield 2-nitro-4-(propylthio)acetanilide

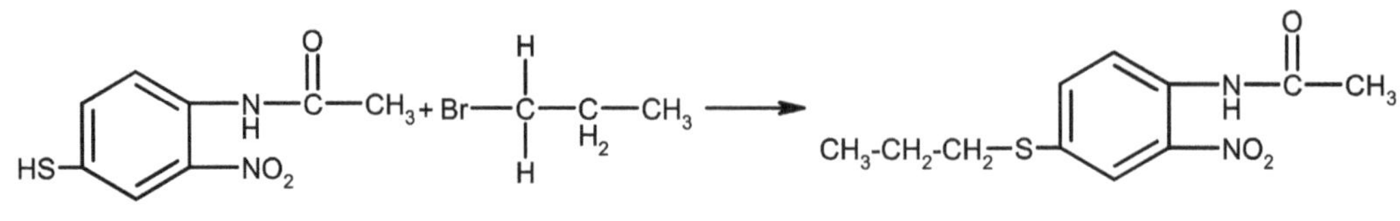

2. 2-Nitro-4-(propylthio)acetanilide is hydrolyzed and reduced($SnCl_2$)

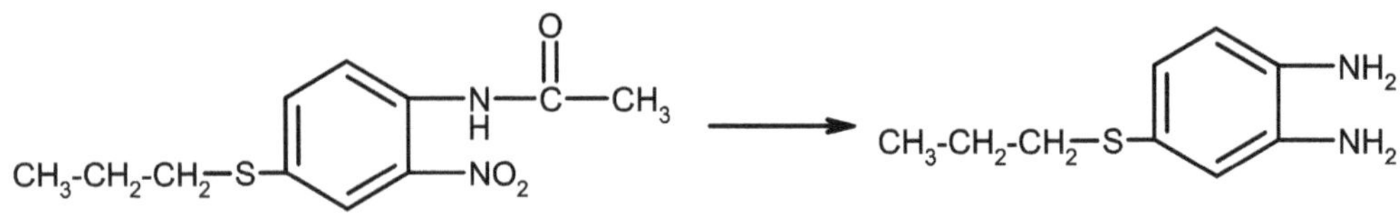

3. The above diamine is converted into albendazole by following reactions

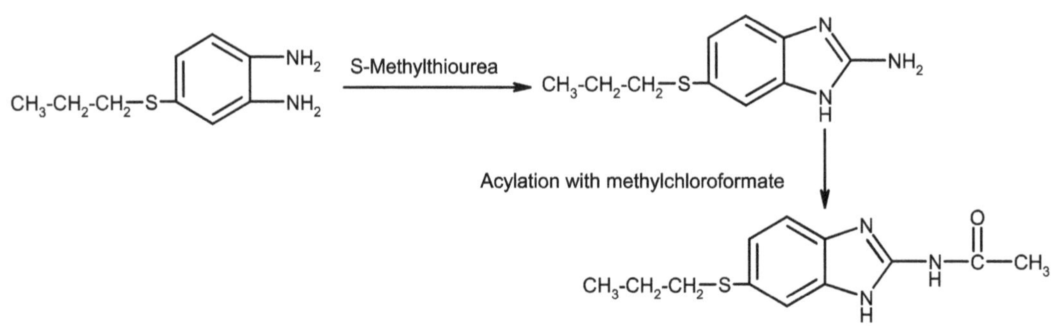

Albendazole is available as white colour powder. It is insoluble in water but freely soluble in dimetuylsulphoxide, strong acids and strong bases. Albendazole is rapidly metabolized to albendazole sulphoxide (active methabolite).

Albendazole is used to treat infections caused by worms such as pork tapeworm and dog tapeworm. It prevents worms from growing or multiplying in body. It is also used as an adjuvant in the treatment of hydatid disease (hydatid disease is caused by the parasite *Echinococcus granulosus* or *Echinococcus multilocularis* and presents as fluid-filled sacs (cysts) that grow in the liver, lungs and brain of infected individuals).

Albendazole works by interfering with proteins of either the worms of intestine or absorptive cells. This leads to the worm not being able to absorb sugars, which are essential for the survival. Therefore the energy stores of the worm are depleted, and this leads to its eventual death within several days (Albendazole interferes with various energy-producing processes of helminths (worms), including impairing the uptake of glucose (sugar) for energy).

Mebendazole

Mebendazole is methyl(6-benzoyl-1H-benzimidazol-2-yl) carbomate. Mebendazole is a drug used to combat pinworms, roundworms and hookworms. It causes slow immobilization and death of the worms by selectively and irreversibly blocking uptake of glucose and other nutrients in susceptible adult intestine where helminthes dowell. Oral dosage is 100 mg

12 hourly for 3 days, although sometimes the dosage is just 100 mg dose, followed by another dose two weeks later if the infection has not cleared up. The dosage may differ depending on which type of worm someone is infected with.

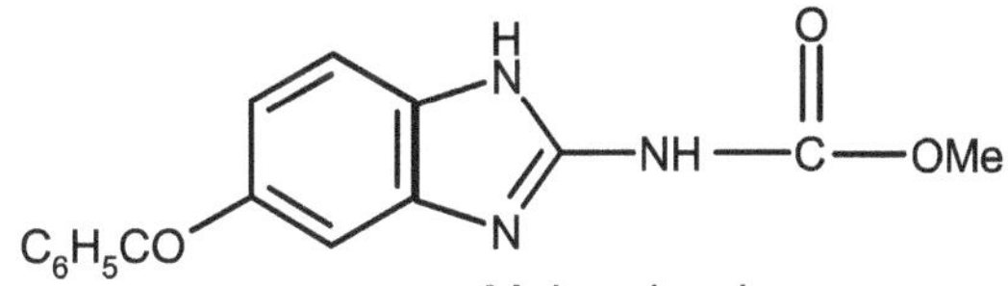

Mebendazole

Thiabendazole

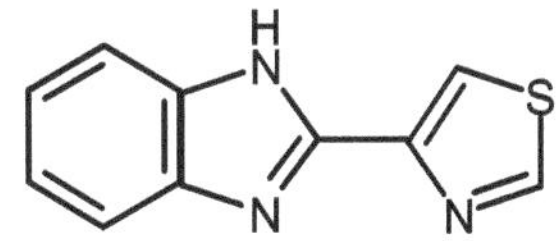

Thiabendazole

Thiabendazole is 2-(4[1]-thiazolyl) benzimidazole. It is a fungicide and parasiticide used primarily to control mold, and other fungal diseases in fruits and vegetables. It is able to control roundworms, hookworms, and other helminth species, which attack wild animals, livestock and humans. Thiabendazole is applied to some bananas, 'to ensure freshness'. It is also a chelating agent, which means that it is used medicinally to bind metals in cases of metal poisoning, such as lead poisoning, mercury poisoning or antimony poisoning.

Niclosamide

Niclosamide is 5-chloro-N-(2-chloro-4-nitrophenyl)-2-hydroxy benzamide. Niclosamide is especially effective against cestodes. It is used specifically to treat tapeworms and is not effective against pinworms or roundworms.

Niclosamide has three major mechanisms of action affecting cestodes: inhibition of glucose uptake, inhibition of energy production by anaerobic metabolism, and inhibition of inorganic phosphate incorporation into ATP. The drug affects the scolex (head) and proximal segments of the cestode leading to detachment of the scolex from the intestinal wall. Once detached, the tapeworm is removed from the intestine by the normal peristaltic action of the host's bowel. Niclosamide is administred orally. Niclosamide is prepared by condensing 5-chlorosalicylic acid with 3-chloro-4-aminonitrobenzene in presence of $SOCl_2$-C_6H_5Cl-pyridine system.

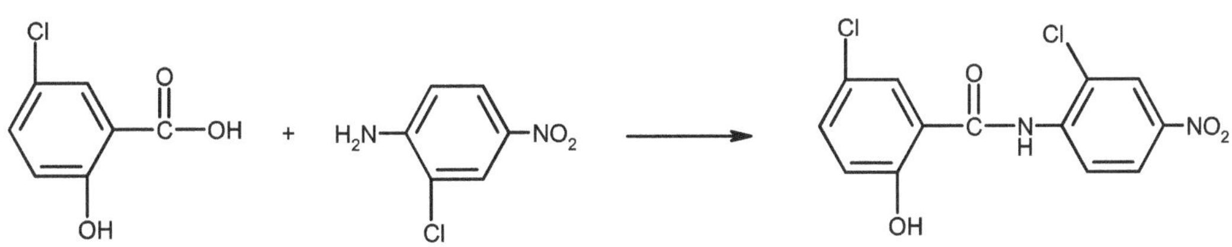

5-Chloro-2-hydroxy benzoic acid

2-Chloro-4-nitro aniline

Nicloxamide

Pyrantel pamoate

Pyrantel pamoate is Trans-1,4,5,6-tetrahydro-1-methyl-2-[2-(2[1]-thienyl)ethenyl]pyrimidine pamoate. Pyrantel is indicated in the treatment of ascariasis caused by *Ascaris lumbricoides*, enterobiasis (oxyuriasis) caused by *Enterobius vermicularis (Oxyuris vermicularis)* (pinworm), multiple helminth infections, hookworm infection (uncinariasis) caused by *Ancylostoma duodenale* (common hookworm; Old world hookworm), *Necator americanus*

(American hookworm; New world hookworm) and trichostrongyliasis caused by *Trichostrongylus* species. It is not vermicidal or ovicidal but acts as a depolarizing neuromuscular blocking agent, thereby causing sudden contraction, followed by paralysis, of helminthes. It is also act as a cholinesterase inhibitor and ganglionic stimulant. Helminths are rendered unable to maintain their position in the intestinal lumen and are expelled from the body in the fecal stream by peristalsis.

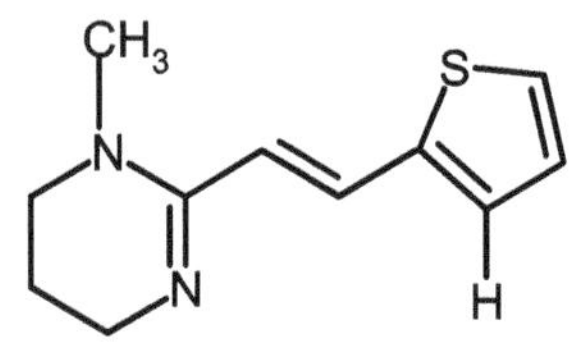
Pyrantel

Pyrantel is poorly and incompletely absorbed from gastrointestinal tract.

Morantel tartrate

Chemically morantel tartrate is [1,4,5,6-tetrahydro-l-methyl-2-[-2-(3-methyl-2-thienyl)vinyl]pyrimidine tartrate]. It is an anthelmintic effective against mature and immature nematodes that infect ruminants. It has been approved for the control of gastrointestinal nematode infections.

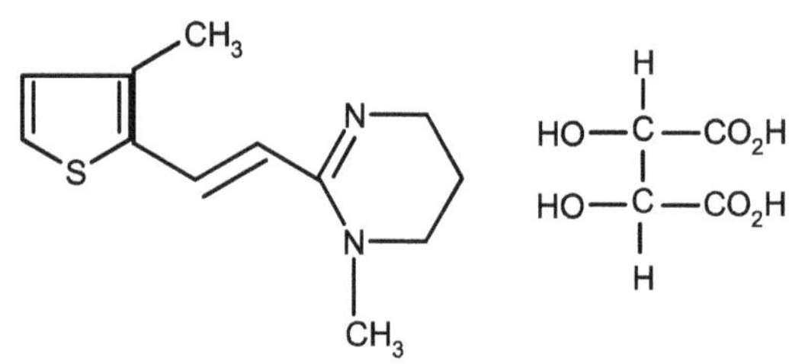
Morantel tartrate

Piperazine

Piperazine is an alternative for the treatment of the nematodes *Ascaris lumbricoides*, and *Enterobius vermicularis*. Piperazine increases the resting potential of the helminth muscle result in parxylsis of ascoris muscles. It has also been shown to block the response of ascaris muscle to acetylcholine. The paralyzed worm is expelled by the normal peristaltic action of the host.

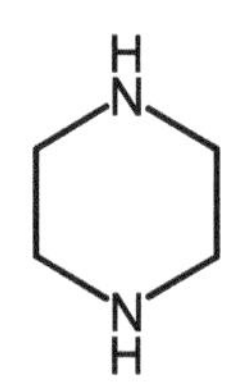
Piperazine

Piperazine is synthesized by condensing ethylene chloride with alcoholic ammonia (Hofmann amine synthesis).

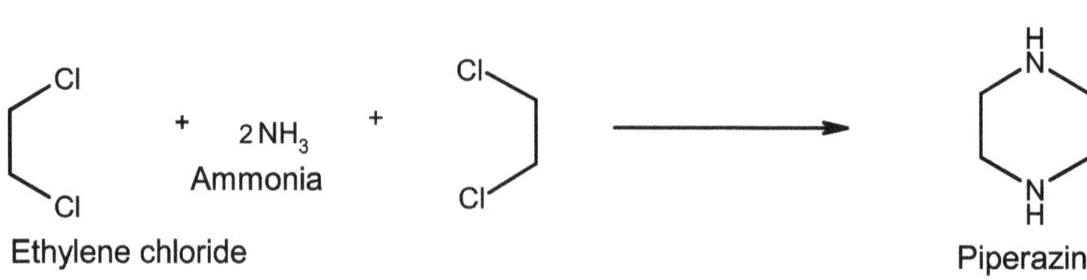

Piperazine is administered orally and is readily absorbed from the intestinal tract. Therapeutic doses do not usually cause adverse side effects, but muscular weakness, vertigo, speech difficulty, confusion, and myoclonic contractions can occur with an overdose or with accumulation in renal insufficiency. These symptoms will usually disappear when the drug is discontinued. Piperazine may induce epileptic seizures hence it is contraindicated in epileptics and in individuals with renal or hepatic insufficiency.

Praziquantel

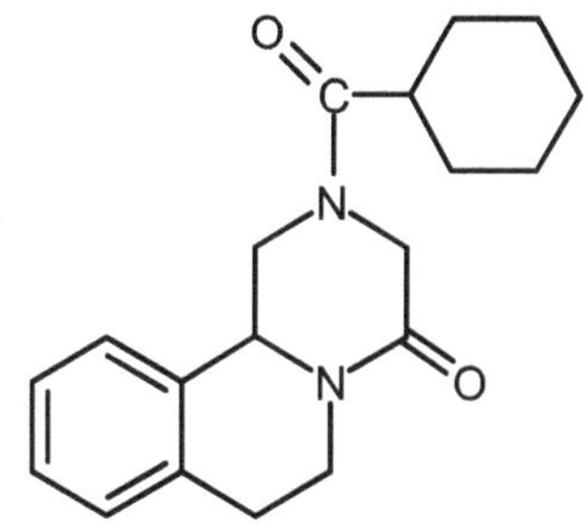
Praziquantel

Praziquantel is 2-(cyclohexylcarbonyl)-1,2,3,6,7,11b-hexahydro-4H-pyrazino[2,1-a]isoquinolin-4-one.
Praziquantel is the drug of choice in the treatment of blood trematodes. It is the latest and most effective drug used in the treatment of schistosomciasis. It is active against all 3 major species: *Schistosoma haematobium, Schistosoma mansoni,* and *Schistosoma japonicum.* Praziquantel may also be the drug of choice in the treatment of beef, pork, fish and dwarf tapeworms.

Mechanism of action

Praziquantel act by causing severe spasms and paralysis of the worms' muscles. This paralysis is accompanied by a rapid Ca^{+2} influx inside the schistosome. Morphological alterations are another early effect of praziquantel. These morphological alterations are accompanied by an increased exposure of schistosome antigens at the parasite surface. The worms are then either completely destroyed in the intestine or passed in the stool.

Diethylcarbamazine

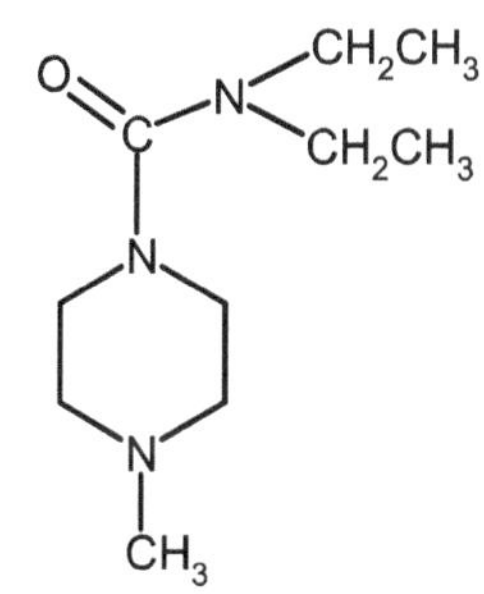
Diethylcarbamazine

Diethylcarbamazine is N,N-diethyl-4_methyl-1-piperzinecarboxamide citrate. Diethylcarbamazine ($C_{10}H_{21}N_3O$) is an anthelmintic drug that does not resemble other antiparasitic compounds. It is a synthetic organic compound, which is highly specific for several parasites and does not contain any toxic metallic elements.

It is prepared by acylating piperazine with diethylcarbamoyl chloride and then methylation at N_4-position(HCHO and HCOOH).

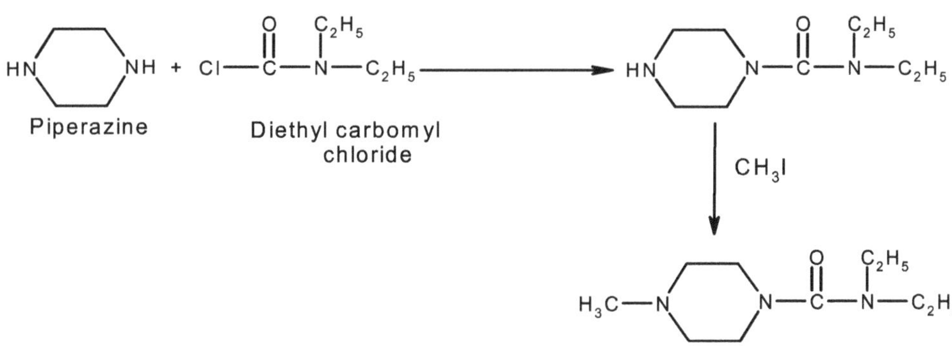

Diethylcarbamazine

Diethylcarbamazine citrate has been used in the treatment and control of lymphatic filariasis (caused by the nematodes *Wuchereria bancrofti*, *Brugia malayi* and *Brugia timori*) since 1947. It is known to interact with the arachidonic acid pathway and also has anti-inflammatory properties, as a result of its interference with arachidonic acid metabolism

Levamisole

Levamisole hydrochloride is (-)-(as)-2,3,5,6-tetrahydro-6-phenylimidazo [2,1-b] thiazole monohydrochloride. It is available as white or almost white crystalline powder and is freely soluble in water. It is quite stable in aqueous acidic media but hydrolyzes in alkaline or neutral solutions.

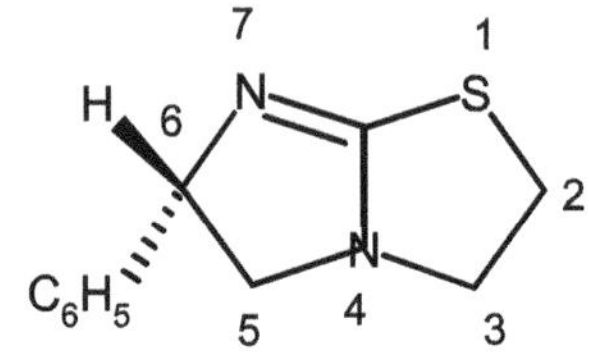

Levamisole

It is active against many nematodes but is restricted to ascaris and ancylostomiasis because action on other worms is poor. Levamisole hydrochloride is an immunomodulator and is also used in the treatment of colon cancer.

20

ANTIFUNGAL AGENTS

Introduction

The true fungi are classified into four groups as *Phycomyceters* (algae like), *Ascmycetes* (Sac-fungi), *Basidiomycetes* (mushrooms) and *Deuksomycetes* (imperfect-fungi). Although thousands of fungal species are found in the environment, only about 50 can produce diseases in humans. The cells of fungi that are pathogenic for animals are non-motile and generally have a rigid cell wall containing chitin and polysaccharide. Fungal cell membranes contain ergosterol and zymosterol (except pneumocysis) whereas animal cell membranes have cholesterol. Fungal infections are spread worldwide due to poor host resistance. These infections are generally resistant to antibiotics used in the treatment of bacterial infections. Fungi may also invade the skin to cause the subcutaneous infections. It is difficult to treat systematic mycoses.

Fungal infections may be classified as 1. Superficial, affecting only skin, hair, nails mucous membranes and 2. Systematic, affecting the body as a whole. The antifungal agents are used to treat superficial, systemic fungal infections.

Classification of antifungal agents

The antifungal agents are classified as follows:

1. Antibiotics - E.g., Amphotericin-B, griseofulvin.
2. Carbanlic acid derivatives - E.g., Tolnaftate.
3. Allylamines - E.g., Naftifine, terbinafine.
4. Azoles - E.g., Ketoconazole, miconazole, fluconazole.
5. Pyrimidine derivatives - E.g., 5-Flurocytosine.
6. Acids and their salts: - E.g., Benzoic acid, salicylic acid, undedecero acid.
7. Miscellaneous - E.g., Chlorphenesin, clotrimazole.

Individual members

Antifungal antibiotics

Antifungal antibiotics are important antibiotics. These include polyenes and griseofulvin.

Amphotericin B

Chemistry

Amphotericin B is a (1R,3S,5R,6R,9R,11R,15S,16R,17R,18S,19E,21E,23E,25E,27E, 29E,31E,33R,35S,36R,37S)-33-{[(2R,3S,4S,5S,6R)-4-amino-3,5-dihydroxy-6-methyloxan-2-yl]oxy}-1,3,5,6,a,11,17,37-octahydroxy-15-16,18-trimethyl-13-oxo-14,39-dioxabicyclo [33.3.1]nonatriaconta-19,21,23,25,27,29,31-heptaene-36-carboxylic acid. Amphotericin B polyene antifungal antibiotic produced by *Streptomyces nodosus*. It consists of seven conjugated double bonds and a highly substituted monocylic lactone as aglycone. It has the following structure.

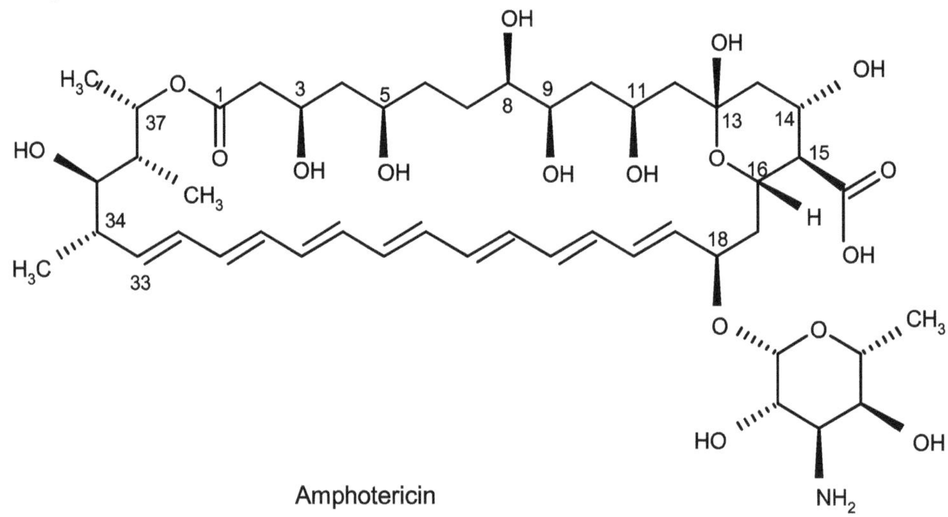

Amphotericin

Properties

It shows the following properties:

1. Amphotericin B is an yellow to orange colored, odorless, water insoluble powder. It is insoluble in ether and alcohol but soluble in DMSO and propylene glycol.
2. It is amphoteric in nature due to the presence of a free amino and a carboxyl group.
3. It is poorly absorbed from gastro intestinal tract hence, it is administered as intravenous infusion.

Mechanism of action

Amphotericin B act by disrupting the cell membrane by binding to ergosterol (in fungi). It produces pores in the cell membrane causes the electrolytes and small molecules to leak from the cell, resulting in cell death. Intermoleculer hydrogen bonding interactions of carboxyl, hydroxyl and amino groups of amphotericin also help in destroying fungal cell membrane to leak cytoplasmic components. It has no antibacterial activity.

Uses

Amphotericin B is used to treat severe systemic mycotic infections like aspergillosis, blastomycosis, candidiasis, cryptococcosis, sporotrichosis either alone or in combination with other antifungals.

Nystatin

It is a polyene antifungal antibiotic complex containing 3 biologically active components A_1, A_2 and A_3 produced by *Streptomyces noursei.* Chemically it is 1*S*,3*R*,4*R*,7*R*, 9*R*,11*R*,15*S*,16*R*,17*R*,18*S*,19*E*,21*E*, 25*E*,27*E*,29*E*,31*E*,33*R*,35*S*,36*R*,37*S*)-33-[(3-amino-3,deoxy rahman

Structure

Nystatin A_1 or A_2 or A_3 composes a macrocylic lactone containing a ketal ring, a polyene system and a mycosamine moiety.

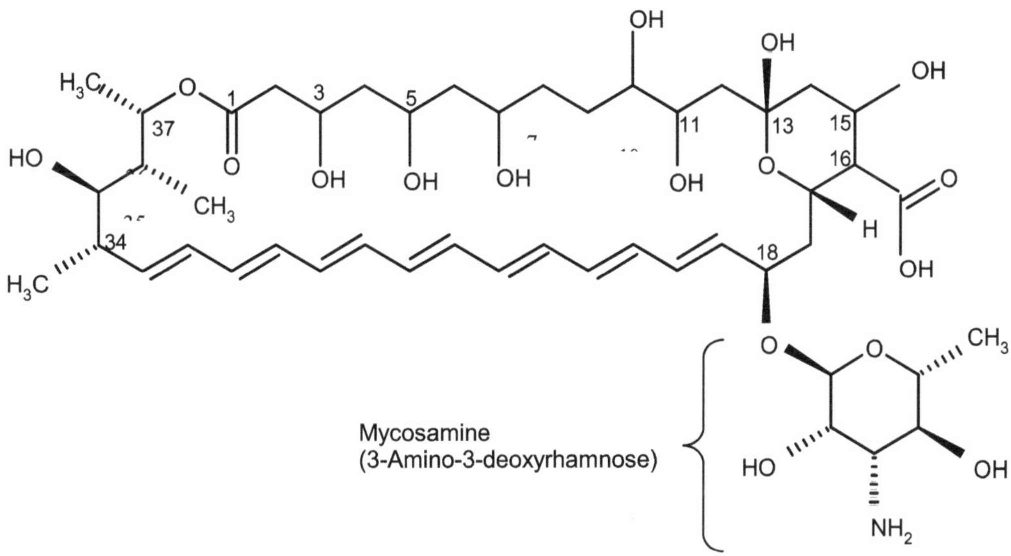

Nystation-A_1

Properties

It is light yellow powder. Gradually decomposes above 160°C.

Uses

Nystatin is used only as a topical agent (It is not absorbed by oral route and is too toxic by parenteral route) for treatment of local and gastro intestinal monilial infections caused by *Candida albicans* and other candida species.

Natamycin

It is polyene antibiotic produced by *Streptomyces natalensis*. Chemically it is 22-[(3-amino-3,6-dideoxy-β-D-mannopyranosyl)oxy]-1,3,26trihydroxy-12-methyl-10-oxo-6,11,28-trioxatricyclo[22,3.1.05,7] octacosa-8,14,16,18,20-pentaene-25-carboxylic acid.

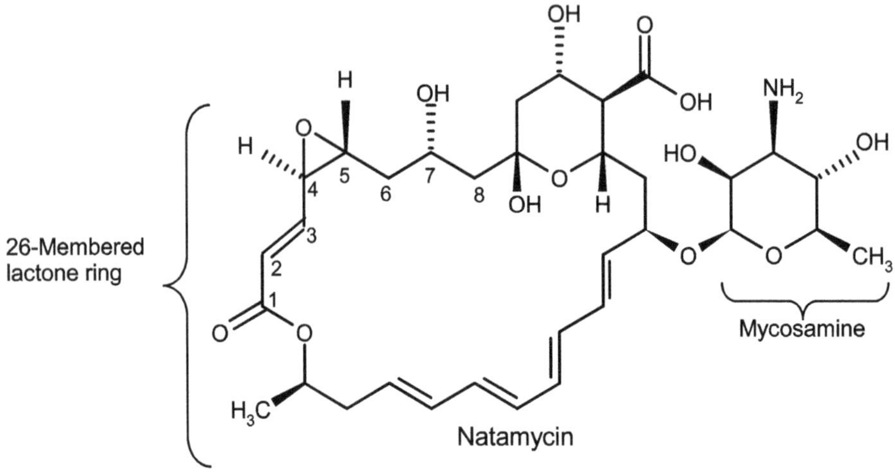

Natamycin

Griseofulvin

Chemistry

Griseofulvin it is a 7-chloro-2^1,4,6,-trimethoxy-6^1,β-methyl spiro[benzofuran-2(3H)-1^1-[2] cyclohexene 3,4'-done. Griseofulvin is an antibiotic produced by *Penicillium griseofulvum* possess the following structure:

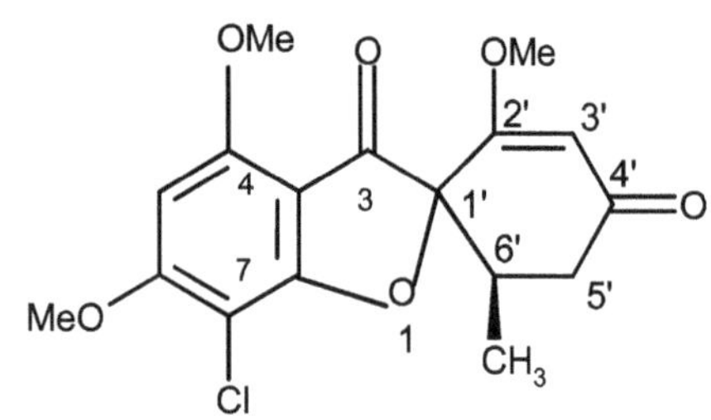

Griseofulvin

The fluoro derivatives of griseofulvin retain the antifungal activity but the bromo and dichloro derivatives are ineffective. The activity of griseofulvin increases by the replacement of methoxy group on cyclohexane ring with propoxy or butoxy group.

Properties

It shows the following properties:

1. Griseofulvin is available as a colorless, bitter taste crystalline solid, water insoluble powder.
2. It is sparigly soluble in water but relatively soluble in alcohol and in nonpolar organic solvents.

Mechanism of action

Griseofulvin inhibits fungal cell division by disrupting the mitotic spindle structure. It may also interfere with DNA production. Griseofulvin also act by inhibiting the synthesis of polysaccharides (chitin and glucan) of cell wall. It has no antibacterial activity.

Uses

1. Griseofulvin is a fungistatic antibiotic and is effective against dermatophytes (Microsporum, epidermophyton and trichophyton).
2. It is used for the systemic treatment of ringworm infections of the body, nails, hair and feet.

Carbonic acid derivatives

Tolnaftate

Chemistry

Tolnaftate is 2-Naphthyl-N-methyl-N-(3-tolyl)thionocarbamide. It is prepared by condensing N-methyl-*m*-tolylamine with 2-naphthyl chlorothionoformate in acetone solvent in presence of sodium bicarbonate.

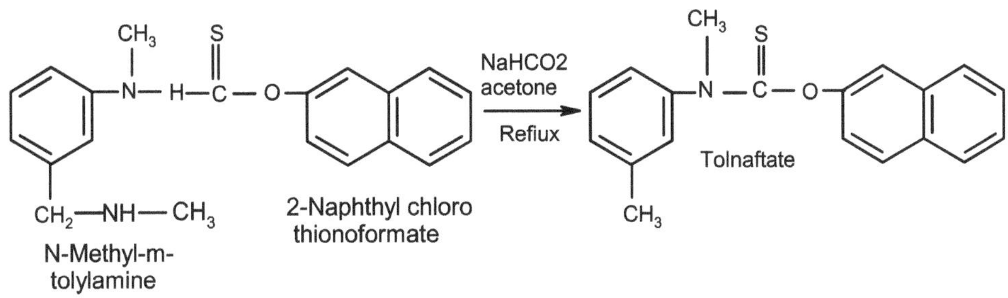

The antifungal activity of tolnaftate is maintained even if the aromatic methyl group is removed or replaced by hydroxy or methoxy or if the entire tolyl group is replaced by an α or β–naphthyl substituent.

The activity is lost if the aromatic methyl group is replaced by halogen or carboxyl or nitro group

The carbamate methyl group is essential for antifungal activity of tolnaftate.

Properties

Tolnaftate is colorless or cream colored, odorless powder. It is insoluble in water and freely soluble in chloroform.

Mechanism of action

Tolnaftate inhibits the enzyme squalene epoxidase which results in a decrease in total sterol content of the fungal cell membrane. Finally leads malfunction of the cell membrane and also leads deposition of squalene (hydrocarbon) which is toxic when present in high amounts.

Tolnaftate is effective against Trychophyton rubrum, Trichophyton mentagrophytes, Trychophyton tonsurans, Epidermophyton floccosum, Microsporum canis but it is in effective against Candida.

Uses

Tolnaftate is used as a topical antifungal agent as 1 % solution or powder or cream in the treatment of tinea infections and Pityriasis versicolour.

Allylamines

Allylamines includes naftifine and terbinafine. These drugs act by interfering with ergosterol biosynthesis i.e by inhibiting the enzyme squalene epoxidase. Inhibition of this enzyme results in decreased synthesis of sterol conbent which alters membrane integrity and loss of cell content. Inhibition of squalene epoxidase also causes the accumulation of squalene which itself shows fungicidal action. Allylamines do not inhibit significantly the mammalian cholesterol biosynthesis.

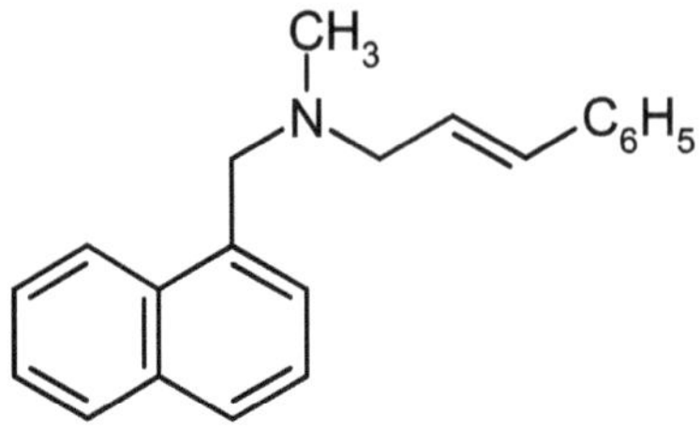

Naftifine

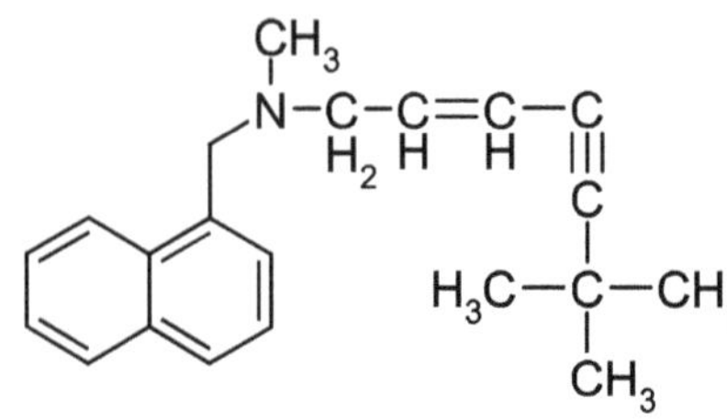

Terbinafine

Naftifine

Naftifine is N-methyl-N-(3(-phenyl-2-)-propenyl)-1-napthalenemethanamine hydrochloride. Naftifine is widely used against various tinea infections of skin.

Terbinafine

Terbinafine is a (E)-N-(6,6-dimethyl-2-hepten-4-ynyl)-N-methyl-1-naphthalene methanamine hydrochloride. Terbinafine is available both in topical and oral dosage forms. It is effective against a variety of dermatophytic infections mainly nail infection (onchomycoses).

Azoles

Azoles are a group of substituted imidazoles or 1,2,4-triazoles possess fungistatic activity (in lower concentration), fungicidal activity (in higher concentrations). They are synthetic antifungal drugs some are primarily used to treat superficial dermatophytic (*Trichophyton, Epidermophyton and Microsporum* spp) and yeast infections (*Candida albicans*) while others are orally administered to treat systemic fungal infections (*Coccidioidesimnoitis, Cryptococcus neoformans, Paracoccidioides brasiliensis, Pterillidium boydii, Blastomyces desmatitidis* and *Histoplasma capsulatum*).

Structure activity relationships

1. Azole derivatives possess a weakly basic imidazole or 1,2,4-triazole ring.

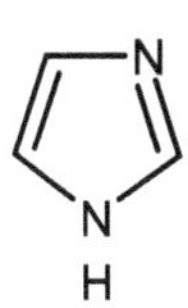

Imidazole

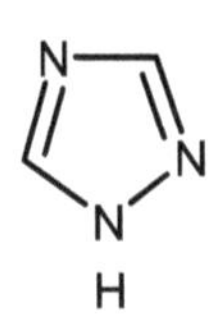

1, 2, 4-Triazole

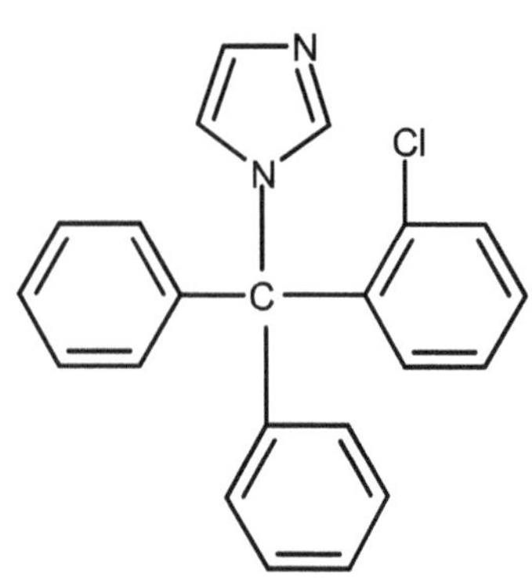

Clotrimazole

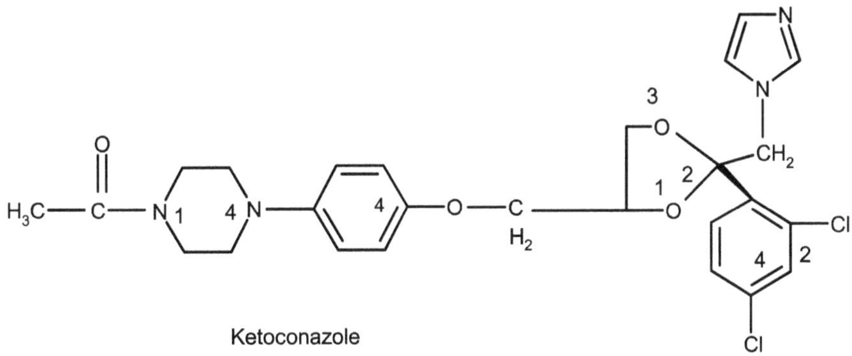

Ketoconazole

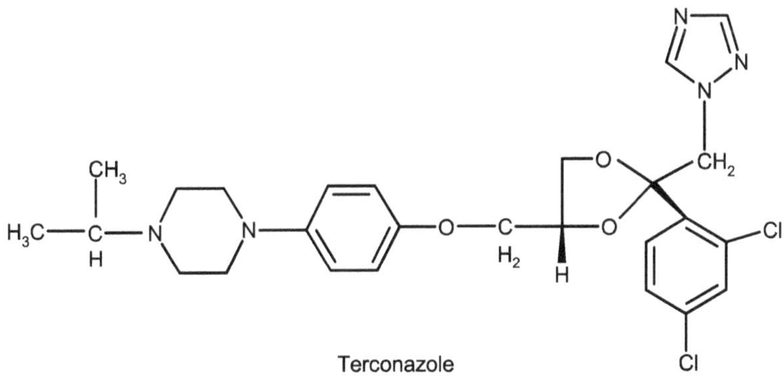

Terconazole

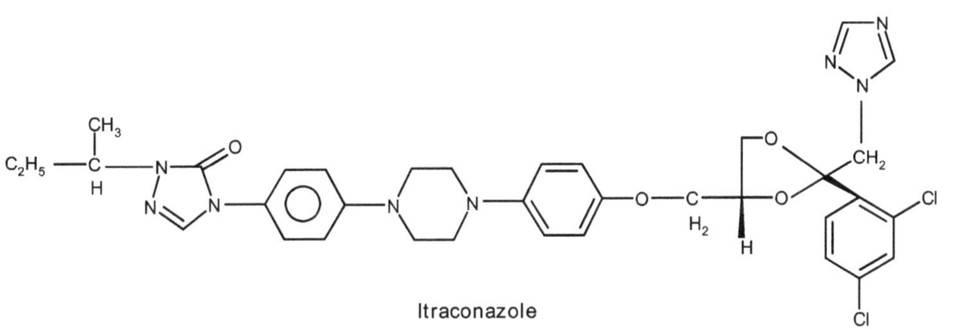

Itraconazole

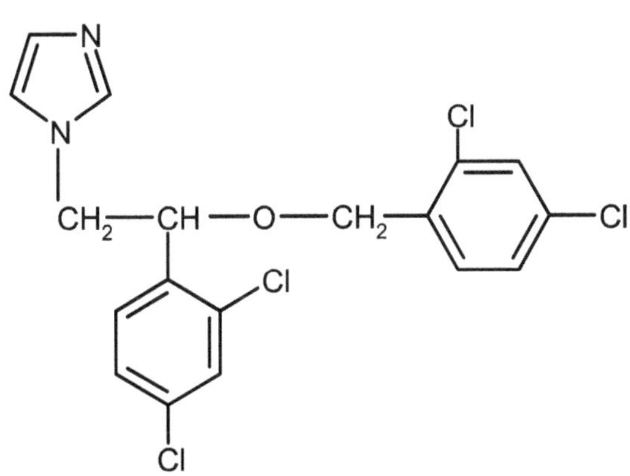

Miconazole

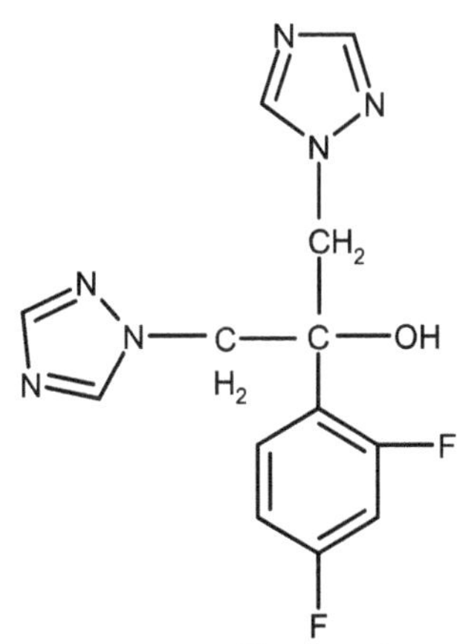

Fluconazole

Clotrimazole

Clotrimazole is 1-(o-chloro-α,α-diphenylbenzyl)-imidazole. Clotrimazole is an imidazole derivative. It is prepared by the reaction between imidazole and 2- chlorotriphenylmethyl chloride using trimethylamine as a base (proton acceptor).

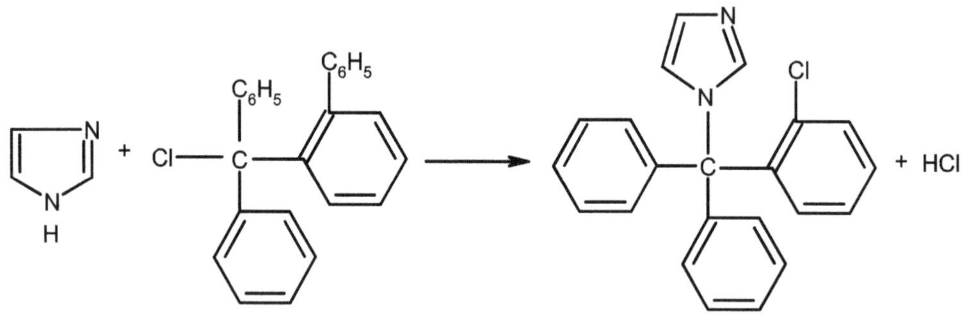

Clotrimazole is a colorless to pale yellow color crystalline powder. It is slightly soluble in water, soluble in alcohol, chloroform and melts at 142°C.

Miconazole

Chemistry

Miconazole is 1-[2-(2,4-dichlorophenyl)-2-[2,4-dichlorophenylmethoxy]ethyl] -1H-imidazole mononitrate. Miconazole is another imidazole derivative. The N-1 atom of five membered azole ring is linked to other aromatic rings via an aliphatic carbon atom or atoms.

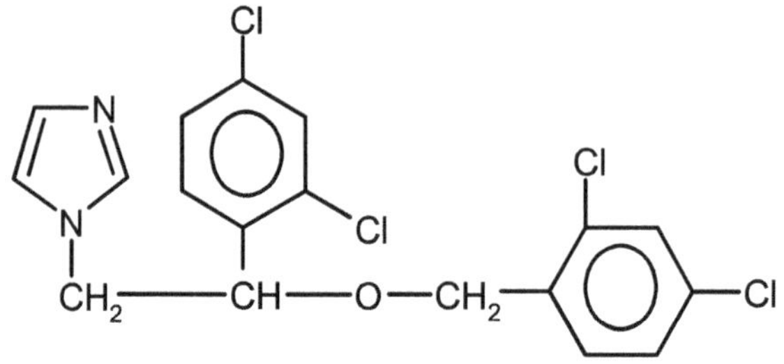

Miconazole

Mechanism of action

Miconazole is a broad spectrum antifungal agent. The antifungal activity of miconazole is by the inhibition of cytochrome P-450 which catalyses lanosterol to ergosterol. The N-3 atom of the azole ring binds to the ferric iron atom in the heme prosthetic group to prevent the activation of oxygen for insertion into lanosterol.

Properties

1. Miconazole is available as miconazole nitrate. Miconazole nitrate is a colorless, odorless, crystalline solid. It melts between 178°C to 184°C.
2. It is slightly soluble in water, ethanol and freely soluble in DMF and DMSO.

Uses

1. It is fungicidal to Aspergillus, Blastomyces, Candida, Cladosporium, Epidermophyton, Histoplasma, Madurella, Microsporum and Trichophyton.
2. Topically, it is used for vulvovaginal candidiasis.

Ketoconazole

Chemistry

Ketoconazole is 1-Acetyl-4-[4-[[2-(2,4-dichlorophenyl)-2(1H-imidazole-1-ylmethyl)-1H-1,2,4-triazole-1-ethanol. Ketoconazole is a synthetic imidazole derivative. It is synthesized from 2,4-dichloroacetophenone through the intermediate preparation of dioxolane. Dioxolane is prepared by the reaction of 2,4-dichloroacetophenone, glycerol and tosic acid. The obtained dioxolane is brominated, esterified, bromine is replaced by imidazole, saponified, and on treatment with mesylchloride and 4-acetyl piperazinyl phenol gives ketoconazole.

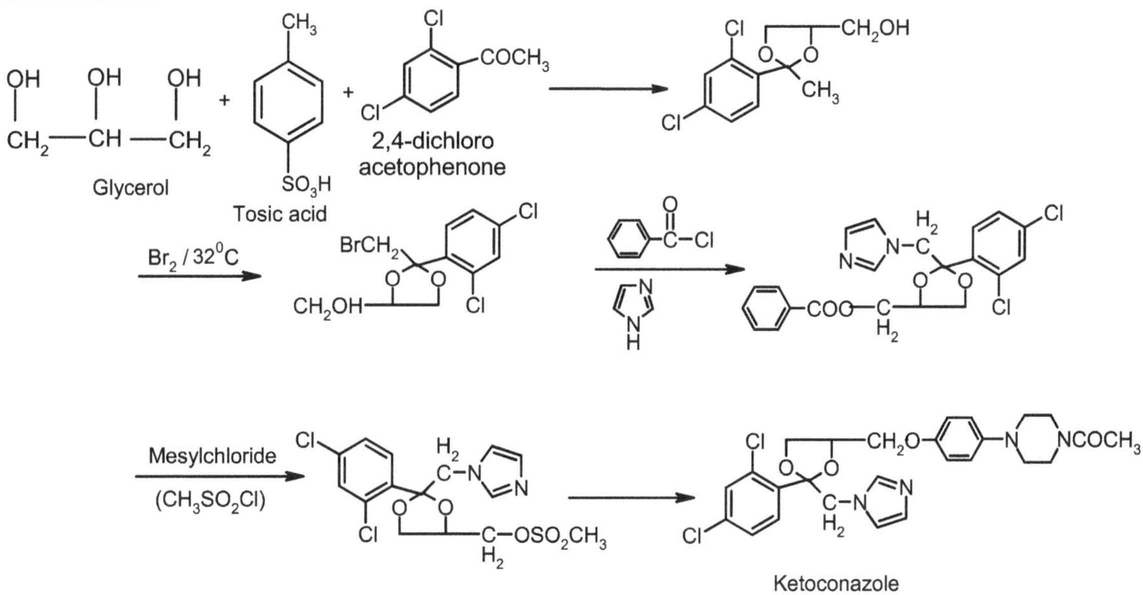

Properties

1. Ketoconazole is a colorless crystalline solid and is slightly soluble in water.
2. It is a weakly basic compound.

Mechanism of action

Ketoconazole is a broad-spectrum antifungal agent. It interferes with ergosterol synthesis and there by alters the permeability of the cell membrane of sensitive fungi. It is administered topically or orally.

Uses

Ketoconazole is recommended for the treatment of the systemic fungal infections like candidiasis, coccidioidomycosis, blastomycosis, histoplasmosis, chromomycosis, and paracocidiodiomycosis.

Fluconazole

Chemistry

Fluconazole is α-(2,4-difluorophenyl)-α-(1H-1,2,4-troazple-1-ylmethyl)-1H-1,2,4-triazole-1-ethanol. It possess two weakly basic triazole rings which imparts sufficient aqueous solubility and 2, 4-difluorophenyl group confers lipophilicity.

Fluconazole is fluorine containing triazole derivative having broad-spectrum antifungal activity. It is synthesized from 2,4-diflurobenzene by the following chemical reactions.

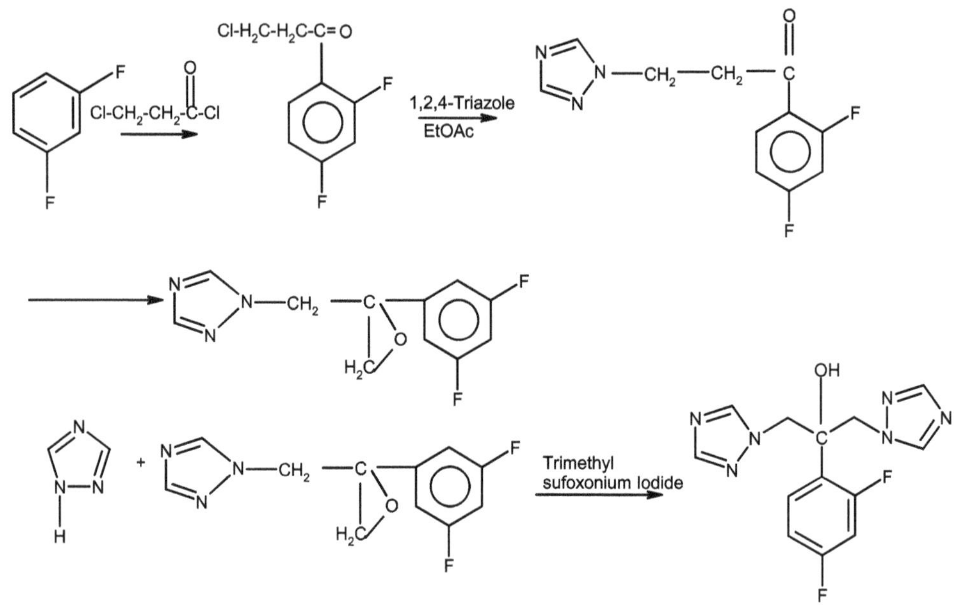

Mechanism of action

Fluconazole inhibits cytochrome P-450 dependent enzymes resulting in impairment of ergosterol synthesis in fungal cell membrane of the fungi. It is active against yeasts, dermatophytes and some mold. It has long elimination half life (27 to 35 hours).

Properties

It is colorless crystalline powder and is insoluble in water. It should be protected from light.

Uses

It is given by mouth or intravenous infusion in the treatment of candidiasis and to control esophageal or oropharyngeal candidiasis, vaginal candidis. It is also used to treat cryptococal meningitis and cryptococcosis in AIDS.

Pyrimidine derivatives

Flucytosine

Flucytosine 4–amino-5-fluoro-2(1H)-pyrimidinone,2-hydroxy-4-amino-5-fluropyrimidine. Flucytosine is a fluorinated pyrimidine. It is prepared from 5-fluorouracil by following chemical reactions. rfc

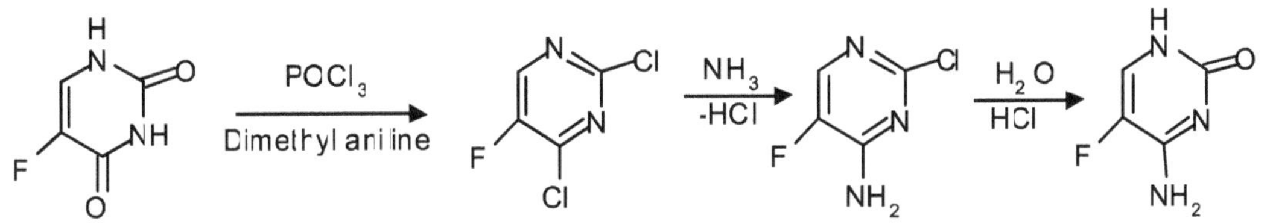

Flucytosine

Mechanism of action

Susceptible fungal cells deaminate S-flurocytosine to 5-fluorouracil. 5-Fluorouracil is metabolized to 5-fluro–2-deoxyuredylic acid which suppresses DNA synthesis by the inhibition of thymidylate synthetase.

Properties

(i) It is a colorless, crystalline powder.
(ii) It is sparingly soluble in water.

Uses

(i) Flucytosine inhibit the strains of Aspergillus, candida, cladosporium and cryptococcus.
(ii) This drug is well absorbed through the GIT, has fine penetration into CSF and is having low toxicity.

Undecylenic acid

Chemistry

Undecylenic acid is Undec-10-enoic acid. It is prepared by pyrolysis of ricinoleic acid (fatty acid of castor oil)

$$CH_3\,(CH_2)_5\,CHOH\,CH_2\,CH = CH\,(CH_2)_7\,COOH \longrightarrow$$
$$CH_2 = CH\,CH_2\,(CH_2)_7\,COOH + CH_3\,(CH_2)_5\,CHO \text{ (n - heptanal)}$$

Undecylenic acid

Properties

Undecylenic acid exhibits the following properties :

(i) It is available as colorless or pale yellow color liquid with bitter taste.
(ii) It is insoluble in water and freely soluble in alcohol, chloroform, ether.
(iii) It is stored in airtight containers at a temperature of 8°C –15°C.
(iv) It is available as zinc undecylenate powder.

Uses

1. It is fungistatic.
2. Undecylenic acid and its zinc salt are used in the treatment of dermatophytosis and tinea capitis fungal infections.

Benzoic acid

Benzoic acid contains not less than 99.5 % and not more than the equivalent of 100.5 % of $C_7H_6O_6$. It occurs as colourless, crystals or needles. Benzoic acid is slightly soluble in water but freely soluble in chloroform and in ether. It melts at 121°C. Benzoic acid is synthesised from toluene or benzaldehyde.

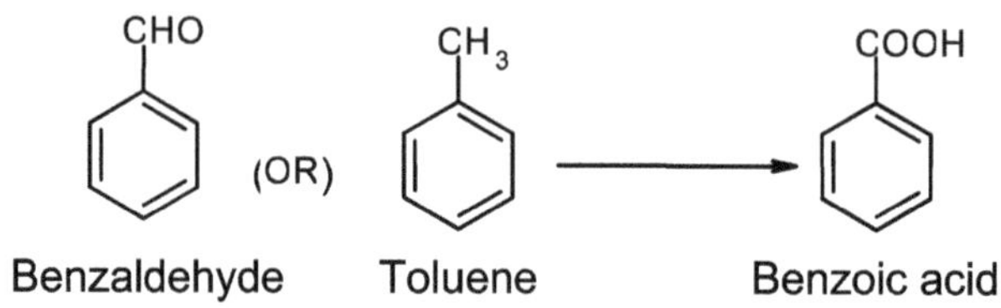

Benzoic acid in combination with salicylic acid used as antifungal agent. It used to treat athlete's foot and ring worm. It is also used as antiseptic in lotions, ointments and mouth washes etc.

Salicylic acid

Salicylic acid is 2-hydroxybenzoic acid. It is available as colorless, crystalline powder. It is slightly soluble in water but freely soluble in alcohol and in ether.

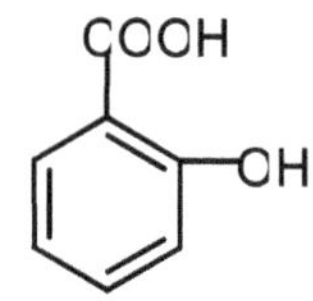

Salicylic acid

Salicylic acid is having antiseptic properties. It also acts as antifungal in 3% to 5% in the form of ointments, creams, lotions.

Phenols

Phenols are believed to destroy cell memb rane which results in loss of cellular components and death of cell.

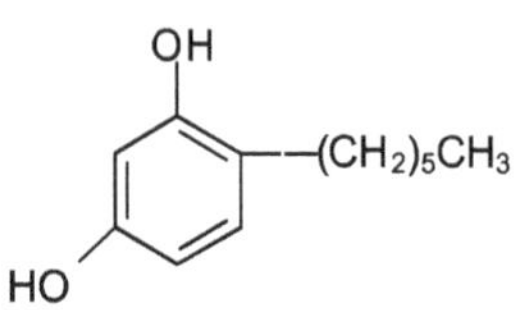

Hexylresorcinol

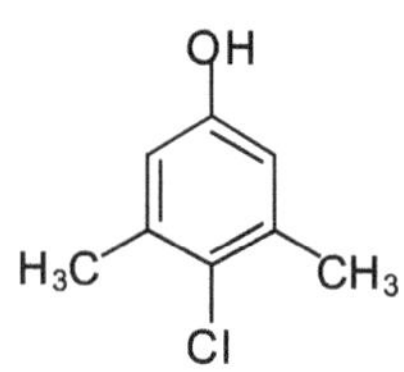

Chloroxylenol

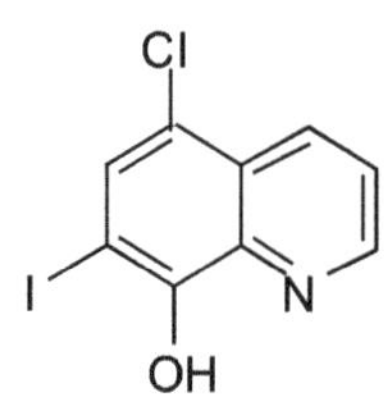

Clioquinol

21

ANTIVIRAL AGENTS

Introduction

Viruses are non-cellular obligate intracellular parasites. They lack both a cell wall and a cell membrane and do not carry out metabolic processes. Viral reproduction uses many of the host's metabolic processes and hence a few drugs are selective enough to prevent viral replication without injury to the host. Antimicrobial agents do not affect them. The drugs used for the prophylaxis (prevention) and therapy (treatment) of viral diseases are called antiviral agents.

Types of viruses

Adult viruses possess only one type of nucleic acid either DNA or RNA. They contain a protein coat that surrounds nucleic acid. The protein coat is known as capsid, which is made of smaller units (capsomers). Depending on virus, envelops may or may not covered with spikes(made of cabohydrate-protein complex).

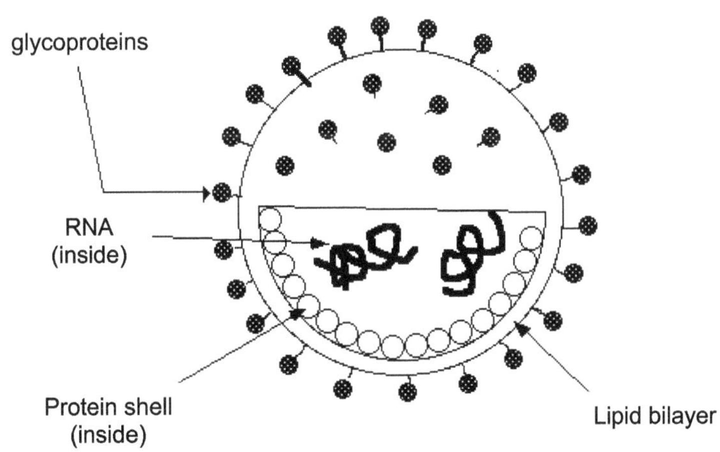

Figure 21.1 Structure of Virus.

Depending up on the nucleic acid content viruses were classified as RNA viruses and DNA viruses. RNA viruses are of two types: RNA viruses and retroviruses.

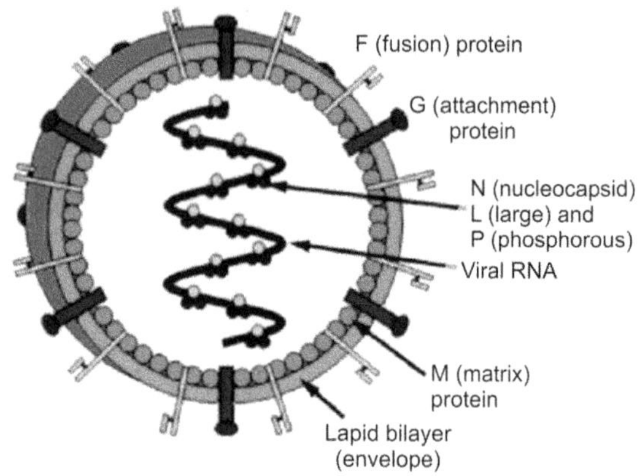

Figure 21.2 Structure of Hemipavirus.

The DNA viruses include the herpesviruses (Herpes simplex 1-eye infections, encephalitis, herpes simplex 2-genital herpes, skin eruptions, varicella zoster-chicken pox, etc), papovaviruses (Warts, upper respiratory tract and eye infections), adenoviruses (upper respiratory tract and eye infections), hepadna virus (Hepatitis), parvovirus(Erythema, hemolytic anemia) and poxviruses(smallpox). The RNA viruses include picornavirus (Polio, commoncold, hepatitis, pneumonia), togavirus (encephalitis, rubella), rhabdovirus (Rabies), orthomyxovirus (influenza), reovirus (gastroentiritis) and retroviruses(humanimmuno deficiency virus-1 and 2 cause AIDS and T-cell leukaemia).

Viral-replication

Viruses multiply inside living cells by using the synthesizing machinery of cell. This growth cycle involves the follwing steps:

1. Attachment of virion to the surface of host cell

Viruses are adsorbed onto the cell surface and penetrate into it and remove their viral coat. The attachment of viral particles occurs through the electrostatic interaction.

2. Release of viral nucleic acid

The viral nuleic acid is released into the host cell.

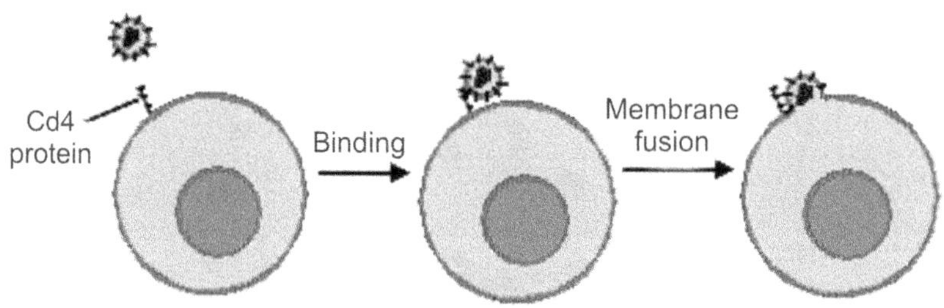

3. Replication of viruses and synthesis of enzymes

Viruses do not multiply without living cells, they depend on the host cell to carry out their metabolic activities. The virus may supply as few as two nonstructural proteins to gain access to the cell, produce the components (viral proteins and viral nucleic acids) of new virions.

4. Assembly of viral particle

The coat and the nucleic acid are synthesized at different parts of the host cell to form new virion.

5. Release of the mature viruses from the cells

The release of the viral cells may often occur by a process known as budding. Released viruses may infect immediately adjacent healthy host cells, where the replication cycle is repeated.

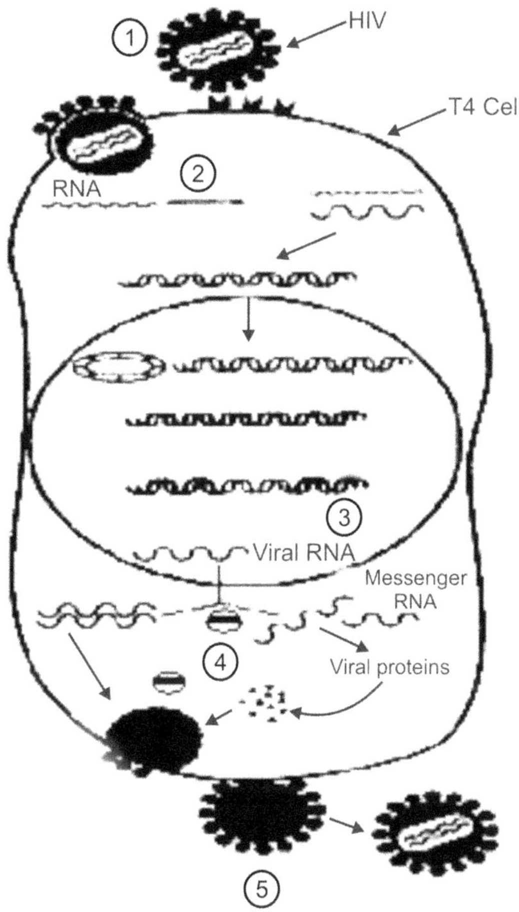

Figure 21.3 Replication of RNA virus.

General approaches for treating viral infections

Viral chemotherapy is quite different from bacterial chemotherapy (bacteria has distinctive metabolic pathways and enzyme systems). Because of the unique properties of viruses and the need for host cell metabolic activities, antiviral agents have been developed to act at various stages in viral replication cycle such as attachment, replication and release of virus. The following are various general approaches for treating viral infections:

(i) Inhibition or interference of virus attachment to host cell receptor, virus penetration and uncoating

(ii) Inhibition of virus associated enzymes such as DNA polymerases and others

(iii) Inhibition of transcription and translation processes
(iv) Interference with viral regulatory proteins and assembly of viral proteins
(v) Interference in release of virus from host cell membrane

The constraints of anti viral drug development are:

(a) Resistance by viral microorganisms to chemotherapeutic agents
(b) Lack of selectivity and hence toxic to host cells; virus share many metabolic processes of the host cell hence it is difficult to find drugs that are selective for the pathogen.
(c) Maintenance of cell-line culture for *in vitro* evaluation
(d) Difficulty in diagnosis of viral diseases

Ideal properties of antiviral drugs

An ideal antiviral drug must meet the following requirements:

(i) It must possess broad spectrum of antiviral properties
(ii) It should completely inhibit viral replication
(iii) It should reach target organ without interfering immune system of patient
(iv) It should have minimum toxicity to host cells
(v) It should be effective against resistant viruses

Nucleic acid synthesis inhibitors or nucleoside antimetabolites

DNA viruses comprise a heterogeneous group composed of DNA. Some of the DNA viruses are simple structures (a single strand DNA + few enzymes, surrounded by a capsule or a protein envelope. Eg: Parovirus, hepatitis B virus) while others are large, complex structures with double strand DNA and several enzymes. DNA viruses contain transcriptases, DNA polymerases and various other enzymes. The nucleic acid synthesis Inhibitors or nucleoside antimetabolites are nucleoside analogues (purine or pyrimidine) which block the replication of DNA viruses by the following mechanisms:

1. The drug converts to corresponding monophosphate by host cell's kinases or by specific viral enzymes. The obtained monophosphate nucleoside interferes with biosynthesis of nucleotides for DNA synthesis.

   Nucleoside Analogue(Drug) —**Cellular Kinases**→ **Nucleoside monophosphate**

2. The above nucleoside monophosphate converts to nucleoside triphosphate by cellular kinases by phosphorylation which competitively inhibits DNA polymerase.

   Nucleoside monophosphate —**Cellular kinases**→ **Nucleoside**
   triphosphate

3. Nucleoside triphosphates are incorporated into growing DNA which is brittle and does not function normally.

Iodoxuridine

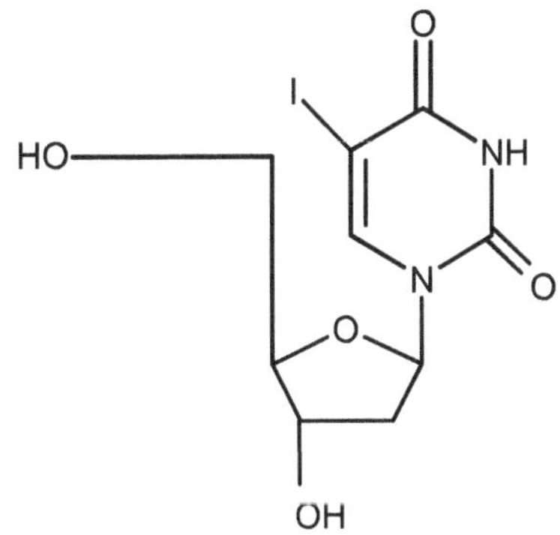

Iodoxuridine

Iodoxuridine chemically it is 2'-Deoxy-5-iodouridine. Iodoxuridine is an iodinated thymidine nucleoside analogue. It is phosphorylated to its active form by cellular kinases, which acts as an inhibitor of DNA polymerase and also acts as chain terminator. Thus iodoxuridine inhibits viral DNA synthesis. The effect of Iodoxuridine results in the inability of the virus to reproduce or to infect/destroy tissue. Iodoxuridine occurs as a pale yellow crystalline solid. It is soluble in water and alcohol but poorly soluble in most organic solvents. It is sensitive to light and heat. It does not possess solubility and inhibit growth of healthy host cells.

Uses

Iodoxuridine is used topicallly to treat herpes and pox viruses (supplied as 0.1% opthalmic solution and 0.5% ophthalmic ointment).

Trifluridine

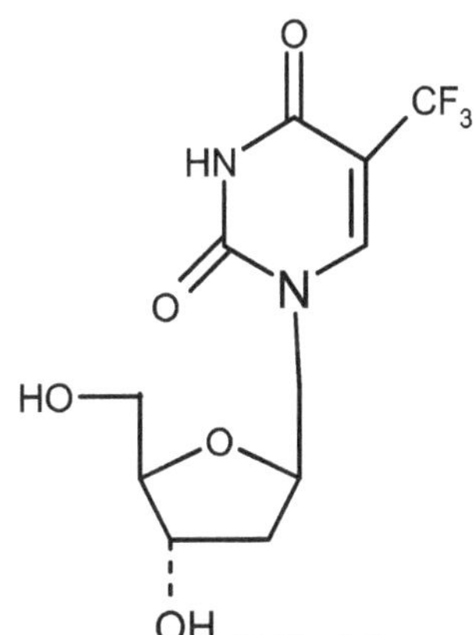

Trifluridine

Trifluridine Chemical it is 2'-Deoxy-5-(trifluoromethyl) uridine. Trifluridine is a halogenated (fluorinated), nucleoside (pyrimidine) analogue. It possesses a trifluoromethyl group at position 5 in pyrimidine nucleus. It is phosphorylated to triphosphate form by cellular kinase and competitively inhibits DNA polymerase. Trifluridine is available as 1% ophthalmic solution.

Uses

Trifluridine is used topically for the treatment of primary conjunctivitis and recurrent keratitis caused by HSV 1 and 2.

Vidarabine

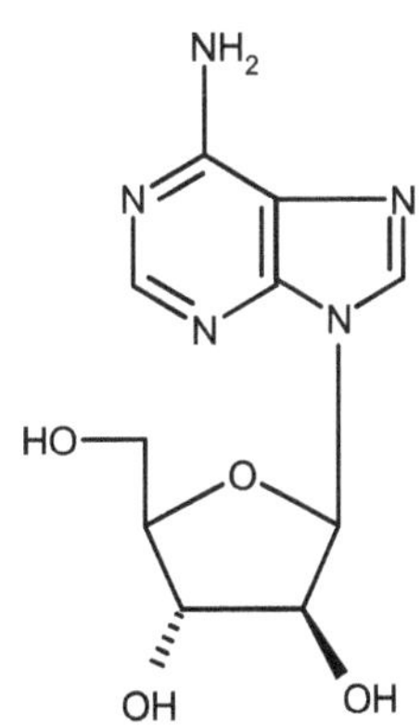

Vidarabine

Vidarabine is a purine nucleoside analogue. It inhits herpes simplex virus type 1 (HSV-1), type-2(HSV-2) and varicella-zoster. Chemically it is 9-β-D-furanosyladenine. Vidarabine has broad spectrum of antiviral activity against DNA viruses. It is phosphorylated to its active triphosphate form, by cellular kinases rather than by viruses induced thymidine kinase so as it is capable of inhibiting thymidine kinase deficient mutants of HSV. Vidarabine triphosphate competes with deoxyadenosine triphosphate for viral DNA synthesis. Vidarabine occurs as a colorless crystalline powder. It is sparingly soluble in water.

Uses

Vidarabine is used in the treatment of HSV encephalitis, neonatal HSV infection and herpes zoster infection. Vidarabine topical solution is used in the treatment of HSV keratitis.

Acyclovir

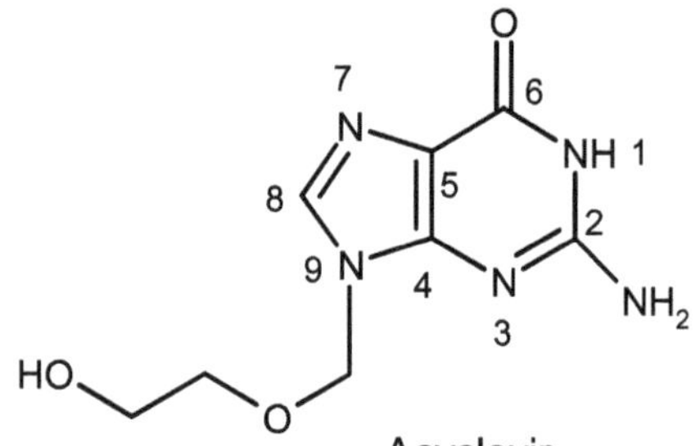

Acyclovir

Chemically acyclovir is 2-amino-1,9-dihydro9-[(2-hydroxyethoxy)methyl]-6H-purin-6-one.

Acyclovir is a guanosine analogue with an acyclic side chain at the 9th position. Acyclovir changes to acyclovir monophosphate in presence of viral thymidine kinase. Acyclovir monophosphate further converts to acyclovir triphosphate under the influence of cellular enzymes. The acyclovir triphosphate inhibits viral DNA polymerases and blocks protein synthesis. Acyclovir is available as colorless crystalline powder. It is slightly soluble in water. Acyclovir is amphoteric in nature hence its solubility is increased by both strong acids and strong bases. It is available in two systematic dosage forms i.e., oral and parenteral (lyophilized sodium salt which is reconstituted before use). Acyclovir is prepared by alkylation of guanine with the chloromethylether, followed by saponification (to remove the protecting group).

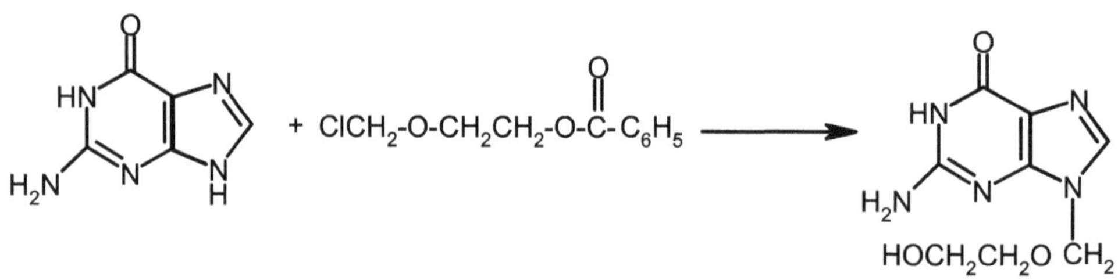

Acyclovir

Uses

1. Acyclovir is available in topical, oral and parenteral preparations.
2. It has been used for both prophylaxis and treatment of herpes virus infections.
3. The intravenous formulation is used for treatment of herpes simplex encephalitis in normal hosts and varicella zoster viral infections.
4. Oral acyclovir is very effective for the suppression of recurrent genital herpes in normal host.
5. It has potent activity against several DNA viruses including herpes simplex type 1 and type 2 viruses, varicella-zoster virus and epstein barr viruses.

Ganciclovir [9-(1,3-dihydroxy-2-propoxymethyl) guanine]

Ganciclovir is structurally similar to acyclovir. Ganciclovir possess an extra hydroxyl group (– OH), which makes it active against cytomegalovirus. It is toxic and is difficult to achieve therapeutic dose orally.

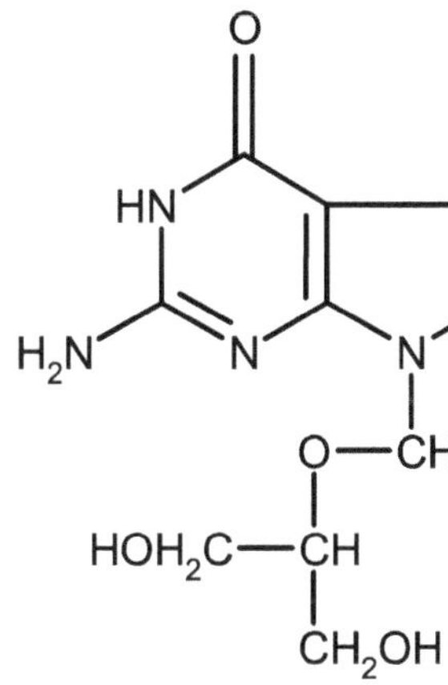

Ganciclovir

Ganciclovir is an acyclic guanosine analogue which is prepared by the following steps:

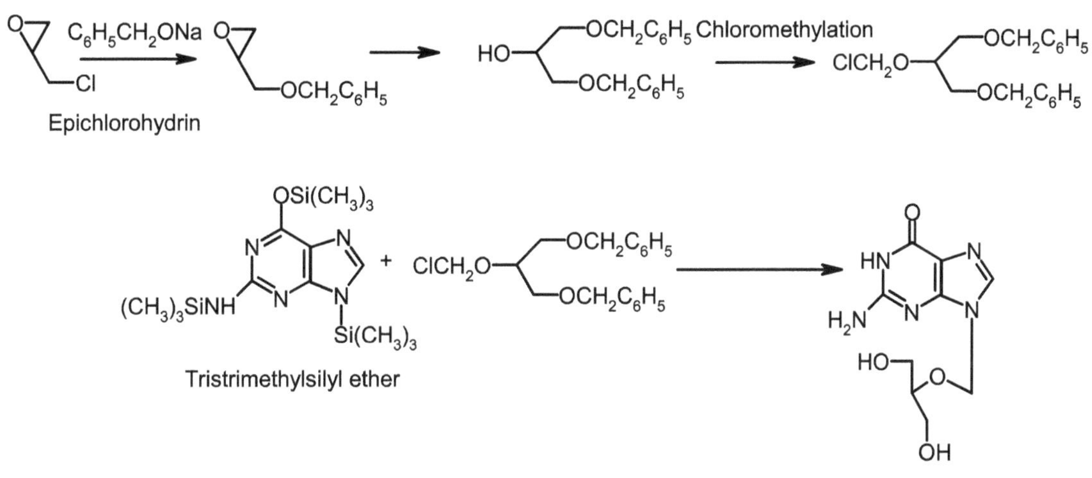

Uses

1. Ganciclovir is useful for the treatment and prophylaxis of cytomegaloviral infections.
2. It is also effective in gastrointestinal disease due to cytomegaloviruses in HIV patient.

Famciclovir

Famciclovir is diacetyl-6-deoxyderivative of penciclovir. It is inactive which readily converts to active penciclovir by deacetylation and oxidation. The mechanism of action of penciclovir is similar to ganciclovir.

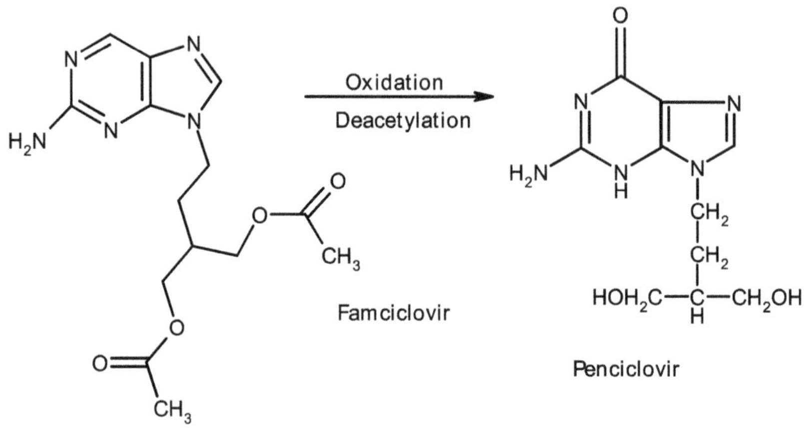

Famciclovir Penciclovir

Mechanism of action

Famciclolvir rapidly converts to penciclovir by oxidation and deacetylation. Penciclovir diffuses in to virus infected cells. In infected cells, penciclovir converts to ponciclovir triphosphate by cellular kinases. Penciclovir triphosphate act against HSV-1, HSV-2 and varicella zoster viruses by inhibiting viral DNA synthesis.

Uses

Famciclovir is used for the treatment of herpes zoster and recurrent herpes simplex virual infections.

Cidofovir

Cidofovir is a phosphonic acid derivative, which has broad spectrum of activity against DNA viruses. It can be administered intravenously and topically by cidofovir implant. Cidofovir is available in monophosphorylated form. The cellular enzymes convert codifovir to the diphosphate form, which is a competitive inhibitor of viral DNA polymerase. The diphosphate also acts as an antimetabolite to deoxycytosine triphosphate. Cidofovir is used to treat cytomegaloviral retinitis.

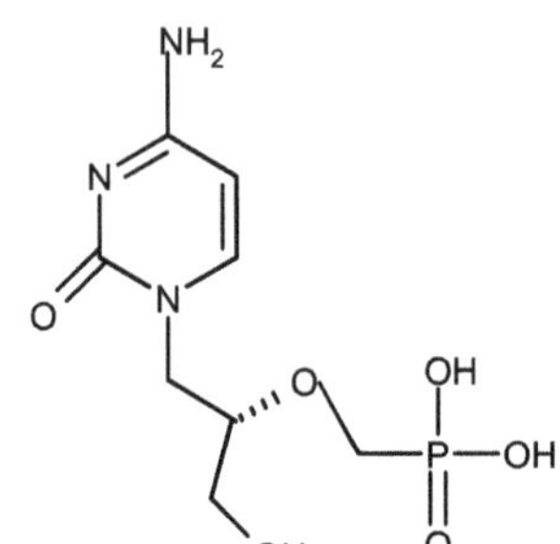
Cidofovir

Foscarnet

Foscarnet is an organic analogue of inorganic pyrophosphate. It exerts antiviral activity by selectively inhibiting the pyrophosphate binding site on virus-specific DNA polymerases.

Foscarnet is active against HSV strains resistant to acyclovir or CMV strains resistant to ganciclovir. The combination of foscarnet and ganciclovir has been shown to have enhanced activity *in vitro*. It is poorly absorbed after oral administration (bioavailability from 12% to 22%).

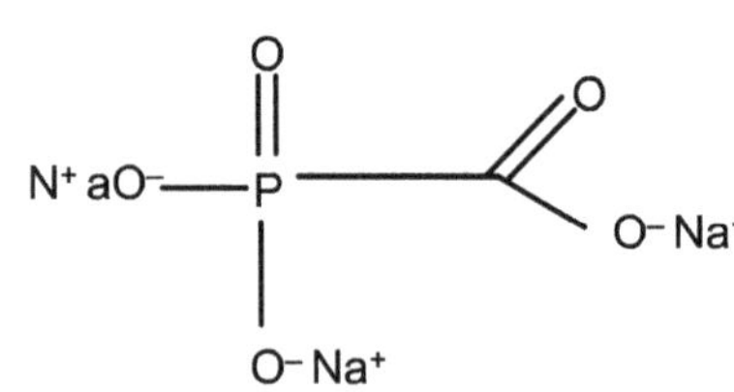
Foscarnet sodium

Host cell penetration inhibitors

Amantadine

Amantadine is an antiviral drug, which also acts as an antiparkinson agent. It is a derivate of adamantine. Chemically it is admantane-1-amine.

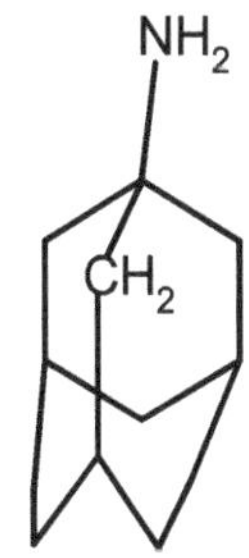

Amantadine

Mechanism of action

Amantadine is well absorbed b oral route. The mechanism of antiparkinsonic effect may be due to release of dopamine from the nerve endings of brain cells. The antiviral mechanism is by interfering with a viral protein (viral protein is needed for viral particle to become uncoated).

It is used for oral prophylaxis against influenza A (but not influenza B) and is a good alternative to the vaccine in immunocompromized patients and the elderly.

Rimantadine

Rimantadine, is also derivative of adamantane, like amantadine. The chemical name is 1-(1-adamantyl) ethanamine.

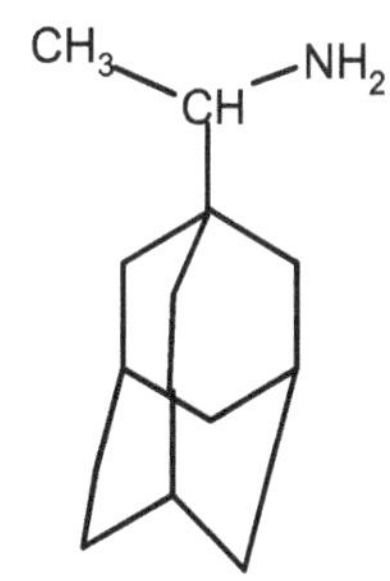

Rimantadine

Mechanism of action

Rimantadine appears to inhibits viral replicative cycle, possibly by inhibiting the uncoating of the virus. It is well absorbed, with the tablet and syrup formulations being equally absorbed after oral administration. Rimantadine is inhibitory to influenza A virus but has little or no activity against influenza B virus.

Reverse transcriptase inhibitors

HIV (Human immunodeficiency virus) is a retro virus (RNA virus) belongs to the family lenti virus (lentus-slow). It may be basically divided into 2 types HIV-1 and HIV-2. HIV infection destroys CD_4 (T) cells which are important to immune system. After a large number of T cells are destroyed, acquired immuno deficiency syndrome develops. HIV-1 reverse transcriptase exists as a heterodimer consisting of tightly associated p^{51} and p^{66} subunits. It is responsible for the synthesis of double stranded viral DNA from proviral RNA.

Reverse transcriptase inhibitors are the agents, which act against the reverse transcriptase enzyme. They have greater affinity for reverse transcriptase than for human DNA polymerase. These are again broadly classified into two classes depending on the structure of the drug:

1. Nucleoside inhibitors
2. Non-nucleoside inhibitors

1. Nucleoside inhibitors

The reverse transcription and other step of viral replication cycle involve nucleic acids. Hence nucleoside derivatives antiviral activity were investigated. They are:

(i) Removal of 3'-hydroxyl group of deoxynucleosides.

(ii) Replacement of 3'-deoxy with an azido group.

Mechanism of action

The triphosphate form inhibits the replication of HIV by interfering with viral reverse transcriptase and elongation of viral DNA chain. The triphosphate, competes with cellular dideoxy-nucleoside-5'-triphosphates and they act as chain terminators in the synthesis of proviral RNA, thereby interfering with elongation of the viral DNA chain. Nucleoside reverse transcriptase inhibitors incorporate into the viral DNA and thus ultimately DNA propagation is blocked due to the lack of 3'-hydroxyl group.

SAR

1. Azido, fluoro, and hydrogen can substitute 3' position of 2', 3'-dideoxy skeleton only when coupled with an appropriate purine or pyrimidine base.
2. Substitution of electronegative atom at 2' or 3' position stabilizes the drug towards acidic pH.
3. Incorporation of cyanide group at 3' position increases the anti HIV activity of AZT.
4. Carbonic nucleosides in which the furanose ring replaced by a cyclopentane ring inhibit the formation of nucleotides from nucleosides and thereby preventing the incorporation of nucleotides into DNA.

Zidovudine

Zidovudine is a thymidine analogue. Chemically it is 1-(3-azido-2, 3 dideoxy-β-D-erythro-pentofuranosyl)-5-methylpyrimidine-2, 4 (1H, 3H)-dione.

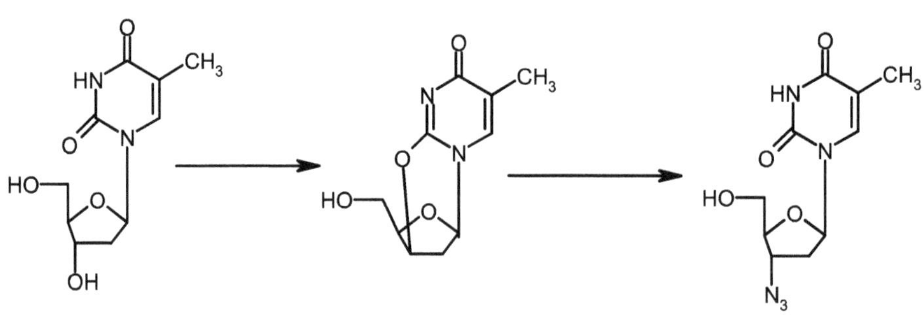

Zidovudine (AZT)

Zidovudine inhibits the activity of HIV-1 reverse transcriptase (RT) both by competing with the natural substrate deoxyguanosine tri phosphate(dGTP)and by its incorporation into viral DNA. This drug is also a chain terminator. It is phosphorylated by a cell kinase so it can be used against viruses without their own thymidine kinase. Reverse transcriptase (RNA-dependent DNA polymerase) is more sensitive to the drug than human DNA-dependent. DNA polymerase accounting for the specificity but there are severe toxicity effects. It is metabolized by glucuronide conjugation to major, inactive metabolite, 3′-azido-3′-deoxy-5′- O-β-D-glucopyranofuranosylthymidine (GZDV).

Uses

Zidovudine is recommended for the management of adult patients with symptomatic human immuno deficiency virus infection.

1. Zidovudine is supplied as 100 mg capsules for oral administration.
2. It is rapidly absorbed from GIT and is well distributed into most body fluids tissues including cerebro spinal fluid.
3. It is a heat and light sensitive drug.

Zalcitabine

Zalcitabine is a reverse transcriptase inhibitor. It has been used as a monotherapy for AIDS or in combination with zidovudine.

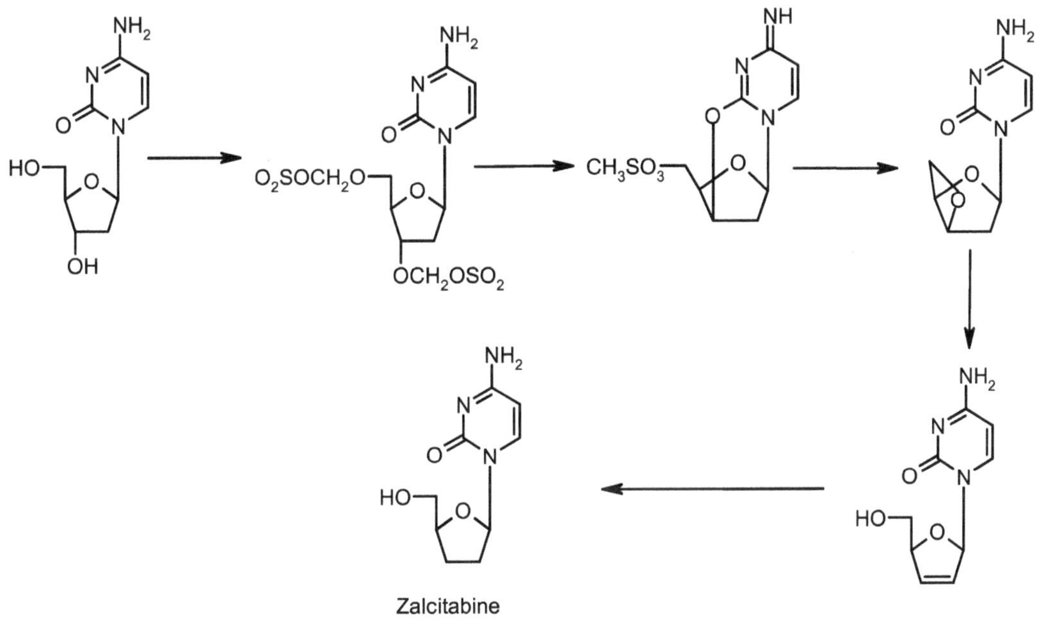

Stavudine

Stavudine is a thymidine analogue. It is an unsaturated derivative (having double bond between 2' and 3' carbons). Stavudine is recommended for the treatment of HIV infections.

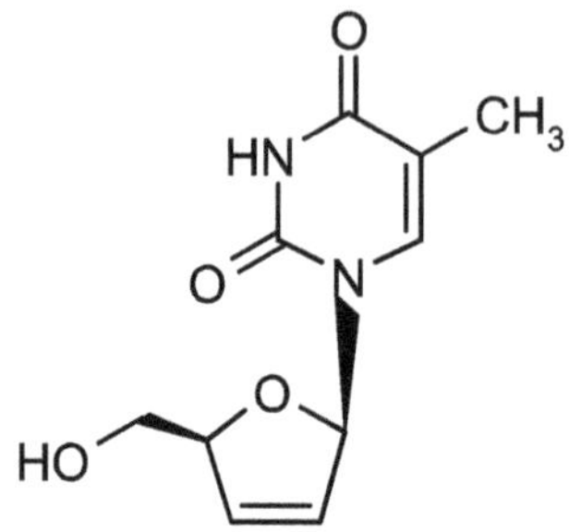

Stavudine [2'.2'-didehydro-3'-deoxy thymidine]

2. Non-nucleoside inhibitors of reverse transcriptase

Because of the problems with zidovudine and the other nucleoside analogues in the treatment of HIV, interest has grown in another approach to inhibit the enzyme, reverse transcriptase. Alternative drugs might be useful in combination therapy since there is a limit to the number of mutations that reverse transcriptase can bear without losing function. Clearly, mutations resistant to a non-nucleoside non-competitive inhibitor of reverse transcriptases would be at a different site in the enzyme from the mutation that makes the enzyme resistant to a competitive nucleoside analog.

Non-nucleoside inhibitors are the most potent and selective reverse transcriptase inhibitors. They have minimal toxicity and have been shown to work synergistically with nucleoside analogs such as AZT. Moreover, they work against nucleoside-analog resistant HIV. Thus, these drugs have high therapeutic index and also show good bioavailability so that anti-viral concentrations are readily achievable. They are non-competitive reverse transcriptase inhibitors.

Nevirapine

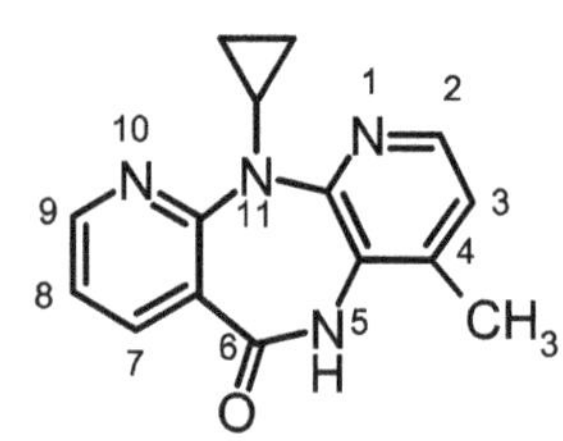

Nevirapine

Chemical name is 11-cyclopropyl-5,11-dihydro-4-methyl-6H-dipyrido [3,2-b:2',3'-e][1,4] diazepin-6-one. Nevirapine is a non-nucleoside reverse transcriptase inhibitor (NNRTI) with activity against human immunodeficiency virus type 1 (HIV-1). HIV-2 RT and eukaryotic DNA polymerases (such as human DNA polymerases α, β, or Σ) are not inhibited by nevirapine. Nevirapine is, in general, only prescribed after the immune system has declined and infections have become evident. The virus can develop resistance to nevirapine if the drug is taken alone, although even if used properly, nevirapine is effective for only a limited time. Nevirapine binds directly to reverse transcriptase (RT) and blocks the RNA-dependent and DNA-dependent DNA polymerase activities by causing a disruption of the enzyme's catalytic site. The activity of nevirapine does not compete with template or nucleoside triphosphates. *In vivo* studies in humans and *in vitro* studies with human liver microsomes have shown that nevirapine is extensively biotransformed via-cytochrome P-450 3A4 metabolism to several hydroxylated metabolites.

Efavirenz

Chemically efavirenz is (4S)-6-chloro-4 -(cyclopropylethynyl)-1,4-dihydro-4-(trifluorometh y)-2H-3, 1-benzoxazin-2-one. Efavirenz used in combination with other drugs, can suppress viral load. It possess benzoxazine nucleus and is the only second generation NNRTI in 2004.

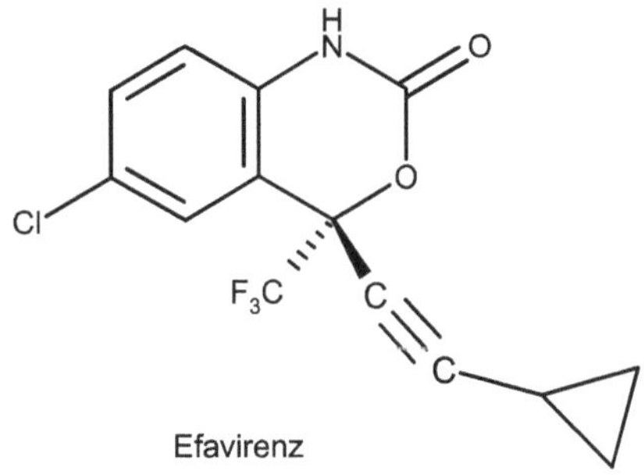

Efavirenz

RNA synthesis inhibitors

Ribavirin

It inhibits influenza RNA polymerase non-competitively *in vitro* but poorly *in vivo*. It may act as a guanosine analogue and inhibit 5' cap formation on mRNA. The cap normally contains methyl guanosine. However, ribavirin is known to inhibit the production of infectious polio virus and this virus does not have a methyl guanosine cap; so there must be alternative mechanisms for ribavirin action. It is likely that this drug introduces multiple mutations into viral RNA rendering it incapable of a new round of cell infection. An aerosol form is used against RSV (respiratory syncytial virus) and the drug is used intravenously against lassa fever. Ribavirin can antagonize the effect of AZT as was found in some initial combination therapy trials against HIV.

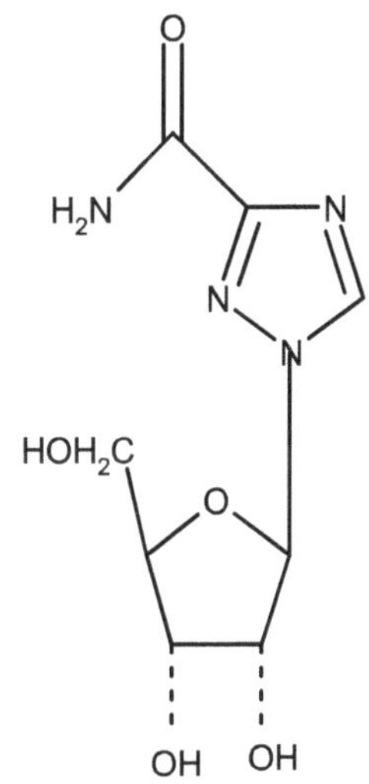

Ribavirin
[1-β-D-ribofuranosyl-1H-1, 2,4,-triazole-3-carboxamide]

Protein processing inhibitors

Protease inhibitors

Many viruses must cleave the proteins that they make. In the case of surface glycoproteins, this is usually carried out by a host protease in the secretory pathway (e.g., in golgi body). In the case of internal proteins, such as the polymerase or the group-specific antigens (GAGs), there is a viral protease that is encoded in the POL gene of retroviruses and by some other viruses. Active site-directed inhibitors of the HIV aspartyl protease have been developed as this enzyme is not similar to known host proteolytic enzymes and therefore the inhibitors should show specificity to viral proteins. The action of the HIV protease is crucial to viral infectivity. Now we have the promise of a drug regimen that can suppress indefinitely the progress of disease.

Eg : Saquinavir, ritonavir, indinavir and nelfinavir. These are all substrate analogues.

Saquinavir

Chamically saquinavir is (S) –N-[(ds)-α-{(1R)-2-[(3S,4as,8as)]-3-(tert-butyl carbamoyl) octahydro-2(1H)isoquinoly]-1-hydroxyethyl}phenethy1-2-quinaldamidosuccina-mide. The design of saquinavir started by considering a viral polypeptide substrate. The peptide line was replaced by hydroxyethylamine transition state of saquinavir which successfully inhibit enzyme. It shows 100-bold selectivity for both HIV-1 and HIV-2 proteases over human proteases. It is the least bioavailable of the present protease inhibitors and is the least effective.

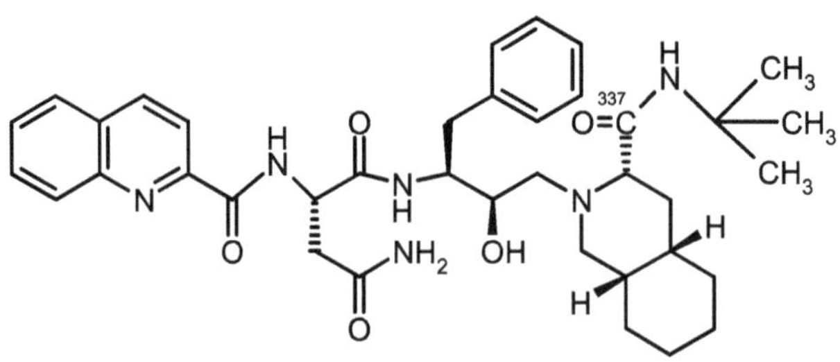

Saquinavir

Ritonavir

Chemically ritonavir is [5S,8S, 10S, 11S]-10-hydroxy-2-methyl-5-(1-methylethyl)-1-[2-(1-methylethyl)-4-thiazolyl]-3,6-dioxo-8,11-bis (phenyl methyl)-2,4,7,12-tetraazatridecan-13oic acid 5-thiazolylmethyl ester. This drug reduces AIDS-defining events and death by 58% compared to placebo. It causes nausea in 25% of patients. It is active against both HIV-1 and HIV-2 proteases and shows selectivity for HIV proteases over mammalian proteases. Despite a high molecular weight and the presence of amide bonds, it has better bioavailability than many other protease inhibitors.

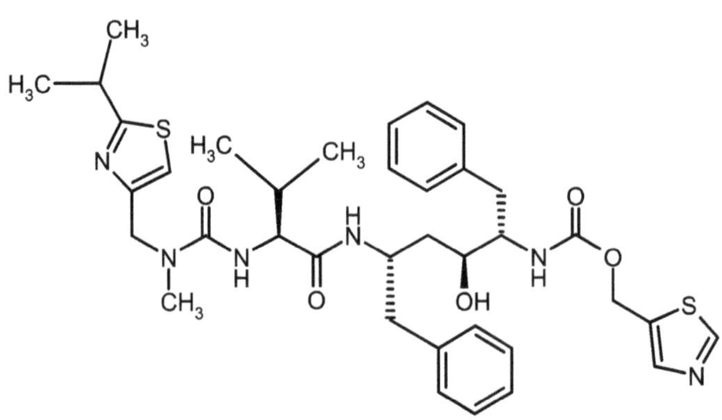

Ritonavir

Indinavir

Indinavir is an anti-RT drug reduces HIV. Unfortunately suffered from poor bioavailability and liver toxicity.

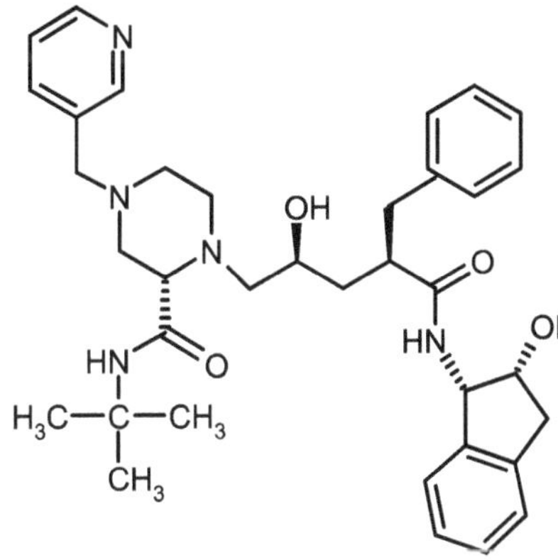

Indinavir

Amprenavir

It is another protease inhibitor used in combination therapy. It is reasonably specific for viral protease and has good oral bioavailability.

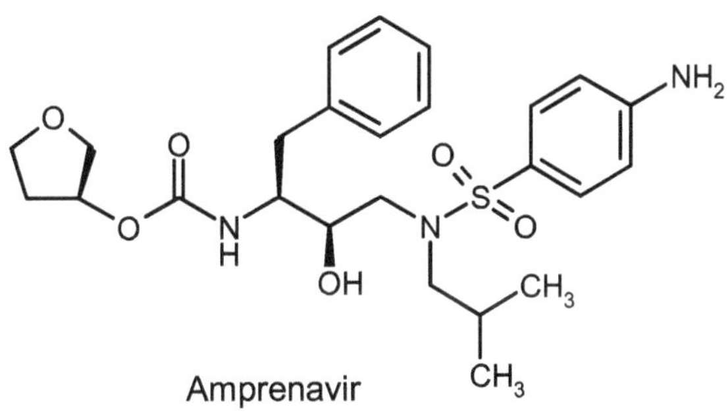

Amprenavir

Interferons

Interferons are the principal compounds that act as inhibitors of protein synthesis. These compounds are members of naturally occurring glycoprotein hormones which are produced by all types of eukaryotic cells. However, no clinically useful compounds have been found for humans, although tilorone is effective in inducing interferon in mice.

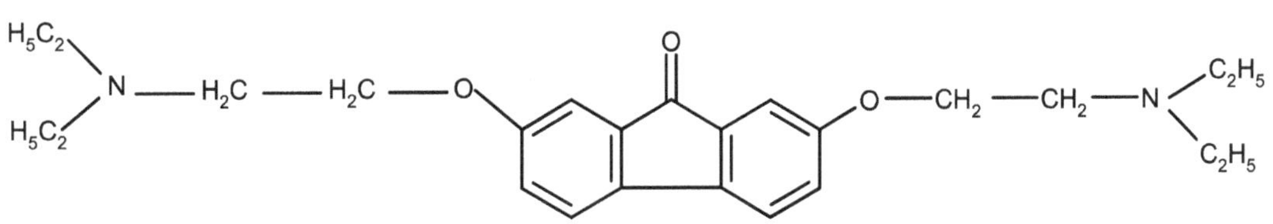

Tilorone

There are three classes of interferons. They are α- β- and γ- interferons. The α and β interferons are cytokines, which are secreted by virus infected cells. They bind to specific receptors on adjacent cells and protect them from infection by viruses. They form part of the immediate protective host response to invasion by viruses. Their presence can be demonstrated in body fluids during the acute phase of virus infection. Recombinant α and β interferons are now available and have been used for the treatment of chronic hepatitis B and C virus infections. However, side effects such as fever, malaise and weight loss have limited the use. *Gamma Interferon* (immune interferon) is a cytokine secreted by TH_1CD_4 cells. Its function is to enhance specific T cell mediated immune responses.

Mechanism of action of the interferons

1. Enhancement of the specific immune response. By increasing the expression of MHC class I molecules on the surface of infected cells, the interferons increase the opportunity for specific cytotoxic T cells to recognize and kill infected cells.
2. Direct antiviral effect (i) degradation of viral mRNA (ii) inhibition of protein synthesis. Prevents the infection of new cells.

22

ANTI-CANCER DRUGS

The term 'cancer' means a relatively autonomous growth of tissue. Tumor is a general term indicating any abnormal mass or growth of tissue which is not necessarily life threatening where as cancerous tumor is a malignant neoplasm, which is highly dangerous. The suffix-*oma* literally means tumor and word with suffix refers to neoplasm. Basing on the embryologic origin, names of cancers can be divided into two categories:a) Sarcoma: A cancer that arises from mesodermal tissue is called sarcoma. b) Carcinoma: Cancer that arises from the ecto-or endodermal cells is called as carcinoma. A cancer of blood involves abnormal increase of leukocytes is called leukemia. On the other hand polycythemia involves increased number of erythrocytes and an increase in total blood volume.

Cancer is a disease of worldwide importance. Its incidence in the developed countries is raising, and its mortality occupies the second rank in the order of death causes. Cancer arises as a result of a series of genetic changes in the cell, the main genetic lesions being: (a) Inactivation of tumour suppressor genes (b) The activation of oncogenes (normal genes controlling cell division).

Characteristics of cancer cells

Cancer cells have four characteristics that distinguish cancer cells from normal cells.

1. ***Uncontrolled proliferation :*** The proliferation of cancer cells is not controlled by the process that normally regulate cell division and tissue growth.
2. ***Loss of function :*** The main characteristic of cancer cell is that they differentiate (poorly differentiated cancers multiply faster).
3. ***Invasiveness :*** Cancer cells are found outside the designated tissue of origin.
4. ***The ability of metastasis :*** Metastasis is secondary tumor formed by cells that have been released from initial or primary tumor.

Cell cycle

Cell growth and division is a continuous process, the cell cycle is divided into 5 stages: G_0, G_1, S, G_2, and M. G_0 is the functional stage of the cell during which it performs its metabolic and synthetic functions. Once a cell is ready to undergo division, it enters the G_1 phase during which the proteins needed for DNA synthesis are produced. Then, the cell enters the S phase in which the DNA is replicated. After a short G_2 phase, the cell then enters the M phase in which the cell undergoes mitotic and cell division. After the M phase, a cell may enter the G_1 phase again or may enter the G_0 phase. In cancer cell cycle, cancer cells continuous dividing in G_0 state. Positive as well as negative forces regulate the cell cycle. These forces can be given as: Positive forces: growth factors and cyclin/cdks. Negative forces gene P_{53} that halts the cycle at check point 1 and triggers apoptosis if the DNA is damaged.

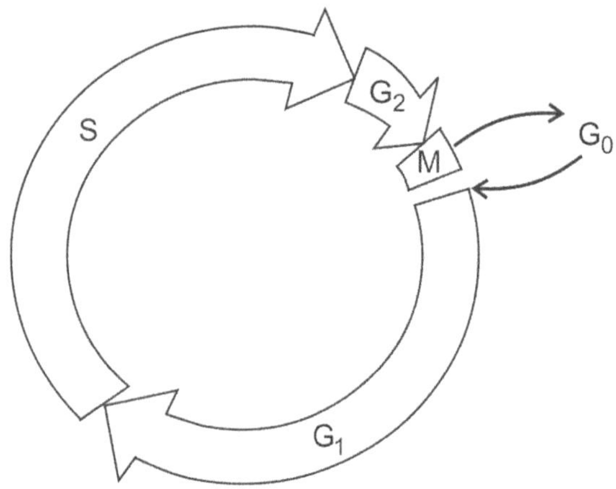

Figure 22.1 Cell cycle.

Causes of Cancer

There are several agents responsible for cancer. They are :

(i) Carcinogenic chemicals : Alkylating agents, polyaromatic hydrocarbons, aniline, arsenic, phenacetin, clofibrate, estrogen, plastics etc.

(ii) Radiation energy : UV rays of sunlight, gamma rays, X-rays, nuclear fission, radionuclides etc.

(iii) Viruses : Oncogenic viruses contain either DNA or RNA genome.

(iv) Environmental factors.

Classification of antineoplastic agents

Antineoplastic agents can be classified in many ways. One of the best methods to classify antineoplastic agent is based on their mechanism of action :

I. DNA alkylating agents
II. Antimetabolites
III. Antimitotics
IV. Antibiotics
V. Hormonal agents
VI. Miscellaneous

I. DNA alkylating agents

The alkylating agents are considered to be cell cycle non-specific. They are also known to be the most cytotoxic to the rapidly proliferating cells.

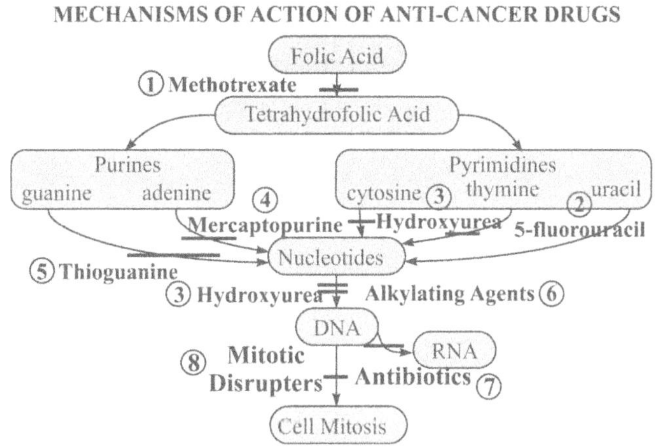

Figure 22.2 Mechanism of action of anticancer drugs.

Mechanism of action

In general alkylating agents form strong electrophiles (carbonium ion intermediates), which forms covalent linkages with various nucleophile moieties (N, O or S of phosphate, carboxyl, hydroxyl, amino and sulphhydryl groups in biological systems). The cytotoxic effects of alkylating agents are due to alkylation of components of DNA.Alkylation of DNA is mainly through the 7th-nitrogen atom of guanine. It is the main molecular target for alkylation of DNA this can interfere with transcription and replication.

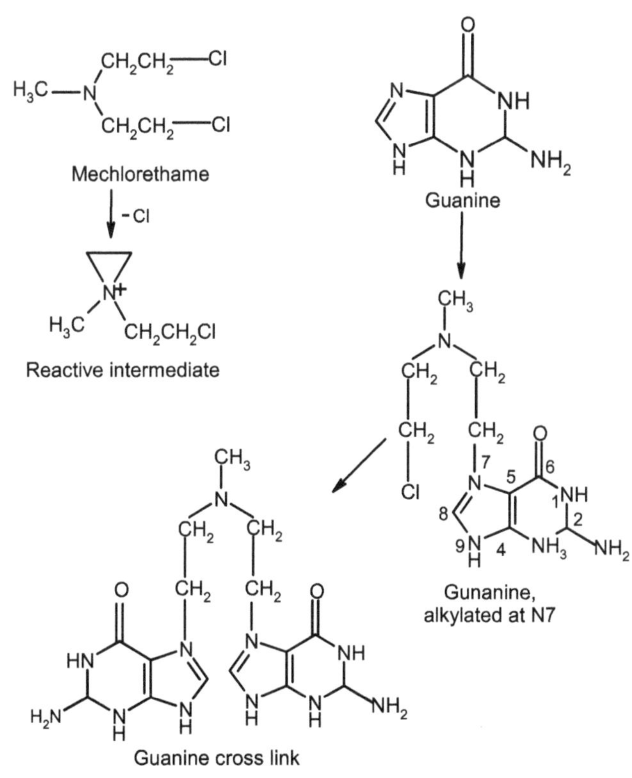

Classification DNA-alkylating-agents

Depending on the structure they can be sub classified as

(i) Nitrogen mustards
(ii) Alkyl sulphonates
(iii) Aziridines
(iv) Nitrosoureas
(v) Miscellaneous

Nitrogen mustards

These are the first alkylating agents, which were used for the treatment of tumors. Though these are unstable their cytotoxic effect towards the proliferating cells insists their use.

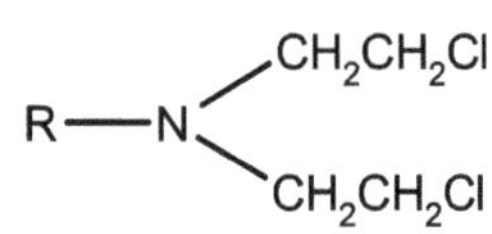

Mechanism of action

These are bifunctional alkylating agents which can undergo a second cyclization of the second side chain and forms a covalent bond with another nucleophilic group. *Eg.:* Cyclophosphamide, chlorambucil, mechlorethamine, and melphalan.

Cyclophosphamide

Cyclophosphamide is N, N-Bis (2-chloroethyl) tetrahydro-2H – 1, 3, 2-oxazaphophorin-2-amino 2-oxide.

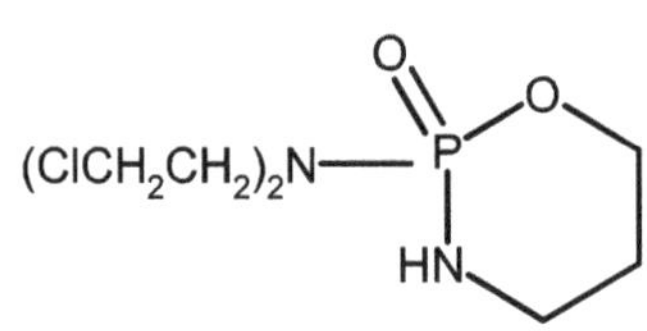

Cyclophosphamide

Properties

Cyclophosphamide is readily soluble in water. It has a melting point of 41°C-45°C. It is slightly soluble in alcohol, benzene, ethylene glycol, carbon tetrachloride and dioxane. It is sparingly soluble in ether and acetone. Cyclophosphamide is available as tablets and injections.

Uses

It is used in the treatment of Hodgkin's disease, acute lymphocytic leukemia and a variety of solid tumors (tumors of breast, cervix, lung and ovary).

Chlorambucil

Chlorambucil is nitrogen mustard. It is chemically 4-[4-Bis(2-chloroethyl)-aminophenyl] butyric acid.

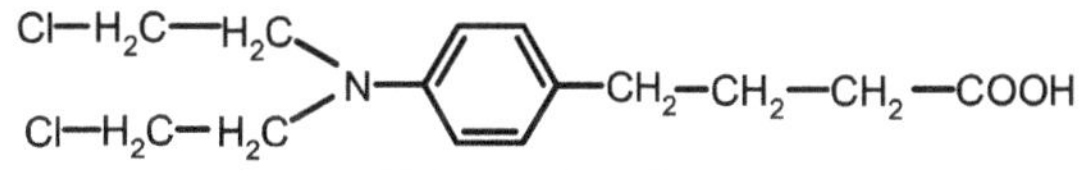

Chloramubucil

Synthesis

Chlorambucil is synthesized by treating 4-phenylbutyric acid with ethylene oxide, followed by thionyl chloride and acidic hydrolysis.

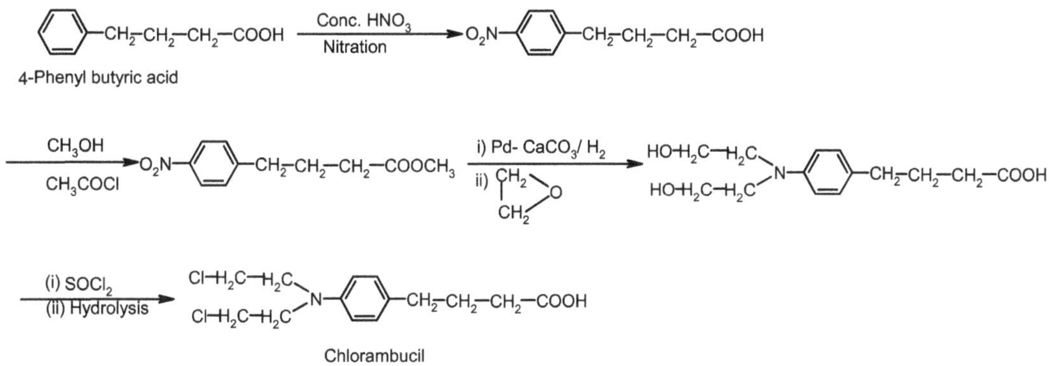

Properties

Chlorambucil is a white crystalline powder having a melting point of 65 °C. It is soluble in ether, chloroform, alcohol and acetone. It is practically insoluble in water. It is absorbed completely by oral route.

Uses

It is used in the treatment of chronic lymphocytic leukemia. It is also used to treat Hodgkin's disease and testicular cancer.

Mechlorethamine

Mechlorethamine is also known as mustine or chlormethethine.It is 2-chloro-N-(2-chloroethyl)-N-methylethanamine. Mechlorethamine is structurally simplest of nitrogen mustards.

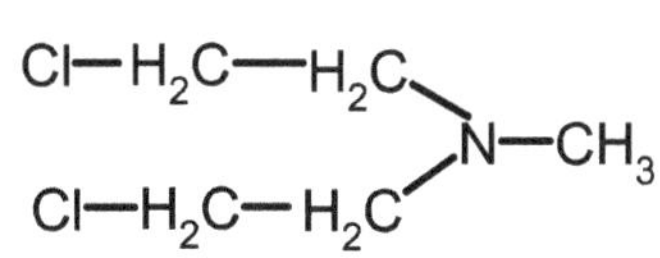

Bis (l-Chloroethyl) methylamine

Synthesis

Mechlormethamine is synthesized by treating 2, 2' - (hydroxy ethylamine) with thionylchloride.

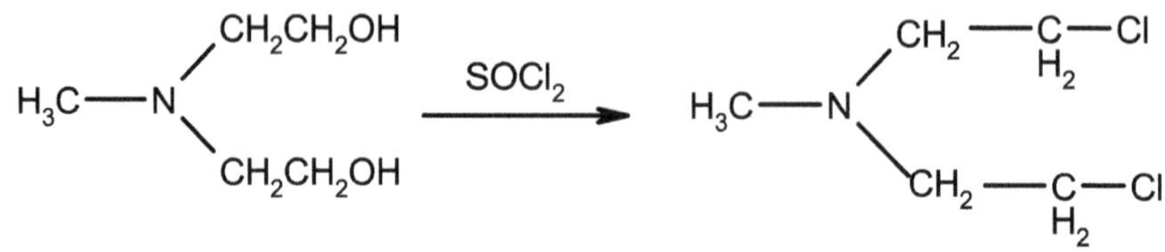

Mechlorethamine

Properties

Mechlorethamine is available as HCl salt. Mechlorethamine HCl is white crystalline powder. It is hygroscopic and is freely soluble in water.

Uses

It is used in the treatment of Hodgkin's disease and other lymphomas.

Melphalan

Melphalan is another nitrogen mustard derivative of natural aminoacid L-phenyl alanine. It is 4-[Bis (2-chloroethyl)-amino]-L-phenylalanine.

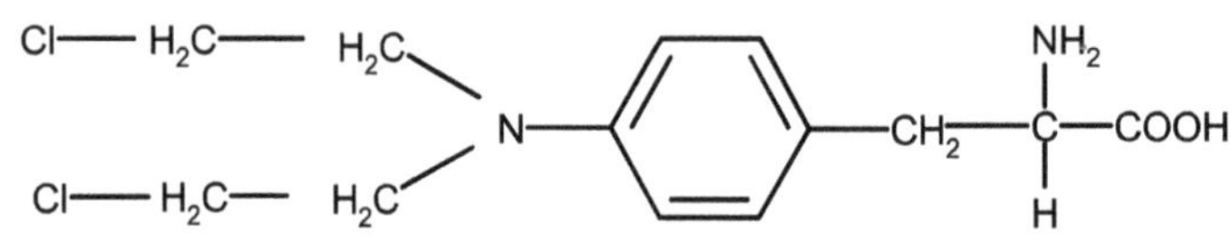

Melphalan

Synthesis

Synthesis of melphalan from phenylalanine involves following steps:

(i) Nitration and esterification of phenylalanine to get 4-nitro-L-phenylalanine ethyl ester

(ii) Protection of amino group and reduction of nitro group

(iii) Heating of the above product with ethylene oxide to introduce hydroxyethyl groups and treatment with sulphonyl chloride to get melphalan.

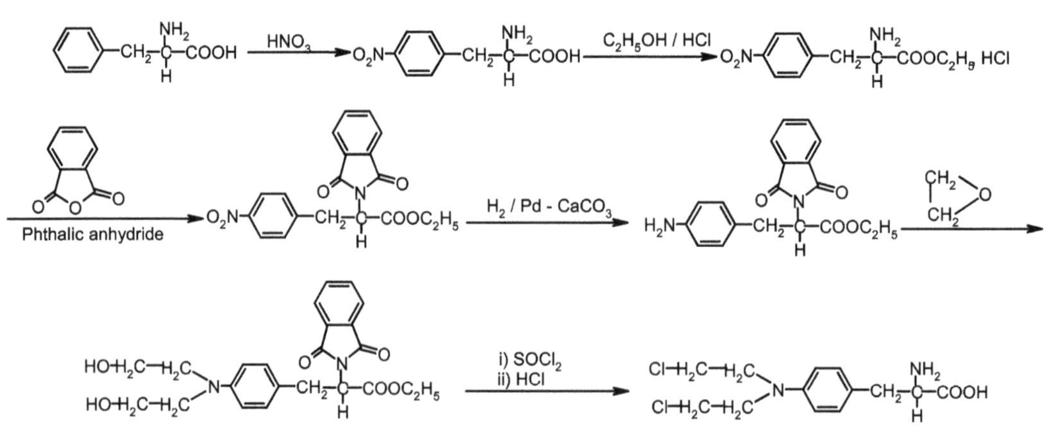

Properties

Melphalan is having a melting point of 186°C. It is soluble in ethanol and propylene glycol.

Uses

It is used in the treatment of multiple myeloma. It is also used to treat breast and ovary cancers.

Aziridines

Aliphatic nitrogen mustards are converted to more stable aziridinium ion at physiological pH in the presence of heterocyclic rings such as purine.

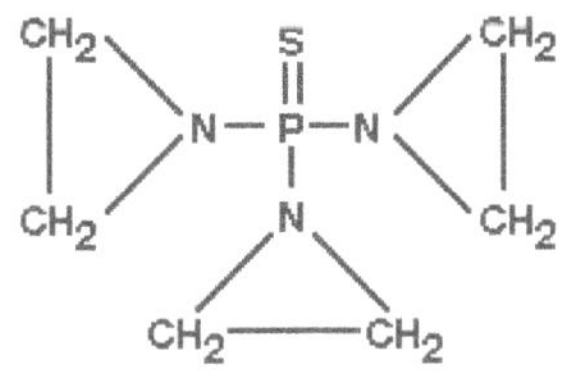

Thiotepa

Thiotepa

Thiotepa is an aziridine derivative. It is N, N', N" - triethylenethiophospharamide.

Synthesis

Thiotepa is synthesized by mixing aziridine with trichloro phosphine chloride.

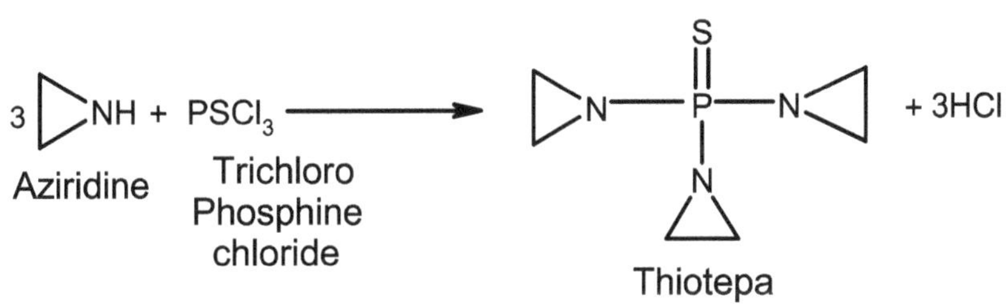

Properties

Thiotepa is a white powder, which is soluble in water. It should be protected from light and should be stored between 2°C - 8°C (High temperature polymerizes thiotepa).

Uses

It is used in the treatment of breast, ovarian and bronchogenic carcinomas and malignant lymphomas.

Nitrosoureas

Nitrosoureas are the alkylating agents. These compounds are converted into the carbonium ion and isothiocyanate non-enzymatically. The carbonium ion is responsible for the cytotoxic effects whereas isothiocyanate is responsible for carbamylation of lysine residues of proteins (by alkylating DNA), isothiocyanate may interact with proteins and account for some of the toxic effects of these drugs. The nitrosoureas are used mainly for the treatment of Hodgkin's disease and meningeal leukemia and brain tumors. Occasionally they are used in the treatment of solid tumors such as lung, carcinoma, G.I. and breast carcinomas in combination with other anticancer agents.

Carmustine

It is chemically N,N'-bis (2-chloroethyl)-N-nitrosourea.

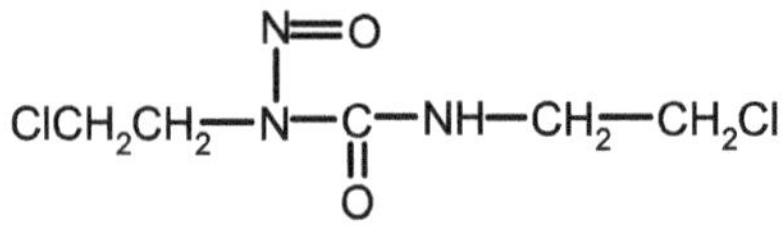

Carmustine

Synthesis

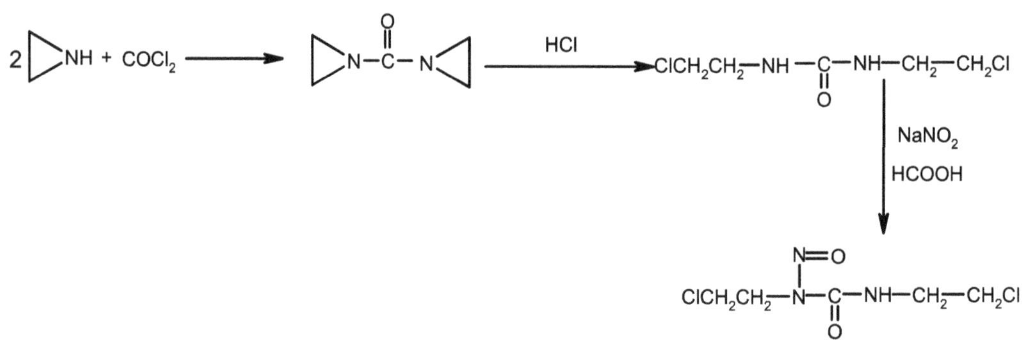

Properties

It is a light yellow color powder that melts to an oily liquid with a melting point of 30 °C - 32°C. It is soluble in water and ethanol.

Uses

It is used in the treatment of Hodgkins disease, meningeal leukemia and brain tumors.

Lomustine

Lomustine is N-(2-chloroethyl)-N[1]-cyclohexyl-1-nitrourea. Lomustine on hydrolysis yield metabolity. The metabolities are responsible for alkylation and cross-linking of DNA.

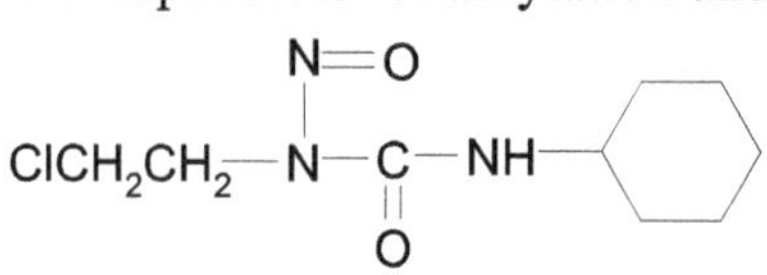

Lomustine

Synthesis

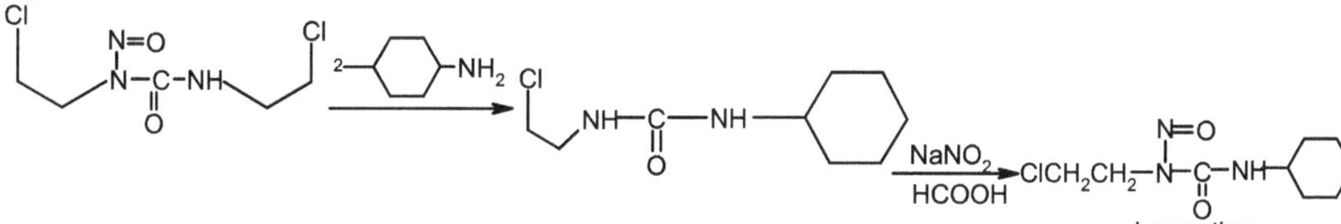

Properties

It is a yellow powder with melting point of 90°C. It is freely soluble in chloroform and soluble in ethanol and acetone.

Uses

It is used in the treatment of Hodgkin's disease, meningeal leukemia and brain tumors.

Procarbazine

It is N-(1-methylethyl)-4-[(2-methylhydrazino)methyl] benzamide. Procarbazine is classified as an alkylating agent. It is a hydrazine derivative. It is a white to pale yellow crystalline powder, which is soluble but unstable in water or aqueous solutions. The structural formula is:

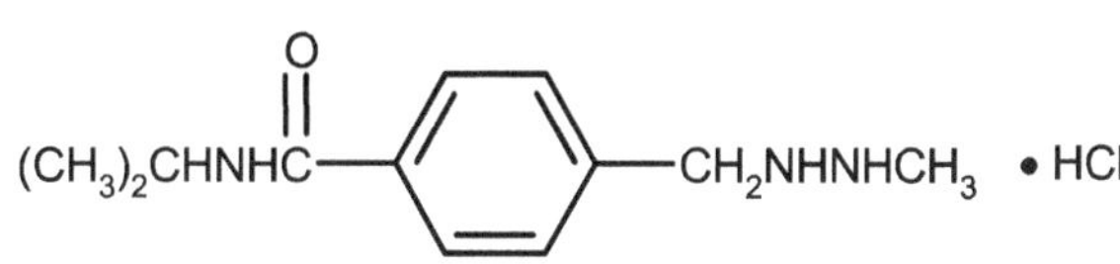

Procarbazine

Mechanism of action

Procarbazine may inhibit transmethylation of methyl groups of methionine into t-RNA. The absence of functional t-RNA could cause the cessation of protein synthesis and consequently DNA and RNA synthesis. In addition, procarbazine may directly damage DNA. Hydrogen peroxide, formed during the auto-oxidation of the drug, may attack protein sulphhydryl groups contained in residual protein.

Properties

These are crystals having a melting point of 226°C.

Uses

It is used to treat Hodgkin's disease.

Dacarbazine

Dacarbazine is a DNA-methylating agent with a broad spectrum antitumor activity in mouse tumor models. It is chemically 5-(3,3-dimethyl-1-triazenyl)-1H-imidazole-4-carboxamide.

Synthesis

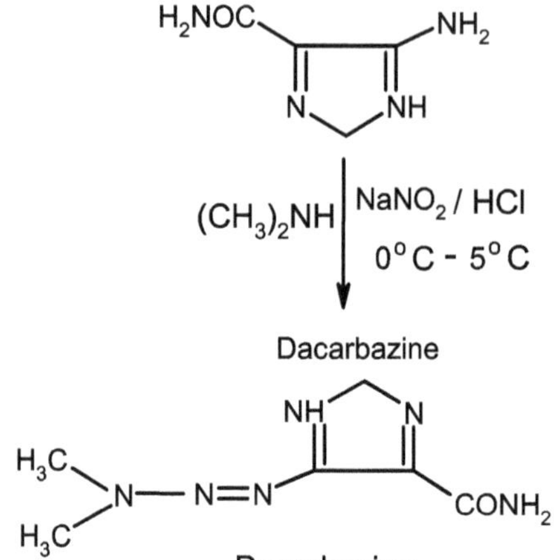

Dacarbazine

Properties

It is an ivory microcrystalline substance with an explosive decomposition temperature of 250°C -255°C.

Uses

It is used in the treatment of malignant melanomas, Hodgkins disease and adult sarcomas.

Uracil Mustard

It is chemically 5-[Bis(2-chloroethyl)-amino]-2,4-(1H,3H)-pyrimidinedione.

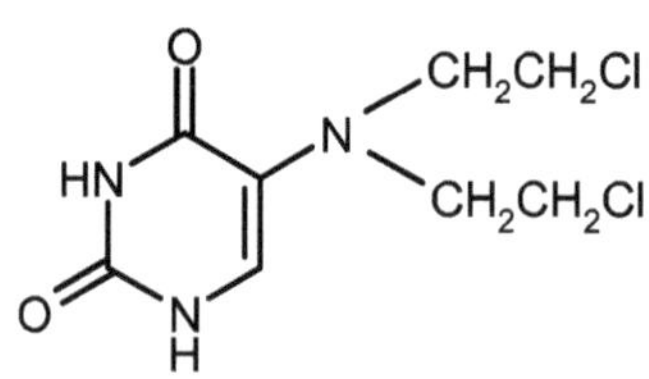

Uracil Mustard

Synthesis

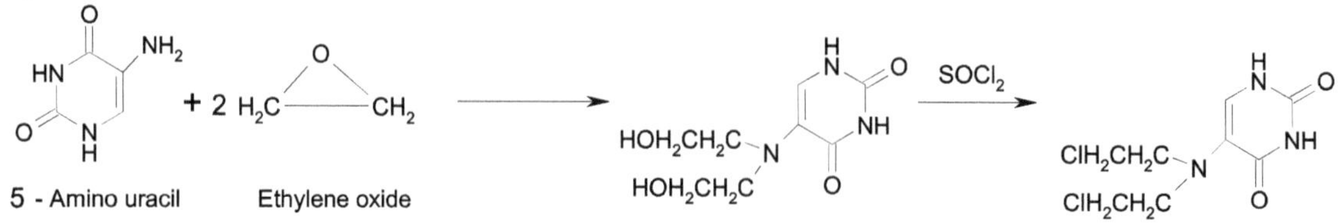

Uracil mustard

Properties

These crystals are having a decomposition temperature of 206 °C, which is sparingly soluble in water.

Uses

It is used as an antineoplastic agent.

II. Antimetabolites

Antimetabolites are structural analogues of naturally occurring compounds (nucleic acids) that block the normal metabolic pathways operating in cells. They inhibit the growth of the most rapidly proliferating cells in the body either by replacing an endogenous substance in the biosynthetic pathway or by inhibiting the enzyme in metabolic pathway in the cell. The structures of antimetabolites are usually very similar to those of normal metabolites used by the cell. There are four categories of antimetabolites:

(i) Folate analogues
(ii) Purine analogues
(iii) Pyrimidine analogues
(iv) Adenosine analogues

(i) ***Folate analogues*:** Folic acid is an essential growth factor for the cells. From the folic acid a series of tetrahydrofolate cofactors are obtained which are essential for the biosynthesis of RNA and DNA precursors such as thymine and purines.

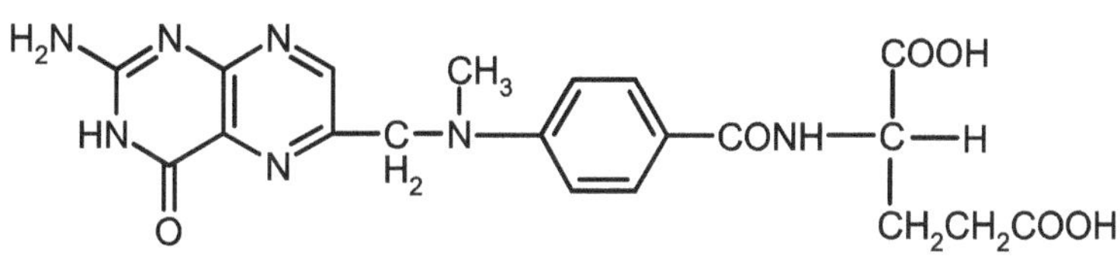

Methotrexate

Folic acid in reduced form (tetrahydrofolic acid) is useful in various metabolic processes. This reduction occurs by the action of dihydrofolate reductase (DHFR) enzyme, which is the primary action site of many folate inhibitors. Folic acid antimetabolites have structures that resemble folic acid.

Folic acid antimetabolites have a stronger affinity for DHFR than folic acid and act by this enzyme at both stages in the conversion of folic acid to THF. This has the effect of inhibiting the formation of purines and thymine required for DNA synthesis. This inhibits cell growth, which prevents replication and ultimately leads to cell death. Methotrexate is the strong inhibitor of tumor cell dihydrofolate reductase enzyme and inhibits the DNA synthesis.

Methotrexate

Methotrexate is the only folate antimetabolite in clinical use. It is N-[4-[[(2,4 diamino-6-pteridinyl)methyl]methylamino] benzoyl]-L-glutamic acid.

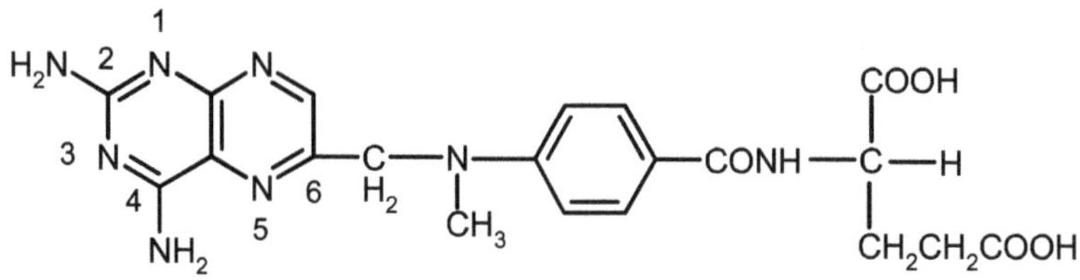

Methotrexate is synthesized by using 2, 4, 5, 6- tetramino pyrimidine.

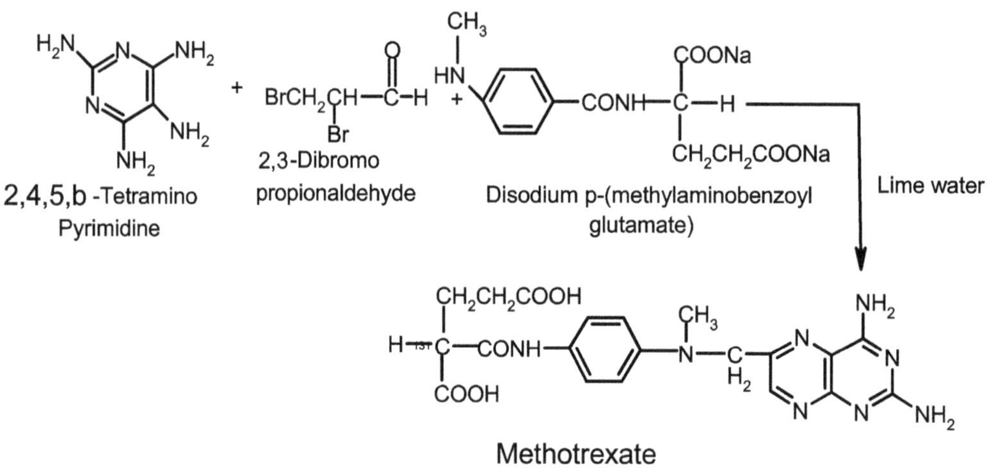

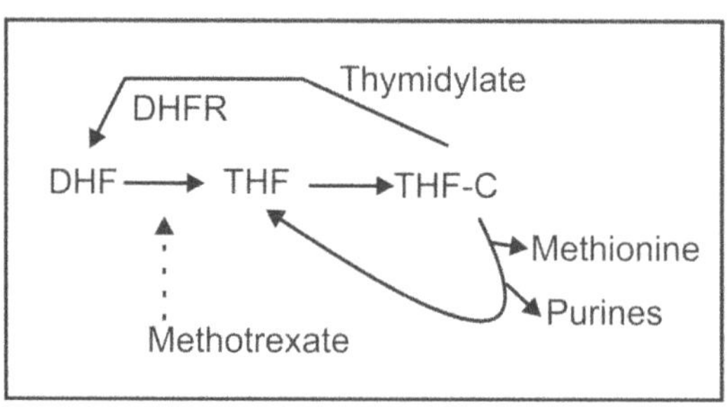

Figure 22.3 Methotrexate inhibits DHFR in both cancer and normal cells. Cancer cells are dividing more rapidly than normal cells and are depleted of THF more rapidly; therefore, they are more susceptible to the effect of MTX (Methotrexate) DHF = Dihydrofolic acid; THF = Tetrahydrofolic acid; THF-C = THF-coenzyme; DHFR = Dihydrofolic acid reductase

Properties

Methotrexate is available as yellow crystals having a decomposition temperature of 204°C. It is soluble in alkaline or acidic solutions and practically insoluble in water.

Uses

It is used as an antineoplastic in the treatment of gestational choriocarcinoma and trophoblastic tumors of women. It is also used to treat acute lymphocytic leukemia in children. It is also used in the treatment of psoriasis, breast, head and lung cancers.

(ii) ***Purine analogues*:** These drugs are structural analogues of hypoxanthine and guanine, which were not only used as anticancer agents but also as antiviral and immunosuppressive agents. These can inhibit both nucleotide and nucleic acid synthesis and be incorporated into nucleic acid.

Mechanism of action

Thiopurines are converted to nucleotide in the presence of phosphoribosyltransferase, which further converts to guanine nucleotide and finally these mononucleotide derivatives converted to triphosphates, which can be incorporated into RNA and DNA. These drugs convert to thioguanine analogue and directly incorporate in to the DNA.

Eg: 6-Mercaptopurine, thioguanine

6-Mercaptopurine

Mercaptopurine is an important purine analogue. Chemically it is 1,7-dihydro-6H-purine-6-thione.

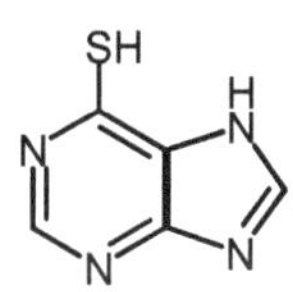

It is prepared from hypoxanthine by following chemical reactions:

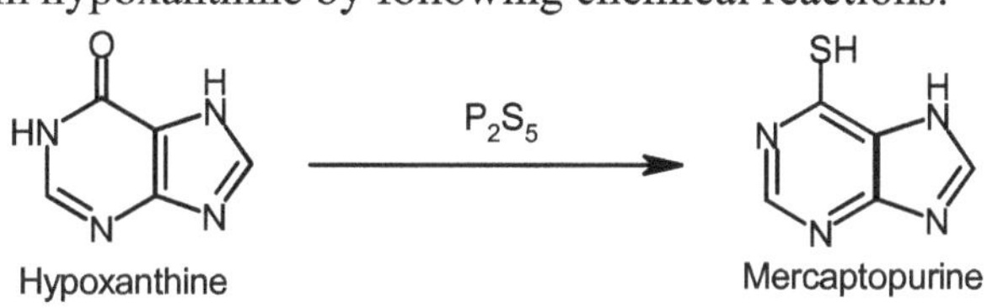

Properties

Mercaptopurine is available as yellow prisms having a decomposition temperature of 313°C. It is insoluble in water, acetone and ether and soluble in hot ethanol. It is soluble in alkali solutions.

Uses

Mercaptopurine interferes with purine synthesis and is a cell-specific drug for S-phase. In addition it has an immunosuppresant action. It is used in the treatment of acute myelocytic leukemia. It is administered by IM or IV injection.

Thioguanine

Thioguanine is a guanine analogue. It is 2-amino-1, 7-dihydro-6H-purine-6-thione.

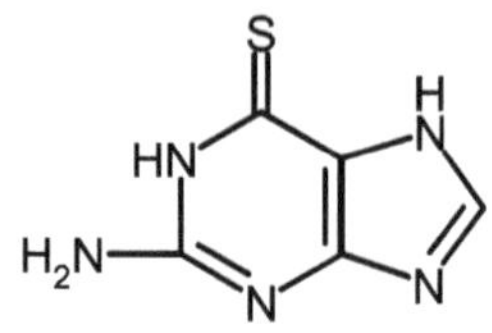

Thioguanine

It is prepared from guanine by following chemical reactions:

Properties

It is available as plae yellow needles. It is insoluble in water but dissolves in alkaline hydroxides.

Uses

Thioguanine is used in the treatment of acute non-lymphocytic leukemia. It has synergistic action with cytarabine to treat adult leukemia. Thioguanine is preferred to mercaptopurine as it causes fewer gastrointestinal reactions.

Azathioprine

It is chemically 6-[(1-methyl-4-nitro-1*H*-imidazol-5-yl) thio]-1H-purine.

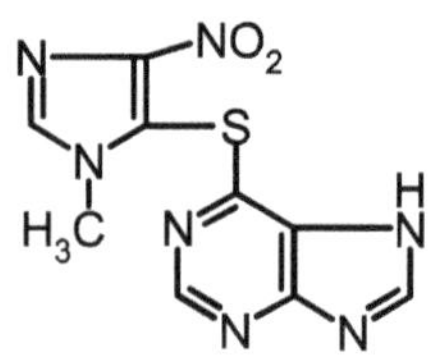

Azathioprine

Azothiopurine is sized from 6-mercaptopurine by following chemical reaction,

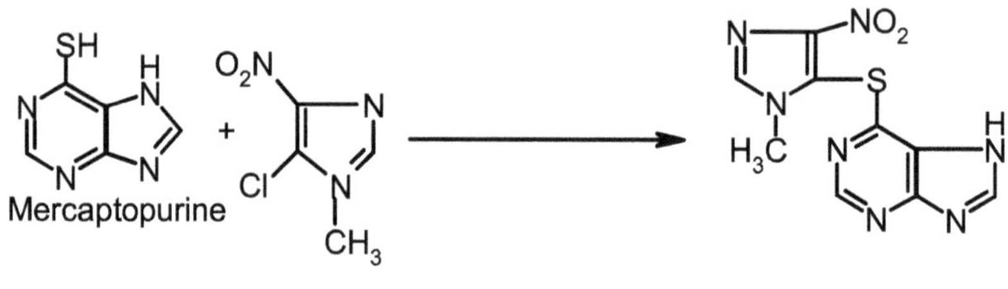

Properties

It occurs as pale yellow crystals. It is slightly soluble in chloroform and ethanol and practically insoluble in water.

Uses

It is used mainly as an adjuvant to prevent the rejection of renal heterotransplants.

(iii) ***Pyrimidine analogues***: The pyrimidine analogues have structures closely resemble to endogenous pyrimidine bases. Fluorine substituted pyrimidine analogues also show very vital action in the treatment of cancer. The most important members of this group are 5-fluorouracil and 5-fluorodeoxyuridine. These are the metabolites whose structures closely resemble to those of endogenous pyrimidine bases.

Mechanism of action

Pyrimidine antimetabolites act by inhibiting one or more of the enzymes that are required for DNA synthesis. They usually act by inhibiting one or more of the enzymes that are required for DNA synthesis.

5-Fluorouracil

5-Fluorouracil is an effective pyrimidine antimetabolite. It is chemically 5-fluoro-2,4 (1H,3H)-pyrimidinedione.

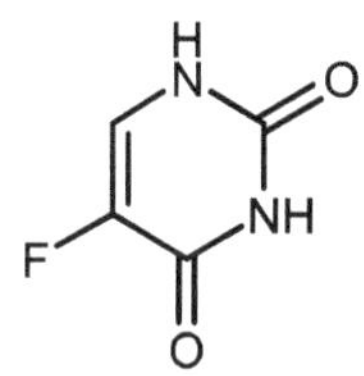

5-Fluorouracil

Fluorouracil is synthesized from uracil by following chemical reaction,

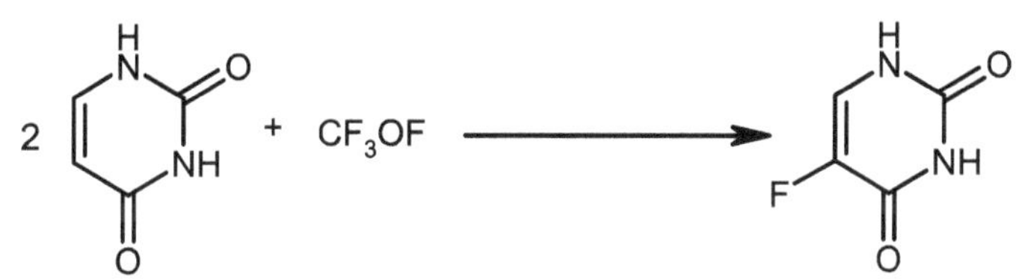

Mechanism of action

Fluorouracil is metabolized to 5-fluoro-2-deoxyuridine. The deoxyuridine act as an antimetabolite by inhibiting the synthesis of 2-deoxy thymidine. The failure to synthesize the thymidine nucleotide results in little or no production of DNA.

Properties

Fluorouracil is white crystalline powder. It is sparingly soluble in water and is a light sensitive compound.

Uses

It is used in the treatment of several common solid tumors and is topically used in the treatment of basal cell carcinomas and premalignant skin keratoses.

Cytarabine

It is 4-amino-1-β-D-arabinofuranosyl-2(1H)-pyrimidinone.

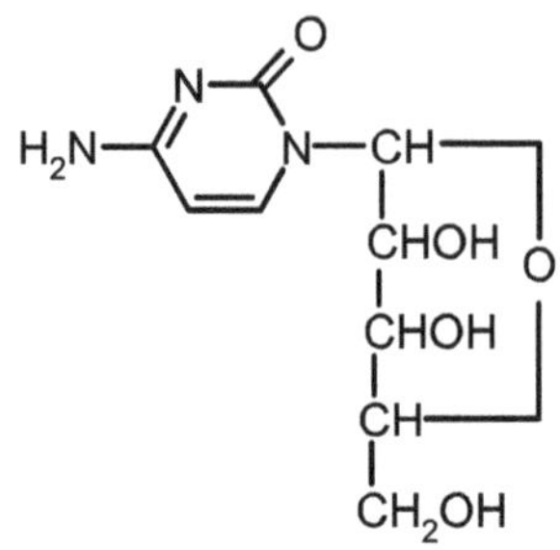

Cytarabine

Cytarabine is synthesized from uracil arabinoside by following chemical reaction,

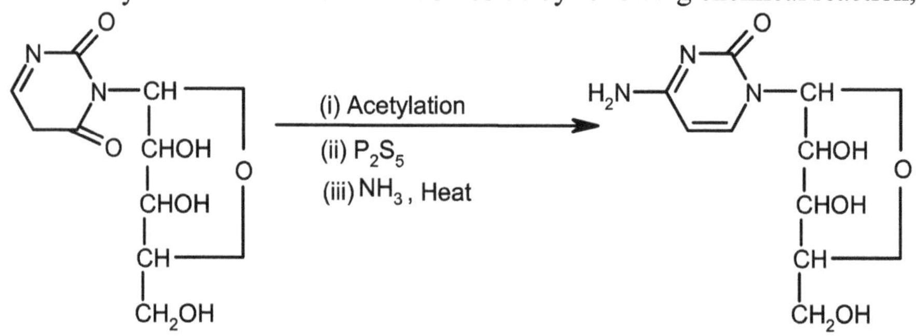

Mechanism of action

Inactive cytarabine is metabolized intracellularly into active triphosphate form (cytosine arabinoside triphosphate). This metabolite then damages DNA by multiple mechanisms, like the inhibition of α-DNA polymerase, inhibition of β-DNA polymerase, and incorporation into DNA. Cytotoxicity is highly specific for the S phase of the cell cycle. It is used in the treatment of acute myelocytic leukemia and in larger doses for non-Hodgkin lymphoma and chronic myelocytic leukemia.

Properties

These are prismatic crystals with a melting point of 212°C.

Uses

It is used in the treatment of acute myelocytic leukemia and in larger doses for non-Hodgkins lymphoma and chronic myelocytic leukemia.

Floxuridine

It is chemically 2'-deoxy-5-fluorouridine. It is used to treat gastrointestinal adenocarcinoma. It is very frequently used with other anticancer drugs in the treatment of acute myelocytic leukemia (AML), lymphomas, and for leukemia and lymphoma affecting the surrounding membranes of the brain and spinal cord (meninges).

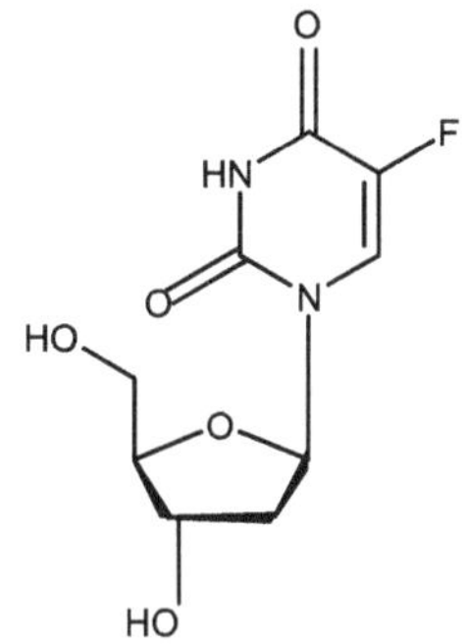

Floxuridine

III Antimitotics

Antimitotics are the drugs acting on the M phase of the cell cycle. These inhibit the mitosis process of cells thereby inhibiting the cancer growth in the cells. Several plants are systematically screened to observe the antitumor activity. About 1,00,000 plants are screened for the antineoplastic activity. The two major antineoplastic activity-exhibiting plants are:

(i) Podophyllum

(ii) Vinca alkaloids

(iii) Taxanes

(i) ***Podophyllum :*** Resin of *podophyllum peltatum* contains podophyllotoxin, which has antineoplastic activity. It inhibits mitosis by destroying the structural organization of mitotic apparatus. Podopyllotoxin is highly toxic but newer analogues such as etoposide and teniposide are much better.

Etoposide

It is chemically 9-[(4,6-o-Ethylidene-β-D-glucopyranosyl)oxy]-5,8,8α,9-tetrahydro-5-(4-hydroxy-3,5-dimethoxyphenyl)furo[3',4':6,7]naphtho[2,3-d]-1,3-dioxo1 6(5αH)-one.

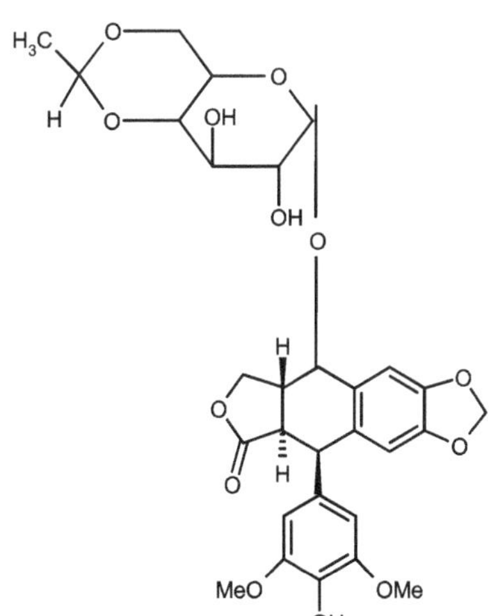

Etoprine

Properties

Etoposide is available as white crystalline powder having a melting point of 236°C-251°C. It is very soluble in methanol, chloroform and slightly soluble in ethanol. It is sparingly soluble in water. It is administered as IV infusion or by oral route.

Uses

It is used to treat small cell lung cancer, refractory testicular tumors, non-lymphocytic leukemia, Hodgkin disease and Kaposi's sarcoma.

(ii) ***Vinca alkaloids*** *:* Vinca alkaloids are the most important antineoplastic agents isolated from the plant periwinkle, *Catharanthus rosea* belonging to the family Apocyanaceae. Alkaloids obtained from this plant are composed of indole containing moiety, catharanthine and an indoline containing moiety, vindoline. The major alkaloids present in the plant are vincristine, vinblastine, vintosidine and vinleurosine.

Vinca alkaloids act by binding to tubulin and inhibiting it's polymerization into microtubules, which prevents spindle formation in mitosing cells and causes arrest at metaphase. Vinca alkaloids act on the dissolution of microtubules in cells. Vinblastine is the most active compound and vincristine causes the irreversible inhibition of mitosis.

Vincristine

It is an antitumor alkaloid isolated from *Catharanthus roseus* family: Apocyanaceae

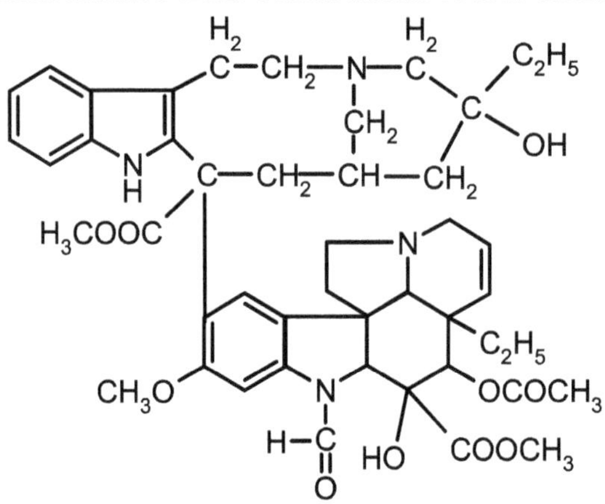

Vincristine

Properties

These are blades having a melting point of 218°C-220°C. It is soluble in water and chloroform and slightly soluble in ethanol.

Uses

It is used as an antineoplastic agent.

Vinblastine

It is antitumor alkaloid isolated from periwinkle, Vinca rosea Family: Apocynaceae.

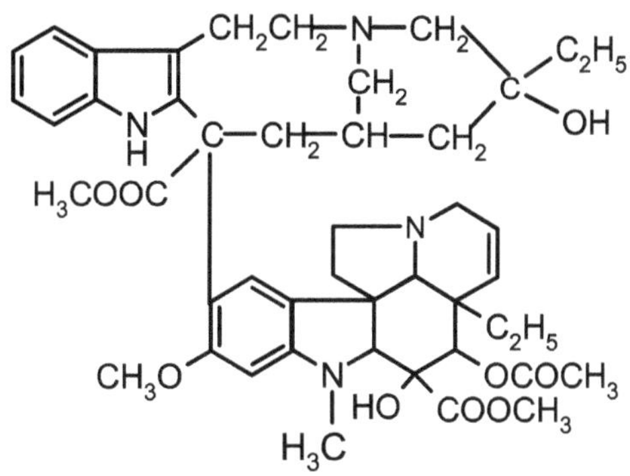

Vinblastine

Properties

These are solvated needles having a melting point of 211°C-216°C. It is practically insoluble in water, petroleum ether and soluble in alcohols, acetone and ethyl acetate.

Uses

It is used as an antineoplastic agent.

Vindesine

It is chemically desacetyl vinblastine amide (2β,3β,4β,5α,15β,19α)-4-(acetyloxy)-6,7-didehydro-3-hydroxy-16-methoxy-1-methyl-aspidospermidine-3-carboxylic acidmethyl ester.

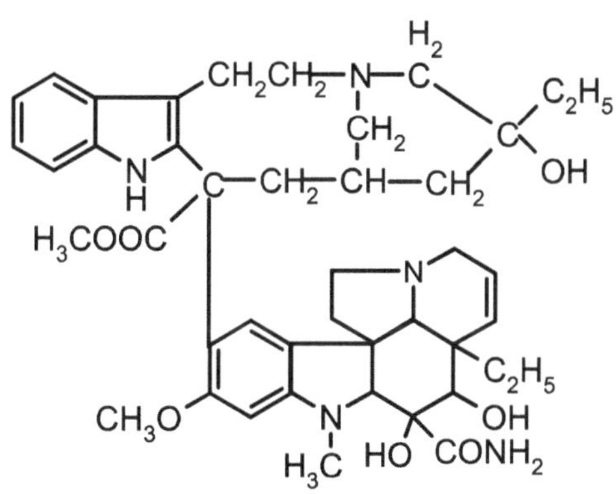

Vindesine

Properties

These are needles having a melting point of 164°C-165 °C.

Uses

It is used as an antineoplastic agent.

(iii) ***Taxanes :*** Taxanes are the plant products, which are of high current interest in chemotherapy of cancer. Paclitaxel was isolated from the bark of the *Taxus brevifolia* and *Taxus baccata*.

Mechanism of action

Paclitaxel inhibits mitosis by acting on mitotic spindle. It acts by promoting the assembly of microtubules and stabilizing them against depolymerization.

Paclitaxel

It is [2aR-[2aα,4β,4aβ,6β,9α(αR*, βS*), 11α,12α,12aα,12bα]]-β-(benzoylamino) -α-hydroxy-benzenepropanoic acid 6,12b-bis(acetyloxy)-12-(benzoyloxy)-2a, 3, 4, 4a, 5, 6, 9, 10, 11, 12, 12a, 12b-dodecahydro-4,11-dihydroxy-4a, 8,13,13-tetramethyl-5-oxo-7,11-methano-1H-cyclodeca [3, 4] benz [1, 2-b] oxet-9-yl ester.

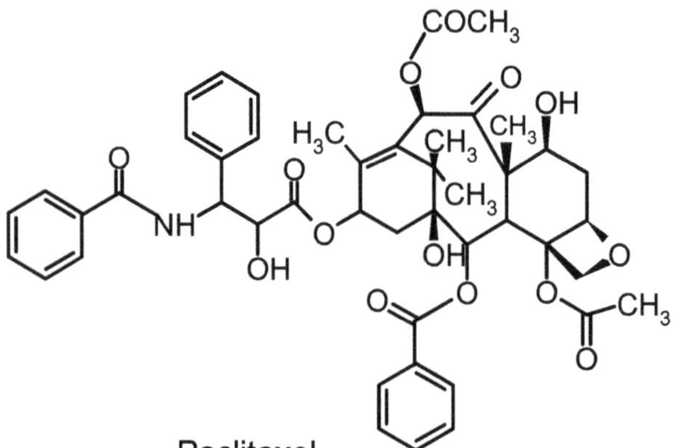

Paclitaxel

Properties

These are needles having a melting point of 213°C-216°C.

Uses

It is used to treat refractory ovarian cancer, metastatic breast cancer, metastatic melanoma and non-small cell lung cancer.

IV Antibiotics

These antibiotics are initially considered as the cytotoxic but later their toxic nature is useful in the treatment of cancer. Antitumor drugs produce their effects mainly by direct action on DNA. The different categories of antibiotics have been used as anticancer agents:

(i) Actinomycins
(ii) Anthracyclines
(iii) Bleomycins
(iv) Mitomycins

(i) ***Actinomycins*:** Actinomycins are comprised of a large group of closely related compounds. These compounds have a substituted 3-phenoxazone-1,9-dicarboxylic acid which is known as actinocin. Carboxylic acids in acitnomycins are attached to pentapeptides. The hydroxyl group in threonine forms the lactone ring with the fifth amino acid, which is generally N-methylvaline. The second amino acid D-valline or alloisoleucine and fourth amino acid is usually sarcosine. The gap highly prone to change amino acid is the third one. It may be L-proline, L-hydroxyproline and L-oxoproline.

Actinomycins which has two identical pentapeptide lactone are called isoactinomycins and those with different pentapeptide lactone are called anisoactinomycins.

Mechanism of action

Actinomycins intercalate into double-helical DNA. The phenoxazone moiety fits between successive base pairs. Adjacent G-C pairs are suitable because the 2 amino groups of guanine can form hydrogen bond with the carbonyl groups of threonines of actinomycins and the interaction between the pentapeptide lactone and DNA adds to the stability.

Dactinomycin

It is also known as actinomycin D. Dactinomycin is produced by the growth of *Streptomyces chrysomallus*. It is chemically actinomycin-[thr-val-pro-sar-meval].

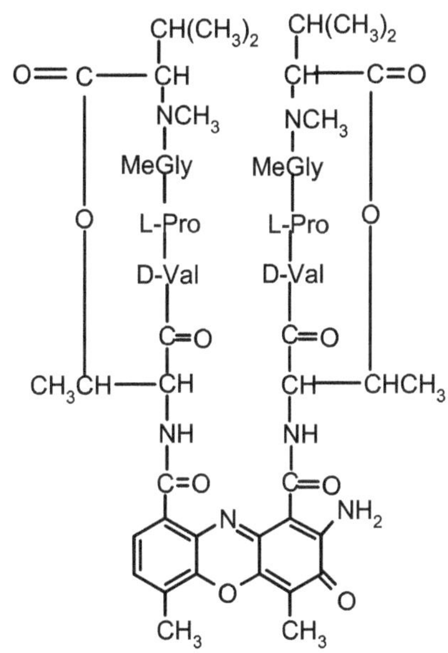

Dactinomycin

Properties

These are bright red rhomboid prisms having a melting point of 241.5°C-243°C. It is soluble in alcohol, propylene glycol and in a mixture of water and glycol.

Uses

It is used against rabdomyosarcoma and Wilm's tumor. It is also used to treat tumors of uterus and testis.

(ii) ***Anthracyclines*:** Anthracyclines are another large group of antibiotics, which are used for cancer therapy. These are the glycosides of the anthracyclinones. Daunorubicin is the first isolated compound from the *Streptomyces coeruleorubidus* and doxorubicin was isolated from *Streptomyces peucetius*. Both are used for the treatment of broad spectrum of tumors. Idarubicin and epirubicin are the drugs belonging to the anthracyclines, which has less cardio toxic effects than the earlier drugs.

Mechanism of action

Anthracyclines intercalate between nucleoside pairs of DNA and further amino sugar of these antibiotics bind tightly to DNA, resulting in decreased synthesis of both DNA and RNA. These compounds inhibit the topoisomerase II. Doxorubicin undergoes reduction and generates hydroxyl groups which attack DNA strand and causes scission of DNA. The other drugs belonging to this category interferes more with RNA synthesis rather than DNA synthesis.

Daunorubicin

This anthracycline antibiotic is the first agent isolated as cytotoxic antibiotics. It is chemically (8Scis)-8-acetyl-10-[(3-amino-2,3,6-trideoxy-α-L-lyxo hexopyranosyl) oxy]-7,8,9,10-tetrahydro-6,8,11-trihydroxy-1-methoxy-5,12-naphthacenedione.

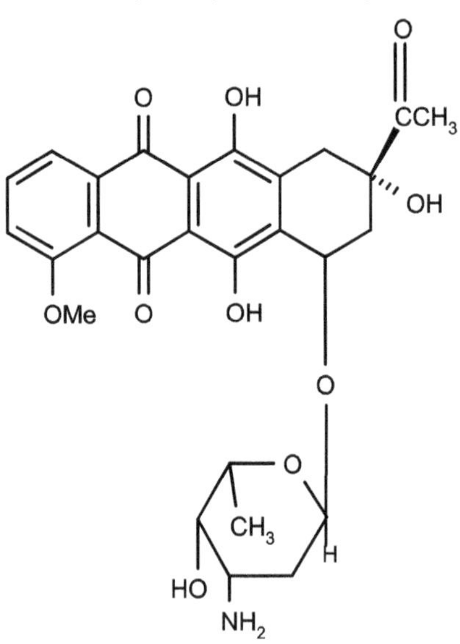

Daunorubicin

Properties

These are thin red needles having a decomposition temperature of 188°C -190°C. It is practically insoluble in chloroform, ether and benzene and soluble in water, methanol and other alcohols.

Uses

It is used in the treatment of acute lymphocytic and granulocytic leukemia.

Doxorubicin

Doxorubicin is one of the most successful antitumor drugs.It is (8S cis)-10-[(3-Amino-2,3,6-trideoxy-α-L-lyxo-hexopyranosyl)oxy]-7,8,9,10-tetrahydro-6,8,11-trihydroxy-8-(hydroxyacetyl)1-methoxy-5, 12-naphthacenedione.

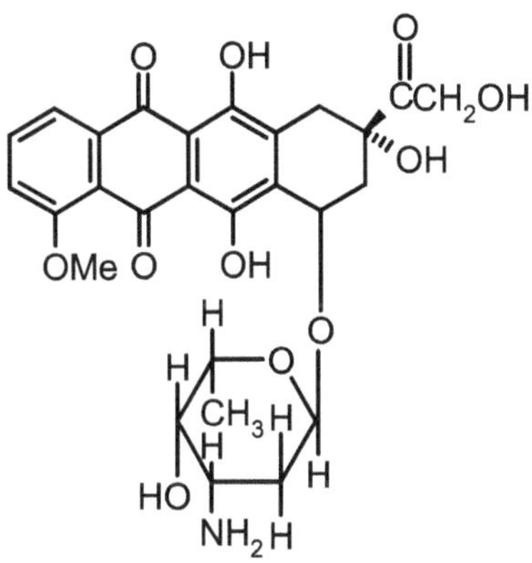

Doxorubicin

Mechanism of action

Doxorubicin elicits anticancer activity by intercalation mechanism (Intercalating agents are compounds that insert themselves between the bases of DNA helix. This insertion causes DNA helix scission and inhibits transcription, which blocks the replication process of the cell). It possess flat aromatic ring system that is responsible for intercalation. However other groups in the structure also contribute to the binding of a drug to DNA (amino group of sugar residue of doxorubicin forms ionic bond with negatively charged oxygen of phosphate groups of DNA chains which effectively locks the drug into place).

Properties

These are orange colored needles having a melting point of 204°C-205°C. It is soluble in water, methanol and aqueous alcohols. It is practically insoluble in acetone, benzene, chloroform, ethyl ether and petroleum ether.

Uses

It is used in the treatment of leukemia, Hodgkin's disease, neuroblastoma, breast and ovarian carcinoma.

Epirubicin

It is chemically (8S,10S)-10-[(3-amino-2,3,6-trideoxy-α-L-arabino-hexopyranosy) oxy]-7,8, 9, 10-tetrahydro-6, 8, 11-trihydroxy-8-(hydroxyacetyl)-1-methoxy-5, 12-naphthacenedione.

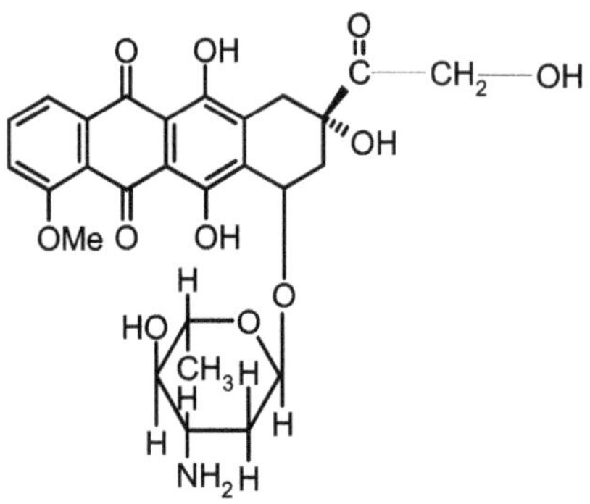

Epirubicin

Properties

These are red orange crystals having a melting point of 185°C. It must be protected from light.

Uses

It is used as antineoplastic agent.

Idarubicin

It is (7S,9S)-9-acetyl-7-[(3-amino-2,3,6-trideoxy-α-lyxo-hexopyranosy)oxy]-7, 8, 9, 10-tetrahydro-6, 9, 11-trihydroxy-5, 12-naphthacenedione.

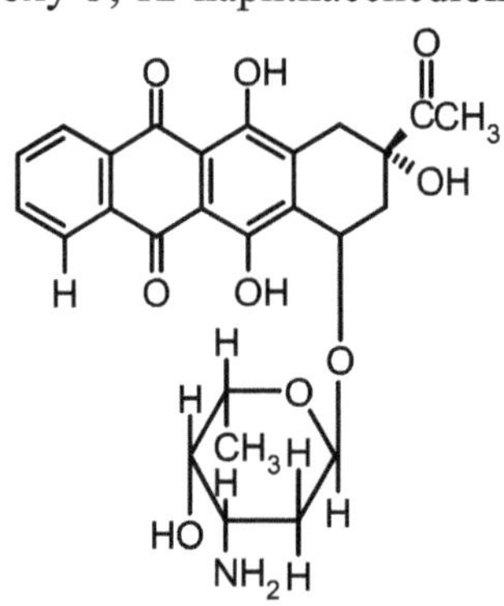

Idarubicin

Properties

It is an orange crystalline powder having a melting point of 183°C-185°C.

Uses

It is used for therapy of acute non-lymphocytic leukemia.

(iii) ***Bleomycins*****:** Bleomycins are glycopeptide antibiotics isolated from *Streptomyces verticillus*. Naturally bleomycins and its analogues occur as copper chelates. Copper-free bleomycin (copper can be removed by chemical reduction) is used for cancer chemotherapy and it has lower toxicity.

E.g : BleomycinA_2, bleomycinB_2

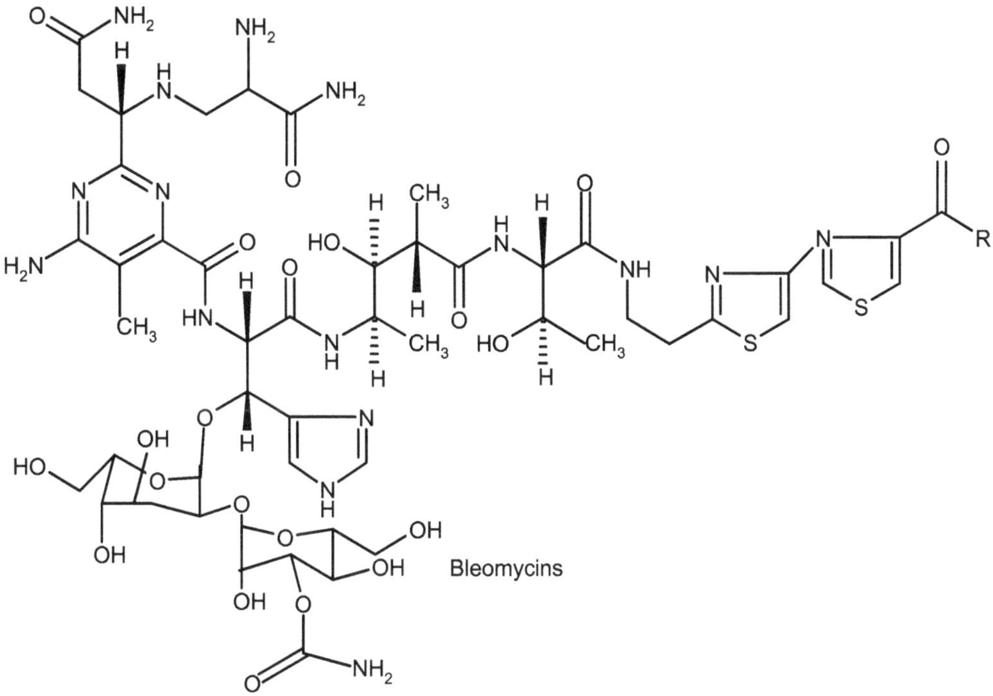

Bleomycins

A_1 : R = $NH(CH_2(_3SOCH_3$

A_2 : R = $NH(CH_2)_3S{+}(CH_3)_2$

Demethyl-A_2 : R = $NH(CH_2)_3SCH_3$

A_2'a : R = $NH(CH_2)_4NH_2$

A_2'b : R = $NH(CH_2)_3NH_2$

A_2'c : R = $NH(CH_2)_2$ 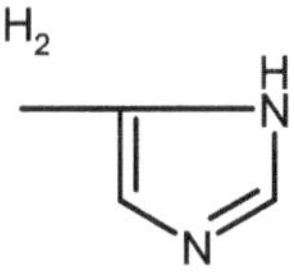

A_5 : R = $NH(CH_2)_3NH(CH_2)_4NH_2$

A_6 : R = $NH(CH_2)_3NH(CH_2)_4NH(Ch_2)_3NH_2$

B_1' : R = NH_2

B_2 : R = $NH(CH_2)_4NH\overset{\overset{NH}{\|}}{C}NH_2$

B_4 : R = $NH(CH_2)_4NH\overset{\overset{NH}{\|}}{C}NH(CH_2)_4NH\overset{\overset{NH}{\|}}{C}NH_2$

Bleomycinic acid : R = OH

Peptomycin R = 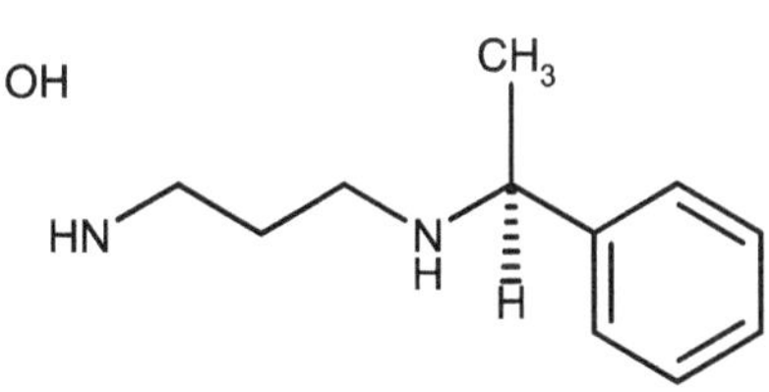

Mechanism of action

The action of bleomycins is not fully understood. Bleomycin posses the bithiazole moiety which intercalates with the DNA. In bleomycin A_2 the resulting adduct is thought to be stabilized by ionic bonding between the phosphate units of DNA and the sulphonium ion of the side chain. The intercalation is believed to be followed by domain Y forming a complex with Fe (II). The complex reacts with oxygen to form free radicals, which cause chain fragmentation

Properties

It is a colorless or yellowish powder, which is very soluble in water and methanol and slightly soluble in ethanol. It is practically insoluble in acetone, ethyl acetate and ether. Bleomycin is inactivated by bleomycin hydrolase (an intracellular enzyme).

Uses

It is used in the treatment of squamous cell carcinomas of head, neck, esophagus, skin and genitourinary tract including penis, cervix and vulva.

Peplomycin

It is chemically N' -[3-[[(1S)-1-phenylethyl]amino]propyl]bleomycinamide.

Properties

It is a pale yellow colored amorphous powder having a melting point of $196^{\circ}C$-$198^{\circ}C$. It is soluble in water, methanol, acetic acid, DMSO, DMF and slightly soluble in dioxane. It is insoluble in ethyl acetate, acetone, ether and benzene.

Uses

It is used as antineoplastic agent.

Mithramycin

It is an oligosaccharide antibiotic produced by *Streptomyces argillaceous*.

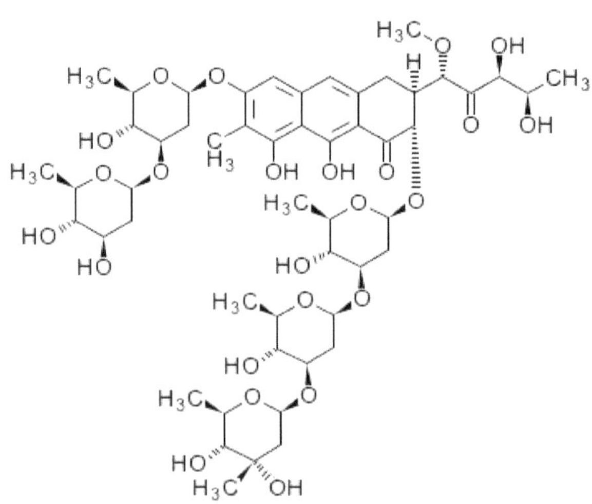

Mithramycin

Mechanism of action

It inhibits DNA -dependent RNA synthesis (similar to dactinomycin).

Properties

It is a yellow solid having a melting point of 180°C -183°C, which is soluble in lower alcohols, acetone, ethyl acetate and water. It is moderately soluble in chloroform and slightly soluble in ether and benzene.

Uses

It is used in the treatment of advanced embryonal tumors.

(iv) ***Mitomycins***: These are the group of antibiotics produced by *Streptomyces caespitosus*. Mitomycins have quinone, carbamate and aziridines in their structures, which inhibit the cancer growth.

Mechanism of action

Mitomycins undergo chemical reduction to form hydroquinone and finally by loosing methanol, it results in the formation of bifunctional alkylating agents indolohydroquinone, which cross-links DNA.

Mitomycin C

It is chemically [1aR-(1aα,8β,8aα,8bα)]-6-amino-8-[[(aminocarbony)oxy]methyl]-1,1a,2,8,8a,8b-hexahydro-8a-methoxy-5-methyl azirino[2',3':3,4]pyrrolo[1,2-a] indole -4-7-dione.

Properties

Mitomycin exists as blue or violet crystals. It is soluble in water, methanol, acetone, butyl acetate and cyclohexanone and slightly soluble in benzene, carbon tetrachloride and ether. It is practically insoluble in petroleum ether.

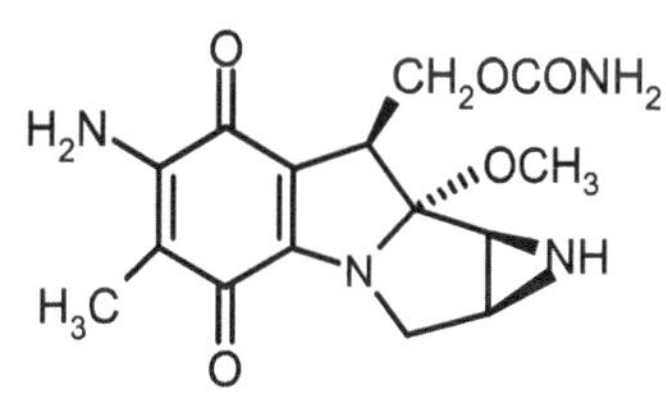

Mitomycin C

Uses

It is used in the treatment of disseminated breast, gastric, pancreatic or colorectal adrenocarcinomas.

Streptozocin

It is 2-deoxy-2-[[(methylnitrosoamino)carbonyl amino]-D-glucopyranose.

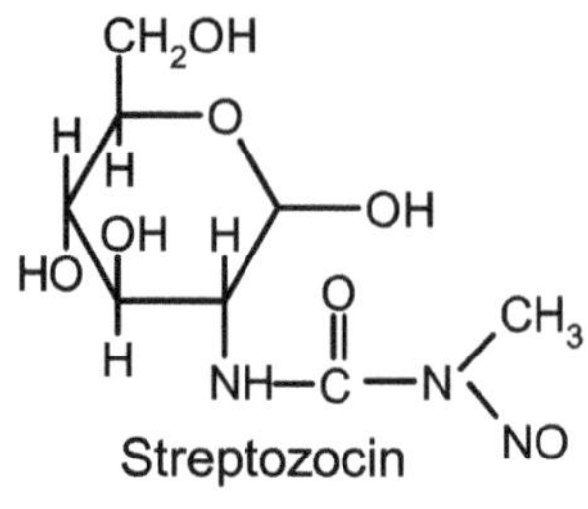

Streptozocin

Properties

These are pointed platelets or prisms having a melting point of 115°C. It is soluble in water, lower alcohols and ketones.

Uses

It is used only in the treatment of metastatic islet cell carcinoma of the pancreas.

(V) ***Hormonal agents*:** Hormones are the major antitumor's used especially in the treatment of solid tumors like breast and prostatic cancers. A normal and neoplastic cell has a number of hormone receptors and depends on the hormonal control. The different groups of hormonal therapy can be given as:

(i) Adrenocortico steroids
(ii) Estrogens
(iii) Progestins
(iv) SnRH analogues
(v) GnRH analogues
(vi) Aromtase inhibitors
(vii) Antiestrogens
(viii) Antiandrogens
(ix) Antiprogestins

(i) *Adrenocortico steroids*

These agents inhibit RNA and protein synthesis, interfere with lymphoid proliferation and have a lympholytic effect. Thus these steroids inhibit growth of mesenchymal tissues and have anti-inflammatory and immunosuppressive activities.

The corticosteroids are used to treat acute and chronic lymphatic leukaemia, Hodgkin's disease, non-Hodgkin's lymphomas, prostatic carcinoma and multiple myeloma.

Prednisone

It is chemically 17α, 21-dihydroxy 1,4 - pregnadiene -3, 11, 20-trione.

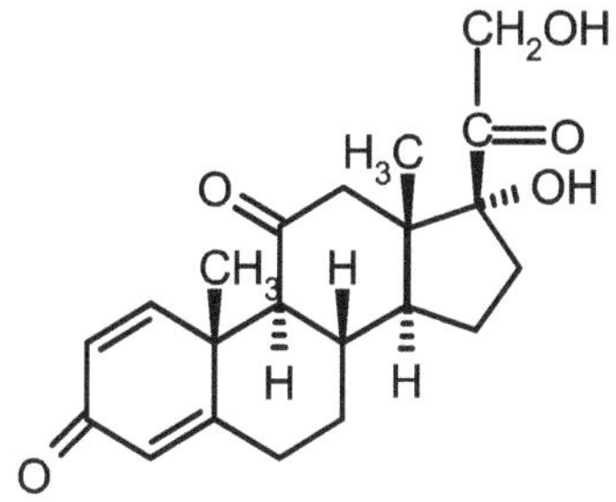

Prednisone

Mitotane

It is 1-chloro-2-[2,2-dichloro-1-(4-chlorophenyl)ethyl]benzene. It is used as antineoplastic agent in the treatment of adrenocortical carcinoma.

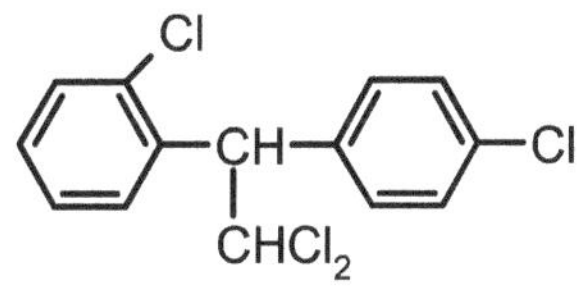

Mitotane

(ii) ***Estrogens***

Estrogens inhibit cell growth and differentiation. They also block the effects of androgen and cause regressive changes in breast in postmenopausal women and in prostatic gland in males

E.g. : Diethylstilbesterol

It is chemically 4,4'[(1E)-1,2-diethyl-1,2-ethenediyl]bisphenol. It is used as an antineoplastic agent.

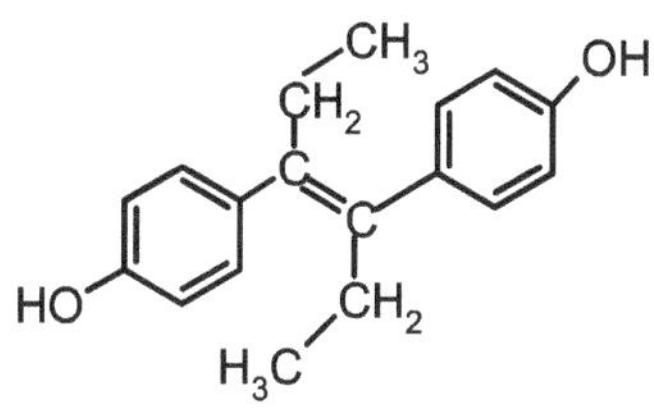

Diethylstilbesterol

It can be synthesized from anethole by the following steps:

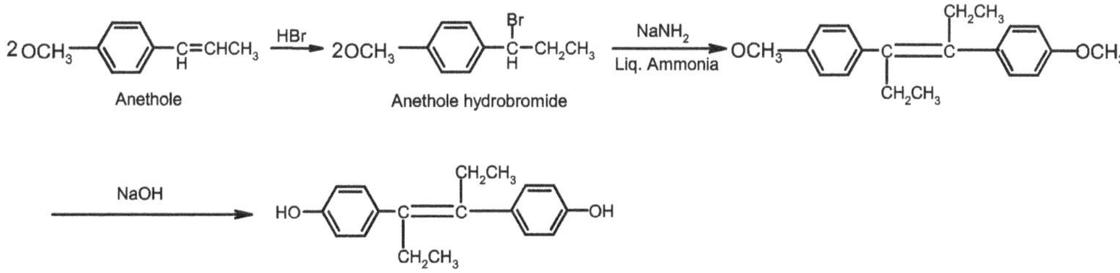

Diethylstilbesterol

(iii) *Progestins*

The progestogens have been employed in the management of endometrial carcinoma, breast cancer, refractory prostatic cancer and rarely carcinoma of kidney and testes

E.g : Hydoxyprogesterone caproate
It is chemically 17-hydroxypregn-4-ene-3,20-dione hexanoate.

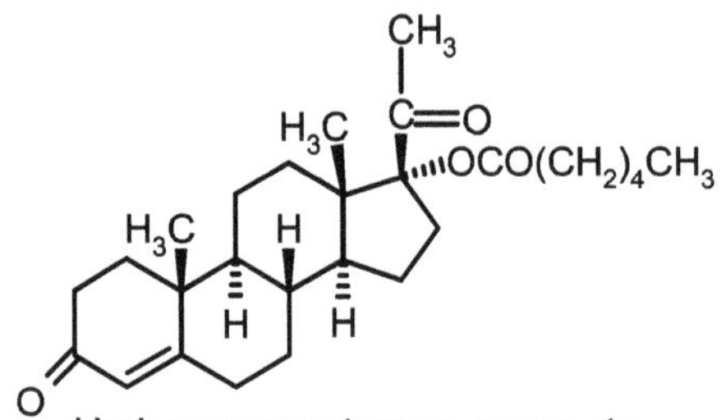

Hydoxyprogesterone caproate

Medroxyprogesterone acetate

It is (6α)-17-acetoxy-6-methylpregn-4-ene-3, 20-dione.

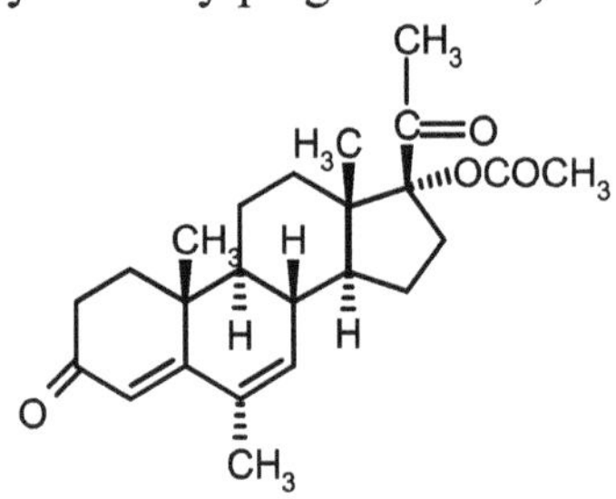

Medroxyprogesterone acetate

Megestrol acetate

It is chemically 17-acetoxy-6-methylpregna-4,6-dien-3,20-dione acetate. It is used in the treatment of advanced breast or endometrial carcinoma.

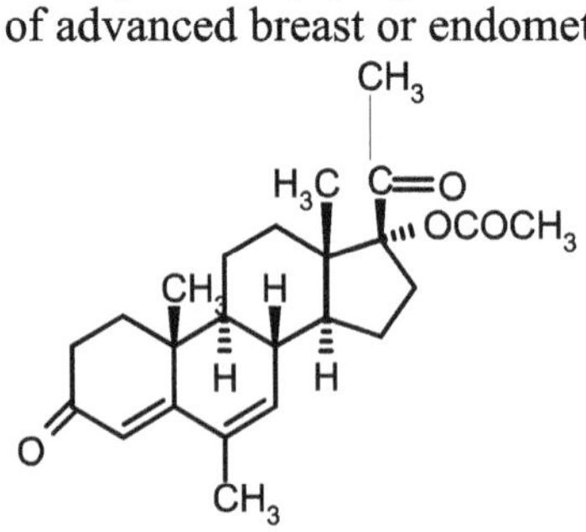

Megestrol acetate

(v) *GnRH analogues*

Gonadotrophin releasing hormone also known as lutenising hormone releasing hormone (LHRH) analogues initially increase the levels of testosterone and later decline in testosterone levels.

Leuprolide

It is chemically 6-D-leucine-9-(N-ethyl-L-prolinamide)-10-deglycinamide.

H-5-oxo Pro-His-Trp-Ser- Tyr-D-Leu-Leu- Arg-Pro-NH - C_2H_5

Leuprolide is a peptide analogue of LH-RH and decrease oestrogen and testosterone production by gonads.

It is used in the treatment of advanced prostatic cancer.

Non-steroidal type

Aminoglutethimide

Aminoglutethimide is an analogue of glutethimide. It inhibits the synthesis of adrenocortical steroids and also effectively block the secretion of cortisol.

It is chemically 3-(4-aminophenyl)-3-ethyl-2, 6-piperidinedione

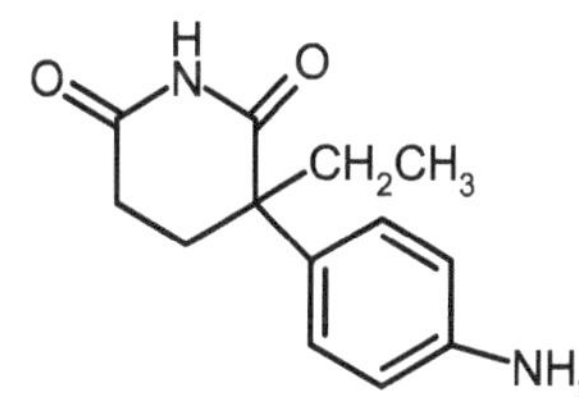

Aminoglutethimide

Properties

It is freely soluble in most of the organic solvents and is poorly soluble in ethyl acetate and absolute ethanol. It is readily soluble in acetone and acetic acid but practically insoluble in water.

Uses

It is used as an adrenocortical suppressant and antineoplastic agent.

(vii) *Antiestrogens*

Estrogen receptors can be identified in tumour cells of 50% of premenopausal women with breast cancer and 75% of postmenopausal women. Antiestrogens bind with estrogen receptors to cause depletion of cytoplasm of free receptor, hence estrogen dependent growth of the tumour. Further antiestrogens bind to estrogen receptors for a longer time than the normal hormone.

E.g : Tamoxifen, clomiphene, nafoxidine

Tamoxifen

It is chemically (Z)-2-[4-(1, 2-dipheny l-1-butenyl) phenoxy] -N, N-dimethyl-ethanamine.

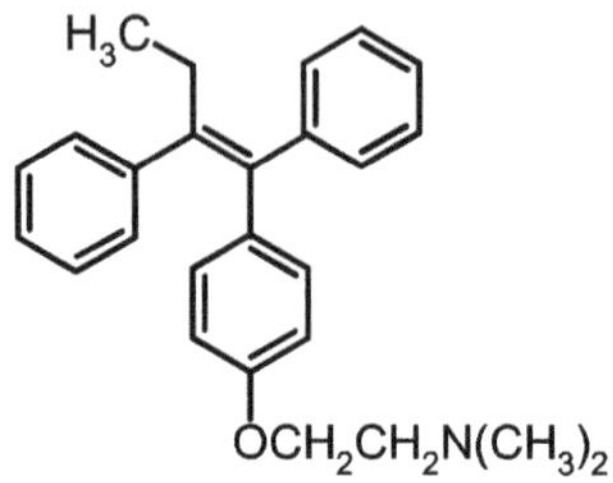

Tamoxifen

Properties

It is a fine, white, odorless, crystalline powder having a melting point of 140°C. It slightly soluble in water and soluble in ethanol, methanol and acetone.

Uses

It is used as an antiestrogen and antineoplastic agent in the treatment of advanced breast cancer.

(viii) *Antiandrogens*

Antiandrogens compete with testosterone for androgen receptor.

E.g : Flutamide, Bicalutamide, testolactone

Flutamide

Flutamide is a non-steroidal antiandrogen which competes with testosterone. It is chemically 2-methyl-N- [4-nitro-3-(trifloromethyl) phenyl] propanamide. It is used to treat prostate cancer.

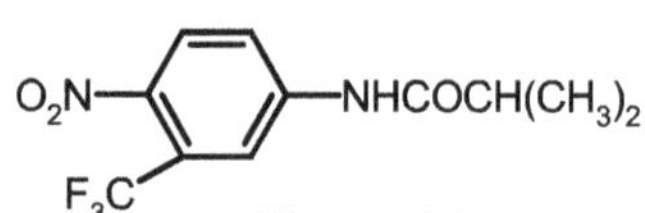

Flutamide

Bicalutamide

It is chemicallyN-[4-cyano-3-(trifluoromethyl)phenyl]-3-[(4-fluorophenyl)sulphonyl]-2-hydroxy-2-methylpropionamide. It is used in the treatment of advanced prostatic cancer.

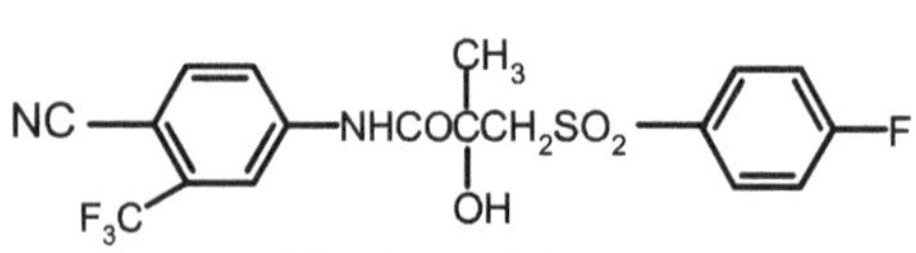

Bicalutamide

Testolactone

It is (4αs,4βR,10αR,10βS,12αS)-3,4,4α,5,6,10α,10β,11,12,12α-decahydro-10α,12α-dimethyl-2H-phenanthro [2,1-b]pyran-2,8(4βH)-dione. It is used in the treatment of advanced or disseminated breast cancer.

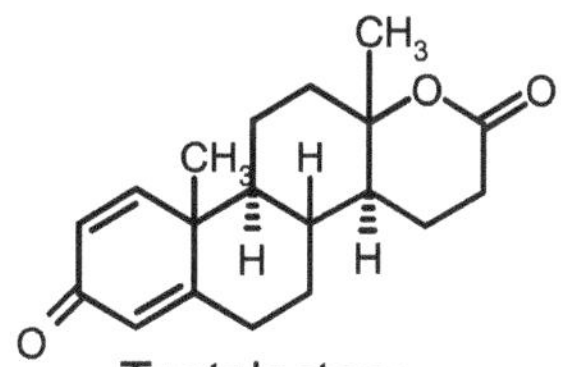

Testolactone

(ix) *Antiprogestins*

Mifepristone

It is chemically (11β,17β)-11-[4-(dimethylamino)phenyl]-17-hydroxy-17-(1-propynyl)estra-4,9-dien-3-one.

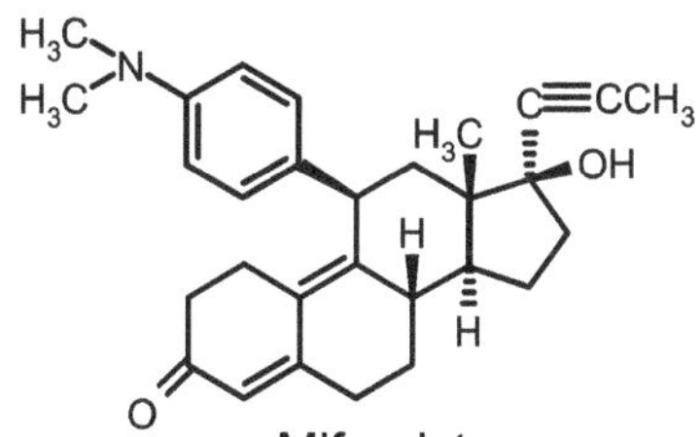

Mifepristone

Mechanism of action of anti cancer drugs

Cisplatin

Cisplatin is mostly used to treat testicular tumors. It destroys the cells by forming cisplatin - DNA adducts by binding with N^7 of guanine whereby transcr iption and replication processes were blocked. DNA mismatch repair protein hMSH2 are over expressed in testicular and ovarian tissues and the tumor in these tissues is treated by cisplatin. High mobility group(HMG) proteins and hMSH2 binds to the cisplatin - DNA adducts and displays the therapeutic action against the tumor.

Hydroxyurea

Hydroxyurea inhibits the reverse transcription process by altering the cellular enzyme ribonucleotide reductase required for the synthesis of deoxyribonucleotide triphosphate (dNTP's).

Proca rbazine

Cytotoxic action of procarbazine is by inhibiting the transmethylation of methyl groups of methionine into t - RNA , required for the synthesis of DNA and RNA. Autooxidation of procarbazine produces the hydrogen peroxiderl-l-Oj) which binds to the sulphydryl,groups of residual proteins causing the damage to DNA.

Mechanism of action of anti - viral agents

Protease inhibitors

In the viral replication cycle, mRNA gets translated to polyproteins (immature budding particles in the HIV virions) by the action of viral protease encoded in the gag - pol gene. This protease enzyme is not available in the host, so HIV aspartyl protease inhibitors are developed which shows specificity to viral protease only and by binding to viral protease enzyme it produces immature non - infectious virions.

RNA synthesis inhibitors

Ribavirin is a guanosine analogue and it inhibits 5^1 cap formation on mRNA containing methyl guanosine. It also produces multiple mutations in viral RNA causing the formation of non - infectious virions.

Nucleoside inhibitors

Nucleoside inhibitors gets converted into triphosphate form which competes with reverse transcriptase enzyme and gets incorporated into viral DNA chain resulting in inhibition of elongation of viral DNA chain.

(vi) *Miscellaneous anti-cancer drugs*

Cisplatin

Cis-Diamminedichloroplatinum (II), or cisplatin, is a chemotherapeutic drug used to treat a variety of cancers. The platinum stereochemistry is very important with the *trans* isomer showing no anti-cancer activity. CISPLATIN is one of the most spectacularly successful of all chemotherapy treatments for cancer, curing nearly 95% of men who develop testicular cancer. But it only works against cancer of the testes and, to a lesser extent, ovaries.

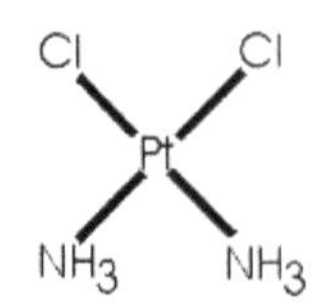

Cisplatin

Cisplatin is used mainly to combat testicular tumors and, with less success, other malignancies. It is not known how platinum (II) compounds kill cells but there is evidence to suggest that its DNA adducts, which block replication and transcription, are the key mediators. It is found that HMG box proteins and the mismatch repair protein hMSH2 in human cells bind tightly to some platinum adducts. Interestingly, the adducts bound were those involved in the toxic response to the drug. Cisplatin forces tumor cells to self-destruct the process known as apoptosis. It begins by binding with the cancer cell's DNA. However, cisplatin has three drawbacks which limit its usefulness: its severe toxicities, it only affects a narrow range of tumors and it causes the development of resistance in the tumor cell.

Hydroxyurea

Hydroxyurea (brand name: Hydrea) has been on the market as an anti-cancer drug for over 30 years. Initially, it was used to treat some types of leukemia, as well as ovarian cancer and sickle cell anemia. However, it has recently been shown to have powerful anti-retroviral properties. Hydroxyurea is classified as an antimetabolite. It is a ribonucleotide reductase inhibitor.

$H_2NCONHOH$

Hydroxyurea

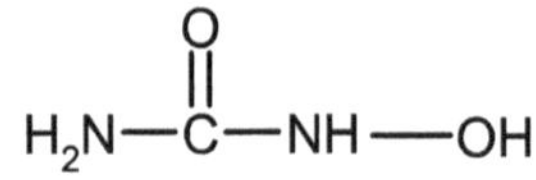

Mechanism

Hydroxyurea alters the cellular enzyme ribonucleotide reductase, which normally facilitates the formation of dNTP's. Without the presence of this enzyme, HIV is unable to reverse transcribe its RNA to DNA. Thus, Hydroxyurea reduces the viral load in some cases to levels, which are undetectable. There is some evidence that this effect may persist for the long term, even when anti-viral therapy is halted. Additionally, hydroxyurea penetrates the brain and lymph tissues, which may make it more effective than other anti-HIV drugs at preventing or treating HIV infection of the CNS.

Procarbazine

Procarbazine is classified as an alkylating agent. It is a hydrazine derivative. Chemically, procarbazine hydrochloride is *N* -isopropyl-(α)-(2-methylhydrazino)-*p*-toluamide monohydrochloride.

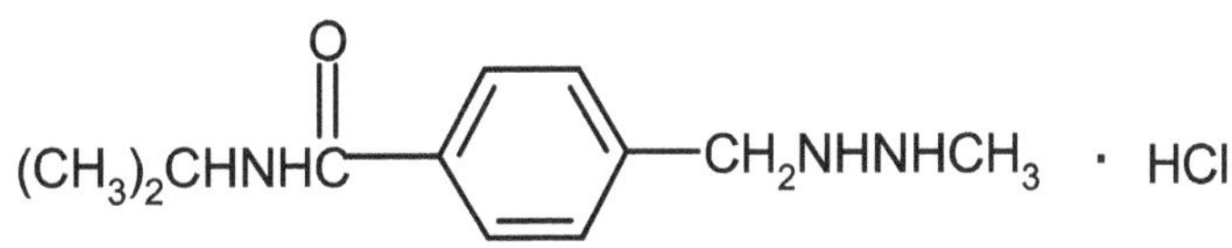

It is a white to pale yellow crystalline powder, which is soluble but unstable in water or aqueous solutions. The structural formula is:

The precise mode of cytotoxic action of procarbazine has not been clearly defined. There is evidence that the drug may act by inhibition of protein, RNA and DNA synthesis. Studies have suggested that procarbazine may inhibit transmethylation of methyl groups of methionine into t-RNA. The absence of functional t-RNA could cause the cessation of protein synthesis and consequently DNA and RNA synthesis. In addition, procarbazine may directly damage DNA. Hydrogen peroxide, formed during the auto-oxidation of the drug, may attack protein sulphydryl groups contained in residual protein which is tightly bound to DNA.

Procarbazine is metabolized primarily in the liver and kidneys. The drug appears to be auto-oxidized to the azo derivative with the release of hydrogen peroxide. The azo derivative isomerizes to the hydrazone, and following hydrolysis splits into a benzyl-aldehyde derivative and methylhydrazine. The methylhydrazine is further degraded to CO_2 and CH_4 and possibly hydrazine, whereas the aldehyde is oxidized to N -isopropylterephthalamic acid, which is excreted in the urine. Procarbazine is rapidly and completely absorbed. Following oral administration of 30 mg of ^{14}C-labeled procarbazine, maximum peak plasma radioactive concentrations were reached within 60 minutes.

Procarbazine is indicated for use in combination with other anticancer drugs for the treatment of stage III and IV Hodgkin's disease. Procarbazine is used as part of the MOPP (nitrogen mustard, vincristine, procarbazine, prednisone) regimen.

23

GASTROINTESTINAL AGENTS

Gastrointestinal agents are the drugs used to treat various diseases of gastrointestinal tract. They are primarily used to treat gastric hyperacidity, peptic ulcers, vomiting, diarrhoea and constipation.

Emetics

Agents or drugs that cause vomiting are known as emetics. They may act directly on the gastrointestinal tract, bringing about emesis through local irritant effects, or indirectly, through their effects on the chemoreceptor trigger zone in the *postremal* area near medulla.

Mechanism of emesis

Receptors on the floor of the fourth ventricle of the brain represent a chemoreceptor trigger zone, stimulation of which can lead to vomiting. The chemoreceptor zone lies outside the blood-brain barrier, can be stimulated by blood-borne drugs that can stimulate vomiting, or inhibit it. Emetics are used for the treatment of poisoning with certain toxins that have been swallowed.

(i) The most commonly used drug for this purpose is ipecac syrup, prepared from the dried roots of *Cephaelis ipecacuanha*, a plant indigenous to Brazil and Central America.

(ii) Apomorphine – an alkaloid derived from morphine by the action of strong acids or zinc chloride. It is the best emetic when swallowing is difficult, but is useless in narcotic poisoning after narcosis has blunted the vagus centre. Apomorphine is (6-α-R)-6-methyl-5, 6,6α, 7-tetrahydro-4H-dibenzoquinoline-10, and 11-diol.

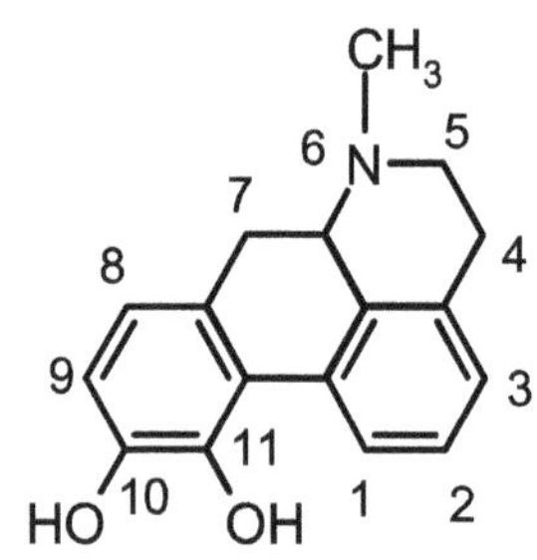

Apomorphine

Antiemetics

An antiemetic is a drug that is effective against vomiting and nausea. Antiemetics are typically used to treat motion sickness and the side effects of opioid analgesics.

Antiemetics Include :

1. ***5-Hydroxytryptamine antagonists :*** Dolasetron, granisetron, ondansetron, tropisetron
2. ***Dopamine antagonists :*** Domperidone, droperidol, haloperidol, chlorpromazine, metoclopramide
3. ***Antihistamines (5HT$_2$ receptor antagonists) :*** Cyclizine, diphenhydramine, dimenhydrinate, cannabinoids

5-HT antagonists

Serotonin (5-hydroxytryptamine or 5-HT) is a monoamine neurotransmitter. It is extensively exist in git and blood. Serotonin is synthesized in serotonergic neurons of CNS and enterochromaffin cells of git. Serotonin believed to play an important role in depression, migraine, anxiety, appetite, sexuality and bipolar disorders.

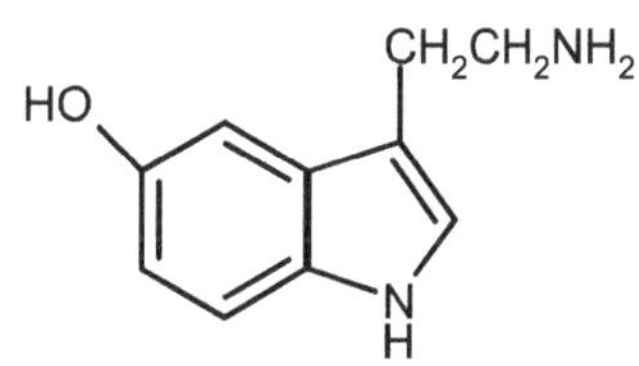

Serotonin

5-HT antagonists such as ondansetron, granisetron and tropisetron are important antiemetic agents. They are particularly important in treating the nausea and vomiting that occur during anticancer chemotherapy using cytotoxic drugs. Another application is in treatment of post-operative nausea and vomiting.

Dolasetron

Dolasetron is a serotonin 5-HT$_3$ receptor antagonist used to treat nausea and vomiting following chemotherapy. Its main affect is to reduce the activity of the vagus nerve, which is a nerve that activates the vomiting center in the medulla oblongata. It does not have much effect on vomiting due to motion sickness. This drug does not have any effect on dopamine receptors or muscarinic receptors.

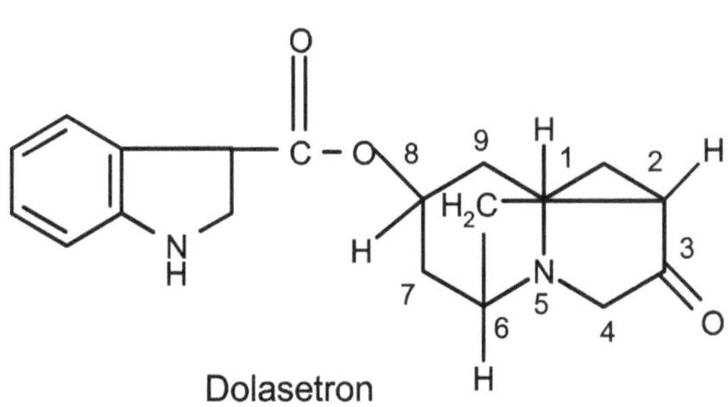

Dolasetron

Dolasetron breaks down slowly, staying in the body for a long time. One dose usually lasts 4 to 9 hours and is usually administered once or twice daily. This drug is metabolised by the liver and kidneys.

Clinical uses

It is used to treat chemotherapy-induced nausea and vomiting, post-operative and post-radiation nausea and vomiting and for nausea and vomiting due to acute or chronic medical illness or acute gastroenteritis.

Granisetron

Granisetron was invented by chemists of British drug company. The drug was approved in the United Kingdom in 1991 and in United States in 1994 by the FDA.

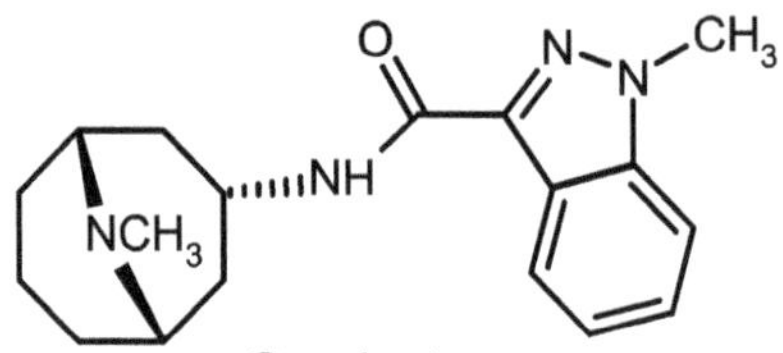

Granisetron

Granisetron is a serotonin 5-HT$_3$ receptor antagonist used to treat nausea and vomiting following chemotherapy.

Ondansetron

Ondansetron is currently marketed by GlaxoSmithKline under the trade name Zofran;

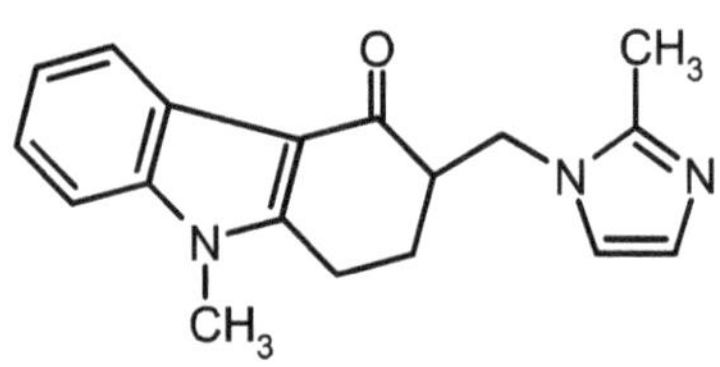

Ondansetron

It is a serotonin (5-HT) receptor antagonist used mainly to treat nausea and vomiting following chemotherapy. Its effects are thought to be on both peripheral and central nerves. This drug does not have any effect on dopamine receptors or muscarinic receptors. Ondansetron is synthesized by the following reaction:

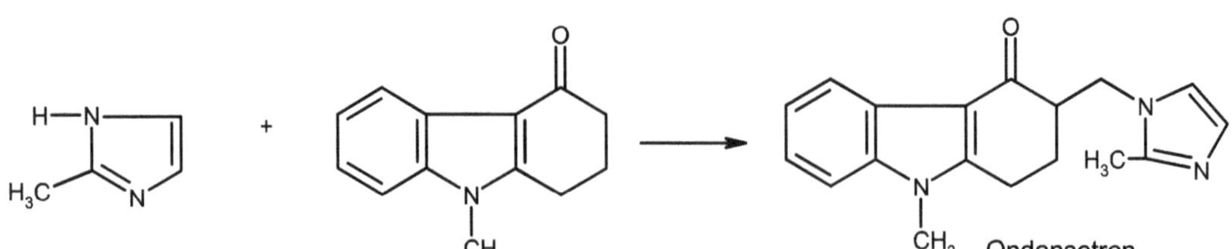

Ondansetron

Ondansetron is metabolized in liver. Its elimination half-life is about 2-3 hours following I.V administration in patients with normal liver and kidney functions. The drug is usually administered once, twice or three times daily, depending on the severity of nausea and/or concentrations. This drug is removed from the body by the liver and kidneys.

Dopamine antagonists

A dopamine antagonist is a drug, which blocks dopamine receptors. There are five subtypes of dopamine receptors in the human body, found in the brain, peripheral nervous system, blood vessels and in the kidney. Some of these drugs are commonly coupled with a serotonin antagonist and are used for treatment of certain kinds of psychosis. Dopamine antagonists used in psychiatry for psychosis include atypical antipsychotics clozapine, risperidone, olanzapine, quetiapine, ziprasidone and aripiprazole. Other dopamine antagonists include antiemetics metoclopramide, droperidol and domperidone.

Domperidone

Domperidone is an antidopaminergic drug used orally or intravenously, generally to suppress nausea and vomiting. It has also been used to stimulate lactation. It is acting at D_2 receptors.

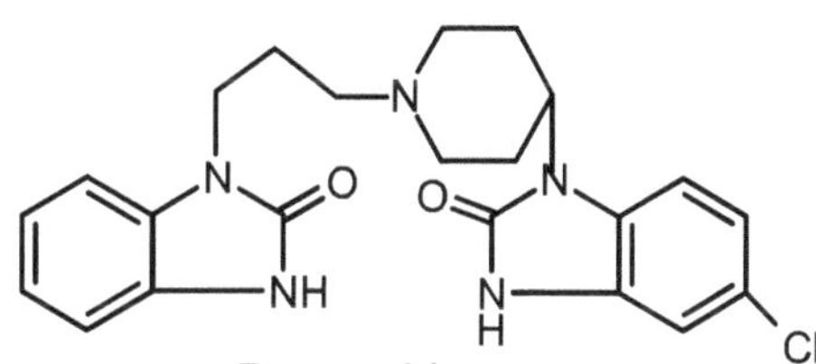

Domperidone

Domperidone is used, together with metoclopramide, cyclizine, and $5HT_3$ receptor antagonists (such as granisetron) in the treatment of nausea and vomiting. It is useful in patients with parkinson's disease because, unlike metoclopramide, domperidone does not cross the blood brain barrier. Domperidone is also prescribed for the treatment of gastroparesis, a stomach motility condition.

Metoclopramide

Metoclopramide molecule of metoclopramide was first described by Dr. Louis Justin-Besancon and Dr. C. Laville in 1964. It was originally developed as an antipsychotic drug, it's main usage is stimulating gastric motility and selectively binds to D_2 receptors, but in higher doses there is also some blocking activity on 5-HT_3 receptors. Metoclopramide acts on D_2 receptors in the CTZ (chemo receptor trigger zone) of the brainstem, thus blocking nausea/vomiting of most etiologies. In metoclopramide, methoxyl group in ortho position to amide functional group is essential for antiemetic activity.

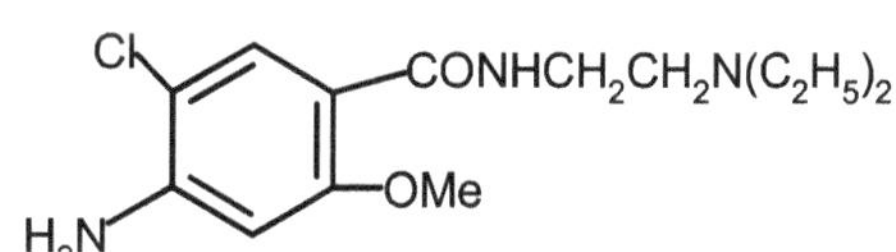

Metoclopramide

It is a potent dopamine antagonist that enters the central nervous system. It is used as an antiemetic and as a prokinetic for gastric emptying in patients with gastric motor failure (gastroparesis, e.g., in diabetic patients). It is also useful for facilitating small bowel evacuation. The most common side effects are somnolence, nervousness, and dystonic reactions.

Antihistamines

Antihistamines reduce or eliminate effects mediated by histamine, in common use, the term antihistamine refers only to H_1-receptor antagonists, also known as H_1-antihistamines. It has been discovered that these H_1-antihistamines are actually inverse agonists at the histamine H_1-receptor, rather than antagonists *per se*.

Diphenhydramine hydrochloride

Diphenhydramine hydrochloride is an overthecounter (OTC) antihistamine and sedative. It is also given in conjunction with typical antipsychotics to prevent tardive dyskinesia. It is a member of the ethanolamine class of antihistaminic agents. It is 2-(Diphenyl methoxy)N, N-dimethyl ethylamine hydrochloride.

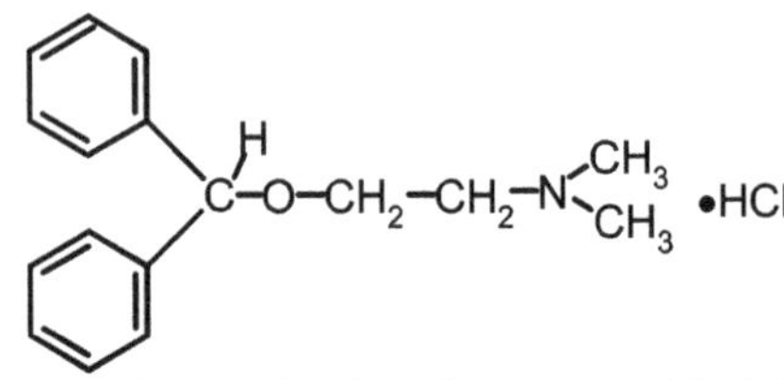

Diphenhydramine hydrochloride

Unlike true antihistamines, which prevent the release of histamine, diphenhydramine works by blocking the effect of histamine at H_1 receptor sites. This results in effects such as, the reduction of smooth muscle contraction, making diphenhydramine a popular choice for treatment of the symptoms of allergic rhinitis, hives, motion sickness, and insect bites and stings.

Cannabinoids

Cannabinoids are a group of chemicals, which activate the body's cannabinoid receptors. Currently, there are three general types of cannabinoids: herbal cannabinoids occur uniquely in the cannabis plant; endogenous cannabinoids are produced in the bodies of humans and other animals; and synthetic cannabinoids are similar compounds produced in the laboratory.

Natural cannabinoids, also called herbal cannabinoids and classical cannabinoids, are nearly insoluble in water but soluble in lipids, alcohols, and other non-polar organic solvents. However, with phenols they form more water-soluble phenolate salts under strongly alkaline conditions. All natural cannabinoids are derived from their respective 2-carboxylic acids (2-COOH) by decarboxylation; that is, catalyzed by heat, light, or alkaline conditions. Natural cannabinoids occur naturally only in the cannabis plant and are concentrated in a viscous resin that is produced in glandular structures known as trichomes. In addition to cannabinoids, the resin is rich in terpenes, which are largely responsible for the odor of the cannabis plant.

Tetrahydrocannabinol($C_{21}H_{30}O_2$, THC), cannabidiol (CBD) and cannabinol (CBN) are the most prevalent natural cannabinoids and have received the most study.

Tetrahydrocannabinol, also known as **THC**, **Δ^9-THC**, **Δ^9-tetrahydrocannabinol** (delta-9-tetrahydrocannabinol), or **dronabinol**, is the main psychoactive substance found in the cannabis plant. In pure form it is a glassy solid when cold and becomes viscous and sticky if warmed. THC has a very low solubility in water, but a good solubility in most organic solvents such as ethanol or hexane.

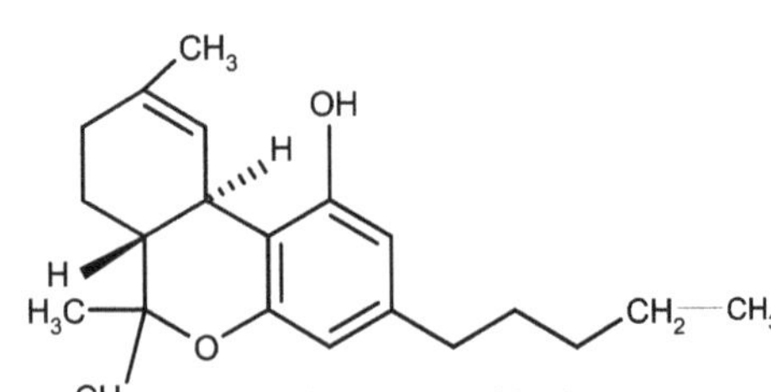

Tetrahydrocannabinol

Cannabidiol, is a non-psychoactive cannabinoid found in the hemp plant *Cannabis sativa*. It is not psychoactive, but it appears to reduce the euphoric effect of THC (which is an isomer of cannabidiol) and add a sedative quality.

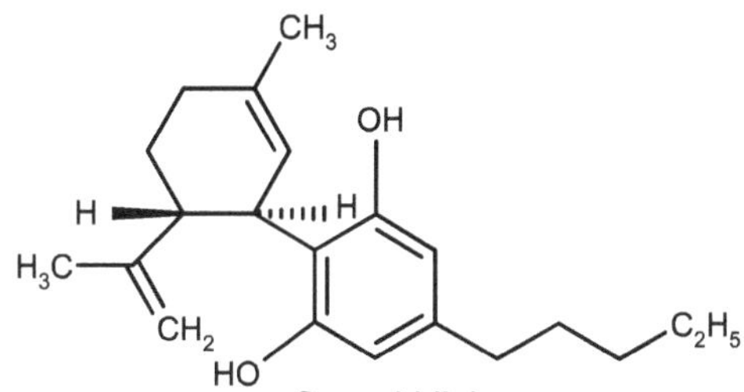

Cannabidiol

Purgatives

Purgatives are the drugs, which promote the evacuation of faeces from the bowel. The terms laxative, cathartic and purgative are considered as synonyms. The purgatives are used in the treatment of constipation. Constipation is a functional disturbance of the gastrointestinal tract. According to their mode of action purgatives may be classified as:

1. Bulk purgatives
2. Stimulant purgatives
3. Lubricant purgatives
4. Saline purgatives

Bulk purgatives

Bulk purgatives absorb water and swell up in GIT. Thus they retain water in the gut lumen and promote peristalsis. These agents are polysaccharide polymers, which are not cleaved by the normal processes of digestion in GIT.

E.g: Methylcellulose, agar, ispaghula husk, sterculia.

Osmotic purgatives

Osmotic purgatives are poorly absorbed solutes. They increase the volume of fluid in human by osmosis. Thus by increasing the bulk of intestine, osmotic purgatives initiate peristalsis and produce watery stools.

E.g: Magnesium sulphate, magnesium hydroxide, lactulose (a semi synthetic disaccharide)

Lubricant laxatives

They are also known as emollient laxatives. These laxatives act by lubricating the faeces and ease the passage. These agents soften the stools by lowering the surface tension.

E.g: Liquid Paraffin, dioctylsodium sulphosuccinate, glycerine.

Stimulant purgatives

They are powerful purgatives and often produce griping. These agents stimulate the nerve endings in intestinal wall. These nerves make the muscles in the intestine and rectum to contract more often and with more force, a process known as peristalsis. This moves the contents of the intestine along so that the bowel can be emptied, and hence relieves constipation.

Phenolphthalein

Phenolphthalein is an indicator, which turns the urine pink if alkaline. It is a synthetic (diphenylmethane derivative) purgative. It irritates the mucosa of small intestine and colon. Some of it is absorbed in the small intestine and is then excreted in the bile. Purgative effect is produced in 6-12 hours.

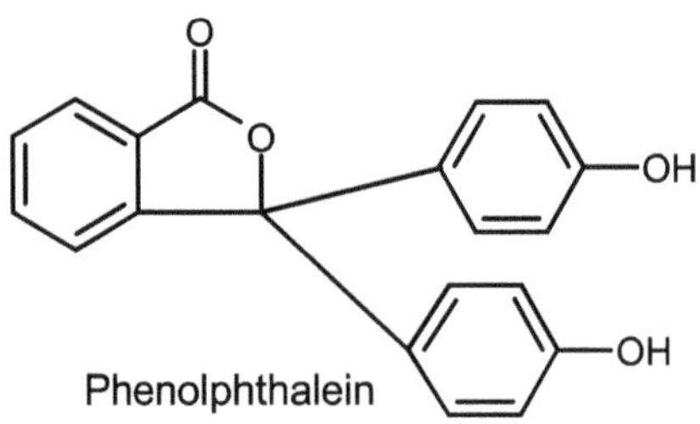

Phenolphthalein

Bisacodyl is a stimulant laxative, which acts on nerve endings in the walls of the intestine and the rectum. It moves the gut contents along faster, thereby relieving constipation. The bisacodyl suppositories produce an effect in about 30 minutes. It is used to empty the bowel prior to surgery or investigative procedures. It is 4,4[1]-(2-pyridyl methylene) diphenol diacetate (ester).

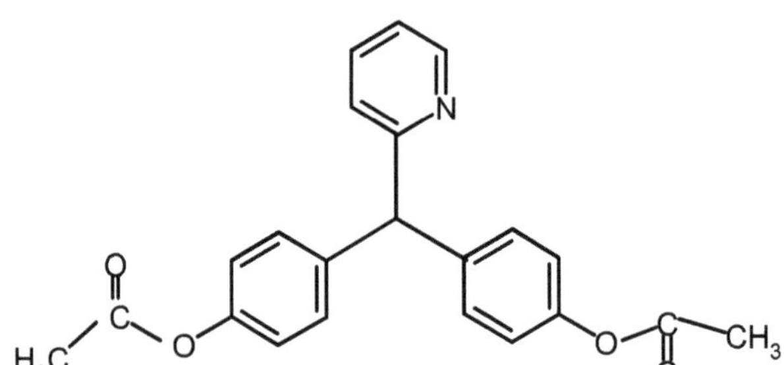

Bisacodyl

Castor oil

Castor oil is a fixed oil obtained from the castor beans *Ricinus communis*. It mainly contains triglyceride of ricinoleic acid, which is a long chain fatty acid.

$$CH_3(CH_2)_6CHOHCH_2CHCH(CH_2)_7COOH$$

Ricinoleic acid

Castor oil is the oldest purgative. The tricyglycerides of ricinoleic acid is hydrolyzed in small intestine (ileum) in presence of bile to yield free ricinoleic acid. The ricinoleic acid is poorly absorbed and mildly irritates the mucosa of intestine and increases peristalsis. The unchanged oil acts as lubricant and softens the stool. Due to structural damage to villi tips, and unpleasant taste and smell, castor oil now has little use as purgative.

Sodium picosulphate

Sodium picosulphate is a new stimulant purgative belongs to phenylmethane group. It has a gentle laxative effect, stimulating the muscles of colon.

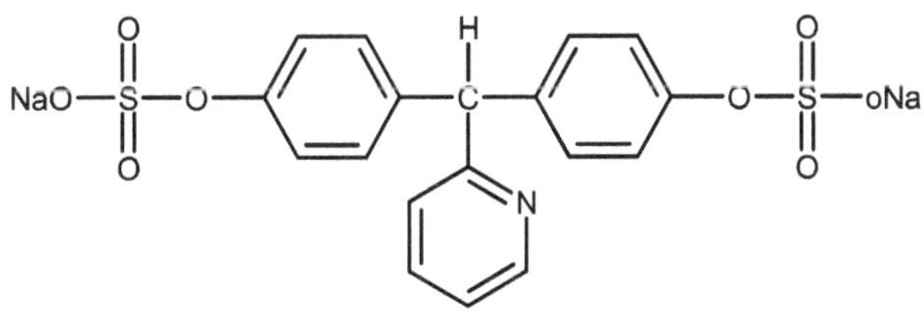

Sodium picosulphate

Mode of action

Sodium picosulphate passes through the stomach and small intestine unchanged. Only when it reaches colon, it converts to an active compound i.e. bis- (p-hydroxydiphenyl)pyridyl methane by arylsulphates enzymes of colonic bacteria. The active component irritates the colon and stimulates the propulsive activity.

Uses

Sodium picosulphate is used to stimulate and emptying of the bowel before surgery. It is also used to treat constipation in patients with cardiovascular disease, hernia etc.

Anthraquinone glycosides

Anthraquinone glycosides are distributed in senna, cascara, rhubarb and aloes. The active principles (emodin chrysophanic acid 1,8-Dihydroxy-3-methylanthraquinone and chrysophanol) are liberated by hydrolysis of parent glycosides in small intestine. The active principles are absorbed and reexecreted into colon. In colon they stimulate the myenteric plexus and induce colonic contractions.

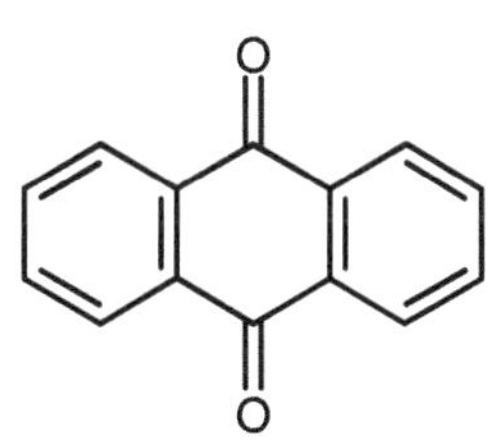

Anthraquinone

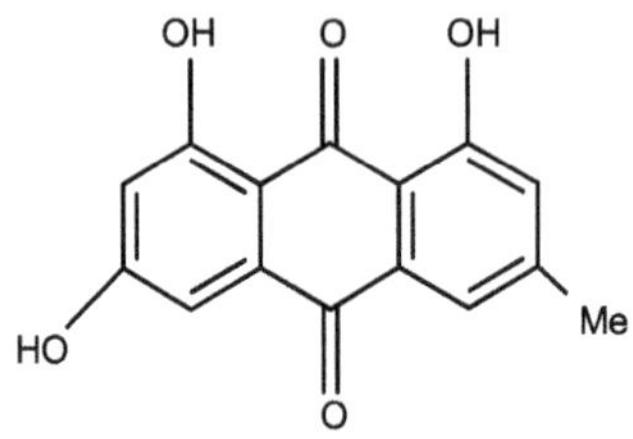

Emodin

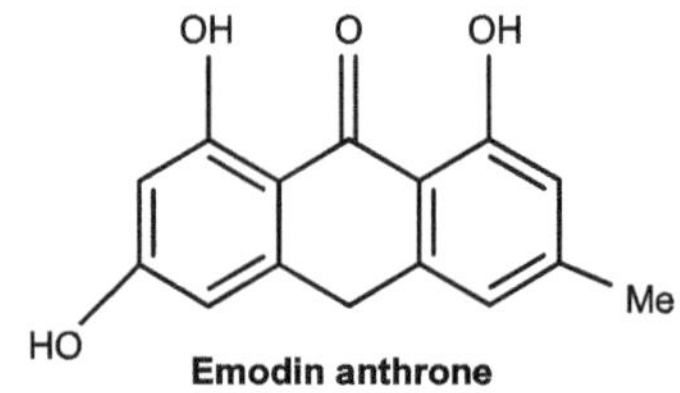

Emodin anthrone

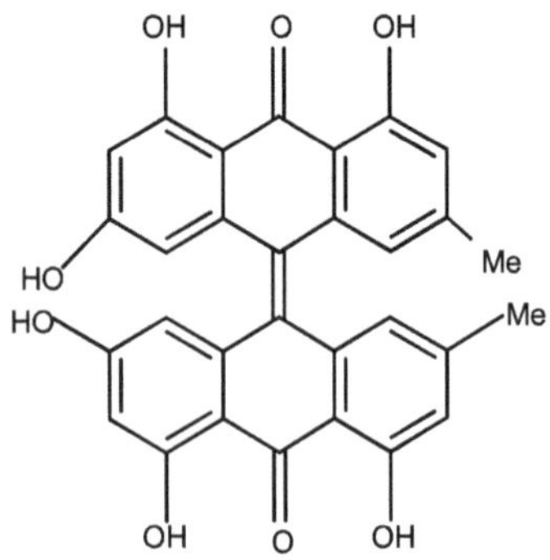

Emodin dianthron

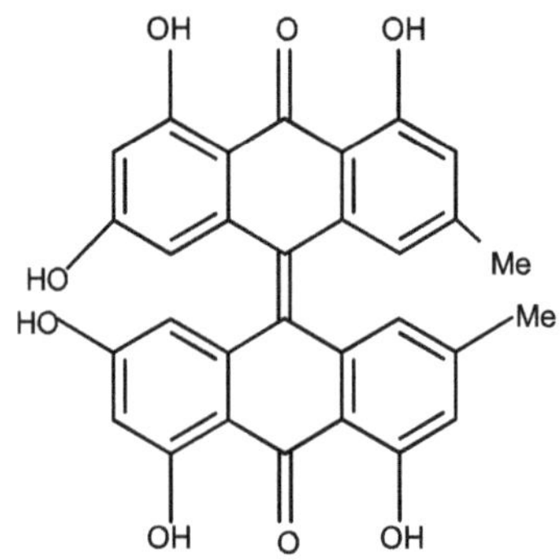

Protohypericin

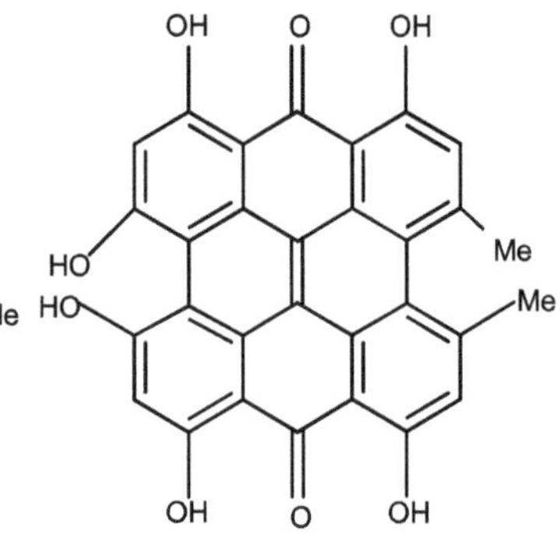

Hypericin (HyH)

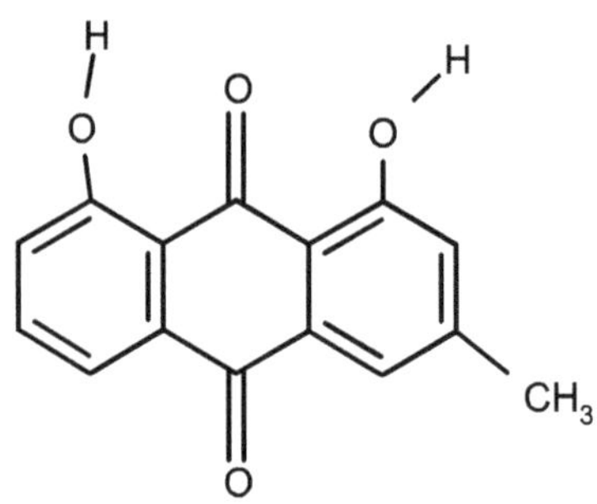

Chrysophanic acid

Diarrhoea

Diarrhoea is termed as gastroenteritis, which means more than three fluid or loose stools in a day. Diarrhoea involves both an increase in the motility of the GIT, along with increased secretion, and a decrease in the absorption of fluid and thus a loss of electrolytes and water. Diarrhoea can be either acute or chronic. Acute diarrhoea occurs suddenly and lasts for a few days whereas chronic diarrhoea is persistent and lasts longer (more than 10 days) with serious inflammatory/irritable bowel diseases.

Pathophysiology

There are numerous causes for diarrhoea including infectious agents, toxins, anxiety, drugs etc.

In the normal gut, the balance between absorption and secretion of fluids is maintained. Diarrhoea is the result of a significant change in this balance, favouring excess fluid reaching the lower colon. Ion transport mechanisms are the primary regulators of this balance, which act in conjunction with various hormones (vasopressin, glucocorticoids) and some neurotransmitters (serotonin). Various diseases affect these regulators which result in diarrhoea. Drugs may act directly (altering osmolarity) or indirectly (antibiotics allowing overgrowth of toxin producing bacteria) giving rise to diarrhoea.

Treatment of diarrhoea

There are two approaches for the treatment of diarrhoea:

(a) Maintenance of fluid and electrolytic balance

(b) Drug therapy

(a) The maintenance of fluid and electrolyte balance by means of oral rehydration is the first priority. The oral rehydration salts (ORS) solution recommended by the WHO contains glucose (20 g) and three salts- sodium chloride (3.5g), trisodiumcitrate dihydrate (2.9 g) or sodium bicarbonate (2.5 g) and potassium chloride (1.5 g) to be mixed in 1litre of water. This oral solution has been used in the treatment of acute diarrhoeal illness for over a decade.

(b) ***Drug Therapy***

Drug Therapy involves usage of :

1. Specific antimicrobial drugs.
2. Non-antimicrobial antidiarrhoeal agents.
3. Antimotility drugs : These are the agents or drugs which decrease propulsive movements of bowel and diminishes intestinal secretions.

(i) Codeine is 7,8- Didehydro-4, 5-epoxy-3-methoxy-17-methyl mophinan-6α-ol.

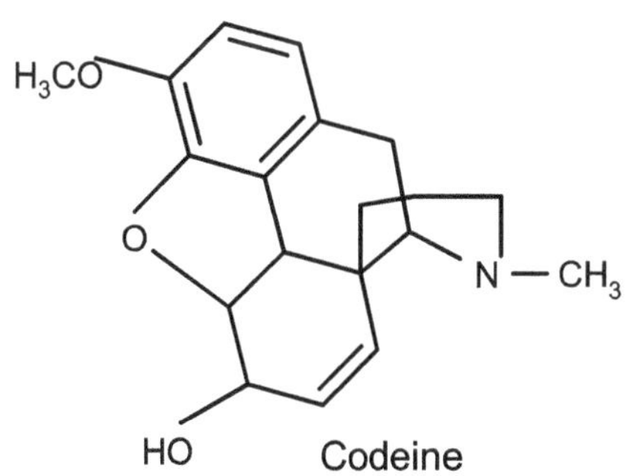

Codeine

(ii) Diphenoxylate is ethyl 1-(3-cyano-3,3-diphenylpropyl)-4-phenylisonipecotate monohydrochloride.

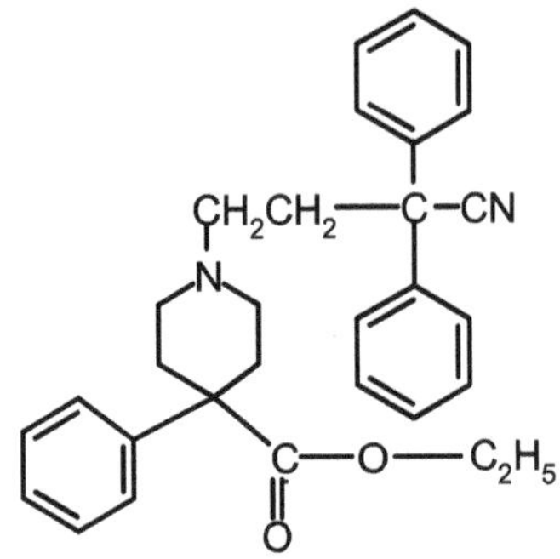

Diphenoxylate

(iii) Loperamide is 4-(4-chlorophenyl)-4-hydroxy-N, N-dimethyl-α,α-diphenyl-1-peperidine butanamide.

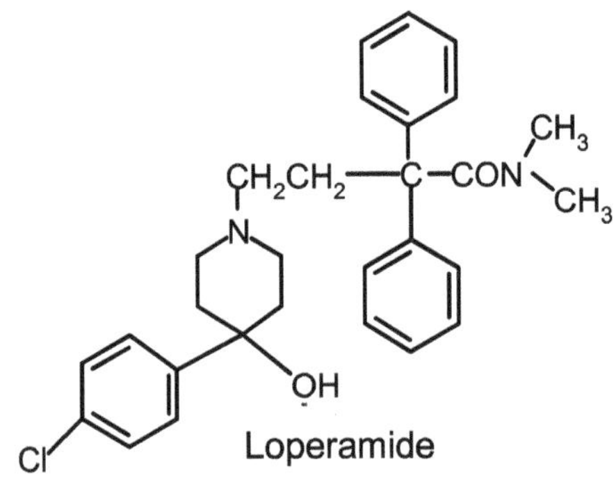

Loperamide

Acute diarrhoea is an often caused by bacteria, viruses and some protozoa and fungi. The acute diarrhoea may be treated with erythromycin, ciprofloxacin, ampicillin, norfloxacin and cotrimoxazole.

Non-antimicrobial antidiarrhoeal drugs : The following are non-microbial antidiarrhoeal agents.

Adsorbents

These are colloidal bulk forming agents, which absorb water and swell. These agents act by adsorbing microorganisms or toxins, by altering intestinal flora or by coating and protecting intestinal mucosa. Many adsorbents have been used, but their value is doubtful. E.g.: Kaolin, pectin, chalk, charcoal, methylcellulose, activated attapulgite.

Anti ulcer drugs

1. The anti ulcer Drugs are used for the treatment of ulcers. Ulcers are sores or raw areas that form in the lining of the stomach or the duodenum (the upper part of the intestine). Those that form in the stomach are called gastric ulcers; in the duodenum, they are called duodenal ulcers. Both types are referred as peptic ulcers.

2. For a long time, physicians thought that stress and certain foods caused the ulcers. Now they came to know that most ulcers are caused either by infection with a bacterium called *Helicobacter pylori* or by long term use of aspirin or other non-steroidal anti-inflamatory drugs (NSAIDs), such as ibuprofen. In either case, something damages the barrier of mucus that normally protects the stomach and duodenum from the powerful acids and enzymes begin to eat away at the unprotected tissue, causing ulcers.
3. Symptoms of a peptic ulcer can be abdominal pain; Hematemesis (vomiting blood); melena (tarry feces due to oxidized iron from ohemoglobin); weight loss; rarely, an ulcer can lead to a gastric or duodenal perforation. This is extremely painful and requires immediate surgery.

Drugs

The three basic types of anti ulcer drugs are H_2-blockers, protein pump inhibitors, and mucosal protective medications.

(a) H_2-blockers blocks the production of histamine, a substance that stimulates acid secretion. By blocking histamine, these drugs reduce the amount of acid production in the stomach.

(b) Proton pump inhibitors completely block the production of stomach acid by stopping the final step in acid secretion.

(c) Mucosal protective medications create a protective barrier that allows the ulcer to heal and prevents further damage to the stomach and duodenum.

An antacid is any substance, generally a weak base, which counteracts stomach acidity. It is taken by mouth to relieve heartburn, sour stomach, or acid indigestion. Most antacids buffer gastric acid, raising the pH to reduce acid damage.

Examples of antacids are : Aluminium hydroxide, magnesium hydroxide, aluminium carbonate gel, calcium carbonate, sodium bicarbonate and hydrotalcite ($Mg_6Al_2(CO_3)(OH)_{16}$. $4(H_2O)$).

Mechanism of gastric acid secretion

Gastric juice contains: HCl, salts, pepsin, mucus, water, intrinsic factor, bicarbonate

(a) ***Mechanism of acid secretion***

The hydrogen ion concentration in parietal cell secretions is roughly 3 million fold higher than in blood, and chloride is secreted against both a concentration and electric gradient. Thus, the ability of the parietal cell to secrete acid is dependent on active transport. The key player in acid secretion is H^+/K^+ ATPase or "proton pump" located in the cannalicular membrane. This ATPase is magnesium-dependent, and not inhibitable by ouabain. The current model for explaining acid secretion as follows:

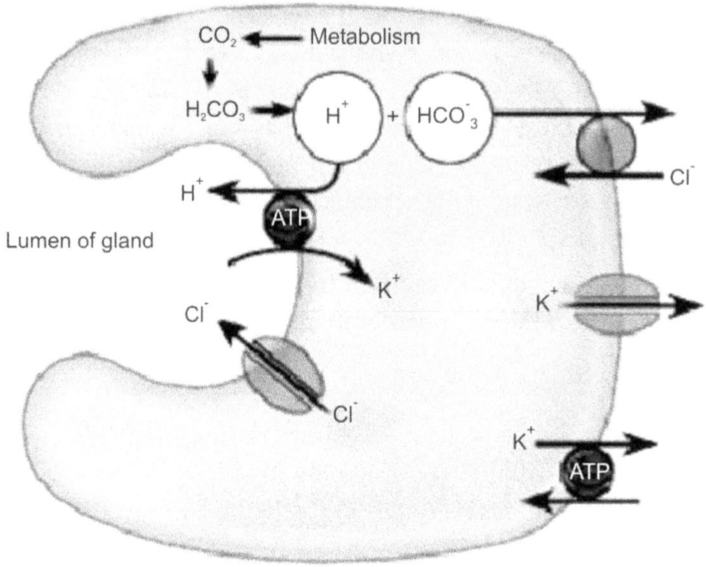

- Hydrogen ions are generated within the parietal cell by dissociation of water. The hydroxyl ions formed in this process rapidly combine with carbon dioxide to form bicarbonate ion. This reaction is catalyzed by carbonic anhydrase. Bicarbonate is transported out of the basolateral membrane in exchange for chloride. The outflow of bicarbonate into blood results in a slight elevation of blood pH in the parietal cells.
- Chloride and potassium ions are transported into the lumen of the cannaliculus by conductance channels, which is necessary for secretion of acid.
- Hydrogen ion is pumped out of the cell, into the lumen, in exchange for potassium through the action of the proton pump; potassium is thus effectively recycled.
- Accumulation of osmoticallly-active hydrogen ion in the cannaliculus generates an osmotic gradient across the membrane that results in outward diffusion of water - the resulting gastric juice is 155 mM HCl and 15 mM KCl with a small amount of NaCl.

Proton pump inhibitors

Proton pump inhibitors are a group of drugs whose main action is pronounced and long-lasting reduction of gastric acid production. Structurally, all these drugs are substituted benzimidazoles. Proton-pump inhibitors reduce the production of acid by blocking the enzyme in the wall of the stomach that produces acid. The reduction of acid prevents ulcers and allows any ulcers that exist in the esophagus, stomach and duodenum to heal.

Mechanism of action

Proton pump inhibitors act by irreversibly blocking the hydrogen-potassium adenosine triphosphate enzyme system (the K^+/H^+ATP ase, or more commonly just proton pump) of the gastric parietal cell. The pump is directly responsible for secreting H^+ ions into the gastric lumen. The proton pump inhibitors are given in an inactive form. The inactive form is neutrally charged (lipophilic) and readily crosses cell membranes into intracellular compartments (like the parietal cell canaliculus) that have acidic environments. In an environment, the inactive drug is protonated and rearranges into its active form. As described above, the above acidic active form will covalently and irrversibly bind to the sulphhydryl group of gastric proton pump and deactivating it.

Examples of proton pump inhibitors

Clinically used proton pump inhibitors are omeprazole, lansoprazole, esomeprazole, Pantoprazole, rabeprazole

Omeprazole

Omeprazole is a proton pump inhibitor used in the treatment of dyspepsia, peptic ulcer disease and Zollinger-Ellison syndrome. Omeprazole is one of the most widely prescribed drugs internationally and is available over the counter in some countries. Omeprazole is a proton pump inhibitor. The inhibition is reversible and is used as its sodium salt. Omeprazole is 5-methoxy-2-[(4 methoxy-3,5–dimethylpyridin-2yl)methylsuphinyl]–1H–benzimidazole.

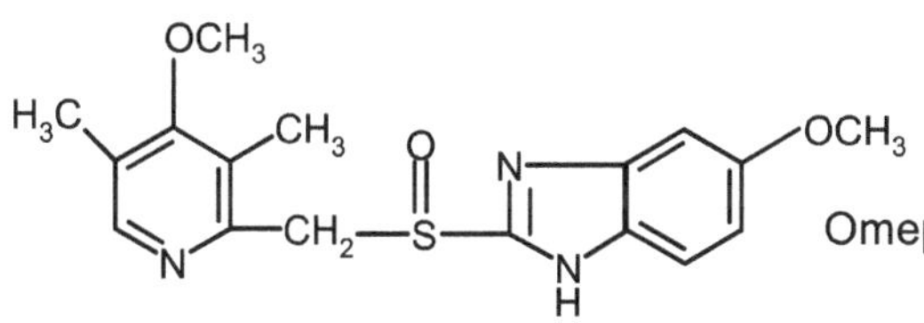

Omeprazole

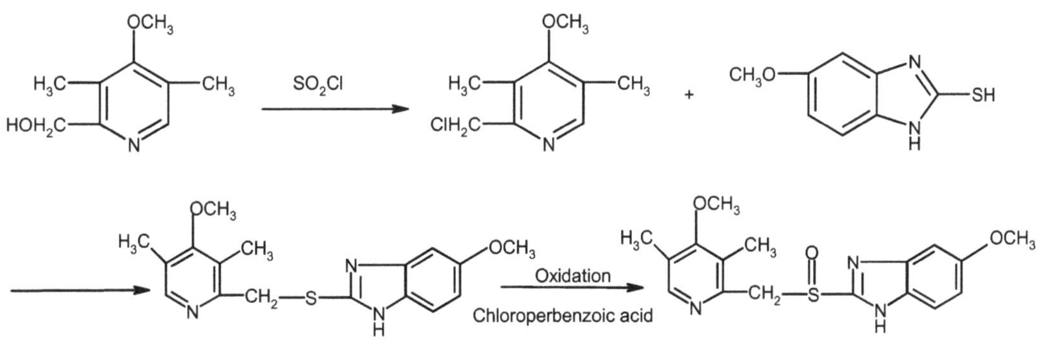

Omeprazole

Lansoprazole

Lansoprazole is a proton pump inhibitor, which prevents the stomach from producing acid. It is 5-methoxy 2-[[[3-methyl-4-(2,2,2-trifluoroethoxy)-2-pyridyl]methyl] sulfinyl] benzimidazole (Prevacid).

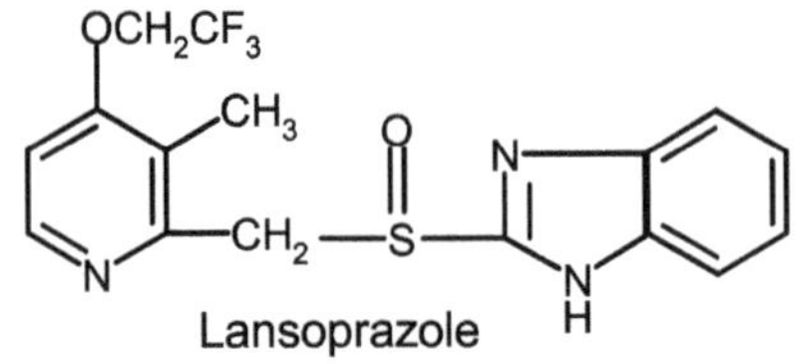

Lansoprazole

Esomeprazole

Esomeprazole is the S-enantiomer of omeprazole. Improved efficacy of this single enantiomer product is more over the racemic mixture of omeprazole has both "left handed" and "right handed" forms of the same molecule, while esomeprazole only having one form. It is S-bis(5-methoxy-2-[(S)-[4-methoxy-3,5-dimethyl-2-pyridinyl)methyl]sulfinyl]-1H-benzimidazole-1-yl)

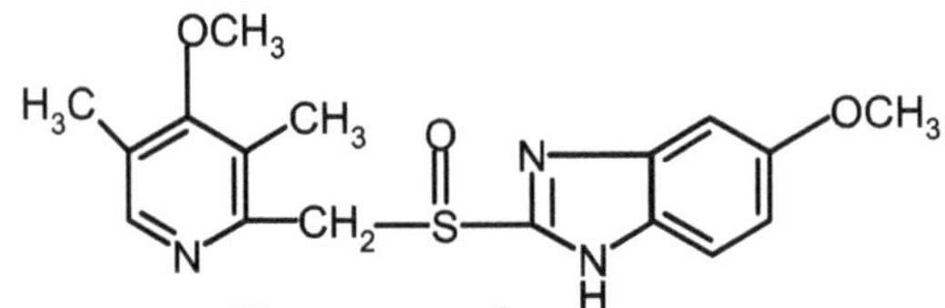

Esomeprazole

Pantoprazole

Pantoprazole is a proton pump inhibitor drug used for short-term treatment of erosion and ulceration of the esophagus caused by gastroesophageal reflux disease. Initial treatment is generally of eight weeks duration, after that another eight week course of treatment may be considered if necessary. It is 5-(difluoromethoxy)-2-[[(3,4-dimethoxy –2-pyridinyl) methyl] sulphinyl]-1H-benzimidazole.

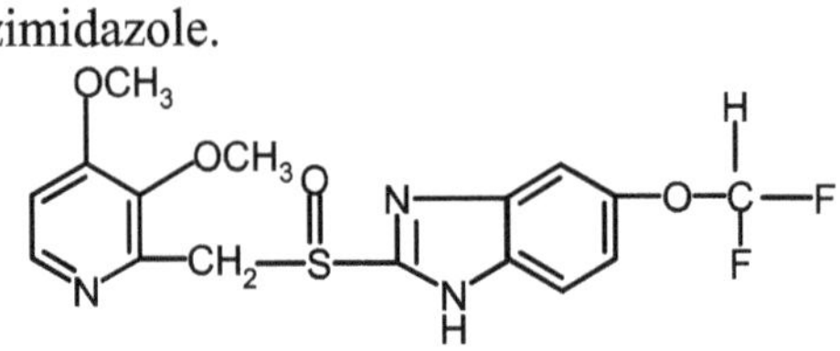

Pantoprazole

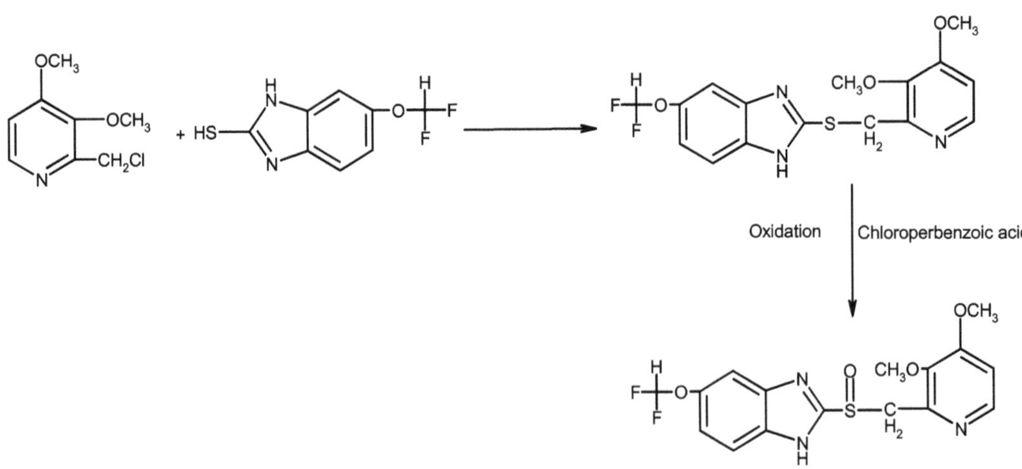

Pantoprazole

Rabeprazole

Rabeprazole is a proton pump inhibitor (as its sodium salt). It is used in the treatment of gastric ulcers and GERD (or heartburn). It is taken once/day along with a full glass of water (preferable 30 min before breakfast). The duration of treatment is usually 4 weeks but could be longer if the symptoms persist. It is 2-[[[4-(3-methoxypropoxy)-3-methyl-2-pyridinyl]methyl]sulphinyl]-1H-benzimidazole.

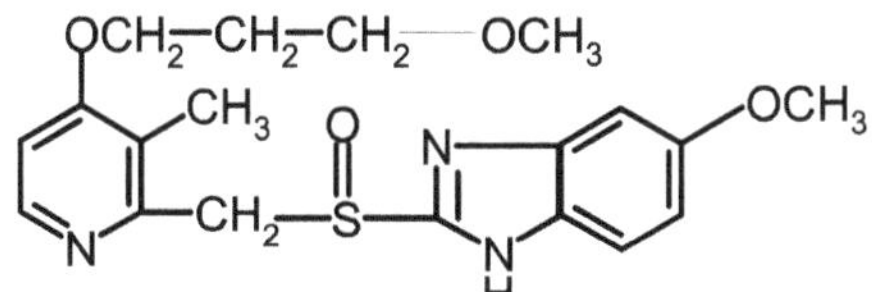

Rabeprazole

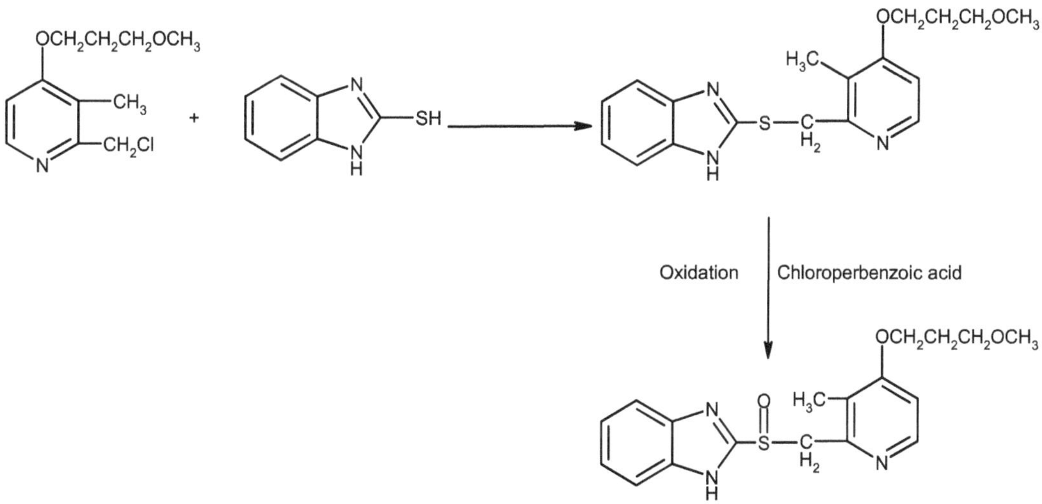

Rabeprazole

H_2 - Blockers

H_2-receptor antagonists are drugs used to block the action of histamine on parietal cells in the stomach, thereby decreasing acid production by these cells. These drugs are used in the treatment of dyspepsia.

H_2 antagonists are competitive inhibitors of histamine at the parietal cell of H_2 receptor. They suppress the normal secretion of acid from parietal cells and the meal-stimulated secretion of acid. They accomplish this by two mechanisms: Histamine released by HCl cells in the stomach is blocked from binding on parietal cell H_2 receptors which stimulate acid secretion, and other substances that promote acid secretion (such as gastrin and acetylcholine) have a reduced effect on parietal cells when the H_2 receptors are blocked.

Cimetidine

Cimetidine was the prototypical member of the H_2 antagonists. Quantitative structure-activity relationships (QSAR) led to the development of newer H_2-blockers with improved tolerability profiles.

Cimetidine inhibits the production of acid in the stomach. It is largely used in the treatment of heartburn and peptic ulcers. Cimetidine was the prototypical histamine H_2 - receptor antagonist from which the later members of the class were developed. Cimetidine is N"-cyano-N-methyl-N'-[2-[[(5-methylimidazole-4yl) methyl]-thio] ethyl] guanidine.

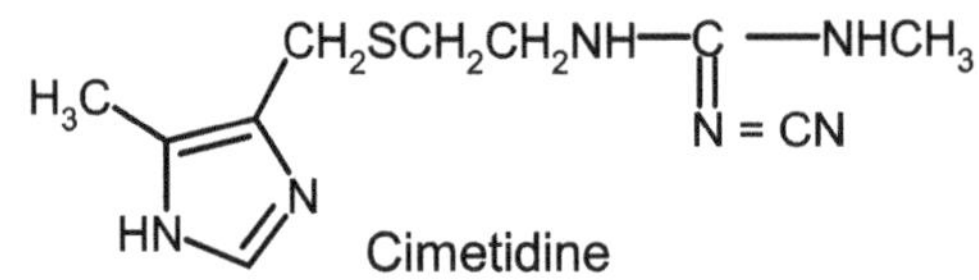

Cimetidine

Ranitidine

Ranitidine is a histamine H_2 - receptor antagonist that inhibits stomach acid production, and commonly used in the treatment of peptic ulcer disease (PUD) and gastroesophageal reflux disease (GERD). It is currently marketed by GlaxoSmithKline under the trade name Zintac. Glaxo refined the model further by replacing the imidazole-ring of cimetidine with a furan-ring with a nitrogen-containing substituent, and in doing so developed ranitidine. Ranitidine was found to have a far improved tolerability profile (i.e., fewer adverse drug reactions), long-lasting action, and ten times the activity of cimetidine.

Ranitidine was introduced in 1981 and was the world's biggest-selling prescription drug by 1988. It has since largely been supresseded by the even more effective proton pump inhibitors, with omeprazole becoming the biggest-selling drug for many years. Ranitidine is N- [2-[[[5-[(dimethylamino) methyl]-2-furanyl] methyl] thio] ethyl]-N^1-methyl-2-nitro-1, 1-ethenediamine.

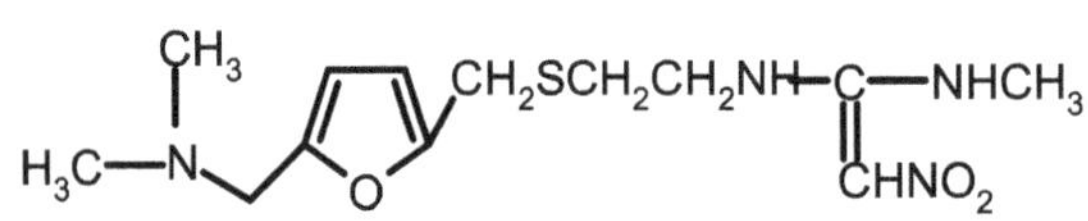

Ranitidine

Famotidine

It is N^1- (aminosulphonyl)-3-[[[2[(diaminomethylene)-amino]-4-thiazolyl] methyl] thio] propanimidamide.

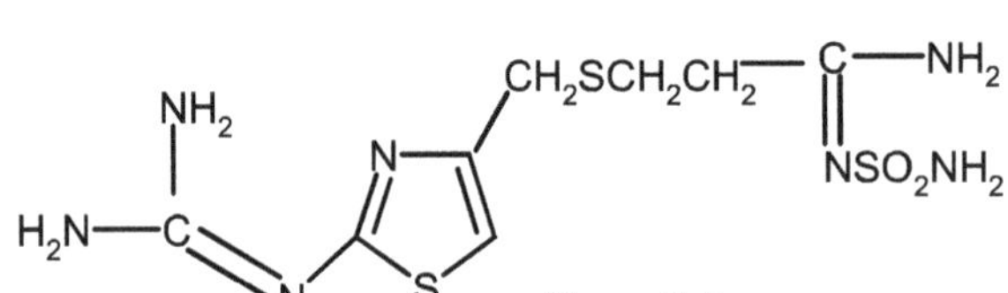

Famotidine

Famotidine was developed by Merck and Co. The imidazole-ring of cimetidine was replaced with a 2-guanidinothiazole ring. Famotidine proved to be 30 times more active than cimetidine. It was first marketed in 1985. On oral administration the onset of action is within 1hr and inhibition of gastric secretion is up to 10-20 hours.

Nizatidine

It was developed by Eli Lilly and is marketed under the trade names Tazac and Axid. It is N- [2-[[[2-[(dimethylamino) methyl]-4-thiazolyl] methyl] thio] ethyl]- N[1]-methyl-2-nitro-1, 1ethenediamine.

It is considered to be equipotent with ranitidine and differs by the substitution of a thiazole-ring in place of the furan-ring in ranitidine. Nizatidine is the newest H_2-receptor antagonist. It has a thiazole ring and a side chain identical to ranitidine.

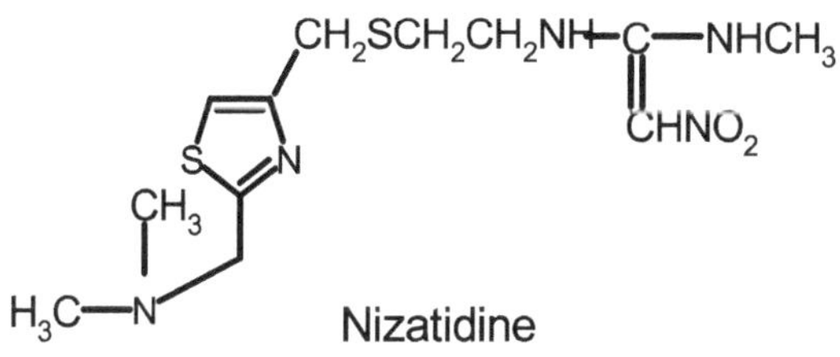

Nizatidine

Herbal medicines

Several herbal medicines have been used for the treatment of ulcers.

1. Liquorice has antiulcer properties due to the presence of glycyrrhizin glycoside (glycorrhetinic acid is aglycone). It has some antibacterial action against *Helicobacter pylori* and protects mucosa.
2. Sylimarin (mixture of silibinin, silichristin and siliianin) obtained from the fruit of *Sylibum marianum* has antiulcer property by reducing histamine concentrations.
3. The aqueous extract of neem tree (*Azadirachta indica*) also has antiulcer activity by inhibiting proton pump.

   (*Helicobacter pylori* survive at the surface of mucus cells and produce proteins and toxins which damage epithelial cells)

Anti-haemorrhoids

Anti-haemorrhoid drugs are medicines that reduce the swelling and relieve the discomfort of hemorrhoids (swellings in the area around the anus).

Purpose

Haemorrhoids are bulges in supply blood to the skin and membranes of the area around the anus. They may form for various reasons. Frequent heavy lifting, sitting for long periods, or straining to have bowel movements may put stress on anal tissues, which can lead to haemorrhoids. Some women develop haemorrhoids during pregnancy as the expanding uterus puts pressure on the anal tissues. Haemorrhoids sometimes result from certain medical problem, such as tumors pressing on the lower bowel.

The main symptoms of haemorrhoids are bleeding from the rectum, especially after a bowel movement, and itching, burning, pain and general discomfort in the anal area. Anti-haemorrhoid products can relieve many of these symptoms. The products contain combinations of four main types of ingredients.

1. Local Anaesthetics such as benzocaine, lidocaine and tetracaine, to temporarily relieve the pain.
2. Vasoconstrictors, such as epinephrine base, epinephrine hydrochloride, ephedrine sulphate and phenylephrine hydrochloride that reduce swelling and relieve itching and discomfort by tightening blood vessels.
3. Astringents (drying agents), such as Witch Hazel, calamine, and zinc oxide. These help to shrink haemorrhoids by pulling water out of the swollen tissue. This, in turn, help to relieve itching, burning, and irritation.
4. Protectants, such as cocoa butter, lanolin, glycerin, mineral oil, and shark liver oil, which soothe irritated tissues and form a protective barrier to prevent further irritation.

Crohn's disease

This is a chronic inflammatory disease which causes stomach pains, diarrhoea, and weight loss. The disease is characterized by periods of activity and remissions. It typically affects the lower part of the small intestine (ileum) or the large intestine (colon), but it can affect any part of the digestive system. The affected areas become red and swollen and ulceration may occur. As the ulcers heal, the formation of scar tissue makes the intestine increasingly narrow, leading to obstruction. There is no cure for Crohn's disease, but the symptoms can be treated and the periods of remission can be made to last several years.

What are the symptoms of Crohn's diseases?

The symptoms vary and depend on the severity and location of the disease. Many patients only have mild symptoms for a long time and have often had the disease for several years before it is diagnosed. Periods of mild fever, sometimes with blood in the stools, and pain in the lower right part of the abdomen, loss of appetite, unintentional weight loss, boils (cavities containing pus) and fistulas (formation of small passages that connect the intestine with other organs or the skin).

How is Crohn's disease diagnosed?

Crohn's disease is suspected in patients who have bad diarrhoea, stomach pains and weight loss for more than three to four weeks. Blood samples, stool specimens, endoscopic examinations of the small and large intestines, and X-ray studies can often confirm or disprove the diagnosis of Crohn's disease.

24

Cardiovascular Agents

Cardiovascular agents are the drugs which modify the functions of cardiovascular system i.e., Heart and the parts of vascular system. The treatment and therapy of cardiovascular diseases have undergone dramatic changes since 1950s. The following classes of cardiovascular agents are used to treat a variety of cardiovascular diseases.

(i) **Cardiotonics :** These drugs increase the force of contraction of heart muscle without increasing heart rate. Cardiac glycosides (digitoxin, gitoxin, gitalin, ouabain), amrinone, losartan, sodium nitropreuside, minoxidil, dobutamine etc.,

(ii) **Anti-arrhythmics :** Anti-arrhythmics are used to treat cardiac arrhythmias quinidine, procainamide, lidocaine, propranolol, verapamil, nifedipine, diltiazem etc.,

(iii) **Antihypertensive agents :** These drugs reduce abnormally raised arterial blood pressure.

(iv) **Antianginal drugs :** The drugs used to treat angina pectoris.

Cardiotonics

Cardiotonics increase the force of contraction of heart. An ideal cardiotonic agent should not increase harart- rate and should be devoid of toxic effects. The following drugs are used as cardiotonics.

(a) Cardiac glycosides : Digitoxin, gitoxin, gitalin, ouabain

(b) Miscellonous cardiotonics : Amrinone, captopril, enalapril, losartan, dobutamine

Cardiac glycosides

The plant steroids possessing the property of stimulating the unsufficient heart muscles are known as cardiac glycosides. They are also known as C23 - glycosides. Cardiac glycosides like digitoxin, gitoxin, gitalin are obtained from *Digitalis purpurea*, digoxin and ouabain are obtained from *Digitalis lanata* leaves and *Strophanthus gratus* seeds.

Each glycoside is a combination of an aglycone or genin with one to four molecules of sugar. The pharmacological activity resides in aglycone, but the particular sugars attached to aglycone modify water solubility, cell permeability and potency of the glycosides. The basic structure is cyclopentanoperhydrophenanathrene nucleus to which is attached an unsaturated lactone ring at C-17 position. Details of different aglycones and sugars of cardiac glycosides are mentioned in the following Table.

	Source	Glycoside	Aglycone	Sugar (number)
1.	*Digitalis purpurea*	Digitoxin	Digitoxigonin	Digitoxose (3)
	(Leaf)	Gitoxin	Gitoxigenin	Digitoxose (3)
		Gitalin	Gitaligenin	Digitoxose (2)
2.	*Digitalis lanata*	Digitoxin	Digitoxigenin	Digitoxose (3)
	(Leaf)	Digoxin	Digoxigenin	Digitoxose (3)
		Gitoxin	Gitoxigenin	Digitoxose (3)
3.	*Strophanthus gratus*	Ouabain	Ouabagenin	Rhamnose

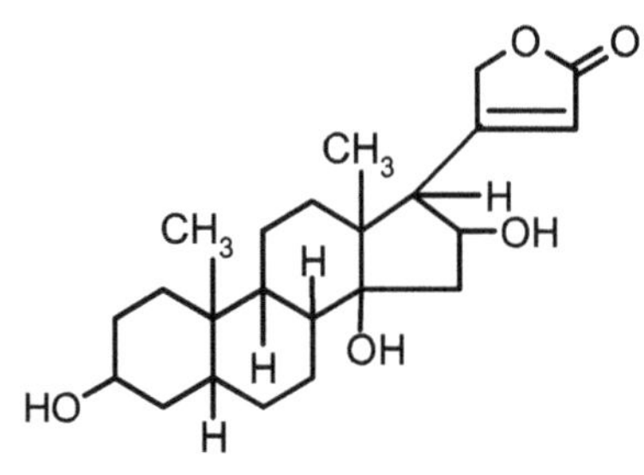

Gitoxigenin

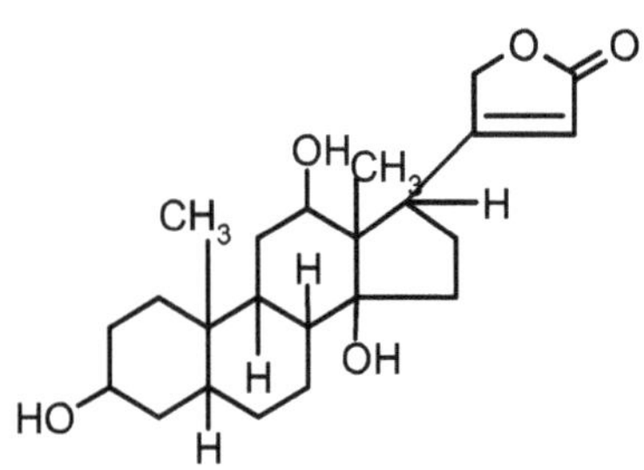

Digoxigenin

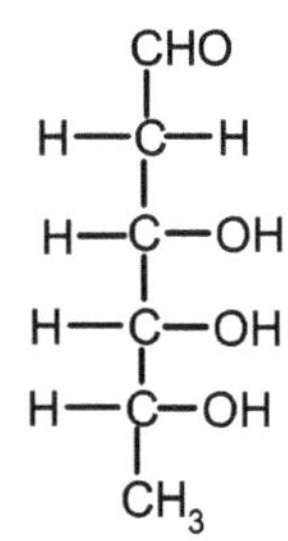

D-Digitoxose

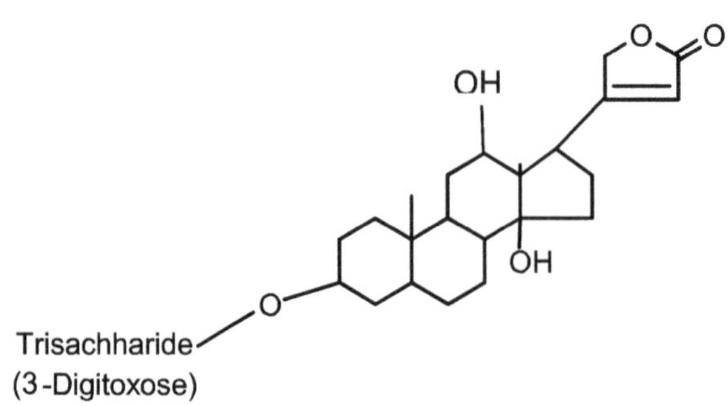

digoxin

Mechanism of action

Cardiac glycosides inhibit Na^+ K^+ ATPase pump and thereby intracellular in Ca^{++} concentration is increased and hence in the force of contraction of heart.

Uses

Cardiac glycosides are used to treat congestive cardiac failure, atrial flutter, fibrillation, and paroxysonal atrial tachycardia.

Amrinone

Amrinone is a bipyridine derivative with positive inotropic and vasodilator effect.

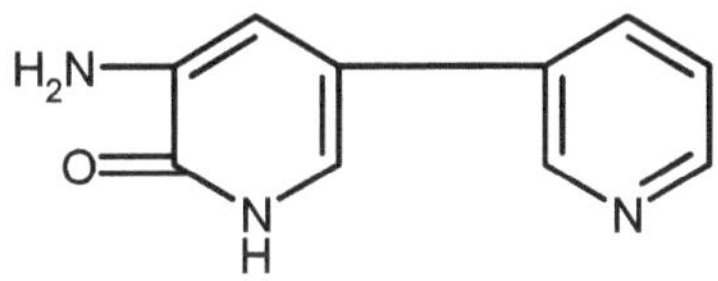

amrinone

Amrinone act by inhibiting phosphodiesterase leading to increase in cyclic AMP concentration in cardiac and vascular muscles. Thus it produces positive inotropic and vasodialation effects.

Electro physiology of cardiac muscles

All cells are electrically polarized, with inside of the cell more negatively charged than the out side. The difference in electrical charge is called resting membrane potential. Nerve and muscle cells are excitable and change the resting membrane potential in response to electrochemical stimuli.

Normally the sinoatrial (SA) node (pacemaker) has highest degree of automaticity which is responsible for sinus rhythm. Sinus rhythm (cardiac impulse) originated from SA node is conducted through the atria, the atrioventricular node (AV node), bundle of His, purkinje fibres and ventricles.

Action potential is an electrical impulse that passes from cell to cell in the myocardium, stimulating the fibres to shorten and causing muscular contraction, which is defined as systole. Diastole is the one, which occurs after the passage of action potential, the fibres relax and return to their resting length. The action potential of an idealized cardiac muscle consists of the following five phases :

Phase 0 – rapid depolarization

Phase 1 – partial depolarization

Phase 2 – plateau phase

Phase 3 – repolarization phase

Phase 4 – pace maker

Phase-0

Rapid depolarization occurs when the membrane potential difference in electrical charge between inside and outside the cell reaches about - 60 mv, the Na^+ ions firing take place from the voltage dependent sodium channels.

Phase-1

Partial repolarization occurs as the Na^+ channels are inactivated and Na^+ ions flow is arrested.

Phase- 2

This phase is also called plateau phase which results from an inward Ca^{+2} ion flow. During this phase the potassium ion conductance falls to low levels.

Phase- 3

It is a repolarization phase, occurs as the Ca^{+2} flow gets inactivated and causing outward K^+ ions flow.

Phase- 4

The pacemaker potential is caused by a combination of increasing inward flow and reduced outward flow during diastole.

Only one impulse can pass along a nerve fiber at any given time. After the passage of an impulse, there is a brief interval before the next impulse can pass along the nerve fiber which is called as refractory period.

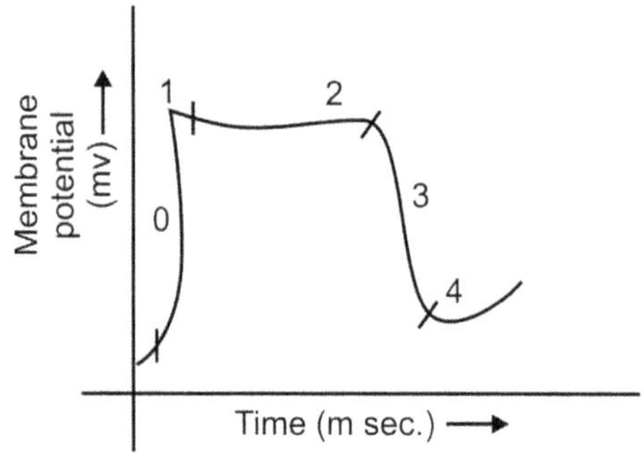

By lengthening the refractory period, the number of impulses travelling along a nerve fiber within a given time is decreased.

Cardiac arrhythmia

A cardiac arrhythmia is a disturbance or irregularity in heart rate, rhythm or both. It may occur as a result of heart disease or from a disorder that affects cardio-vascular function. Conditions such as emotional stress, hypoxia, electrolyte imbalance can trigger an arrhythmia. Some cardiac arrhythmias are caused by the generation of an abnormal number of electrical impulses. These impulses may come from the SA node or may be generated in other areas of the myocardium. Ischaemia, electrolyte and pH imbalance, mechanical injury, stretching, neurogenic and some of the drugs can cause arrhythmias by altering electrophysiological properties of cardiac fibres.

Antiarrhythmic drugs

The antiarrhythmic drugs are primarily used to treat cardiac arrhythmias. They are exclusively used to restore normal cardiac function to prevent life–threatening arrhythmias. Antiarrhythmic drugs are classified according to their effects on the action potential of cardiac cells.

Class-I, Antiarrhythmic drugs

These have a membrane stabilizing or anesthetic effect on the cells of the myocardium. Their actions differ slightly, hence they are sub classified into classcs I-A, I-B and I-C

Class I-A

Class I-A drugs block the sodium channels and slows phase 0 depolarization. *e.g.,* Quinidine, procainamide, disopyramide. They suppress A-V conduction and prolong P-R, QRS, QT and action potential duration.

Class I-B

These drugs also affect the sodium channels in both activated and inactivated states but they shorten phase o repolarization. *e.g.,.* Lidocaine, mexelitine, tocainide.

They do not depress A-V conduction or prolong action potential duration, effective refractory period and Q-T.

Class I-C

Class I-C drugs block the sodium channels with marked slowing of phase 0 depolarization. They markedly delay conduction, prolong P-R, broaden QRS complex but have variable effect on action potential duration. *e.g.,.* Flecainide and propafenone.

Class II

Class II antiarrhythmic drugs include beta–adrenoceptor blocking drugs. These drugs decreases myocardial response to epinephrine and nor epinephrine because of their ability to block beta-receptors of the heart. *e.g.,* Propranolol, esmolol and acebutolol.

Class III

This class of antiarrhythmic drugs prolong repolarization, prolongs refractory period and increase the ventricular fibrillation threshold. These drugs are in general potassium channel blockers acting on phase 3 of action potential. *e.g.,* Bretylium and amiodarone.

Class IV

Class IV drugs are calcium channel blockers acts by inhibiting the movement of calcium through channels across the myocardial cell membranes and vascular smooth muscle by reducing the Ca^{+2} flow, conduction through SA node and AV node is slowed and the refractory period is prolonged resulting in suppression of arrhythmia. *e.g.,* Verapamil and diltiazem.

Uses

In general these drugs are used to treat cardiac arrhythmic such as premature ventricular contractions (PVC's), ventricular tachycardia, premature atrial contractions (PAC's), paroxysmal atrial tachycardia, atrial fibrillation.

Class I-A Drugs

Procainamide

It is a structural analogue of procaine, which is chemically 4-amino-N-[2-(diethylamino) ethyl] benzamide belonging to class IA antiarrhythmic drug.

Structure

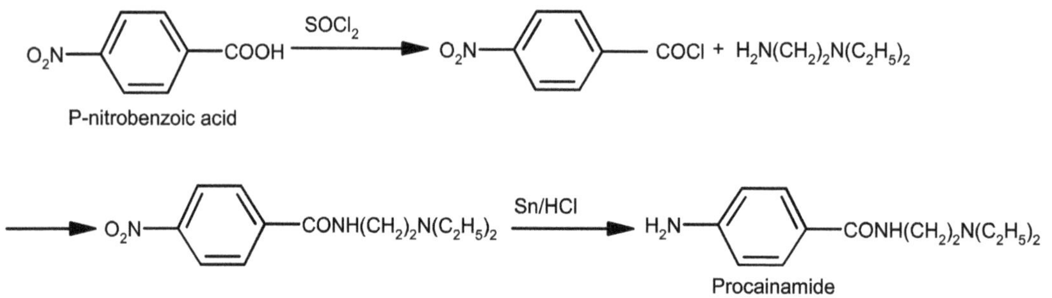

Procainamide is orally active and is resistance to both chemical and enzymatic hydrolysis but procaine is not active orally because of its short duration of action (Enzymatic and chemical hydrolysis) Procainamide is synthesised by condensing p-nitrobenzoyl chloride with N, N-diethyl ethylene diamine followed by reduction.

Mode of action

Procainamide diminishes excitability, decreases conduction velocity, and porlongs the effective refractory period to a greater extent in arteries than ventricles.

Properties

Pracainamide is also available as procainamide hydrochloride. Procainamide hydrochloride is white crystalline, very soluble in water. Procainamide is completely absorbed by oral route. In case oral route is not suitable procainamide hydrochloride is given by IM injection.

Uses

It is a second-choice of antiarrhythmic agent to treat life-threatening ventricular arrhythmias. It is effective against atrial arrhythmias.

Disopyramide

Disopyramide is a newer antiarrhythmic drug. It is chemically [4-[bis(1-methyl ethyl)amino]-2-Phenyl-2-(pyrid-2-yl) butyramide belongs to class IA antiarrhythmic drugs. Disopyramide decreases automaticity, diminishes conduction velocity and increases refractory period of cardiac cells. Disopyramide is completely absorbed by oral route. It is synthesized from phenylautoritrile by the following chemical reactions.

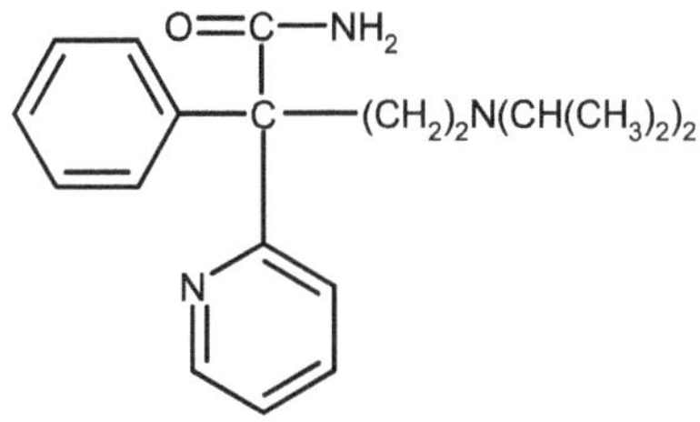

Disopyramide

It is used as an antiarrhythmic agents to suppress and treat sustained ventricular or supraventricular arrhythmias.

Lidocaine

It is an anilide, which is chemically 2-(diethylamino)-N-(2, 6-dimethylphenyl) acetamide, has long-acting membrane stabilizing agent against ventricular arrhythmias. Lidocaine shortens phase 3 repolarization and decreases the duration of action potential. It supresses the automaticity of both normal and abnormal arrhythmias.

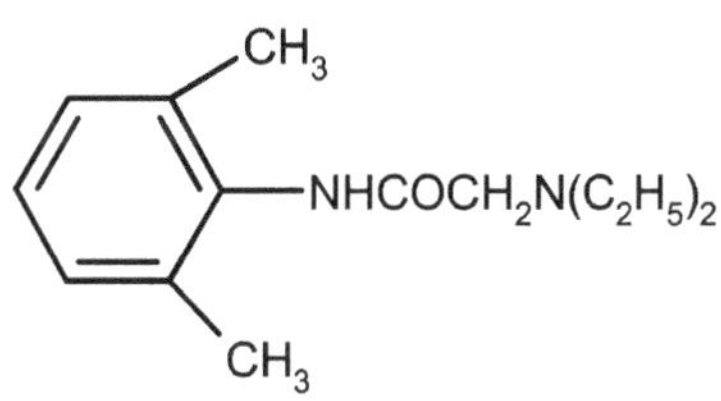

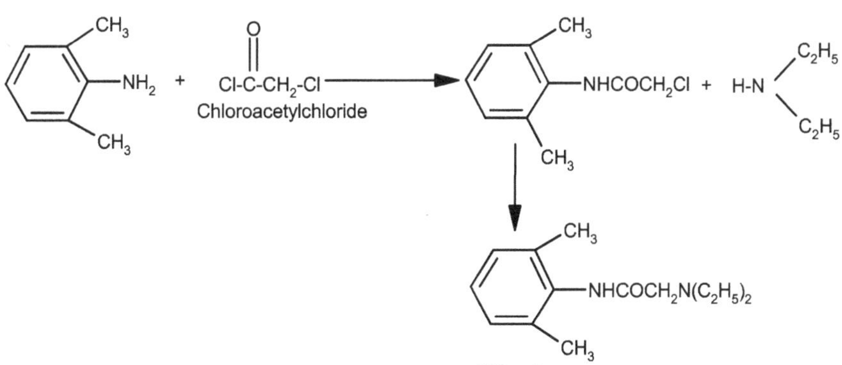

Lidocaine

Lidocaine is colorless, odorless, slightly bitter taste crystalline powder. It is used as an antiarrhythmic agent belonging to class IB to treat ventricular arrhythmias.

Mexiletine

Mexiletine is a structural analogue of lignocaine. Unlike lignocaine it undergoes first-pass metabolism. It is an orally effective drug. Mexiletine is readily and completely absorbed from GIT.

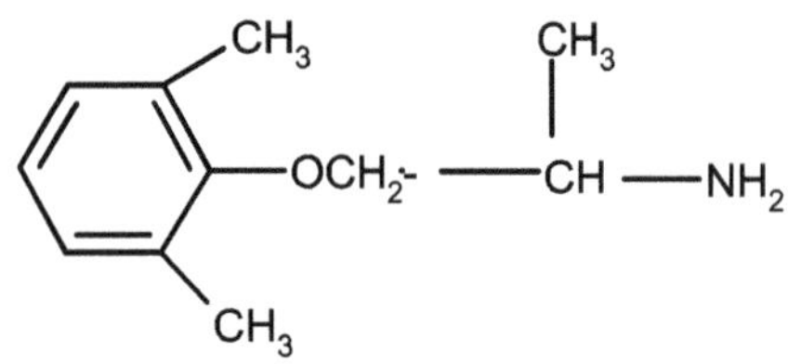

Mexiletine

Properties

It is white to off white crystals having a melting point of 203 °C. It is having slightly bitter taste and is freely soluble in water and alcohol.

Tocainide

Tocainide is another close structural analogue of lidocaine.

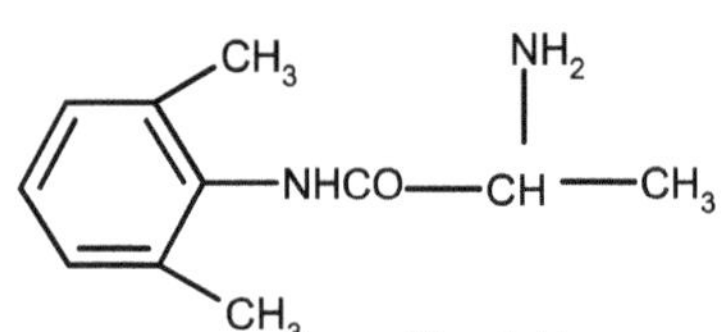

Tocainide

It is an anilide analogue, which is chemically 2-amino-N-(2, 6 dimethylphenyl) propanamide.

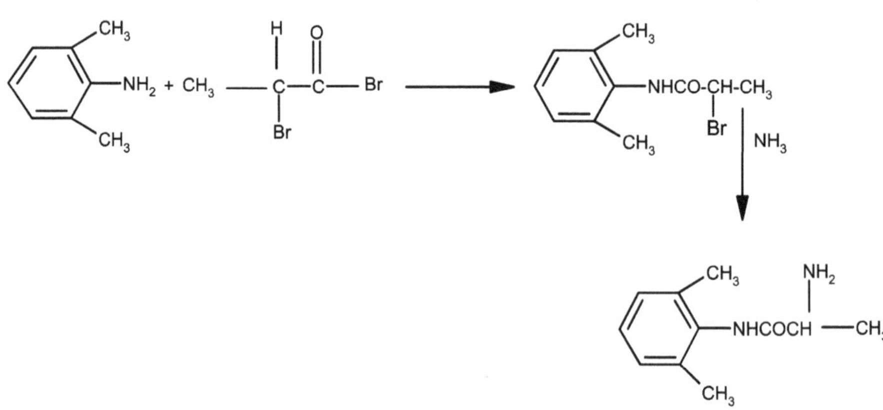

Tocainimide

Uses

Tocainide is used to treat premature ventricular contractions and ventricular tachycardia.

Encainide

It is chemically 4-methoxy-N-[2-[2-(1-methyl-2-piperidinyl) ethyl] phenyl] benzamide. Encainide exists as crystals. It is freely soluble in water and is slightly soluble in ethanol.

Uses

It is used as class I-C antiarrhythmic agent.

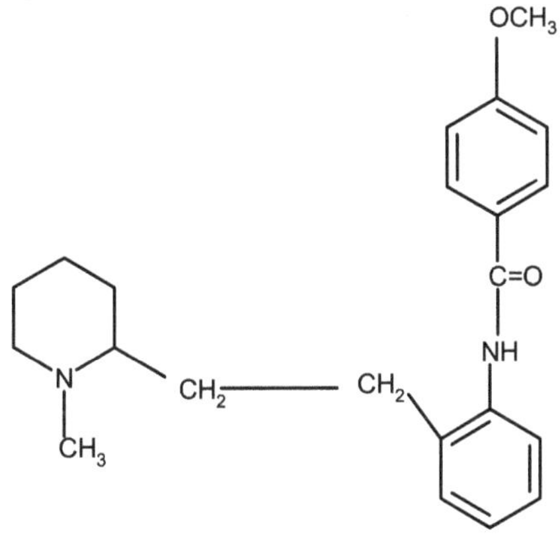

Encainide

Synthesis

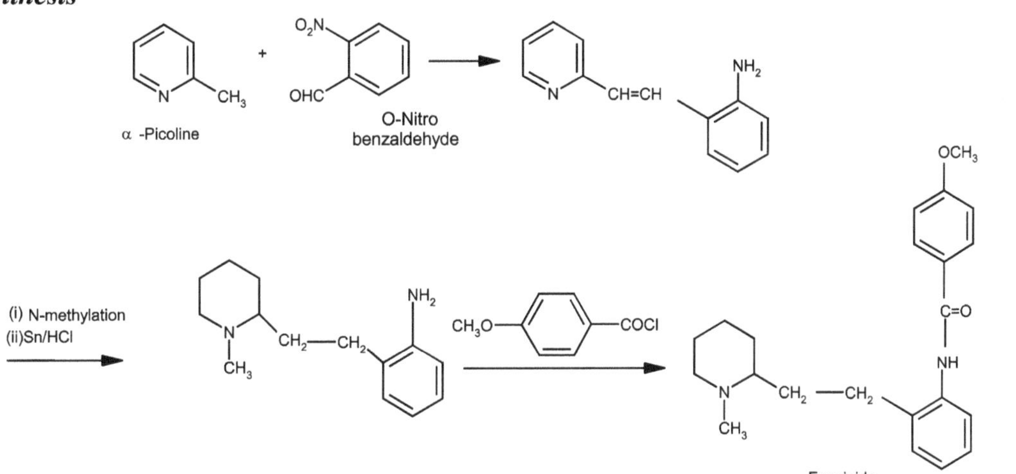

Flecainide

Flecainide is an important I-C antiarrhythmic drug. It is chemically N-(2-piperidinylmethyl)-2,5-bis (2, 2, 2-trifloroethoxy) benzamide. Flecainide act by suppressing ventiricular ectopic beats and reducing the frequency of extopic beats.

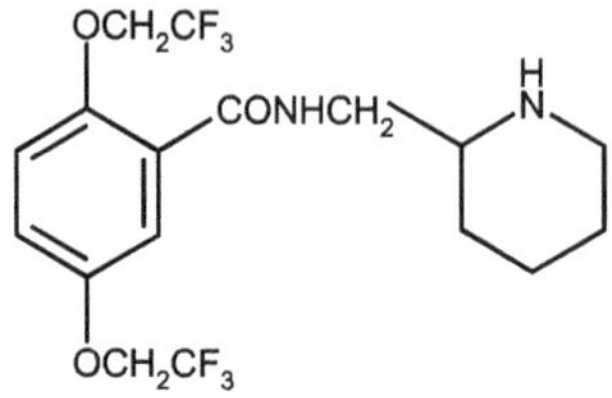

Flecainide

Synthesis

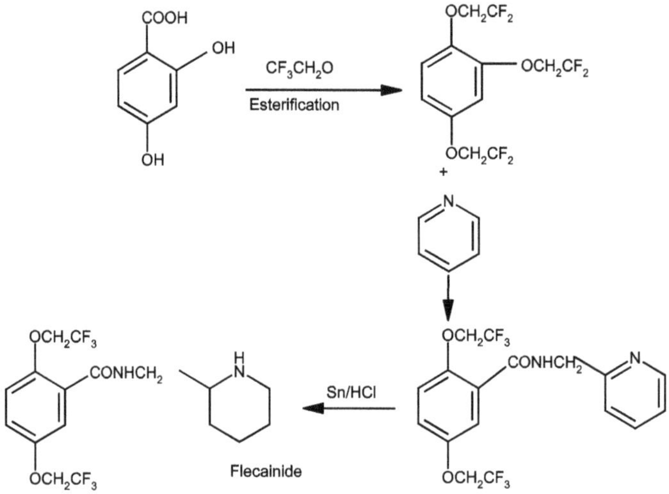

Lorcainide

It is chemically N-(4-chlorophenyl)-N-[1-(1-methylethyl)-4-piperdinyl] benzeneacetamide. It is used as class I-C antiarrhythmic agent.

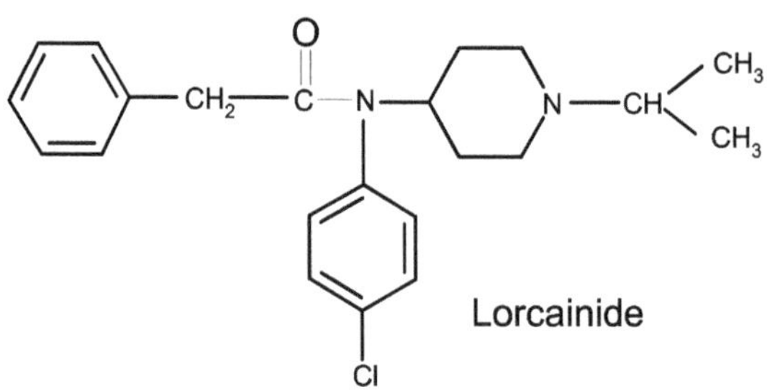

Lorcainide

Class II Drugs

The β-blockers competitively antagonize the action of adrenergic agents, specially on heart i.e., β_1 receptors. As a result sinus rate is slowed, AV conduction is depressed, contractivity is decreased, and the automaticity of SA node and ectopic pacemakers is decreased.

Propranolol

Propranolol exhibits optical isomerism. The levo isomer is 100 times more active than dextroisomer. It is chemically 1-(isopropyl amino)-3-(1-naphthyloxy)-2-propanol. It is prepared from 1-naphthol on reaction with epichlorhydrin followed by treatment with isopropyl amine.

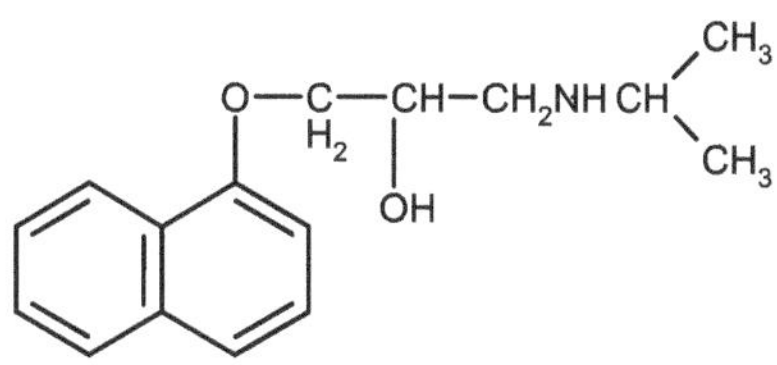

Propranolol

Properties

Propanolol is a secondary amine. It is available as hydrochloride salt. Propanolol hydrochloride is soluble in water.

Uses

It is used to treat cardiac arrhythmias, angina pectoris, hypertension, essential tremor, myocardial infarction, migraine headache.

Acebutotol

It is chemically N-[3-acetyl-4-[2-hydroxy-3-[(1-methyl ethyl) amino] propoxy] phenyl] butanamide, a selective beta-blocker. It is used to treat ventricular arrhythmias and hypertension. It is discussed under antihypertensives.

Esmolol

It is chemically 4-[2-hydroxy-3-[(1-methyl ethyl) amino] propoxy] benzene propanoic acid methyl ester, also a selective beta-blocker. It is described under antihypertensives.

It is used for rapid short term treatment of ventricular rate in supra ventricular arrhythmia and sinus tachycardia.

Class III Drugs

Amiodarone

It is a (2-butyl-3-benzofuranyl) [4-(2-(diethylamino) ethoxy]3,5-diiodophenyl] methanone, which has multiple electro physiological effects.

Properties

It is a crystalline powder having a melting point of 156°C. It is soluble in chloroform, methylene chloride, methanol, ethanol, tetrahydrofuran, acetonitrile,water and ether. It is sparingly soluble in propanol and slightly soluble in acetone, dioxane and carbon tetrachloride.

Uses

It is used as class III antiarrhythmic agent to treat life-threatening ventricular arrhythmias. This drug is highly toxic and should be used only by cliniciars familiar with its actions.

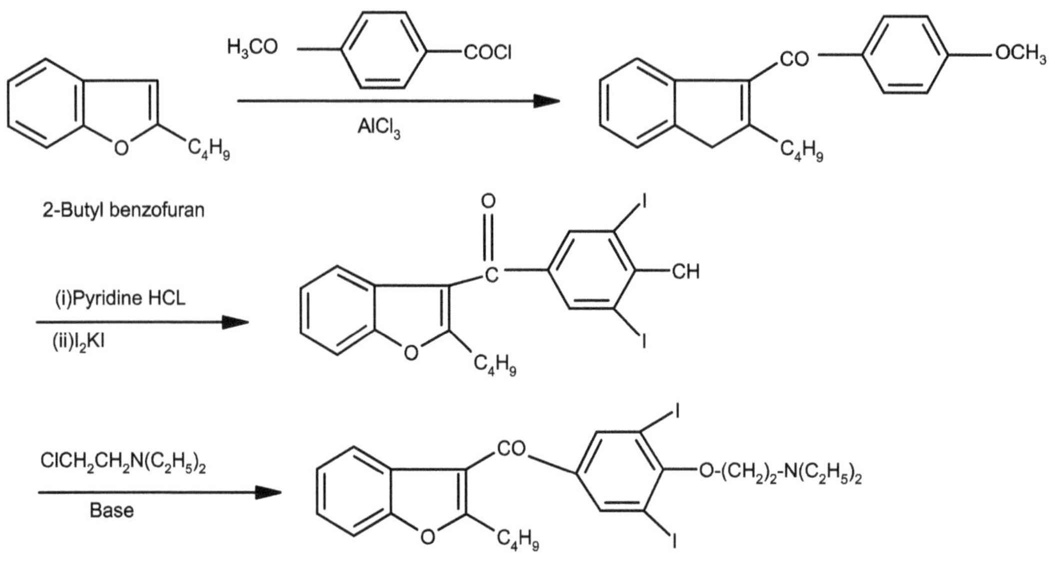

Amiodarone

Bretylium

It is chemically 2-bromo-N-ethyl-N, N-dimethylbenzenemethanaminium. It is a crystalline powder having a melting point of 97°C. It is extremely bitter to taste. Freely soluble in water, methanol and ethanol. Practically insoluble in ether and ethylacetate. It is used as class III antiarrhythmic agent to treat as well as prophylaxis of ventricular fibrillation.

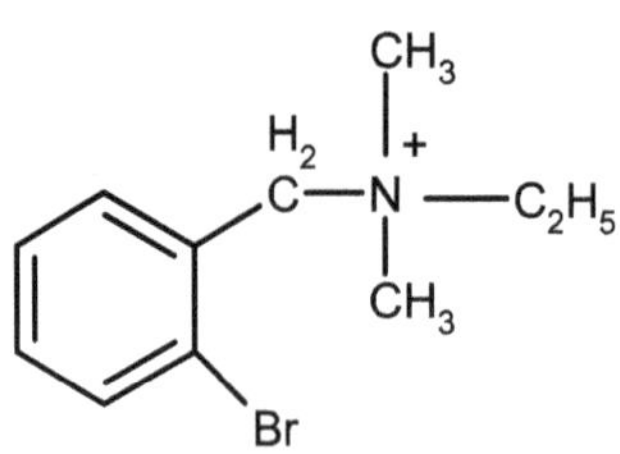

Bretylium

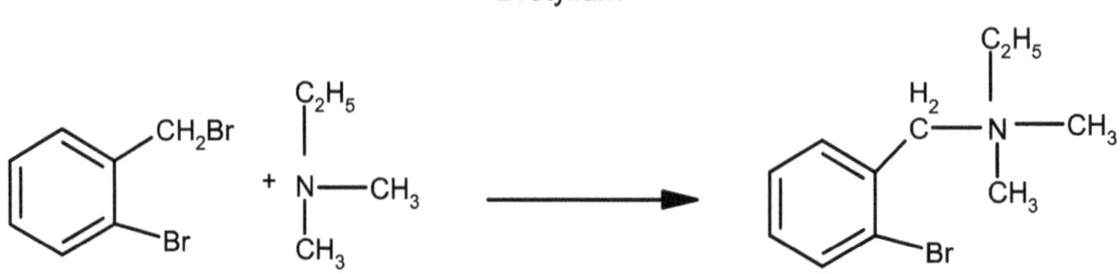

O-Bromo benzyl bromide

Bretylium

Class IV Drugs

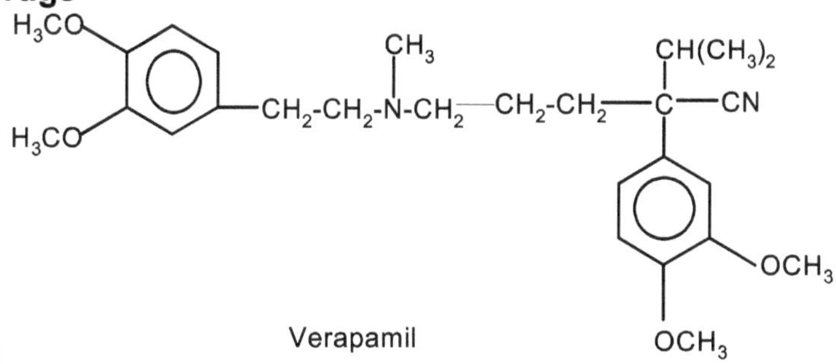

Verapamil

Verapamil

It is chemically [3-[[2-(3,4-dimethoxyphenyl)ethyl]methylamino]propyl]-3,4-dimethoxy (1-methylethyl) benzeneacetonitrile, a prototype calcium antagonist having vasodilating activity resided primarily in the S-isomer. It is viscous pale yellow oil having a boiling point of 243°C-246°C. Practically immiscible with water. Sparingly miscible with hexane. Miscible with benzene and ether. Freely miscible with the lower alcohols, acetone, ethyl acetate and chloroform.

It is used as antihypertensive, antianginal (unstable), antiarrhythmic for the treatment of super ventricular tachyarrhythmias, temporary control or rapid ventricular rate in atrial flutter or fibrillation.

Chemistry of verapamil is described in calcium channel blockers.

Diltiazem

It is (2S-cis)-3-(acetyloxy)-5-[2-(dimethylamino)ethyl]2,3-dihydro-2-(4-methoxyphenyl)-1, 5-benzothiazepin-4 (5H)-one.

It occurs as fine needles having a melting point of 207°C. It is odorless having bitter taste, freely soluble in water, methanol, chloroform and formic acid. Slightly soluble in absolute alcohol. Practically insoluble in benzene. It is used as antianginal, antihypertensive and antiarrhythmic.

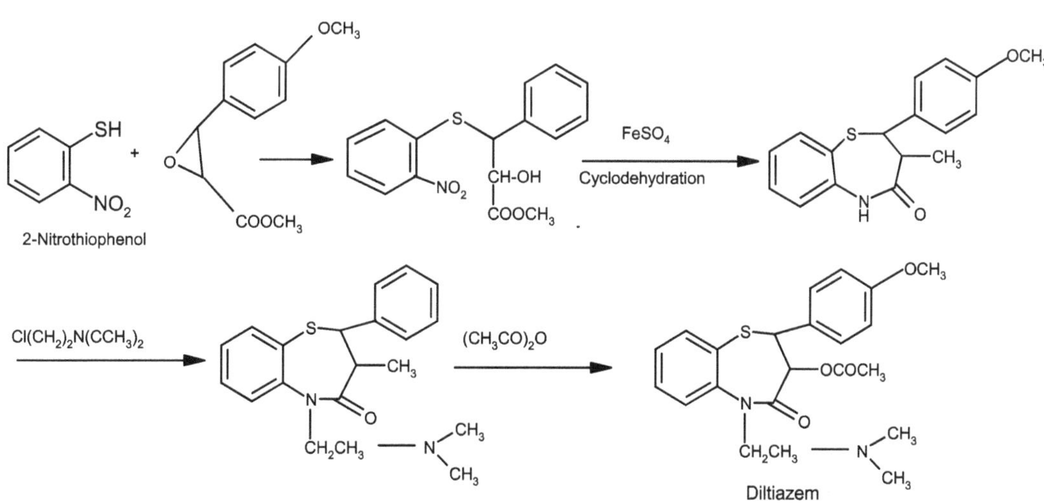

Antihypertensive agents

Hypertension is defined as the level of diastolic or systolic blood pressure at which treatment is required. Blood pressure (BP) is commonly expressed as both systolic pressure (peak pressure at the time of cardiac contraction) and diastolic pressure (minimum pressure at the time of cardiac relaxation). According to WHO, hypertension is the state of the body in which systolic BP is 150 mmHg or more and diastolic BP is 95mm Hg or more.

Category normal hypertension	Systolic (mm of Hg) < 130	Diastolic (mm of Hg) < 85
Stage I (mild)	140 - 159	90 – 98
Stage II(moderate)	160 - 179	100 – 109
Stage III (severe)	180 - 209	110 – 119
Stage IV (very severe)	> 210	>120

Hypertension is divided into primary or essential hypertension where the etiology is unknown and secondary hypertension where etiology can be identified. The secondary hypertension is due to renal disease, adrenal disease, toxemia of pregnancy, centrally mediated neurogenic causes (encephalitis, increased intracranial pressure, thyrotoxcosis, and oral contraceptives). Antihypertensive drugs are used to treat hypertension i.e., to lower blood pressure.

Classification

Antihypertensives are classified basing on mechanism of action or primary site of action as given below:

1. ***Centrally acting drugs :*** *e.g.,* Methyldopa, clonidine, guanabenz, guanfacine
2. ***Agents affecting peripheral sympathetic nerves :*** *e.g.,* Rauwolfia alkaloids-reserpine, guanethedine, guanadrel
3. ***Alpha adrenergic blockers :*** *e.g.,* Prazocin, terazocin
4. ***Beta adrenergic blockers :*** *e.g.,* Propranolol, atenolol
5. ***Vasodialators***
   (i) Directly acting:
      (a) Arterial : *e.g.,* Hydralazine, diazoxide, minoxidil
      (b) Arterial and venous vasodilators : *e.g.,*Sodium nitroprusside
   (ii) Calcium channel blockers : *e.g.* Verapamil, diltiazem, nifedipine, amlodipine, isradipine
6. ***Angiotensin converting enzyme (ACE) inhibitors :*** *e.g.,* Captopril, lisinopril, enalapril, benazepril, quinapril, ramipril.
7. ***Diuretics :*** *e.g.,* Chlorothiazide, hydrochlorothiazide, furosemide, amiloride

Ideal characteristics of antihypertensive agents

An ideal antihypertensive must have following characteristics:

1. It should have specific site of action.

2. It should control blood pressure of alone.
3. It should not alter the heart rate and sexual function.
4. It should not have interaction with other commonly used drugs.
5. It should be stable in light and heat.
6. It should not cause cardial, renal or cerebral damage.
7. It should be inexpensive.

Drugs acting centrally

These are the drugs that act centrally on the vasomotor centers of the brain and activate the alpha 2 receptors. The drugs that come under this category are: Methyldopa, clonidine, gaunabenz and guanfencine

Methyldopa

It is tyrosine derivative. Methyldopa is chemically L-3-(3,4-dihydroxy phenyl) 2-methyl alanine. It is also available as HCl salt.

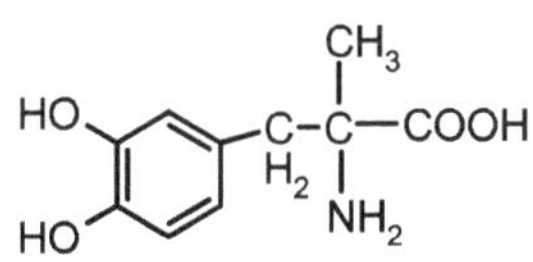

Methyldopa

Methyldopa is synthesized from 4-hydroxy-3-methoxy phenyl acetone by following chemical reactions.

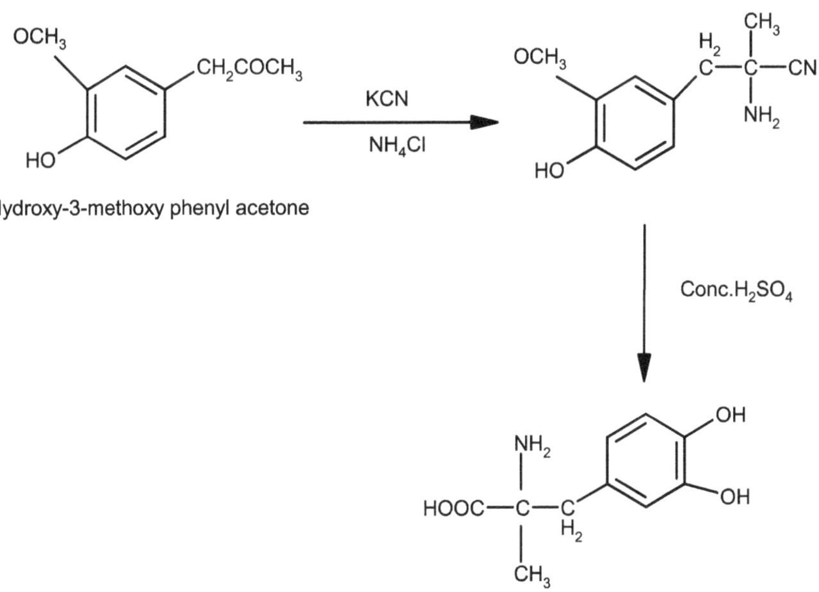

Mechanism of action

Methyldopa selectively stimulates α_2 receptor because of the presence of alpha methyl group. Thus the stimulation ultimately decreases the concentration of dopamine, norepinephrine, epinephrine and serotonin in the CNS and periphery and produces antihypertensive effect. It inhibits DOPA decarboxylase there by decreases noradrenaline synthesis. It also inhibits renin release by the kidneys and has some direct action on blood vessels.

Properties

Methyldopa is white colored hygroscopic powder and decomposes at 300 ^{O}C. Methyldopa HCl is soluble in water, but it is practically insoluble in the common organic solvents.

Uses

It is used to treat moderate to severe hypertension along with diuretics.

Clonidine

It is an imidazoline derivative, which selectively acts on α_1 receptors (α_{2A} subtype) in brain stem. Chemically clonidine is 2-[(2,6-dichlorophenyl) amino]-2-imidazoline.

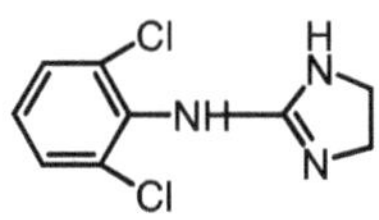

Clonidine

Clonidine is synthesized by following chemical reaction.

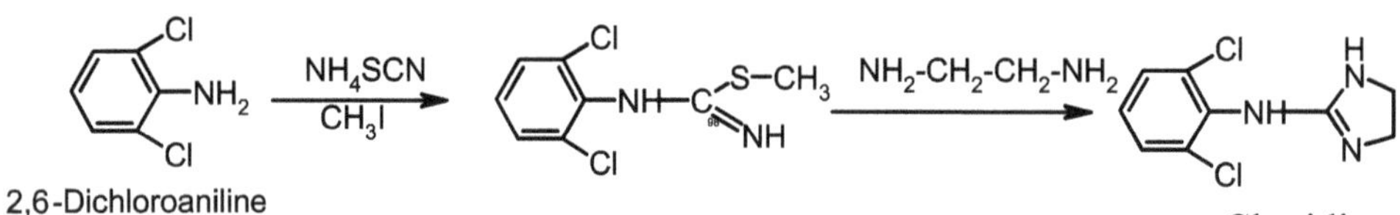

Mechanism of action

Clonidine is more selective towards α_2 receptor. When clonidine is administered, it exhibits mild vasoconstrictive activity due to the stimulation of peripheral adrenergic receptors. Later it enters the CNS and stimulates the α_2 receptors, which decreases sympathetic outflow, and finally it decreases the blood pressure.

Properties

It is soluble in absolute alcohol and slightly soluble in chloroform. The hydrochloride salt is freely soluble in water.

Uses

It is a moderately potent antihypertensive to treat all grades of hypertension.

Guanfacine

Guanfacine chemically – N- (aminimno –methyl) –2,6 – dichloro benzene acetamide.

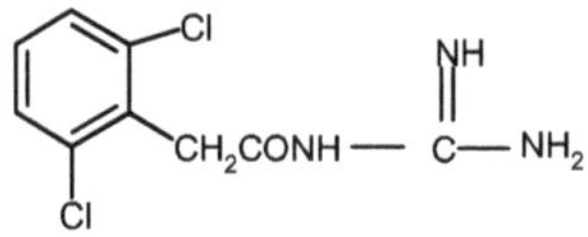

Guanfacine

Guanfacine is synthesized by following chemical reaction.

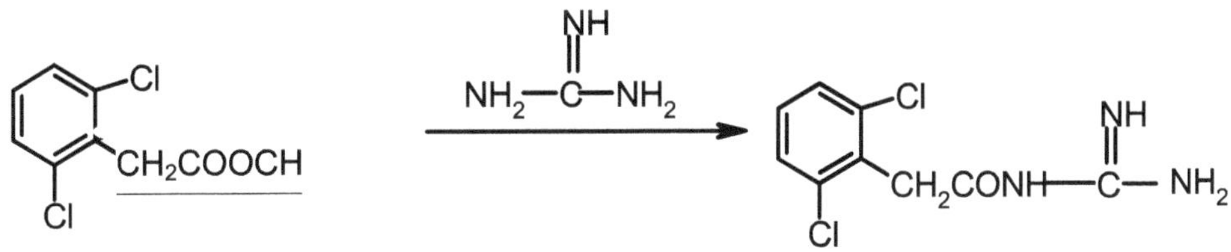

2, 6-dichloro phenyl acetate

Guanafacine

Mechanism of action

Guanfacine is the structural analogue of clonidine which acts centrally by binding to α_2 receptor and results in the blockade of the synaptic impulses. It is related to clonidine but has longer duration of action.

Uses

It is used as an antihypertensive agent.

Guanabenz

Guanabenz is [(2,6 - dichloro benzylidine) amino] guanidine.

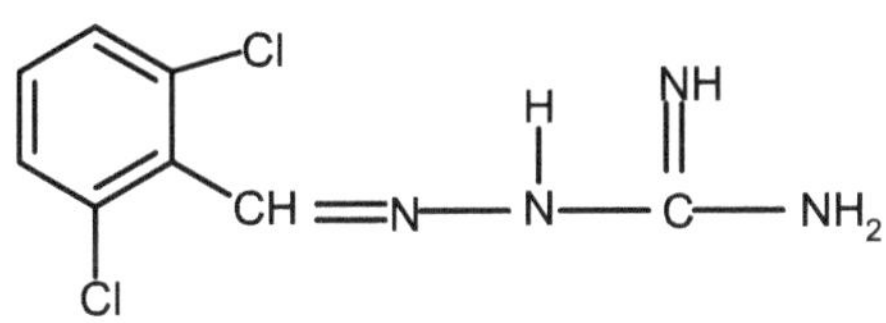

Guanabenz

Guanabenz is synthesized by following chemical reaction.

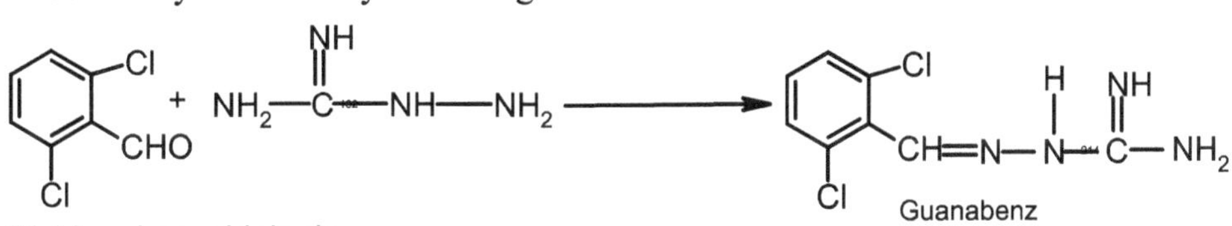

2,6- Dichloro benzaldehyde

Guanabenz

Uses

It is a short acting antihypertensive agent.

Sympathetic nerve blockers

Drugs grouped under this category acts by inhibiting the sympathetic function through interfering with chemical mediation at nerve endings.

Reserpine

Reserpine is an indole alkaloid isolated from the roots of *Rauwolfia serpentina*.

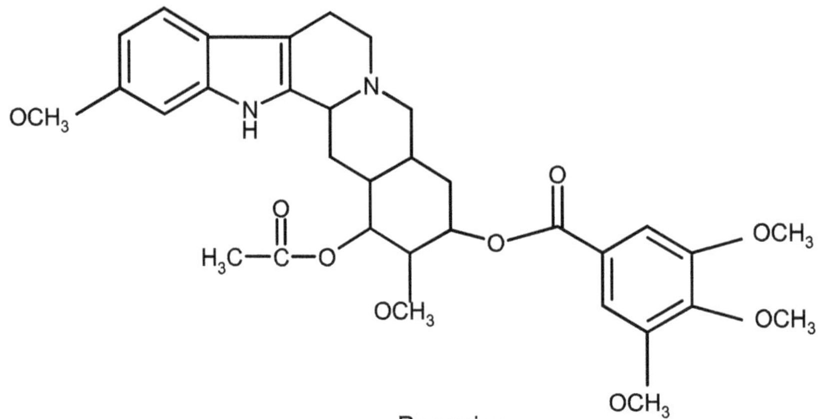

Reserpine

Mechanism of action

Reserpine depletes norepinephrine in sympathetic neurons and epinephrine in the adrenal medulla by acting on hypothalamus and midbrain reticular formation. It also depletes the storage sites of serotonin and dopamine. Thus reserpine decreases sympathetic tone and there by decrease in sympathetic activity is responsible for antihypertensive action.

Properties

It is very sparingly soluble in water. It is freely soluble in chloroform, glacial acetic acid. It is soluble in benzene and ethyl acetate. Slightly soluble in acetone, methanol, alcohol and ether. Upon standing it acquires a yellow color and pronounced fluorescence.

Uses

It is used as antihypertensive and tranquilizer. Reserpine is seldom used as antihypertensive because it produces a wide range of adverse reaction.

Guanethidine

Guanethidine is a synthetic adrenergic neuron blocker. It is a selective sympathetic blocker. Guanethidine is 1-[2-(perhydroazocin-1-yl) ethyl] guanidine. Guanethidine possesses a hexahydro azocinyl ring linked to guanidine by ethyl group.

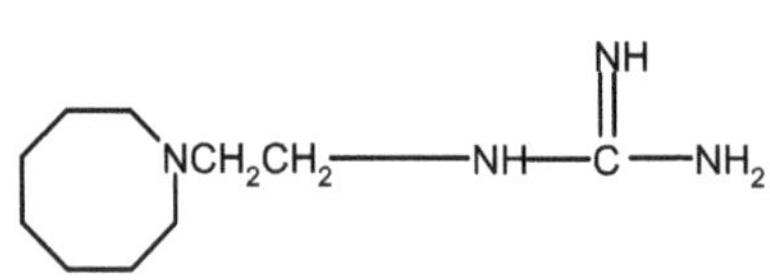

Guanethidine

Guanethidine is prepared from azocine through an intermediate 1-(2- aminoethyl) perhydro azocine by following chemical reaction.

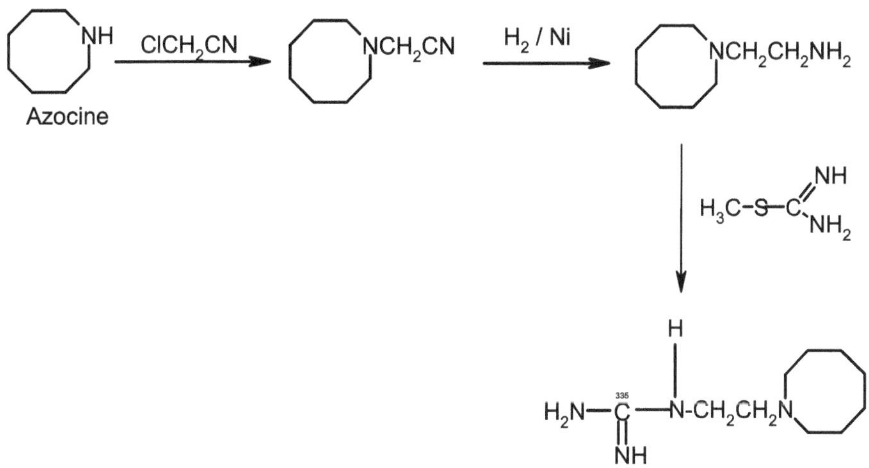

Mechanism of action

Guanethidine is a neuronal blocking agent acts by preventing the release of neurotransmitter, norepinephrine (NE) from peripheral adrenergic neurons. On long-term administration this can deplete storage sites of NE in sympathetic neurons.

Properties

This is colorless, crystalline and odorless powder. It is soluble in water, very slightly soluble in alcohol and practically insoluble in ether and chloroform.

Uses

It is used in the treatment of hypertension and glaucoma.

Guanadrel

Guanadrel is chemically (1,4 dioxaspiro [4.5] dec – 2-yl methyl) guanidine. It possess a dioxaspirodecyl ring system linked to guanidine by a methyl group.

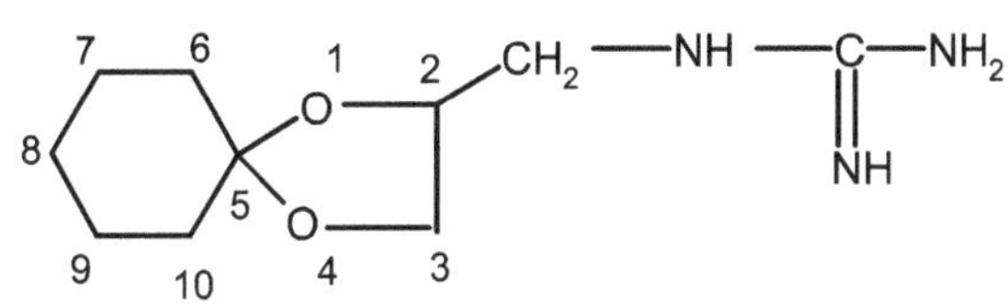

Guanadrel

Guanadrel is prepared by following chemical reactions,

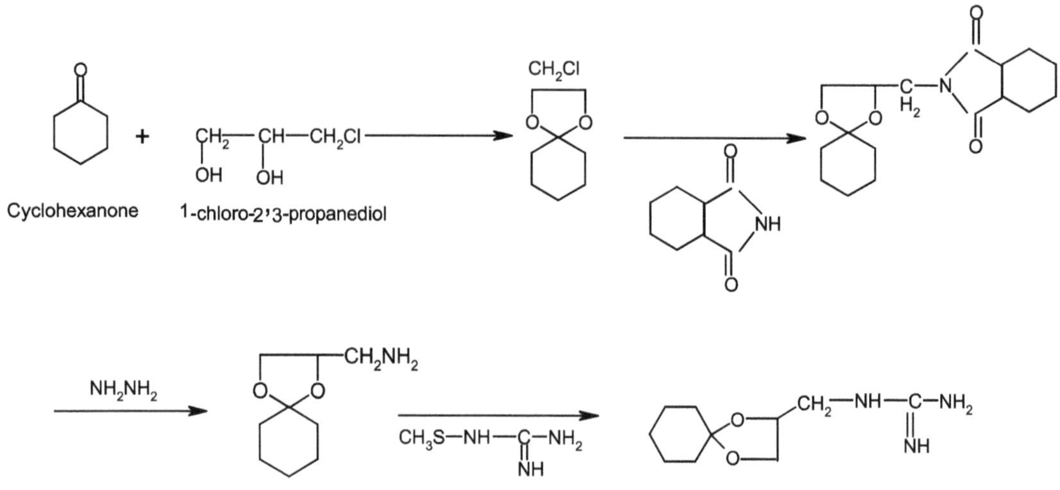

Guanadrel

Mechanism of action

It is similar to guanethidine, acts by inhibiting the release of neurotransmitter from peripheral nerve endings.

Uses

It is used to treat mild to moderate hypertension.

Vasodilators

Directly acting

They act directly on arteries or veins to reduce the blood pressure and are further classified as:

Arteriolar vasodilators

Arteriolar and venular vasodilators

Arteriolar vasodilators

These agents directly relax arteriolar smooth muscle, which results in decrease of peripheral resistance and blood pressure.

Hydralazine

Hydralazine is 1-hydrazinophthalazine.

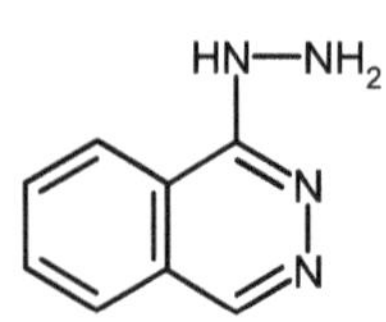

Hydralazine

It is synthesized from half-aldehyde of phthalic acid by the following scheme:

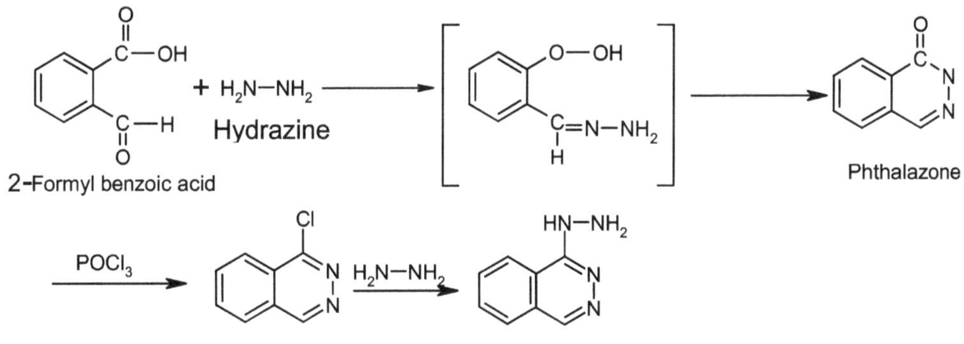

Hydralazine

Hydralazine reduces peripheral resistance and blood pressure by a direct vasodilating effect on vascular smooth muscle by opening ATP-modulated potassium channel. Activator of potassium channel increases the efflux of K^+ ions from the cells, causing hyperpolarisation of smooth muscle cells and vasodilatation on arterioles.

Uses

It is used as arteriolar vasodilator in the treatment of hypertension. Hydralazine is recommended to be used in combination with a diuretic and another hypotensive drugs.

Diazoxide

Diazoxide is a non-diuretic thiazide. It is a benzothiadiazine derivative which is 7 -chloro - 3 - methyl - 2H - 1, 2, 4-benzothiadiazine 1, 1 - dioxide.

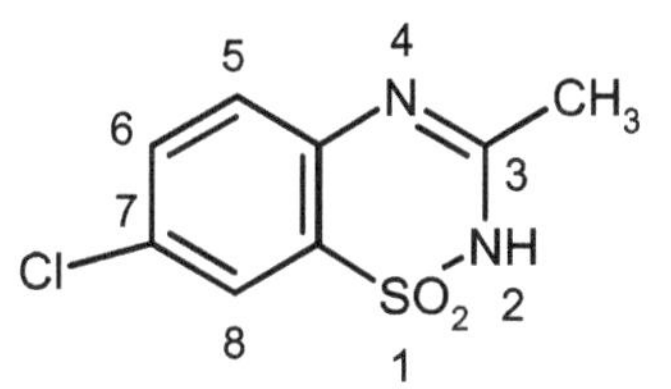

Diazoxide

It is prepared by following chemical reaction,

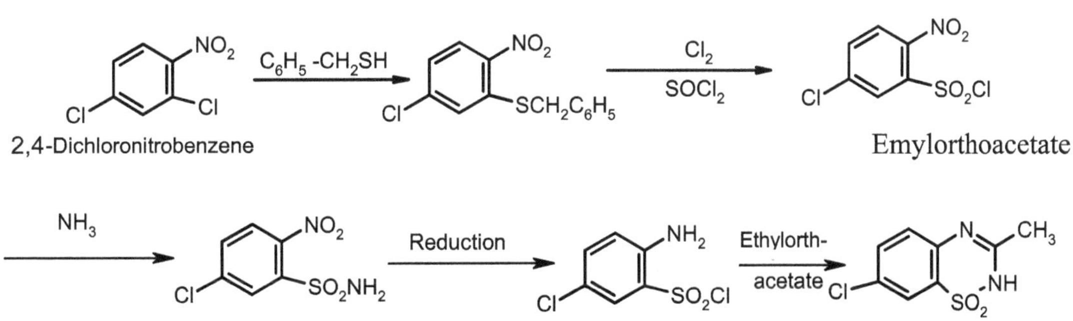

Diazoxide

Diazoxide act directly on arterioles and lower the total peripheral resistance thus decreases blood pressure similar to hydralazine. It is a K channel opener, which leads to a decrease of intracellular Ca^{2+} and releases smooth muscle. If efflux K^+ ions from the cell, results in hyper polarization, which decreases excitability and develops vasodialation.

Uses

It is used for arteriolar vasodilation. It has hyperglycemic and sodium-retention properties.

Minoxidil

Chemically minoxidil is 2, 4 - diamino - 6 - piperdino pyrimidine - 3 - oxide. Minoxidil and its active metabolite (minoxidil–o-sulphate) exert antihypertensive effect similar to hydralazine.

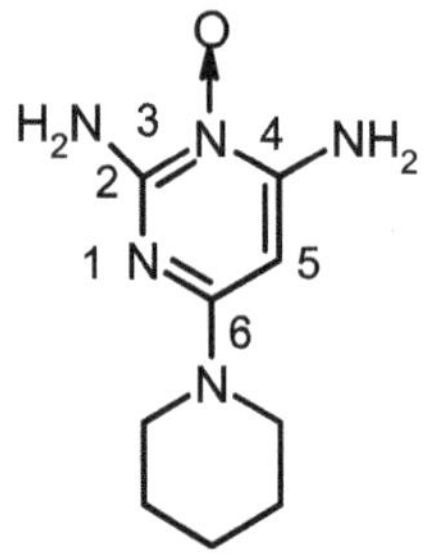

Minoxidil

It is prepared by following chemical reaction.

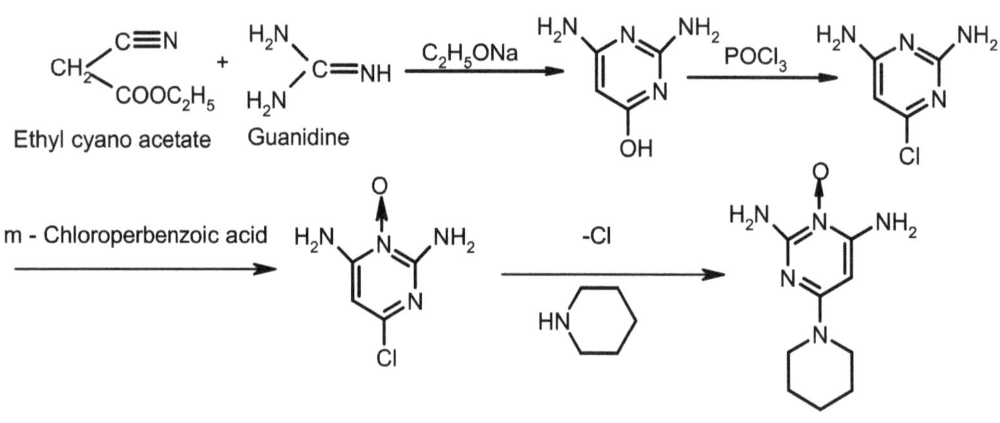

Uses

It is used as arteriolar vasodilator to treat severe hypertension. It is topically applied to promote hair growth in male pattern baldness. The increased hair growth may be by increasing microcirculation around hair follicles. It is used with a diuretic (minoxil) causes sodium and water retention.

Arterial and venular vasodilators

Sodium nitroprusside

Sodium nitroprusside has very fast onset of action and lasts only for short duration of time.

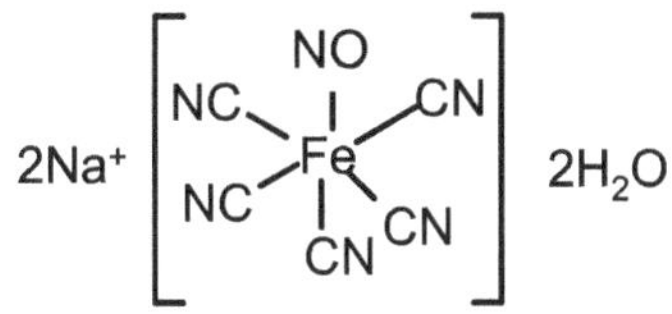

Sodium nitroprusside

It is prepared by following chemical reaction.

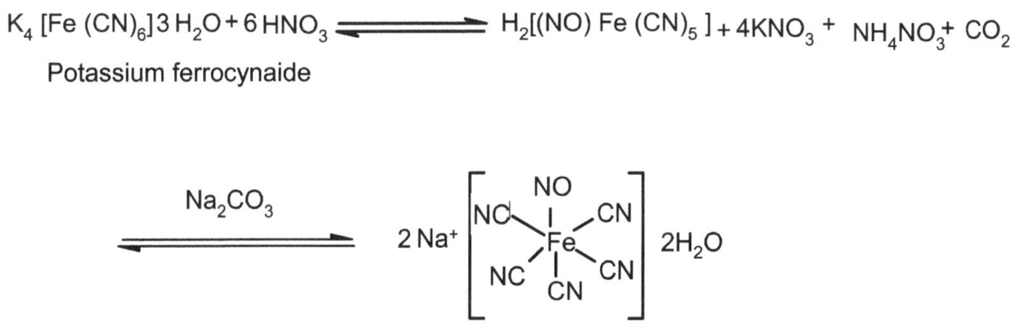

Potassium ferrocynaide

Sodium nitroprusside

Mechanism of action

Sodium nitroprusside forms an active nitricoxide (NO) with glutathione in vascular endothelium that increases cGMP and causes vasodilation.

Properties

These are ruby red colored odorless transparent crystals. It is soluble in water and slightly soluble in alcohol.

Uses

It is used as antihypertensive agent when required for fast reduction in blood pressure.

α-adrenergic blockers

The main action of alpha adrenoreceptor blocking agents is to produce peripheral vasodilation. (The α_1- adrenoreceptors are located at postsynaptic sites on tissues innervated by adrenergic neurons; the α_2-adrenoreceptors have presynaptic location).

The alpha-receptors stimulation causes the movement of intracellular Ca^{++} ions from their stores. Increase in Ca^{++} concentration causes contraction of smooth muscles through the activation of Ca^{++} sensitive protein kinases.

The inherent mechanism involved can be explained as the stimulation of alpha receptors activated phospholiopase C (PLC) through G proteins. PLC gets hydrolysed to inositol triphosphate (IP_3) and diacylglycerol (DAG). IP_3 stimulates the Ca^{++} from intracellular stores and DAG activates the protein kinase C. Finally the phosphorylation of cellular proteins occurs and produces response.

Prazosin

Prazosin is 1 - (4 - amino - 6,7 -dimethoxy - 2 - quinazolinyl) - 4 - (2 - furoyl) piperazine. It is selective α_1 blocker.

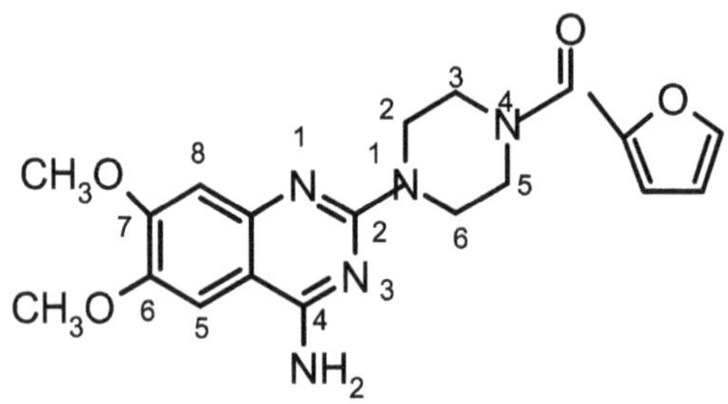

Prazosin

Prazosin synthesized from 3,4 dimethoxy benzaldehyde by following chemical reaction,

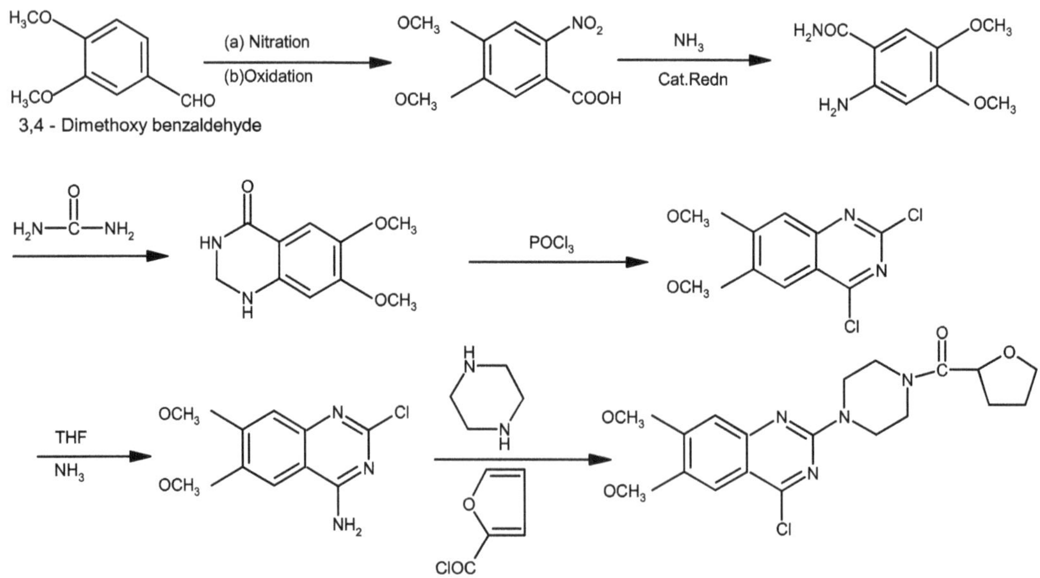

Prazosin acts by a competitive postsynaptic α_1- adrenoreceptor blocking. It dilates both arterioles and veins and produces falling B.P. It does not release noradrenaline due to absence of α_2 blockade. It also inhibits phosphodiesterase which degrades cAMP (cAMP could contribute to its vasodilator action).

Uses

Prazosin is effective orally. It is used to treat essential hypertension and chronic congestive heart failure.

Terazosin

Terazosin is 1-(4-amino-6,7-dimethoxy-2-quinazolinyl)-4-[tetrahydro-2-furanyl), Carbonyl) piperazine. Terazosin is a long acting selective α_1- adrenoreceptor blocker. It reduces total peripheral resistance. Chemically and pharmacologically it is similar to prazosin but it has higher bioavailability and longer plasma $t_{1/2}$ 12 hrs).

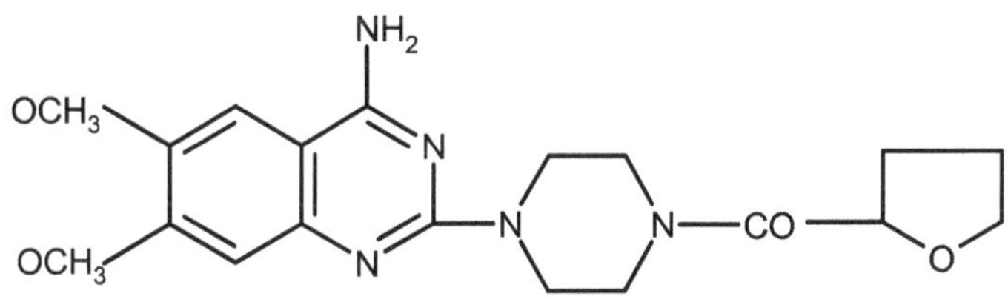

Terazosin

Terazosin is prepared by following chemical reactions,

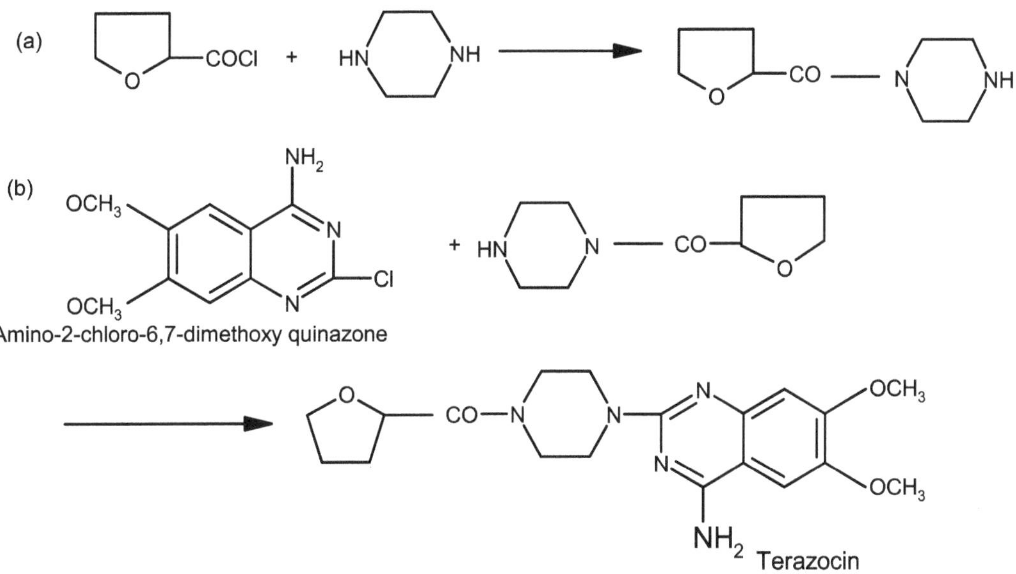

Uses

It is used in the treatment of benign prostatic hyperplasia. It is used alone or with a diuretic to treat mild to moderate hypertension.

β-Blockers

β-adrenergic receptors activate adenyl cyclase through G protein which leads to the accumulation of cyclic-AMP dependent protein kinase which will phosphorylate the cellular proteins and produces hypertension. Beta adrenoreceptors are located predominantly in heart (β_1), arteries, arterioles of skeletal muscle (β_2), and in bronchi (β_2), where their stimulation induces cardiac excitation, peripheral vasodilation and bronchial relaxation respectively.

The beta-blockers bind to the receptors and block their activity and reduce the hypertension.

All β-adrenoreceptor blocking agents (β-blockers) are synthetic compounds and completely inhibit the action of adrenergic agonists on β-receptors. Blockade of β_1 receptors reduces heart rate, myocardial contractivity and cardiac output. Consequently the blood pressure is reduced.

Propranolol

It is a non-selective beta-blocker drug. It is chemically 1-(isopropyl amino)-3-(1-naphthyloxy)- 2-propanol. The levo isomer is 100 times more active than dextro isomer. Propranolol is highly lipophilic and is completely absorbed from gastrointestinal tract. It blocks β_1 and β_2-receptors equally by competitive mechanism. Propranolol is metabolized to 4-hydroxypropranolol which has sympathonimetic acitivity.

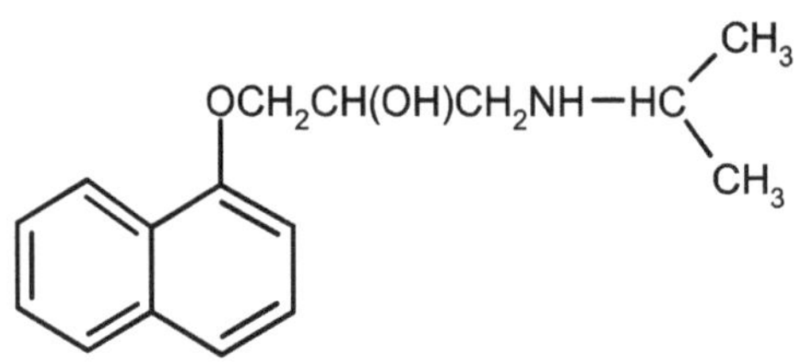

Propranolol

Propranolol is synthesized from α-naphthol by following chemical reaction,

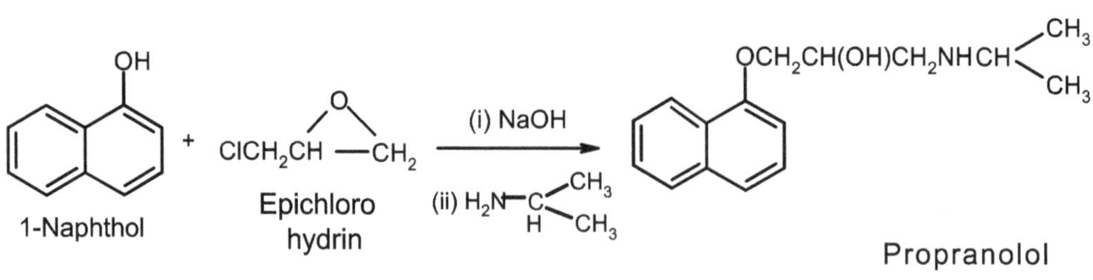

Uses

It is used to treat cardiac arrhythmias, angina pectoris, hypertension, essential tremor, myocardial infarction, migraine headache.

Timolol

It is (s)-1-(tert-butylyamino)-3-[(4-morpholino-1, 2, 5-thiadiazol-3-yl] oxy]-2-propanol.

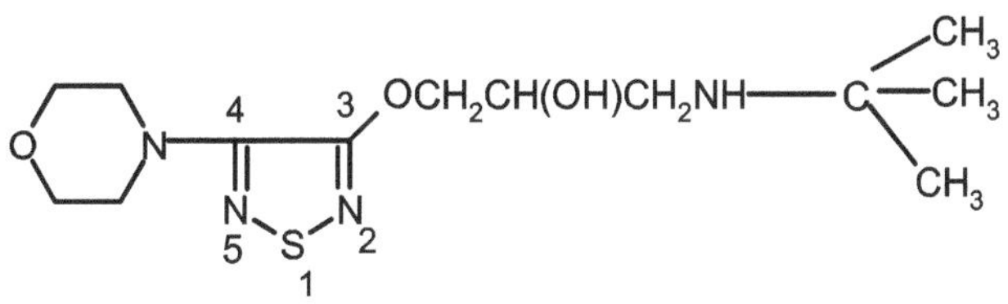

Timolol

Timolol is synthesized from 4-chloro-3-hydroxy thiazole by following chemical reactions,

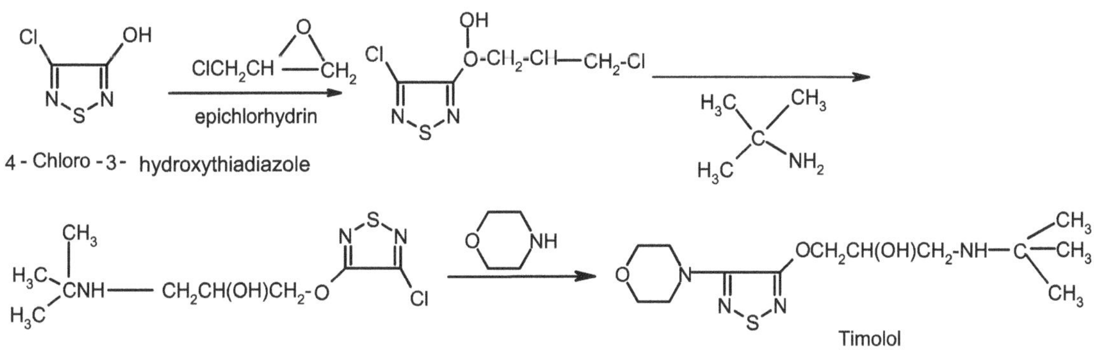

Properties

Timolol exists as white crystals having a melting point of 202 ^{O}C. It is soluble in water, ethanol and methanol. It is sparingly soluble in chloroform and insoluble in ether.

Uses

It is used as an antihypertensive, antiarryhthmic agent and especially in the treatment of glaucoma.

Pindolol

Pindolol is 1-(1H-indol-4-yloxy)-3-[(1-methyl ethyl) amino]-2-propanol.

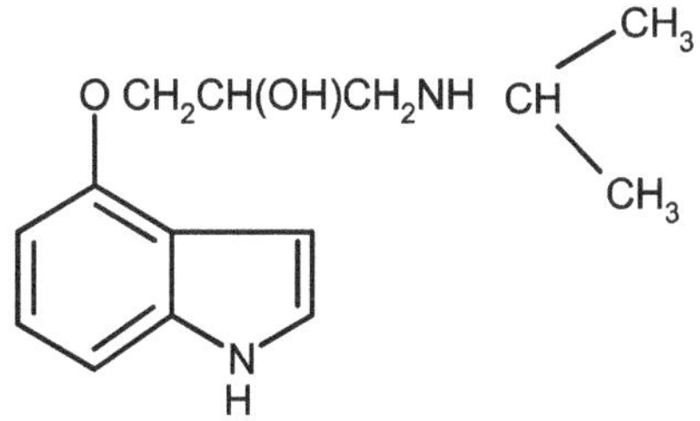

Pindolol

Pindolol is synthesized from 4-hydroxy indole by following chemical reaction,

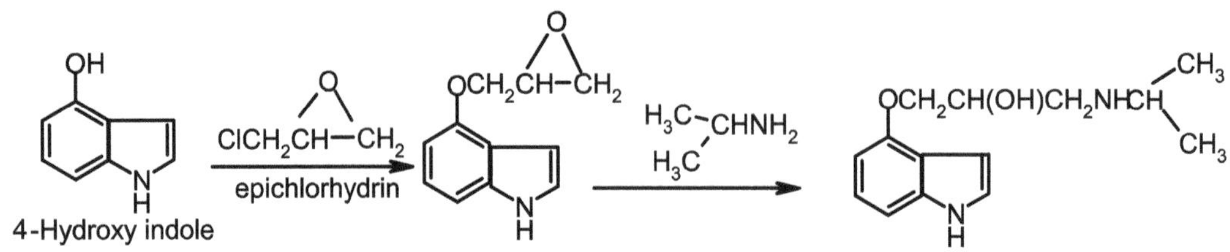

4-Hydroxy indole

epichlorhydrin

Pindolol

Uses

It is used as antihypertensive agent, antiarrhythmic agent and used to treat glaucoma.

Atenolol

It is 4-[2-hydroxy-3-[[(1-methyl ethyl) amino] propoxy] benzacetamide.

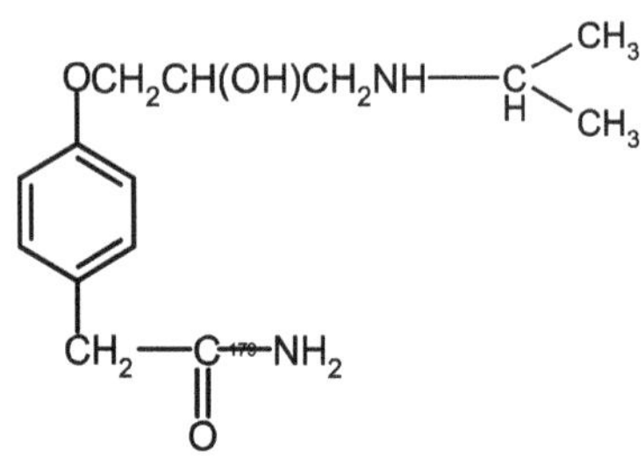

Atenolol

Atenolol is synthesized by following chemical reaction.

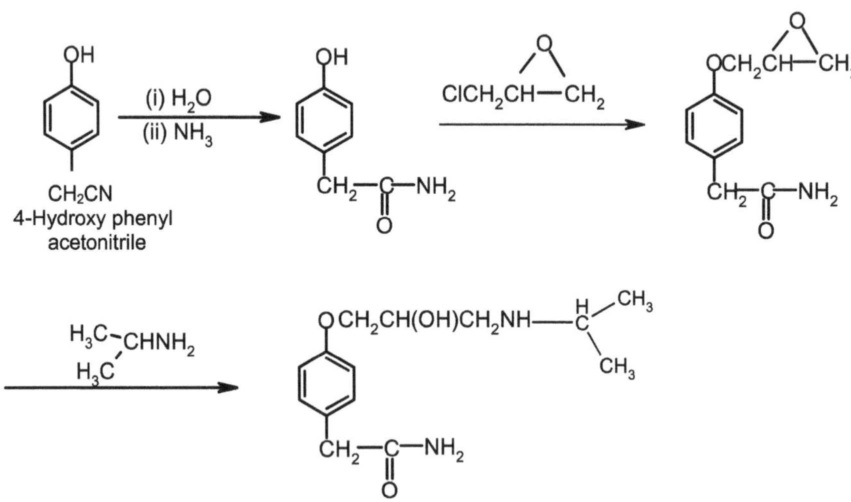

4-Hydroxy phenyl acetonitrile

Atenolol

Uses

Atenolol is a selective β_1 blocker having low lipid solubility. It is used as antihypertensive, anti arrhythmic and anti anginal agent.

Acebutolol

It is N-[3-acetyl-4-[2-hydroxy-3-[(1-methyl ethyl) amino] propoxy] phenyl] butanamide, which is selective beta-blocker with partial agonistic activity.

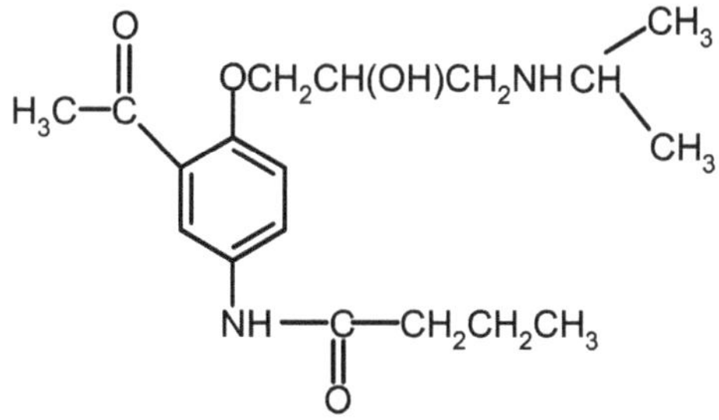

Acebutolol

Acebutolol is synthesized from 4-butyraminophenol by following chemical reaction.

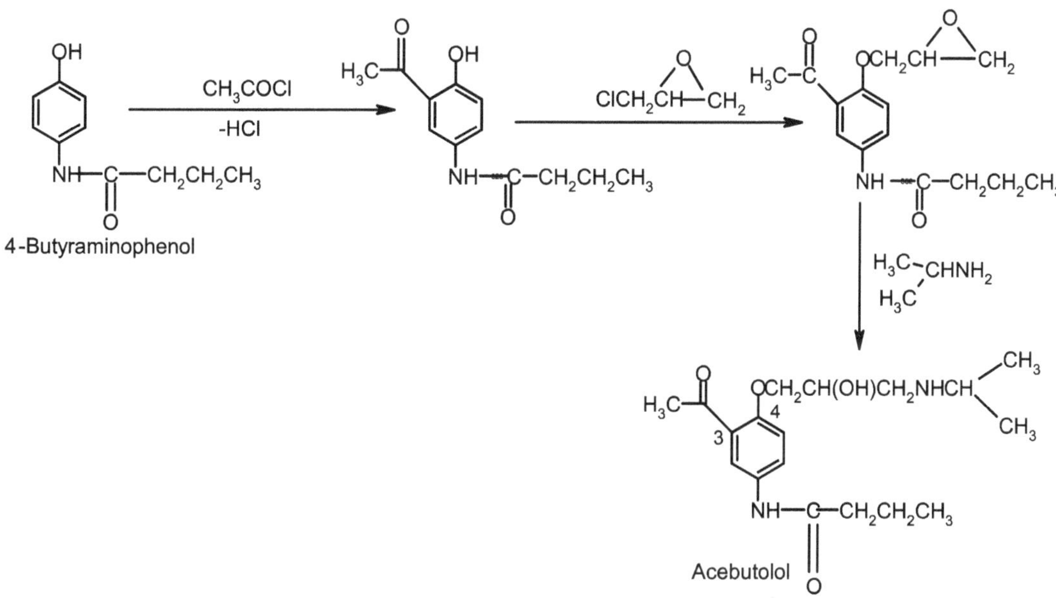

Uses

Acebutolol is another cardio selective agent with significant partial agonistic and membrane stabilizing properties.

These are used to treat :

- Ventricular arrhythmias,
- Hypertension.

Acebutolol is metabolized to diacetolol which is also a selective β_1-receptor antagonist.

Esmolol

It is 4-[2-hydroxy-3-[(1-methyl ethyl)amino] propoxy]benzene propanoic acid methyl ester, also selective beta-blocker.

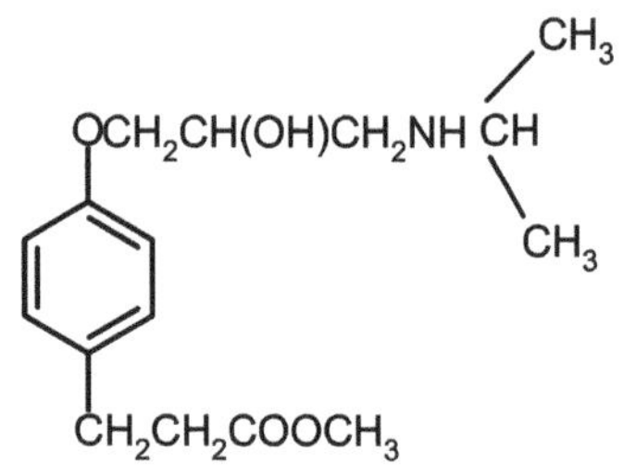

Esmolol

Esmolol is synthesized by following chemical reaction,

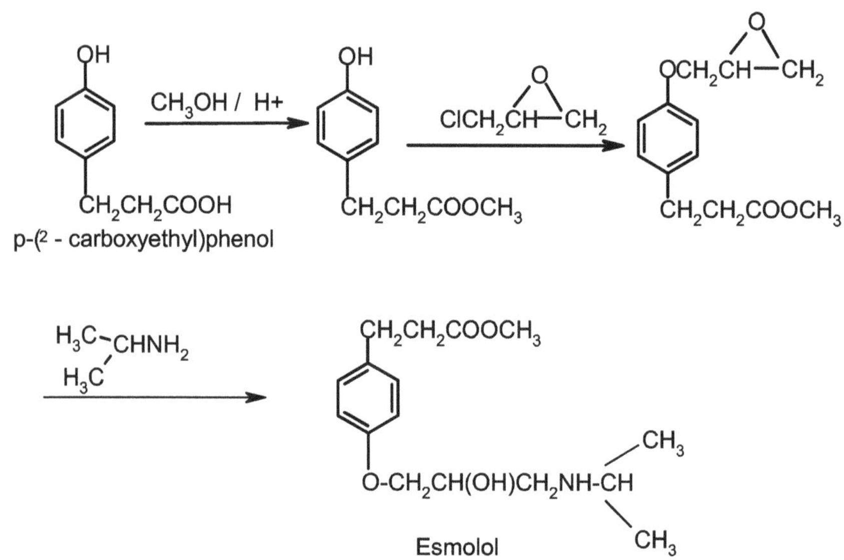

Uses

Esmolol is an ultra short acting β_1 blocker. It is inactivated by esterases in blood. It is used for rapid short term control of ventricular rate in supra ventricular arrhythmia and sinus tachycardia.

Angiotensin converting enzyme (ACE) inhibitors

Renin angiotensin system

Responding to the stimuli renin (a protease enzyme) secreted by the kidneys which influences the conversion of angiotensiongen to angiotensin I. Angiotensin I is converted to angiotensin II by the action of angiotensin converting enzyme (ACE). Angiotensin II by its arterial vasoconstriction helps to maintain blood pressure. It also stimulates the aldosterone, which increases the plasma volume by salt and water retention.

The major stimulus for renin release is renal hyperfusion, caused by volume depletion or low cardiac output. It is activated therefore in response to dehydration, haemorrhage and heart failure.

These drugs are introduced in order to treat hypertension. They reduce the angiotensin II synthesis by inhibiting the ACE.

ACE also involves in the breakdown of bradykinin. ACE inhibitors increase the activity of vascular peptide and contribute to its vasodilating effects.

Caution

The most significant side effect of ACE inhibitors is dry cough, which vanishes up on drug withdrawal, and it is contraindicated in patients with aortic stenosis.

Uses

Hypertension: The ACE inhibitors are one of the first choice drugs in all grades of essential as well as renovascular hypertension.

These are highly effective antihypertensive agents that lower blood pressure. Efficacy of ACE inhibitors can be increased by co-prescription with diuretics. ACE inhibitors together with diuretics, are first line drugs in symptomatic heart failure. These drugs are observed to improve long-term prognosis in heart failure.

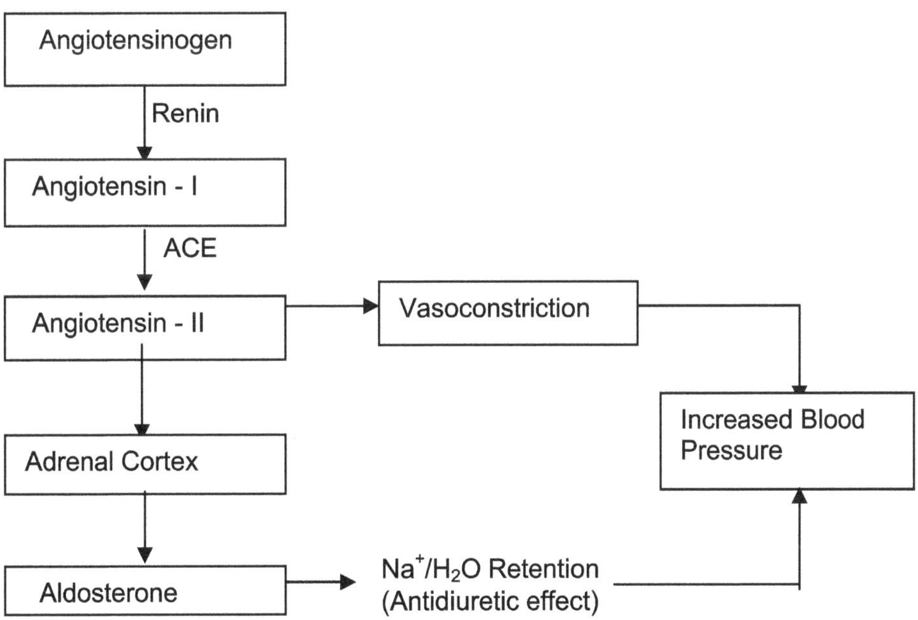

Acute myocardial infarction

These drugs have direct effect on the atherosclerotic process and susceptibility to plaque events there by reducing the risk of recurrent infarction.

Diabetes

These are showing their grounds in the treatment of diabetes particularly in nephropathy and retinopathy. There are evidences that these may be protective against macrovascular complications and enabling their use for treatment of diabetic coronary artery disease.

Captopril

Captopril is 1-[(2S)-3-mercapto-2-methyl-1-oxo propionyl]-L-proline. This is the first orally active angiotensin converting enzyme inhibitor. The carboxylic acid group binds to arginine residue and mercapto group with zinc of ACE. However captopril develops rashes and loss of sense of taste due to the presence of mercapto group.

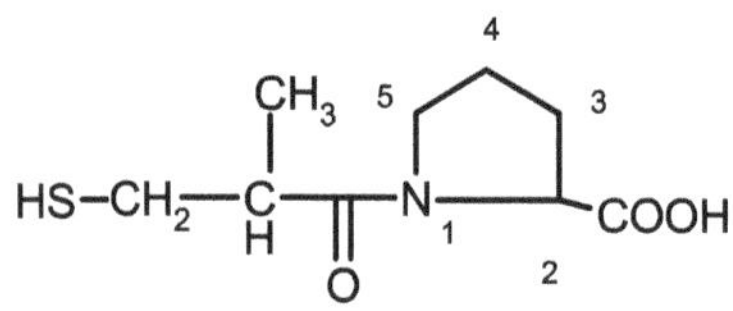

Captopril

Captopril is synthesized by following chemical reaction,

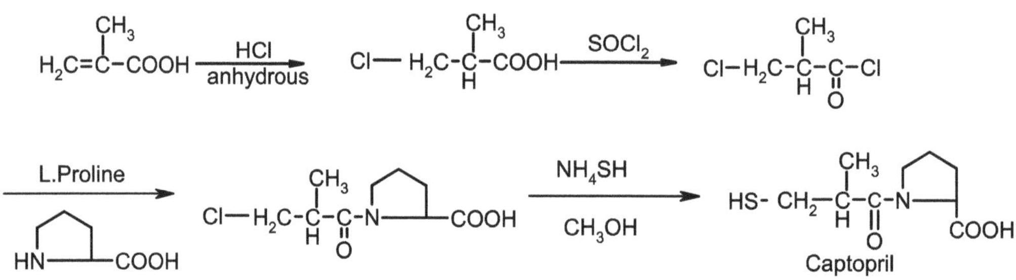

Uses

It is used either alone or in combination with other drugs to treat hypertension, heart failure, myocardial infarction and diabetic nephropathy.

Enalapril

Enalapril is N-[(1S)-1-(ethoxycarbony)-3-phenyl propyl]-L-alanyl-L-proline. It is de-esterified *in vivo* to its active diacid metabolite, (enalaprilat) and is a non-thiol containing ACE inhibitor.

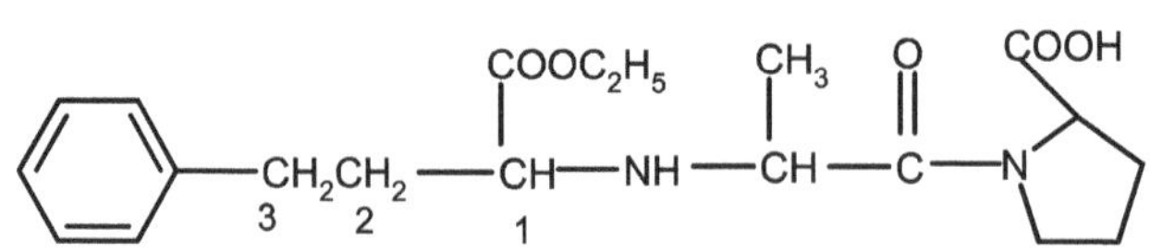

Enalapril

Enalapril is synthesized from 2-oxo-4-Phenyl butyrate by following chemical reaction,

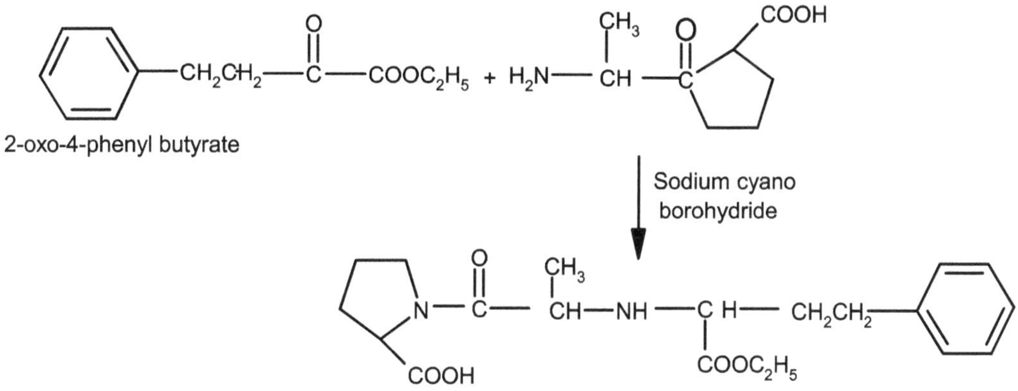

Enalapril

Properties

It is white to off white powder having a melting point 144 °C. It is soluble in water, alcohol and methanol.

Uses

It is a long acting ACE inhibiting drug and used as antihypertensive.

Fosinopril

Fosinopril is (4S)-4-cyclohexyl-1-(4S)-1-hydroxy-2-methylpropoxy)(4-phenylbutyl) phosphinyl)-acetyl– L-proline propionate. It is a phosphor containing ACE inhibitor. It is hydrolysed by intestinal and liver enzymes to the active form.

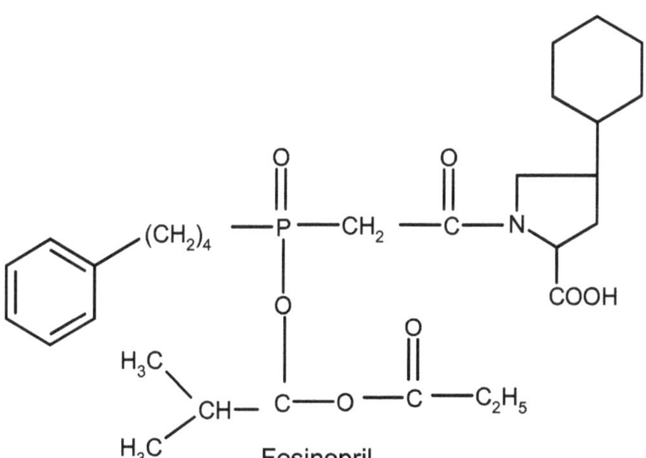

Fosinopril

Properties

It has melting point of 140 °C-153°C.

Uses

It is used as antihypertensive

Angiotensin antagonists

Angiotensin antagonists can inhibit angiotensin II competitively to produce a vasodilatory effect. These drugs are observed to be imidazole 5 acetic acid derivatives, which can inhibit angiotensin II.

Losartan

Losartan is 2-butyl-4-chloro-1-[2-(1H-tetratzol-5-yl)[1,1-biphenyl]-4-yl]methyl-lH-imidazole–5-methanol. It is a recently introduced non-peptide angiotensin II receptor antagonist. Losartan undergoes first pass metabolism to an active metabolite (5- carboxylic acid metabolite). The metabolite has greater pharmacological activity than losartan. It is used to treat hypertension.

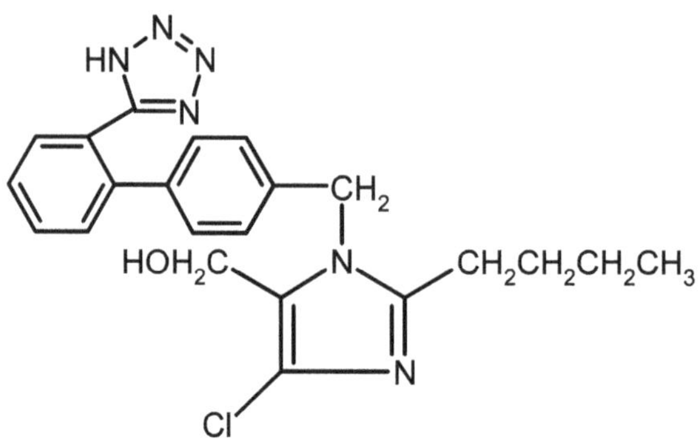

Losartan

Calcium channel blockers

Introduction

Movement of calcium ions across cell membranes is crucial for the functioning of muscle in the heart and blood vessels as well as the electrical conduction system of the heart. Calcium channel blockers, as the name implies, block the influx of calcium into cells of heart and arteries. This relaxes the muscle in the walls of arteries, resulting in dilation of arteries. This, in turn, lowers the blood pressure and improves the blood supply to the heart. They also relax the heart muscle. All of these effects allow the heart to decrease the force of contraction of the myocardium (muscle of the heart), and help treat the symptoms of angina. This is known as the negative inotropic effect of calcium channel blockers. It is because of the negative inotropic effects of most calcium channel blockers are avoided (or used with caution) in individuals with cardiomyopathy (weak muscle of the heart). Many calcium channel blockers also slow down the conduction of electrical activity within the heart, by blocking the calcium channel during the plateau phase (of the action potential) of the heart. This causes a lowering of the heart rate and may cause heart blocks. The negative chronotropic effects of calcium channel blockers make them a commonly used class of agents in individuals with atrial fibrillation or flutter in whom control of the heart rate is an issue.

Mechanism of action

Calcium channel blockers work by blocking voltage-sensitive calcium channels in the heart and in the blood vessels. This prevents calcium levels from increasing as much in the cells when stimulated, leading to less contraction. This decreases total peripheral resistance by dilating the blood vessels, and decreases cardiac output by lowering the force of contraction. Because resistance and output drop, so does blood pressure. With low blood pressure, the heart does not have to work as hard, this can ease problems with cardiomyopathy and coronary disease.

Classification of calcium channel blockers : Calcium channel blockers are classified as follows:

(a) **Dihydropyridine calcium channel blockers**: Amlodipine besylate, felodipine, nicardipine, nifedipine, nimodipine, nisoldipine, nitrendipine, lercanidipine

(b) **Phenylalkylamine calcium channel blockers**: Gallopamil, verapamil hydrochloride,

(c) **Benzothiazepine calcium channel blockers**: Diltiazem hydrochloride,

(d) **Others**: Menthol (mint oil)

Characteristics of calcium channel blockers: The following characteristics are observed by the calcium channel blockers:

1. They exhibit excitation-contraction in isolated vascular smooth muscle.
2. They inhibit calcium uptake into vascular smooth muscle.
3. They inhibit contractile force of cardiac tissue.
4. They increase coronary blood flow *in vivo*.

(a) **Dihydropyridine Type:** These are the most widely used calcium channel blockers. These agents act on the dihydropyridine receptors that are present in the myocardium. E.g. Nifedipine, nitrendipine, nicardipine, felodipine, amlodipine, nimodipine, nisoldipine, lercanidipine

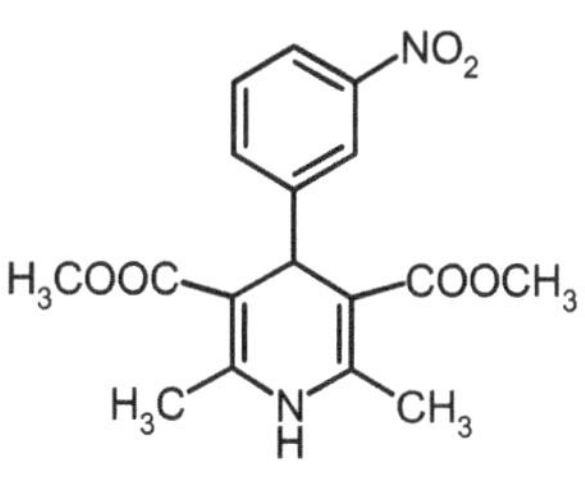

Nifedipine

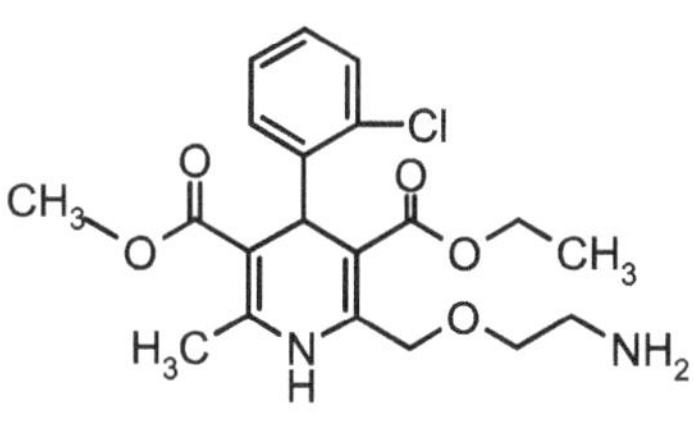

Amlodipine

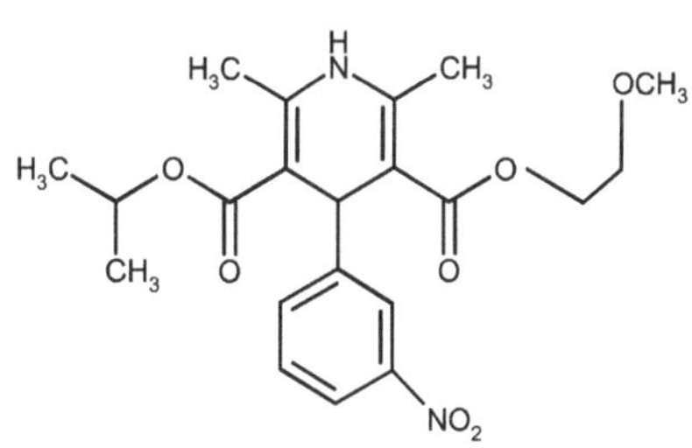

Nimodipine

SAR

1. These compounds contain an aryl 1,4-dihydropyridine ring with an unsubstituted nitrogen as a core structure.
2. Lower alkyl substitution was preferred on 2nd and 6th position
3. Introduction of ester group enhances the duration of action.

4. Presence of asymmetric centers at 3rd and 5th positions give more potent compounds. E.g. Nitrendipine.
5. Introduction of nitro group for alkyl group at position 4 yields a compound with good Ca^{+2} channel blocking activity.

Nifedipine

It is 1,4-dihydro pyridine analogue. It is chemically dimethyl, 1,4 dihydro-2,6-dimethyl-4-(o-nitrophenyl)-3,5-pyridinedi carboxylate.

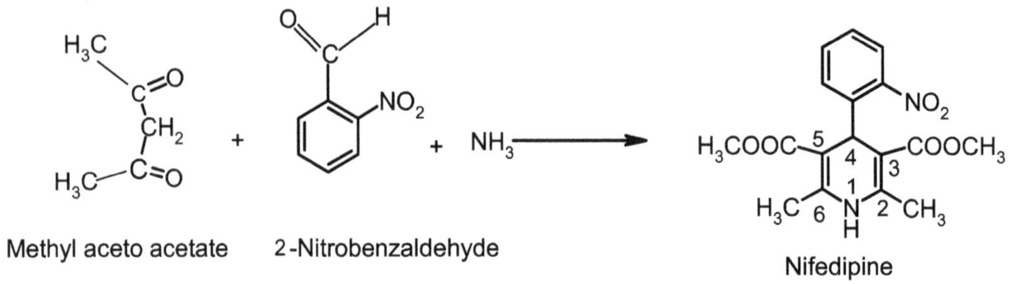

It exists as yellow crystals having a melting point of 172°C -174°C. It is soluble in acetone methylene chloride, chloroform, ethyl acetate, methanol and ethanol.

It is used as antianginal, anti hypertensive. It is also used to treat Raynaud's phenomenon, premature labor, and painful spasms of the esophagus in cancer patients.

Amlodipine

Amlodipine (as besylate or malleate) is a long-acting calcium channel blocker used as an anti-hypertensive and in the treatment of angina. Amlodipine acts by relaxing the smooth muscle in the arterial wall, decreasing peripheral resistance and hence improving blood pressure; in angina it improves blood flow to the myocardium. Chemically it is 3-ethyl-5-methyl-2-(2-aminoethoxymethyl)-4-(2-chlorophenyl)-1,4-dihydro-6methyl3, 5pyridi nedi carboxylate.

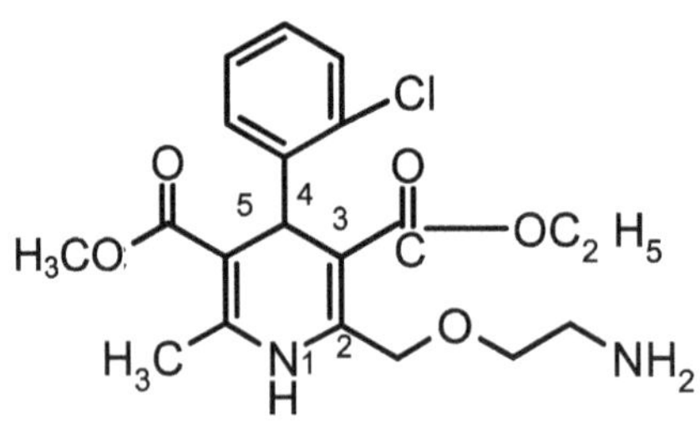

Amlodipine

Nimodipine

Nimodipine is a calcium channel blocker originally developed for the treatment of high blood pressure. Chemically it is 1,4-dihydro-2,6-dimethyl-4-(3-nitrophenyl)-2-methoxyethyl

1-methylethyl ester 3,5-pyridinedicarboxylic acid

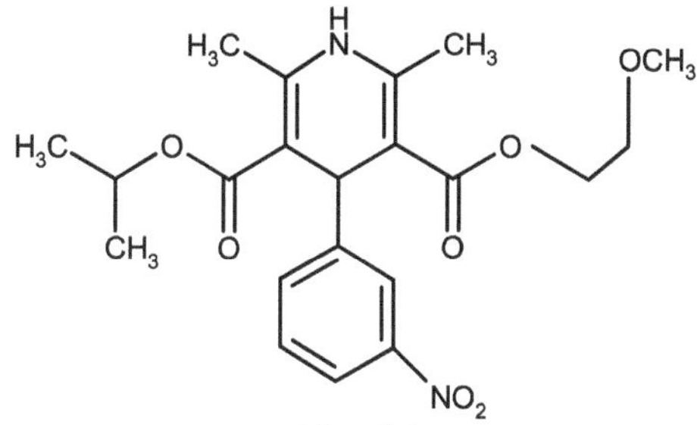

Nimodipine

Nimodipine binds specifically to L-type voltage-gated calcium channels. There are numerous theories about its mechanism in preventing vasospasm, but none are conclusive.

Usage:

Nimodipine has some selectivity for cerebral vasculature, its main use is in the prevention of cerebral vasospasm and resultant ischemia, a complication of subarachnoid hemorrhage (a form of cerebral bleed). Its administration begins within 4 days of a subarachnoid hemorrhage and is continued for three weeks. If blood pressure drops by over 5%, dosage is adjusted. There is still controversy regarding the use of intravenous nimodipine on a routine basis.

Diphenyl alkylamines

Verapamil is the diphenyl alkyl amine derivative that lowers the vascular resistance and increases myocardial blood flow with an increase in sinus oxygen content. It shows it's major action through slowing the cardiac conduction.

Verapamil

It is chemically 5-[(3,4-Dimethoxyphenethyl) methylamino]-2-(3,4-dimethoxyphenyl)-2-isopropylvaleronitrile. Verapamil acts as an L-type calcium channel blocker.

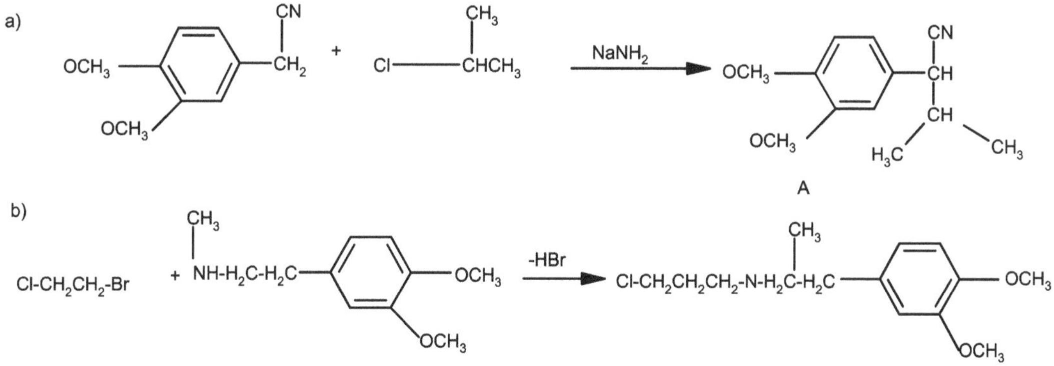

c)

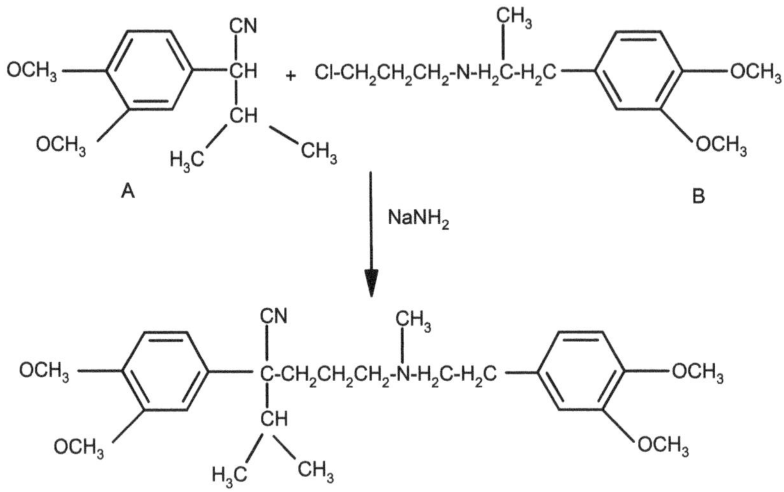

Verapamil

q

It is viscous pale yellow oil having a boiling point of 246 °C. Practically insoluble in water. Sparingly soluble in hexane. Soluble in benzene and ether. Freely soluble in the lower alcohols, acetone, ethyl acetate and chloroform. Verapamil is available as verapamil HCl, which is white crystalline powder. It is used as antihypertensive, antianginal (unstable), antiarrhythmic for the treatment of super ventricular tachyarrhythmias and temporary control or rapid ventricular rate in atrial flutter or fibrillation.

Benzothiazepines : The benzothiazepine analogue which decreases the peripheral resistance and arterial pressure is diltiazem.

Diltiazem

It is chemically (+)-cis-3-(acetyloxy)-5-[2-(dimethylamino) ethyl] 2,3-dihydro-2-(4-methoxyphenyl)-1, 5-benzothiazepin-4 (5H)-one.

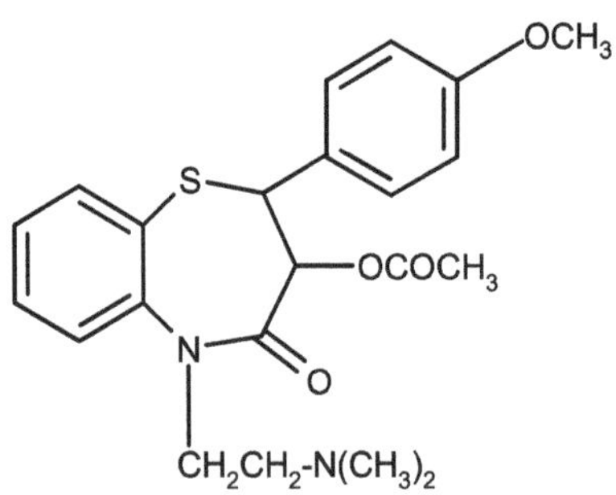

Diltaiazem

It occurs as fine needles having a melting point of 212°C. It is odorless having bitter taste, freely soluble in water, methanol, chloroform and formic acid. Slightly soluble in absolute alcohol. Practically insoluble in benzene. It is rapidly absorbed on oral administration and undergoes first-pass metabolism. It is used as antianginal, antihypertensive, and antiarrhythmic.

Antianginal drugs

Angina pectoris is a symptom of ischemic heart disease caused by a relative insufficiency of blood flow to myocardium. Angina pectoris develops when the blood supply is inadequate to meet myocardilal demand. Angina is characterized by a sudden severe pressing substernal pain radiating to the left arm.

Types of angina

Angina pectoris (chest pain) is of three types

1. *Stable or essential angina* (*classical angina*)

   It is characterized by predictable precipitating factors – Exercise, emotion or heavy mental tension and retrosternal chest pain. It is usually lasts for only few minutes following rest. It is due to atherosclerotic obstruction to common blood flow.
2. *Unstable angina* - It is new or sudden worsening of previous angina occuring at rest or minimal effort.
3. *Variant or prinzimetal angina* - It is less common form of angina; its symptoms are due to coronary vasospasm and can occur during night.

Mechanism of smooth muscle relaxation

Organic Nitrates relaxes vascular smooth muscle by their intracellular conversion to nitrate ions and then to nitric oxide (NO). This nitric oxide activates guanylate cyclase and increases the cells cyclic GMP. Elevated cGMP causes the dephosphorylation of the myosin light chain which results in vascular smooth muscle relaxation

Amyl Nitrate

Angina pectoris is a clinical condition which manifests itself as a severe retrosternal pain which radiates to the chest, left shoulders, upper arm and neck. Initially pain develops in retrosternum.

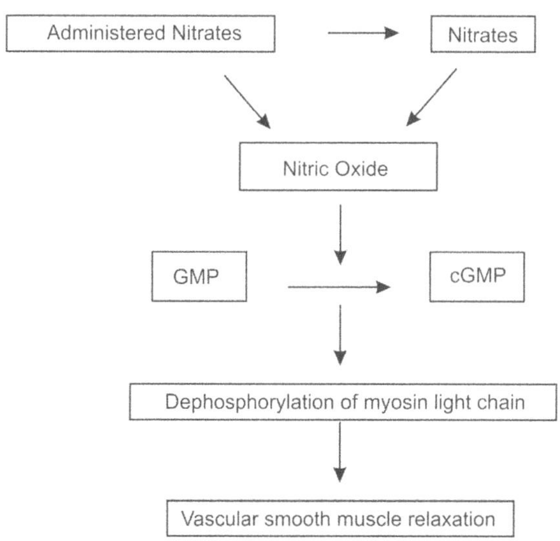

Figure 24.1 Mechanism of nitrovasodilators.

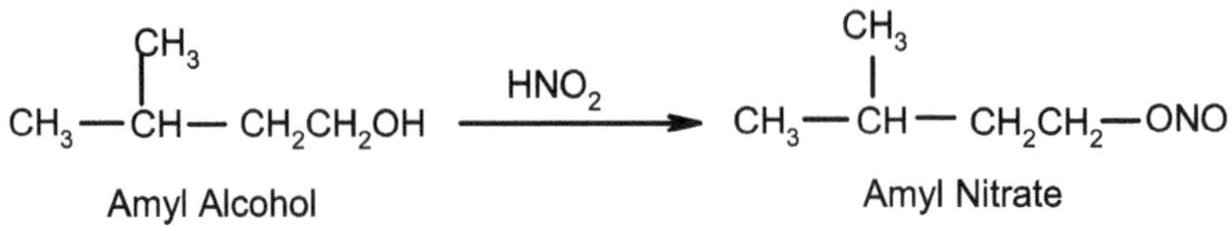

Nitro glycerine

It is chemically 1, 2, 3 propanetriol trinitrate

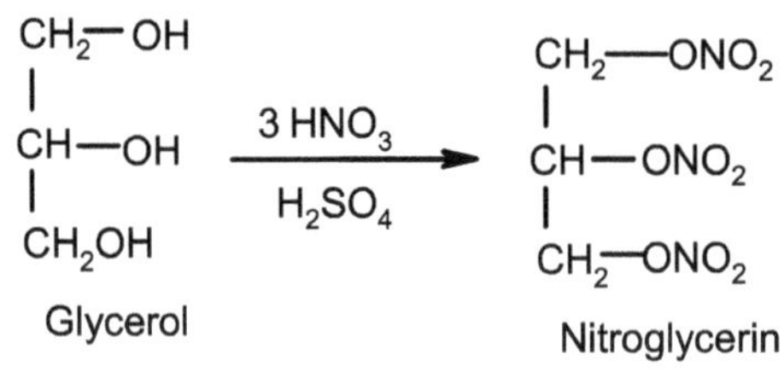

Properties

It is a pale yellow, oily liquid having a sweet burning taste. It produces headache on tasting. Explodes on heating or on combustion. It crystallizes in two forms: labile form, melting point of 2.8°C and stable form, melting point 13.5°C. It is soluble in water, ethanol, methanol and carbon disulfide. Miscible with ether, acetone, glacial acetic acid, ethyl acetate, benzene, nitro benzene, pyridine, chloroform, ethylene bromide and dichloro ethylene. Sparingly soluble in petroleum ether, liquid petroleum and glycerol.

Uses

It is used in the treatment of angina and acts as coronary vasodilator

Isosorbide Dinitrate

It is nitrated isosorbitol which is chemically 1, 4:3, 6 – dianhydro-D-glucitol-2,5-dinitrate.

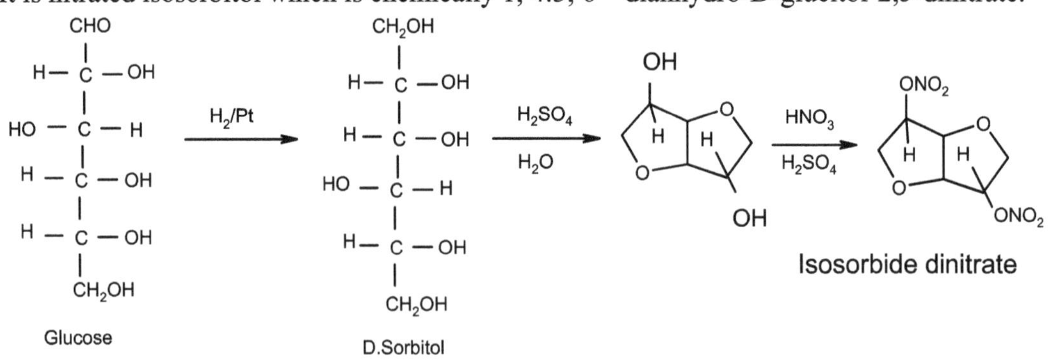

Properties

It exists as hard colorless crystals having a melting point of 70 °C. It is sparingly soluble in water. Freely soluble in organic solvents, such as acetone, alcohol and ether.

Uses

It is used as an antianginal agent.

Erythrityl tetra nitrate

It is chemically (2R, 3S)-1, 2, 3, 4 butanetetroltetranirate. It is used as a coronary vasodilator

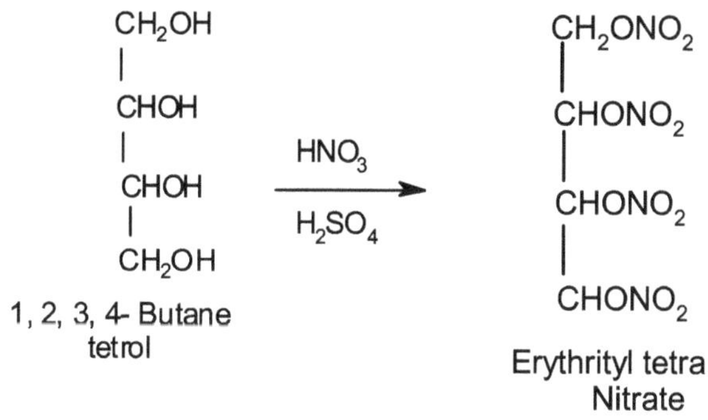

Penta erythritol tetra nitrite

It is chemically 2, 2-bis-[(hydroxy)methyl]-1, 3 propanediol tetranitrate.

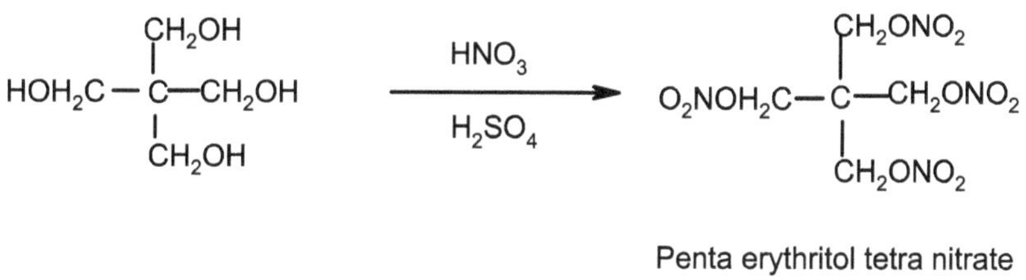

It has a melting point of 140°C. It is soluble in acetone. Practically insoluble in water. Sparingly soluble in alcohol and ether. It does not reduce Fehling's solution. It is used as a coronary vasodilator.

25

Coagulants and Anticoagulants

Blood coagulation

Blood coagulation is an important host defense mechanism. It also termed as haemostasis (cessation of blood loss from damaged blood vessel). Immediately after a blood vessel injury, platelets of blood circulation adhere to macromolecules of subendothelial tissues and then aggregate to form a primary haemostatic plug. Platelets stimulate plasma coagulation factors which results to form a fibrin clot. Later as wound healing starts, the platelet aggregate and fibrin clot are disintegrated. Mechanisms which restrict platelet aggregation and fibrin clots at the sites of injury are essential to maintain the fluidity of the blood.

Coagulation factors

The phenomenon of blood coagulation is very complex. The coagulation factors are involved in blood coagulation which are generally indicated by Roman numerals, with a lowercase *a* appended to indicate an active form. The coagulation factors are generally serine enzymes (some exceptions for example, FVIII and FV are glycoproteins and Factor XIII is a transglutaminase).

- Factor I (fibrinogen)
- Factor II (Prothrombin)
- Factor III (Thromboplastin, tissue factor)
- Factor IV (Calcium)
- Factor V (Labile factor)
- Factor VI (Accelerin)
- Factor VIII (Antihemophilic factor [AHF], antihemophilic globulin [AHG], antihemophilic factor A, Factor VIII: C)
- Factor IX (Plasma thromboplastin component [PTC], Christmas factor, antihemophilic factor B)
- Factor X (Stuart factor, prower factor, Stuart-Prower factor)
- Factor XI (Plasma thromboplastin antecedent [PTA], antihemophilic factor C)

- Factor XII (Hageman factor, surface factor, contact factor)
- Factor XIII (Fibrin stabilizing factor [FSF], fibrin stabilizing enzyme, fibri-nase)
- Other factors: (Prekallikrein [Fletcher factor], high molecular weight kininogen [Fizgerald]).

The coagulation mechanism can be summarised as follows :

Tissue factor pathway

Following damage to the blood vessel, endothelium tissue factor (TF) is released, forming a complex with FVIIa (FVIIa circulates in a higher amount than any other activated coagulation factor) (TF-FVIIa), which activates FIX and FX. FVII itself is activated by thrombin, FXIa, plasmin, FXII and FXa. The activation of FXa by TF-FVIIa is almost immediately inhibited by tissue factor pathway inhibitor (TFPI). FXa and its co-factor FVa form the prothrombinase complex which activates prothrombin to thrombin. Thrombin then activates other components of the coagulation cascade, including FV and FVII (which activates FXI which in turn activates FIX), and activates and releases FVIII from being bound to vWF. FVIIIa is the co-factor of FIXa and together they form the "tenase" complex which activates FX and so the cycle continues.

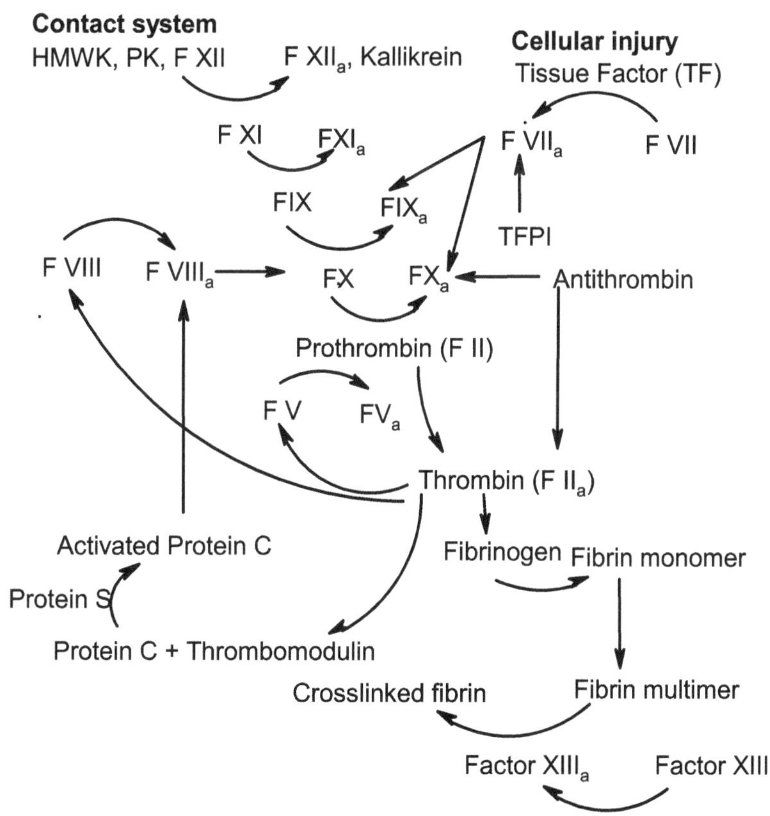

1. ***Contact activation pathway :*** There is formation of the primary complex on collagen by high molecular weight kininogen (HMWK), prekallikrein and FXII (Hageman factor). Prekallikrein is converted to kallikrein and FXII becomes FXIIa. FXIIa converts FXI into FXIa. Factor XIa activates FIX, which with its co-factor FVIIIa form the tenase complex which activates FX to FXa. The minor role that the contact activation pathway has in initiating clot formation can be illustrated by the fact that patients with severe deficiencies of FXII, HMWK and prekallikrein do not have a bleeding disorder.
2. *Thrombin* has a large array of functions. Its primary role is the conversion of fibrinogen to fibrin, the building block of a haemostatic plug. In addition, it activates factors VIII and V and their inhibitor protein C (in the presence of thrombomodulin), and it activates factor XIII, which forms covalent bonds that crosslink the fibrin polymers that form from activated monomers.

Anticoagulants

An anticoagulant is a drug that helps to prevent the clotting (coagulation) of blood. These drugs tend to prevent new clots from forming or an existing clot from enlarging. They don't dissolve a blood clot. They are used in treatment and prophylaxis of thrombo-embolic occlusive vascular diseases such as venous thrombosis, pulmonary embolism and cardiac infarction. The following anticoagulants are used in clinical practice:

Heparin

An anticoagulant stored in, and released from the mast cells lying beneath the vascular endothelium. Commercial heparins are extracted from animal tissues, purified, concentrated and have molecular weights of 3,000 to 57,000.

Heparin is a heterogeneous group of straight-chain anionic mucopolysaccharides, called glycosaminoglycans having anticoagulant properties. Although others may be present, the main sugars occurring in heparin are:

1. α-L-Iduronic acid 2-sulphate,
2. 2-Deoxy-2-sulphamino-α-D-glucose 6-sulphate,
3. ß-D-Glucuronic acid,
4. 2-Acetamido-2-deoxy-α-D-glucose, and
5. α-L- Iduronic acid.

These sugars are present in decreasing amounts, usually in the order (2) > (1) > (4) > (3) > (5), and are joined by glycosidic linkages, forming polymers of varying sizes. Heparin is strongly acidic because of its content of covalently linked sulfate and carboxylic acid groups. In heparin sodium, the acidic protons of the sulfate units are partially replaced by sodium ions.

Structure of Heparin sodium (representative subunits):

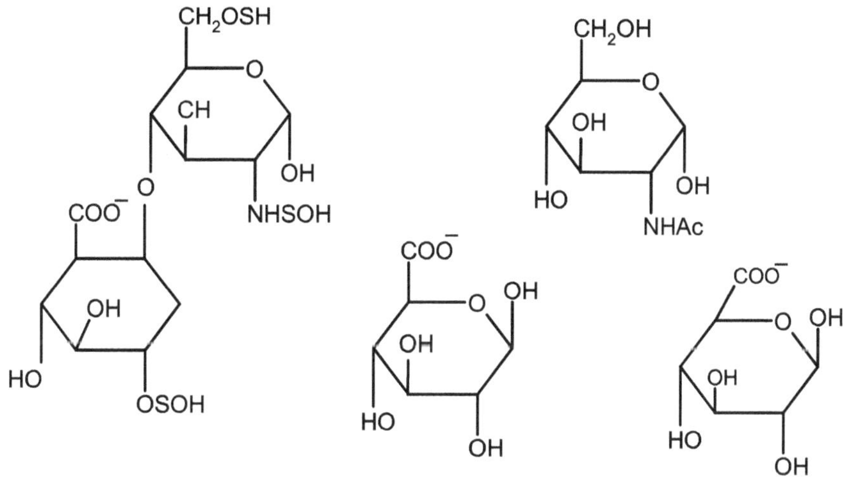

(1) (2) (3) (4) (5)

Pharmaceutical grade heparin is commonly derived from mucosal tissues of slaughtered meat animals such as porcine intestine or bovine lung. Heparin is not absorbed after oral administration and is never given by intramuscular injection because of the risk of haematoma. The common routes of administration are intravenous and subcutaneous.

Low molecular weight heparin (LMWH)

Heparin with a mean molecular weight of about 5,000 Daltons. They are commercially prepared by chemical or enzymatic degradation of heparin to produce more regular polysaccharide chains of about one third the length of standard heparin porcine heparin. LMWH does not prolong the APTT as much as high-molecular weight heparin and binds less to platelets. Low molecular weight heparin is superior for preventing venous thrombosis in patients undergoing hip replacement.

Heparinoids

Heparinoids are compounds with heparin-like properties which may be useful in patients developing adverse effects to other heparin preparations e.g., Danaparoid.

Mechanism of action

Heparin chains contain binding sites to antithrombin III scattered along their length. When antithrombin III binds to these sites, its activity increases allowing it to inactivate certain clotting factors (2a, 9a, 10a). The chain lengths with LMW heparin are mostly insufficient to allow factor 2a inactivation and therefore the activity of LMW heparins relies on inactivation of the other clotting factors. This differential effect on clotting factors has important implications for monitoring the intensity of anticoagulation. LMWH also interacts less with platelets, Von Willebrand factor and endothelial cells than standard heparin, resulting in reduced risk of bleeding.

Protamine sulphate

Protamine is a heparin antagonist. Protamine sulphate is a drug that reverses the anticoagulant effects of heparin by binding to it. Protamines are simple proteins of low molecular weight that are rich in arginine and strongly basic. Protamine sulphate occurs as fine white or off-white amorphous or crystalline powder. It is sparingly soluble in water. The pH is between 6 to 7. The cationic hydrogenated protamine at a pH of 6.8 to 7.1 reacts with anionic heparin at a pH of 5.0 to 7.5 to form an inactive complex. Protamine sulfate is administered intravenously.

Protamine is isolated from the sperm of various fish, and is a highly cationic peptide. It binds to heparin to form a stable ion pair which does not have anticoagulant activity. This complex is then removed and broken down by the reticuloendothelial system.

Phenindione

An indandione that has been used as an anticoagulant. Chemically it is 2-phenylindane-1,3(2H)-dione. Phenindione has actions similar to warfarin, but it is now rarely employed because of its higher incidence of severe adverse effects. It is an anticoagulant.

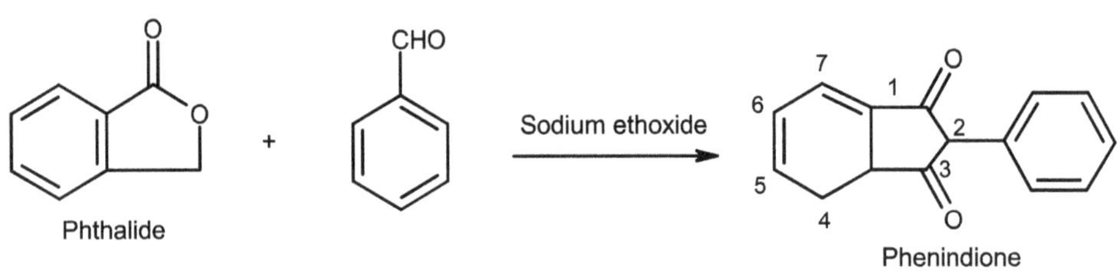

Phenindione is an anticoagulant, used to prevent blood clots which can be damaging to the body. The formation of blood clots involves a complicated interaction of substances. Phenindione prevents the normal formation of factors II, VII, IX and X, and this prevents blood clots formation.

Uses

It is used for prophylaxis of embolisation in rheumatic heart disease and atrial fibrillation.

Warfarin

Warfarin is a synthetic derivative of coumarin, (a chemical found naturally in many plants, notably woodruff at lower levels in licorice, lavender and various other species). The drug is commercially available as a racemic mixture of the two optical isomers of the sodium salt. Warfarin sodium occurs as a white, crystalline powder that has a slightly bitter taste and is very soluble in water and freely soluble in alcohol.

Warfarin has high bioavailability, predictable onset and duration of action and its lower association with serious hypersensitivity reactions. It is administered orally, warfarin is the mainstay for long-term anticoagulation.

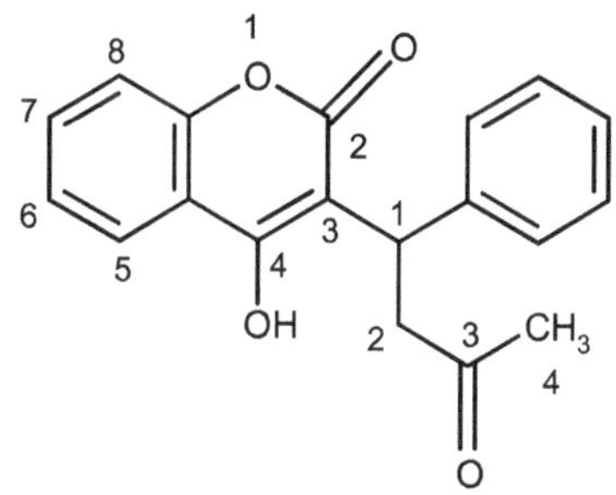

Warfarin

(RS)-4-Hydroxy-3-(3-oxo-1-phenylbutyl)-2H-chromen-2-one

Mechanism of action

Both warfarin and phenindione produce their anticoagulant effect by inhibiting the hepatic production of clotting, factors II, VII, IX and X. The synthesis of these proteins involves the conversion of reduced vitamin K to its epoxide. The oral anticoagulant blocks the conversion of the epoxide back to vitamin K.

The onset of action of these drugs is delayed until pre-existing coagulation factors disappear from the circulation through normal catabolism; this may take from 1-3 days. The anticoagulant effect of warfarin and phenindione can be reversed by vitamin K because this can be converted to reduced vitamin K by enzymes not affected by these drugs. Recovery is delayed with some correction of the prothrombin time noted within 6 hours of an IV dose and full correction within 24 hours. Large doses of vitamin K may make patients resistant to the effect of oral anticoagulants for several days.

Warfarin is only administered orally. It is absorbed rapidly and has 100% bioavailability but its onset of action depends on the rate of disappearance of clotting factors rather than the plasma level of the drug. The drug is highly protein bound, with a relatively small volume of distribution. It is metabolised slowly by the liver (capacity-limited elimination) with a half-life averaging about 36 hours. Warfarin consists of equal parts of two optically active isomers (R and S) which differ in activity (S isomer is 5 times as potent as R) and both are metabolised through different hepatic enzyme systems. This pattern of pharmacokinetic properties leads to a number of important clinical sequelae.

Warfarin is an effective oral anticoagulant for clinical conditions like atrial fibrillation, artificial heart valves, deep venous thrombosis and pulmonary embolism.

Anisindione

The 1,3-indanediones have been known to be anticoagulant since 1940s. A commercially available indandione is anisindione. The molecule has a weakly ionizable proton on C-2 that is extracted in alkaline solutions to confer mildly soluble properties (equation below).

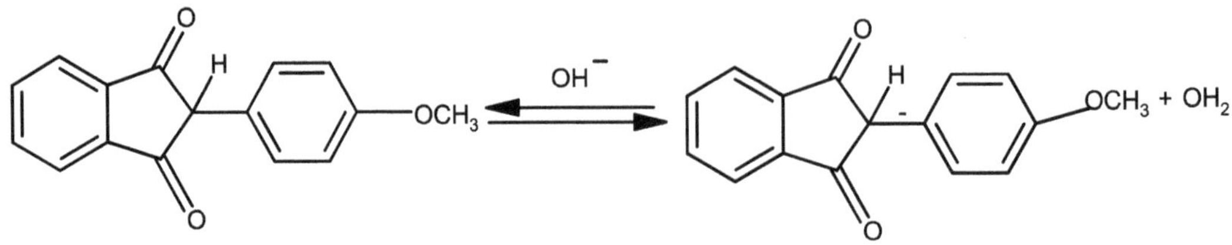

The anion so formed in alkaline solutions is reddish-orange. Thus patients on anisindione treatment may be alarmed to see reddish colored urine. This phenomenon may be easily distinguished from hematuria by acidification of the urine which should remove the red color.

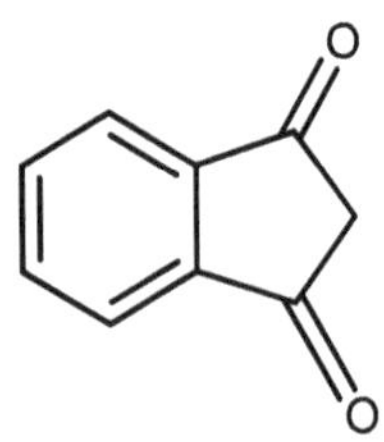

1,3-Indandione

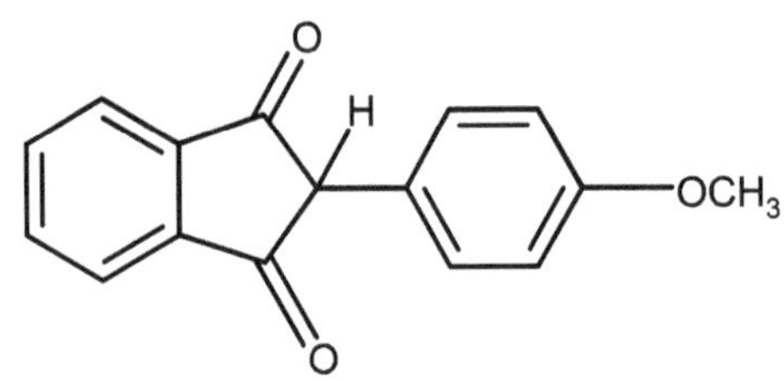

Anisindione

It is a long acting oral anticoagulant. It is used to prevent and treat blood clots in the veins. It is also used in the prevention and treatment of pulmonary embolism (a clot lodged in an artery serving the lungs), and in the treatment of certain serious heart conditions. The onset and duration of action of anisindione are similar to those for coumarins. The chief disadvantage of indandiones is their side effects. Some patients are hypersensitive to it and develop a rash, pyrexia, and leukopenia. Coumarins would be the drug of choice.

Just as coumarins, 1,3-indandiones are competitive inhibitors of vitamin K in the biosynthesis of prothrombin and follow the same biochemical mechanism of action.

26

DIAGNOSTIC AGENTS

Diagnostic agents do not have any therapeutic value but they are used to detect impaired function of body organs or diagnosis of disease. These chemical substances are helpful to identify normal and pathological products in urine, blood, faeces and other body fluids. The organic diagnostic agents are classified into the following groups.

(i) ***Radiopaque agents :*** Iopanic acid, propyliodone

(ii) ***Drugs used for organ function tests*** *:* Sulphobromophthalein sodium

(iii) ***Agents used to determine blood volume :*** Evans blue, fluorescein sodium

(iv) ***Miscellaneous diagnostic agents :*** Cango red, fluorescein sodium

Radiopaque agents

Radiopaque agents are drugs used to diagnose certain medical problems. These agents contain iodine, which blocks X-rays. Up on administration of radiopaque agents, they get localized in certain parts of the body. The particular body part consisting of radiopaque agent appears white on X-ray. This creates the needed distinction, or contrast, between one organ and other tissues. This will help the physician to diagnose any special conditions that may exist in that organ or part of the body.

The radiopaque agents are used in the diagnosis of:

- Biliary tract problems E.g., Diatrizoates, iodipamide, iohexol, iothalamate
- Blood vessel diseases E.g., Diatrizoates, iohexol, iopamidol, iothalamate, ioversol, Ioxaglate, Metrizamide
- Blood vessel diseases of the brain E.g., Diatrizoates, iohexol, iopamidol, Iothalamate, ioversol, ioxaglate
- Blood vessel diseases of the heart E.g., Diatrizoates, iohexol, iopamidol, Iothalamate, ioversol, ioxaglate, metrizamide
- Brain diseases and tumors E.g., Diatrizoates, iohexol, iopamidol, iothalamate, ioversol, ioxaglate, metrizamide
- Breast lesions E.g., Diatrizoates
- Heart disease E.g., Diatrizoates, iohexol, iopamidol, iothalamate, ioversol, ioxaglate, metrizamide

- Impaired flow of cerebrospinal fluid in brain E.g., Iohexol, iopamidol, metrizamide
- Kidney diseases E.g., Diatrizoates, iothalamate, ioversol, ioxaglate
- Joint diseases E.g., Diatrizoates, iohexol, iothalamate, ioxaglate, metrizamide
- Liver diseases E.g., Diatrizoates, iohexol, iothalamate, ioversol, ioxaglate
- Pancreas disease E.g., Diatrizoates, iohexol, iothalamate, ioversol, ioxaglate
- Spinal disk diseases E.g., Diatrizoates
- Spleen diseasese E.g., Diatrizoates, iothalamate
- Stomach and intestinal problems E.g., Diatrizoates, iohexol
- Urinary tract problems E.g., Diatrizoates, iohexol, iopamidol, iothalamate, ioversol, ioxaglate, metrizamide

Radiopaque agents are taken by mouth or given by enema or injection. Some radiopaque agents, such as iohexol, iopamidol, and metrizamide are given by injection into the spinal canal. The doses of radiopaque agents will be different for different patients and depend on the type of test. The strength of the solution is determined by how much iodine it contains. Different tests will require a different strength and amount of solution depending on the age of the patient, the contrast needed, and the X-ray equipment used. Radiopaque agents are to be used only by or under the direct supervision of a doctor.

Sodium diatrizoate

Sodium diatrizoate is the sodium salt of diatrizoic acid (3,5diacetamido-2,4,6-triiodobenzoic acid)

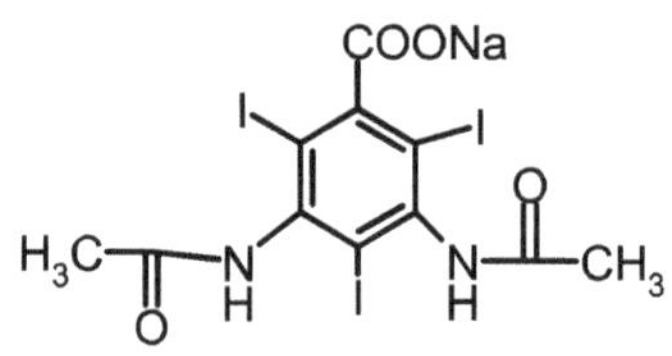

Sodium diatrizoate

Uses

This is used before an X-ray or similar tests (E.g., Tomography) to help doctor to view, to throat (Esophagus), stomach, and intestines more effectively. It may be used with other injectable products (IV contrast).

Sodium diatrizoate is used as a density gradient reagent in blood cell separation. The use of sodium diatrizoate in a discontinuous gradient protocol for neutrophil separation in whole blood has been described. It has also been utilized as a radiological contrast agent. Several studies have examined the effects of diatrizoate on mammalian cell viability, such as on cultured human vascular smooth muscle cells.

Preparation instructions

This product is soluble in water (350 mg/ml), yielding a clear to slightly hazy, colorless to faint yellow solution. The pH of a 50% solution is 7.0 - 7.5. Solutions of this product may be sterilized by autoclaving.

Storage/stability

Solutions should be protected from light.

Iodipamide

Iodipamide consists of two 3-amino-2,4,6-triiodobenzoic acid units linked through an adipoyl(-$COCH_2$-CH_2-CH_2-CH_2-CO-) group. Chemically it is 3,3(adipoyldiimino) bis[2,4,6-triiodobenzoic acid]. It is very slightly soluble in water. This agent is used for examination of biliary tract.

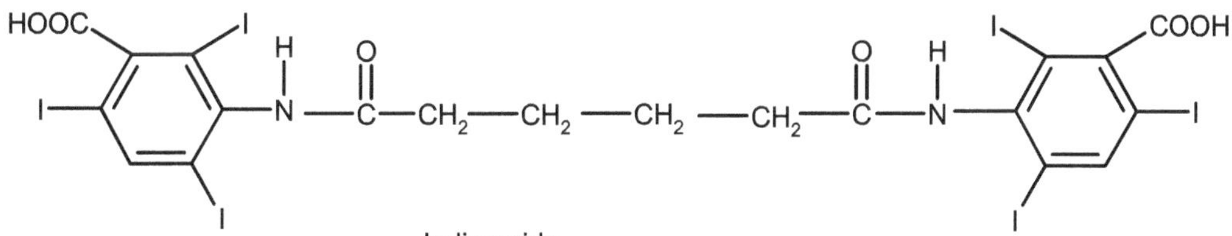

Iodipamide

Propyliodone

Propyliodone is the propyl ester of diodone. It occurs as a white crystalline, odourless, water insoluble powder. This water-insoluble X-ray contrast medium is used for examination of biliary tract

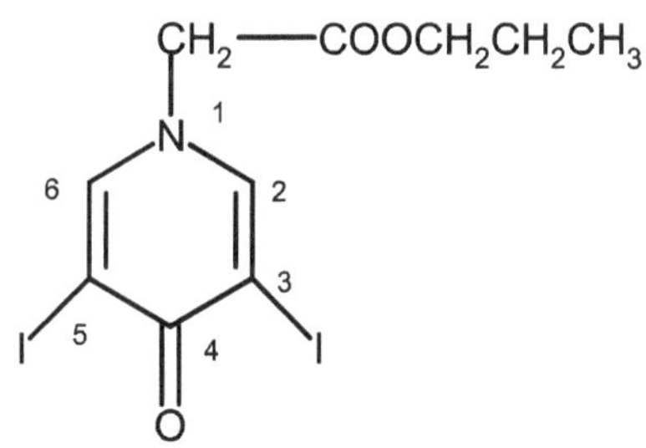

Propyliodone

Iopanoic acid

Iopanic acid 3-amino - α -ethyl-2, 4, 6-triiodohydrocinnamic acid. It is prepared from m-nitro benzaldehyde by Perkin condensation reaction as below :

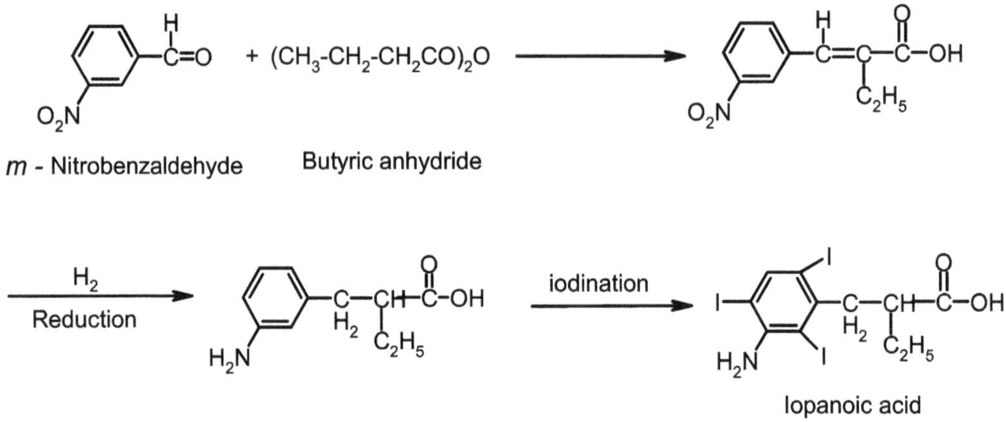

Iopanoic acid is water insoluble cream colored compound. It is used as radiopaque medium for examination of biliary tract.

Agents used for organ function tests

These chemical compounds are used to test the functioning of various body organs such as liver, kidney, cardiovascular system, gastrointestinal system, hypothalamus, pitutary gland, thyroid gland, etc.,

E.g., Sulphobromophthalein sodium
Fluorescein sodium
Phenolsulphonaphthalein
Histamine acid phosphate

Histamine acid phosphate

Histamine is 2-(4-imidazolyl) ethylamine. Histamine acid phosphate is a light sensitive solid. It is used as diagnostic agent to test the secretary function of stomach.

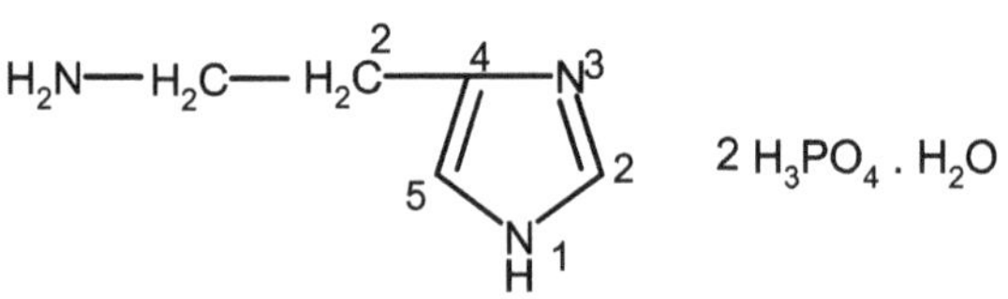

Sulphobromophthalein sodium

Sulphobromophthalein sodium is 5,5(4,5,6,7tetrabromo-1,3-dihydro-3-oxo-Isobenzofuran-1, 1-diyl) bis (2-hydroxybenzene sulphonate). It occurs as a water soluble, colourless, hygroscopic, white crystalline powders. It exhibits purple colour in alkali but disappears in acidic medium. Sulphobromophthalein sodium is administered intravenously. It is used as a diagnostic agent for testing functional capacity of liver.

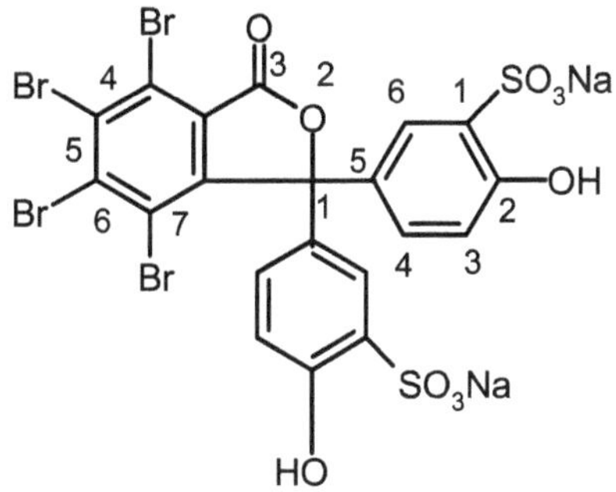

Sulphobromophthalein sodium

***Fluorescein sodium*:** Fluorescein is an orange coloured dye of phthalein group. It is prepared by melting phthalic anhydride with resorcinol in presence of anhydrous zinc chloride (condensing agent).

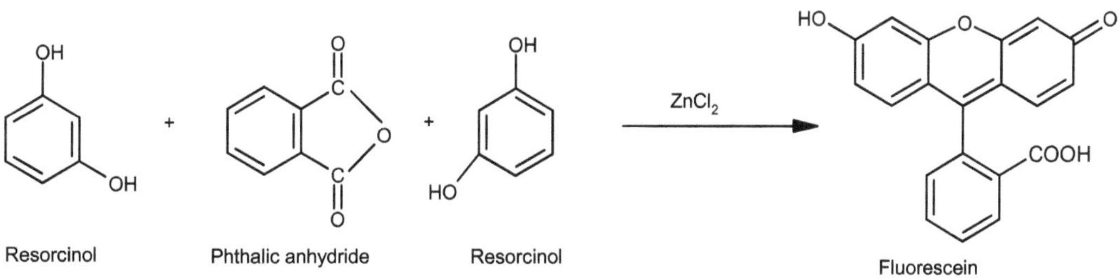

It is available as sparingly soluble crystals which imparts yellow-red colour and intense yellowish-green fluorescence. The fluorescence disappears when the solution is made acidic and reappears when the solution is again made neutral or alkaline. It is administered by rapid intravenous injection or measuring circulation time. It is also used to visualize the gall bladder and bile ducts.

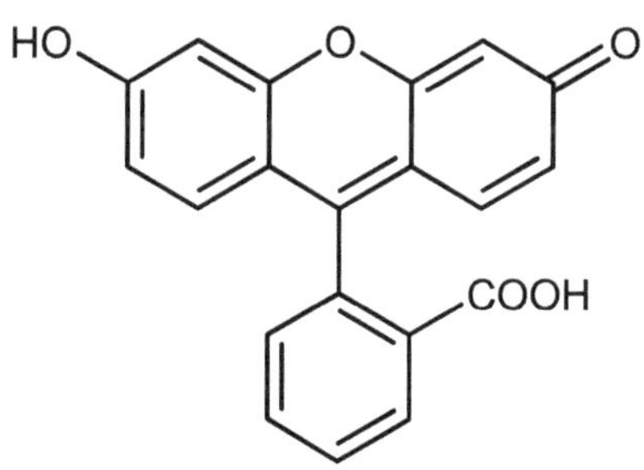

Fluorescein

27

CHEMISTRY OF VITAMINS

Introduction to Vitamins

Many enzymes cannot catalyze a reaction without the help of a cofactor. Cofactors assist enzymes in carrying out a variety of reactions that cannot be carried out solely by the amino acid side chains of the protein. Some cofactors are metal ions and some are organic molecules. Cofactors that are organic molecules are called enzymes. Coenzymes are derived from organic compounds that are commonly known as vitamins.

Vitamins can be defined as naturally occurring organic substances which are required in minute amounts to maintain normal health of the organism and which have to be supplied in food as they can not be synthesized by the organism. In 1912, Cosimir Funk coins the word 'Vitamin', an amine necessary for life.

Classification

All vitamins are broadly classified into the following two groups basing on their solubility in water. They are :

1. Fat–soluble vitamins : E.g. : Vitamins A, D, E and K
2. Water soluble vitamins: E.g. : Vitamin B_1 (Thiamine)
   Vitamin B_2 (Riboflavin)
   Vitamin B_3 (Nicotinic acid)
   Vitamin B_5 (Pantothenic acid)
   Vitamin B_6 (Pyridoxine)
   Biotin,
   Folic acid,
   Inositol and
   VitaminB_{12} or (cyanocobalamin)

Difference between fat-soluble and water-soluble vitamins

Fat-soluble vitamins	Water-soluble vitamins
1. These are soluble in fats.	1. These are soluble in water
2. These require bile salts and fats for their absorption	2. These are easily absorbed.
3. Normally these are not excreted in urine.	3. These have a threshold for urinary excretion.
4. These are generally stored in liver.	4. These are not stored in body except vitamin B_{12}
5. These do not act as coenzymes.	5. These act as co–enzymes.
6. Examples - Vitamin – A, D, E and K.	6. Examples - Vitamin B complex and Vitamin – C.

Vitamin A (Retinol, axerophthol)

1. ***General properties :*** Vitamin A is also usually referred as Vitamin A_1. Vitamin A_1 occurs either as free or as esters in fats, in fish liver oils (halibut liver oil, cod liver oil) and in blood. It is a pale yellow crystalline water insoluble powder. It is soluble in most organic solvents, fats and oils.

2. ***Chemistry :*** This vitamin is a diterpenoid. Structurally vitamin A is closely related to plant pigment carotene, ($C_{40}H_{56}$) which exists in different isomeric forms. They act as precursors of vitamin A. β-carotene is most active precursor which forms two molecules of vitamin A. β-carotene is found in yellow-orange fruits and vegetables such as apricots, mangoes, carrots and sweet potatoes.

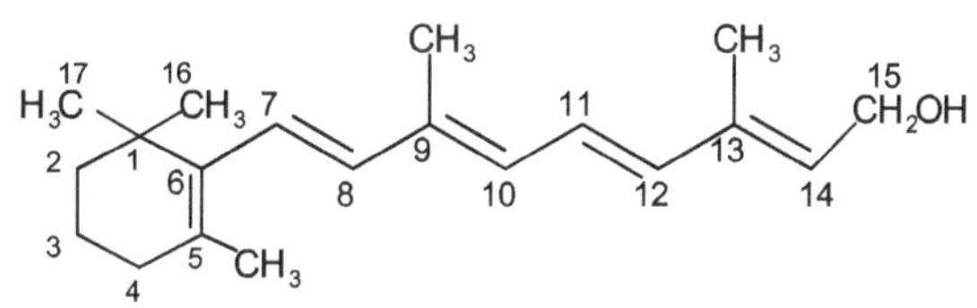

VITAMIN A_1 or RETINOL

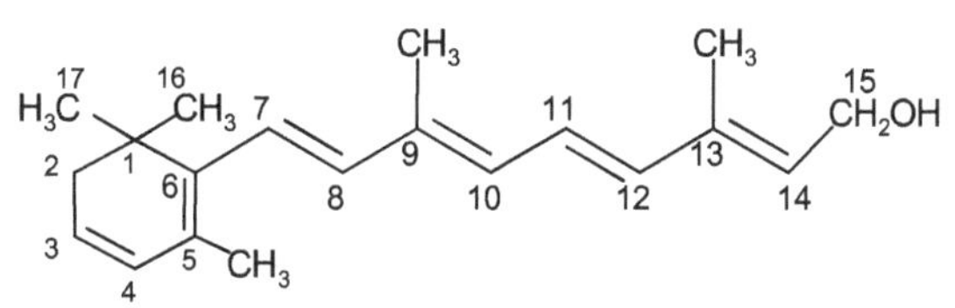

VITAMIN A_2 or DEHYDRORETINOL

3. ***Synthesis of vitamin A :*** The vitamin A of commerce is now almost exclusively synthetic. A procedure of synthesis from citral is described below:

   (i) Citral is condensed with acetone to give ψ-ionone, which on treatment with acid gives β-ionone.

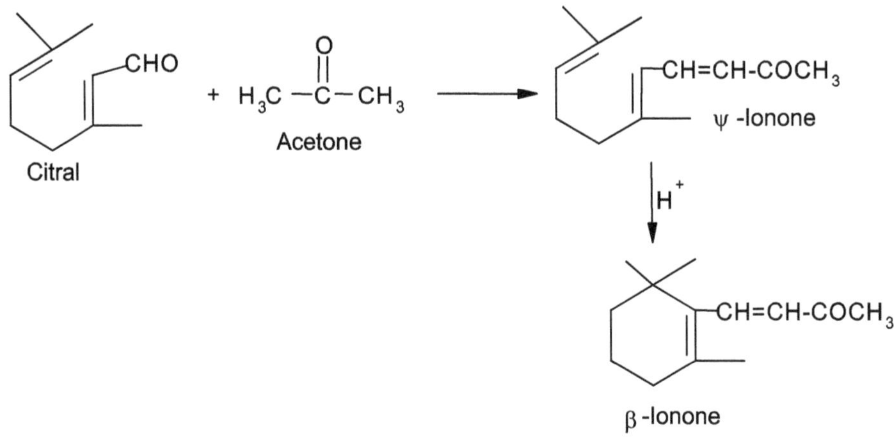

(ii) A Grignard reagent is prepared by treating with two molecules of Grignard reagent.

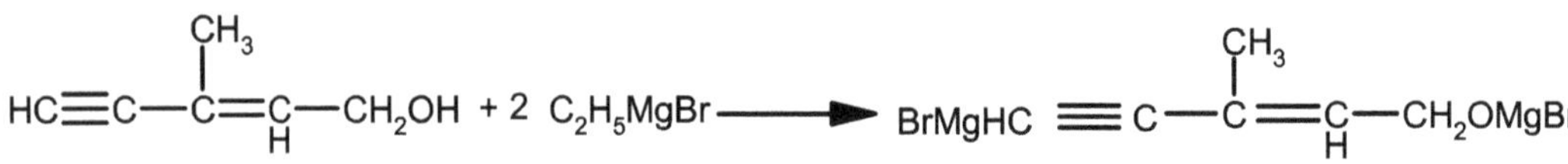

(iii) Retinol is synthesized finally by the condensation of intermediates of i and ii reactions by the following reactions.

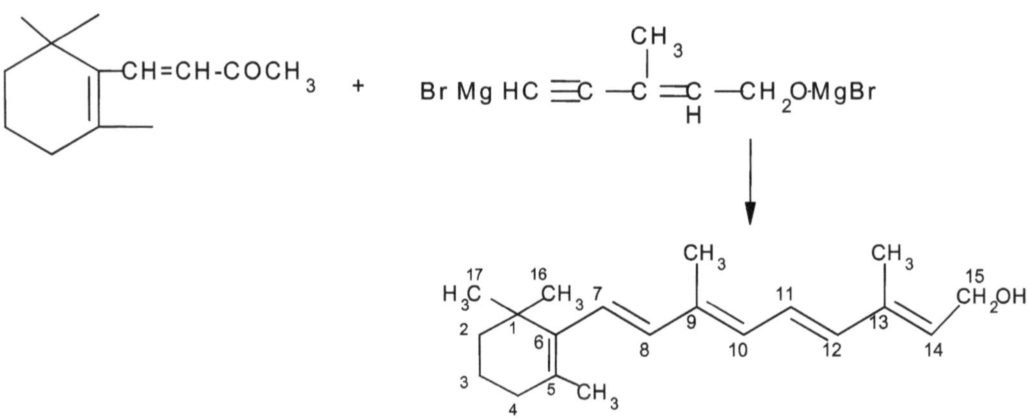

VITAMIN A_1 or RETINOL

4. ***Biological functions*** :

(i) Vitamin A performs the following important functions in the body. It is required for development and maintenance of epithelial tissue.

(ii) It enhances the function of immune system.

(iii) Vitamin A is responsible for vision: The retina of the eye contains cone cells and rod cells. The cone cells are responsible for color vision and for vision in bright light. The rod cells are responsible for vision in dim light. In rod cells vitamin A is oxidized to an aldehyde.

(iv) It is also essential for growth.

5. ***Defficiency*** **:** Prolonged deficiency may result in xerophthalmia, the initial symptom of which is night blindness and may lead to blindness.

6. ***Official drugs*** **:**

   (i) Vitamin A, I.P.: The vitamin A consists of an ester or a mixture of esters of vitamin A alcohol.

   (ii) Synthetic vitamin A concentrate BNP in powder form.

   (iii) Synthetic vitamin A concentrate BNP in oily form.

   (iv) Synthetic vitamin A concentrate BNP in water-dispersible form.

Vitamin E Group

1. ***General properties:*** The term 'Vitamin E' refers to a group of closely related compounds, which occur naturally and are anti-sterility factors. Eight compounds (α, β, γ, δ, E, $\S_1$, $\S_2$ and η - tocopherols) are collectively called tocopherols. However, the most biologically active compound is α -tocopherol. The main source o α-tocopherol is wheat germ oil.

2. ***Chemistry :*** α -Tocopherol is a benzopyran derivative. Chemically it is 5,7,8 – trimethyl derivative, which has the highest activity.

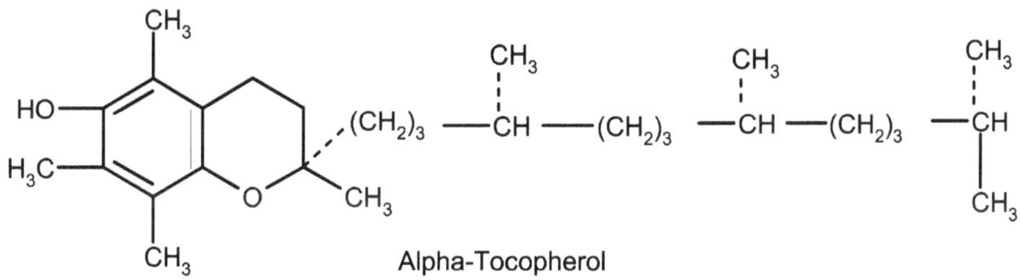

Alpha-Tocopherol

3. ***Biological functions :***

   (i) The primary role of vitamin-E is to prevent oxidation of polyunsaturated fatty acids.

   (ii) It stabilizes cellular membranes.

   (iii) It prevents hepatic necrosis and cerebral disorders.

4. ***Deficiency :***

   (i) The deficiency syndromes of vitamin-E are development of myopathic and neurological disorders.

   (ii) Anaemia, edema and hepatic necrosis are developed by the deficiency of vitamin-E.

5. ***Official drugs :***

   (i) Alpha tocopherol B.P.

   (ii) Tocopheryl acetate I.P.

   (iii) Alpha tocopheryl succinate.

Vitamin D (Calciferol-or-Anti-rachitic factor)

1. ***General properties :*** Vitamin – D, also called as 'calciferol', is a group of steroid hormones. It is rich in egg yolk, milk, butter, fish liver oils and the livers of animals. Sunlight is the cheapest source of Vitamin D. The Vitamin D group are more stable and are not lost by ordinary cooking and preserving processes.

2. ***Chemistry :*** Ergocalciferol (Vitamin D_2) and cholecalciferol (Vitamin D_3) the most important calciferols. Ergocalciferol does not occur naturally. It is produced artificially by the action of UV-light on ergosterol (provitamin – D_2). Cholecalciferol, occurring in animals, is produced by the irradiation of 7-dehydrocholesterol present in the epidermal cells of the skin to the sunlight.

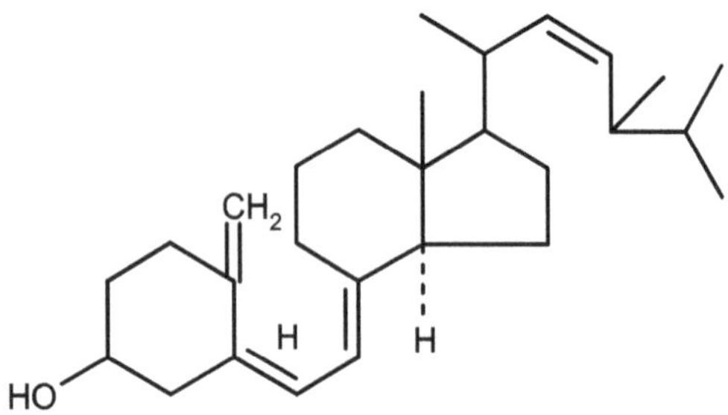

Ergocalciferol or Vitamin-D_2

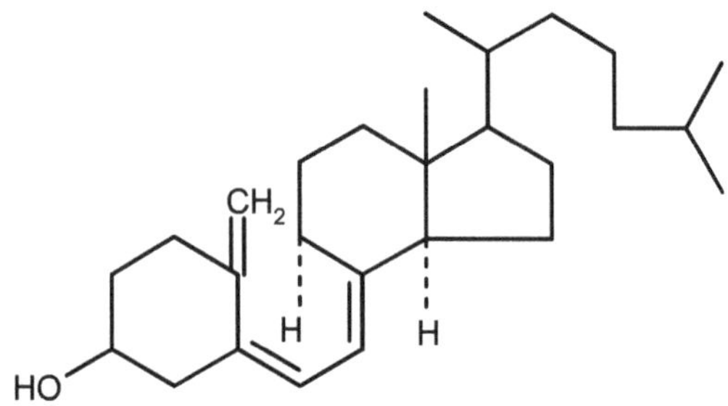

Cholecalciferol or Vitamin-D_3

3. ***Biological functions:***
   - (i) Vitamin – D is responsible to increase the availability and retention of calcium and phosphorus and their utilization for proper mineralization of the skeleton.
   - (ii) The major function of Vitamin D is to stimulate transcription of mRNA for calcium transport. Thus, its ultimate effect is very much related to the concurrent activity of parathormone and calcitonin.
   - (iii) It increases the excretion of phosphate by kidney and decreases concentration of serum phosphate.
   - (iv) It decreases the pH in the lower intestinal tract which helps in increasing the absorption of calcium and phosphorus.
   - (v) It is required for the development of bones and normal growth of the body.
   - (vi) It stimulates calcification of bones in both the adults and growing children.
   - (vii) It increases the citrate level of blood, bone, kidney and heart tissues and also excretion of citric acid.
   - (viii) It stimulates the activity of phytase which catalyses the hydrolysis of pytic acid in the intestine.

4. ***Deficiency manifestations :***

   (i) ***Rickets :*** The deficiency of vitamin-D results in rickets due to inadequate deposition of calcium salts in newly formed bone matrix. This results in the irregularity in the zone of provisional calcification. The minerals may be reabsorbed away from the shaft of long bone making it soft.

(ii) ***Osteomalacia :*** It may occur in fully developed bones in adults, due to defective mineralization of osteoid tissue (Softening of bones). The formed bones get demineralized and soft. This deficiency occurs in pregnant and lactating women and also in women wearing purdah or in climates where sunshine is scanty.

Vitamin K (Antihaemorrhagic factor)

1. ***General properties :*** Vitamin K is also known as 'antihaemorrhagic factor' or 'coagulation' factor. Vitamin K has two important derivatives i.e. vitamin K_1 (phylloquinone) which occurs in all green leaves and vegetables, and vitamin K_2 (famoquinone) which is found in bacteria.
2. ***Chemistry :*** Vitamin-K. consists of 'naphthaquinone' structure.

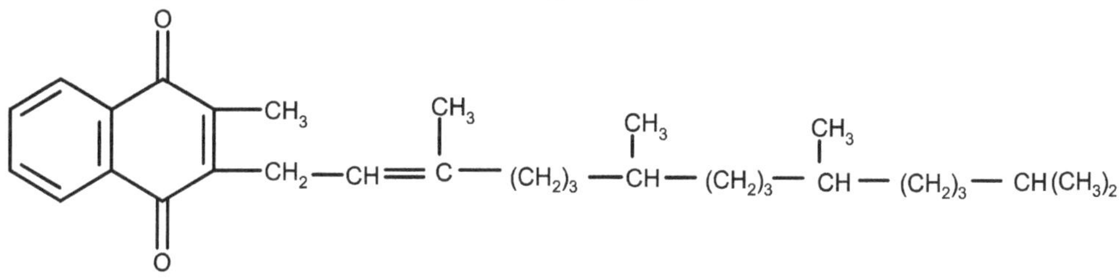

VITAMIN-K_1

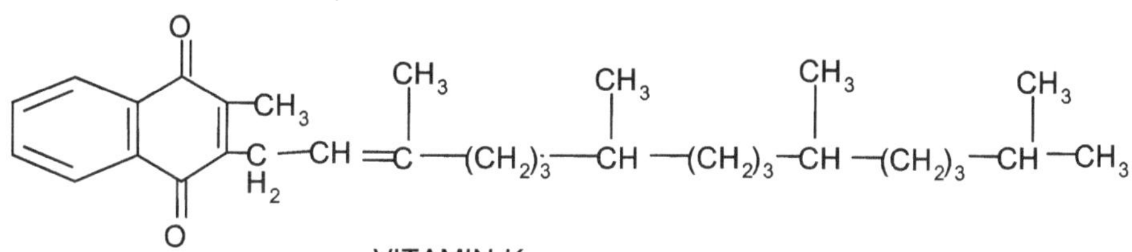

VITAMIN-K_2

3. ***Biological functions :***
   - (i) It catalyses the synthesis of 'prothrombin' by the liver.
   - (ii) It reduces prothrombin time.
   - (iii) It regulates the synthesis of clotting factors viz. factor VII, IX and factor X.
   - (iv) It is involved in the oxidative phosphorylation of animal tissues.
   - (v) It maintains the normal level of blood clotting factors. – II, VII IX and X.
   - (vi) It is used therapeutically to poisoning by dicoumarol – type drugs.

4. ***Deficiency manifestations :*** The deficiency of Vitamin K results in:
   - (i) Lowering of prothrombin level.
   - (ii) Increased clotting time of blood.
   - (iii) Haemorrhagic conditions.
   - (iv) Haemorrhagic diseases of the newborn.

5. *The Vitamin B – Complex*: Water-soluble vitamins of B-complex group are necessary for the action of certain enzymes. Water soluble vitamin are converted into their active form in the body, and called as 'co-enzymes'. Thus, the co-enzymes are derived from vitamins.

Vitamin B1 or Thiamine or Aneurin

1. ***General properties :*** Vitamin B_1 is also known as, anti-beri beri substance' or 'antineuritic vitamin' or 'aneurine'. It is a colorless, water-soluble, odorless, crystalline solid. The richest sources of thiamine are rice polishings, wheat germ and yeast. The other good sources include – cereals, pulses, nuts, oil seeds, meat, fish, eggs, milk, vegetables and fruits.

2. ***Isolation :*** The material rich in vitamin B_1 is agitated with acidulated water at pH 4.5. When vitamin B_1, goes into aq.solution, then this solution shaken with Fuller's earth, which only allows vitamin B_1 to be adsorbed on Fuller's earth. The later, when eluted with quinine sulphate solution releases vitamin B_1.

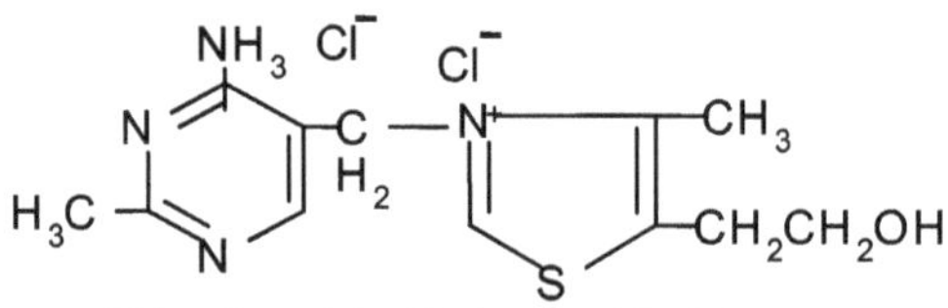

Thiamine chloride hydrochloride

Synthesis of thiamine :

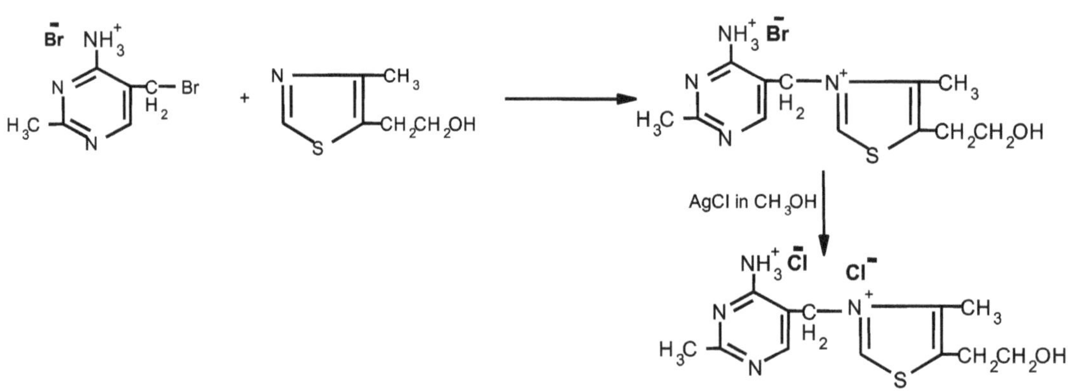

Thiamine chloride hydrochloride

3. ***Biological functions :***
   - (i) Thiamine is essential for growth.
   - (ii) Thiamine is essential for maintaining the nerves in normal conditions.
   - (iii) The coenzyme TPP, is involved in oxidative decarboxylation in carbohydrate metabolism. Thiamine is therefore referred to as 'co-carboxylase'.
   - (iv) The coenzyme TPP is also involved in the HMP shunt.

4. ***Deficiency manifestations:*** The deficiency of vitamin B_1 causes 'beri-beri' and neurological manifestations.

   The beri-beri is of two types :

   1. ***Wet beri-beri:*** Symptoms of wet beri-beri are :
      (i) Oedema
      (ii) Palpitation and breathlessness
      (iii) Fast pulse
      (iv) Weak heart
   2. ***Dry – beri-beri :*** Symptoms of dry beri-beri are:
      (i) Weak and wasted muscles
      (ii) Difficulty in walking
      (iii) Required stick to stand and walk
      (iv) Finally, bedridden

   The disease beri-beri can be prevented by administering thiamine intramuscularly.

Riboflavin (Vitamin B$_2$) or Lactoflavin

1. ***General properties*** **:** Riboflavin is an orange-yellow colored compound containing D-sorbitol, (a ribose alcohol) and heterocyclic nucleus, iso-alloxazine (Flavin). It is a crystalline, water-soluble substance. The richest source of vitamin B_2 is anaerobic fermenting bacteria. Other good sources are milk, liver, kidney, heart, fish, and cereals and roots germination wheat.
2. ***Isolation***: The material rich in vitamin B_2 is agitated with concentrated HCl followed by filtration. The filtrate contains vitamin B_2 is adsorbed on Fuller's earth. The later, when treated with water, loses HCl and after the vitamin B_2 is eluted by basic solvents like pyridine – methanol – water mixtures, ammonia, caustic solution. Then vitamin B_2 is precipitated from elute as sparingly soluble thallium salt. Finally vitamin B_2 is crystallized from aqueous acetone – petroleum ether mixture in which thallium salt of vitamin B_2 has been dissolved.

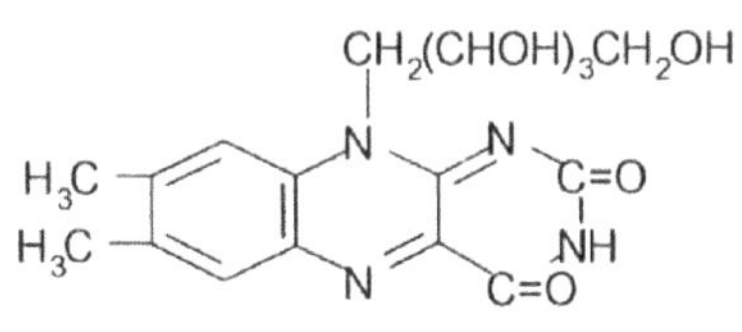

Structure of Riboflavin

Synthesis of riboflavin:

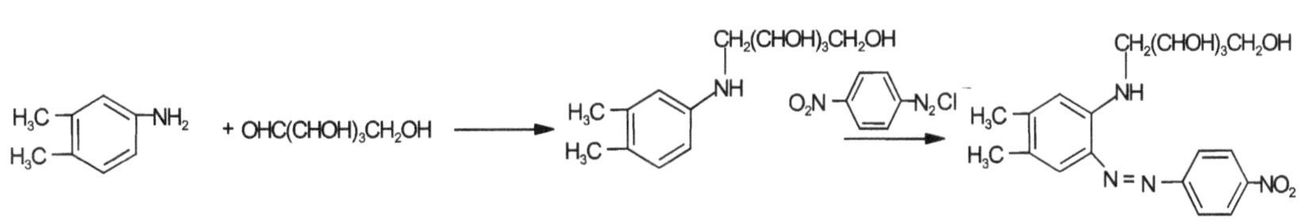

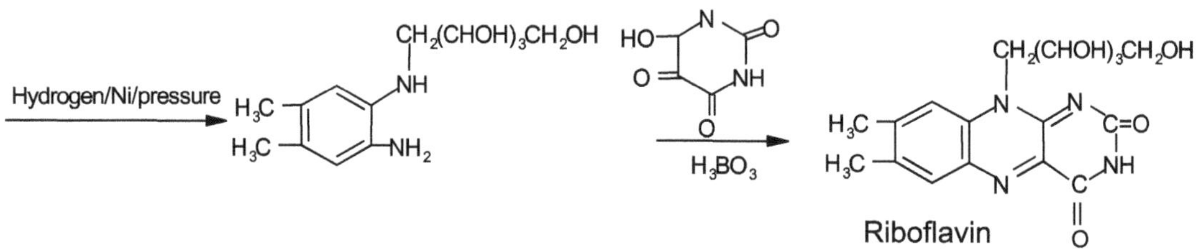

3. ***Biological functions***:

   (i) It involves in the regulatory functions of some hormones connected with carbohydrate metabolism.

   (ii) The free riboflavin present in the retinol is converted by light to a compound involved in stimulation of the optic nerve.

   (iii) It involves in the electron transport system in the mitochondria.

   (iv) It involves in intermediate metabolism as an enzyme called 'flavoproteins'.

   (v) It is also the prosthetic group of acyl-CoA dehydrogenase, which is involved in the oxidation of fatty acids.

4. ***Deficiency manifestations***: The deficiency of riboflavin results in:

   (i) Lesions of the lips.

   (ii) Fissures at the angles of the mouth.

   (iii) Dermatitis of the face.

   (iv) Magneta tongue.

   (v) Functional and organic disorders of the eye.

Pantothenic acid

1. ***General properties :*** In 1930, R.J. Williams and his collaborators identified and synthesized pantothenic acid. It also has been called Vitamin B_5. It is an yellow coloured water soluble oily substance. It is unstable to heat, acid and alkali. The sources of vitamin B_5 are liver, eggs and cereals. This Vitamin is synthesized by most green plants and micro organisms. The precursors are α, γ-dihydro-by-β, β-dimethly butyric acid (or) Pantoic and β-alanine. This Vitamin is found in the form of co-enzyme A.

2. ***Chemistry :*** Pentothenic acid consists of β-alanine and pantoic acid units which are joined through a peptide bond. Chemically pantothenic acid is α, γ-dihydroxy-β, β-dimethyl butyric acid-β-alanine.

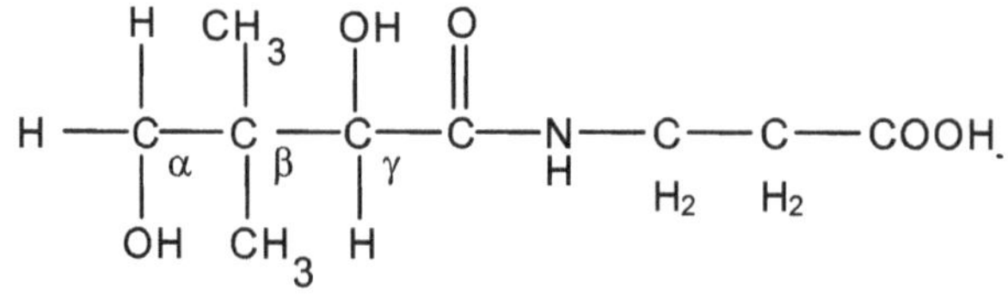

Pentothenic acid

3. ***Biological functions :***

   (i) Pantothenic acid is a structural component of CoA. CoA is essential for many important metabolic processes.

   (ii) It plays an important role in the metabolism of fats and carbohydrates.

4. ***Deficiency manisfestations :*** The deficiency of pantothenic acid results in:

   (i) Inadequate growth.

   (ii) Gastrointestinal disorders, nausea, vomiting.

   (iii) Irritability.

   (iv) Failure in gaining weight.

   (v) Graying of hair and loss of hair.

Vitamin B6

1. ***General properties :*** Vitamin B_6 refers to a group of pyridoxine, pyridoxal and pyridoxamine compounds having similar biological activity. Vitamin B_6 is readily soluble in water which can be readily destroyed in presence of light in basic solution. It is widely distributed in foods like vegetables, fruits, cereals, eggs, fish, liver, meat etc. The daily requirement is about 2 mg for healthy adults.

2. ***Chemistry :*** Vitamin B_6 refers to pyridoxine, pyridoxal and pyridoxamine compounds. Chemically pyridoxine is 3-hydroxy-4,5-dihydroxymethyl2-methyl pyridine.

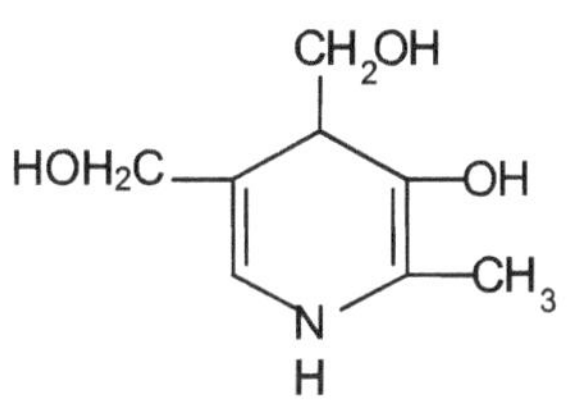

Pyridoxine

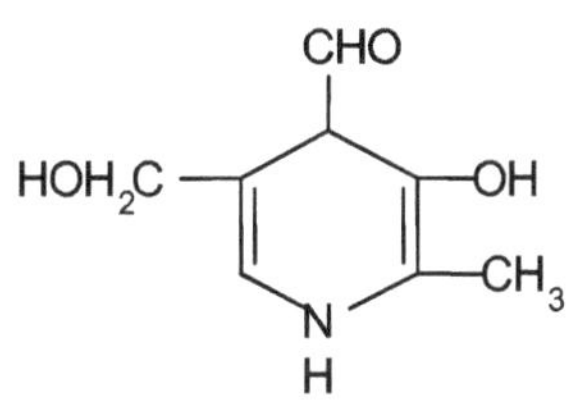

Pyridoxal

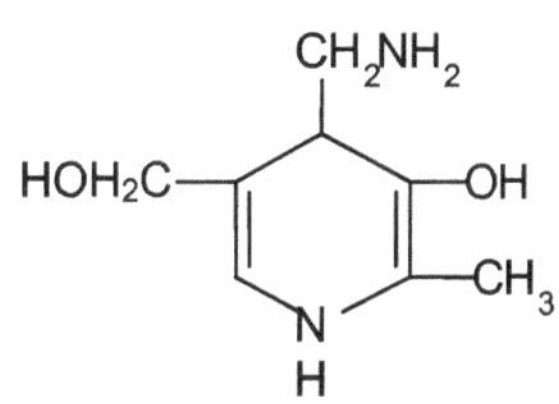

Pyridoxamine

3. ***Biological functions :***

   (i) Pyridoxine containing enzymes are important for amino acid and protein metabolism.

   (ii) Pyridoxine acts as co-enzymes for decarboxylation reactions.

   (iii) It acts co-enzyme in transamination, desulphuration and transulphuration reactions.

4. ***Deficiency :*** The deficiency of pyridoxine causes peripheral neuritis, metabolic disorders and dermatisis.

Biotin

1. ***General properties :*** In 1930 biotin was identified and isolated. It was also known as Vitamin H. This vitamin is found in highest concentrations in liver, kidney, eggs, yeast, vegetables, grains and nuts. Microorganisms synthesize biotin from oleic acid.
2. ***Chemistry :*** Biotin consists of two condensed five-membered heterocyclic systems.

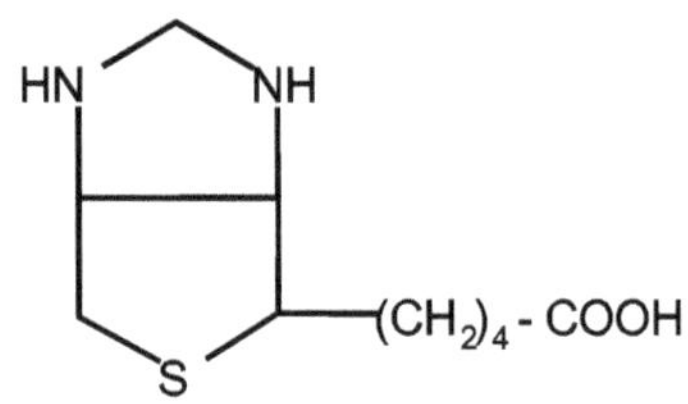

BIOTIN

3. ***Biological functions :***
   (i) Biotin is involved in the CO_2 transfer reactions i.e., in carboxylation reaction or CO_2 fixation.
   (ii) Biotin acts as co-enzyme in the conversion of propionic acid to succinic acid.
   (iii) Biotin catalyses β-methylcrotonyl – CoA carboxylase for the conversion of β-methylcrotonyl – CoA to β-methylglutaconyl – CoA.
4. ***Deficiency manifestations :***
   (i) The deficiency of biotin may result from the destruction of intestinal bacteria by drugs like sulphonamides or antibiotics.
   (ii) The deficiency of biotin may develop nausea, anorexia, anaemia, muscular pain and dermititis of extrimities.

Folic acid

1. ***General properties :*** Mitchell, Snell and Williams coined the term folic acid. Folic acid is found in leafy vegetables and from other sources like yeast, kidney, meat, fish, milk and fruits. Folic acid is a yellow to orange colour yellow crystalline powder. It is practically insoluble in water but soluble in dilute acids and in alkaline solutions. Folic acid should be stored in well-closed containers and protect from light.
2. ***Chemistry :*** Folic acid is a compound made up of pteridine nucleus, p-amino benzoic acid and glutamic acid and hence pteroyl-glutamic acid chemical name is given to folic acid.

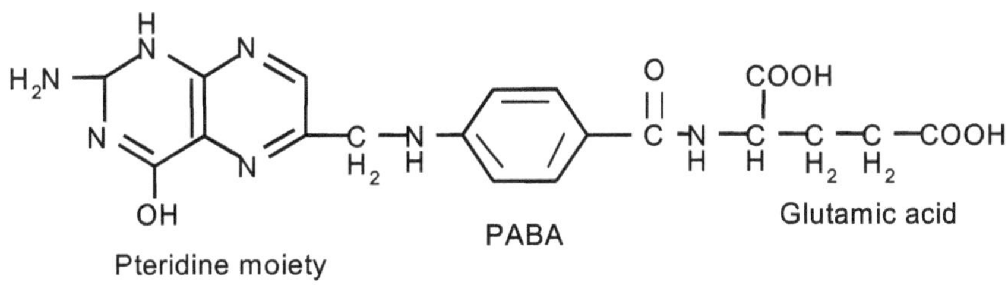

Structure of folic acid

3. ***Biological functions :***

   (i) In living cell, folic acid is reduced to dihydrofolic acid and tetrahydrofolic acid. The tetrahydrofolic acid consumes one carbon moiety from formyl, methyl, and formate groups at 5 or 10 position of pteroyl structure and converts to coenzyme. The coenzyme of tetrahydrofolic acid is responsible for biosynthesis of purines, nucleic acids, histidine, methionine, serine and nicotinamide.

   (ii) Folic acid is responsible for the catabolism of histidine. It is required for the synthesis of red blood cells.

4. ***Deficiency manifestations :*** The deficiency of folic acid may lead to megaloblastic anaemia.

Inositol

Inositol is a growth factor for animals and microorganisms. The status of inositol as a vitamin is also not certain. Inositol is widely distributed in plants and animals. It has been isolated from heart muscle and liver.

1. ***Chemistry :*** Chemically inositol is a hexahydrocyclohexane. There are nine isomers for inositol. Inositol is a meso-isomer and is optically active having the configurations as shown in the structure:

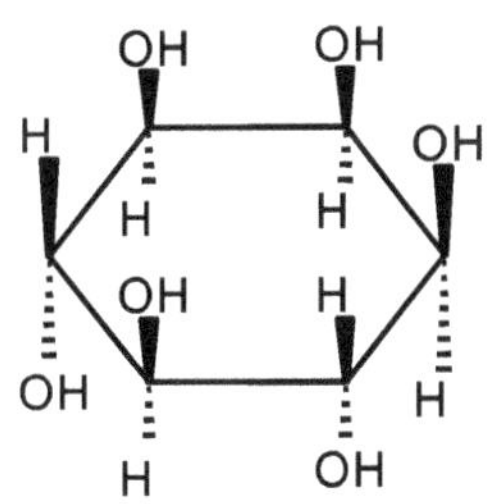

Structure of Inositol

2. ***Biological functions :***

   (i) Inositol has rachitogenic effect (decresing the absorption of magnesium and calcium elements).

   (ii) Inositol is responsible for the growth of yeast and fungi.

Cyanocobalamin (Vitamin B_{12})

1. ***General properties :*** In 1948, the Merck Laboratories and Glaxo Laboratories designated the red crystalline compound as vitamin B_{12}. The vitamin B_{12} is present in liver, kidney, meat, fish, eggs, milk, cheese. It has also been obtained from *Streptomyces griseus*, *Streptomyces aureofaciens* by fermentation.

   Cyanocobalamin is a deep red colored crystalline compound. It is soluble in water and is stable to heat. Cyanocobalamin is destroyed in acidic or alkaline solution. It should be stored in an airtight container and protect from light.

2. ***Chemistry :*** The structure of vitamin B_{12} was established by X-ray analysis. Cyanocobalamin is a cobalt containing complex substance that has a modified porphyrin unit called corrin ring, coordinating a trivalent cobalt ion. A cyanide ion is also coordinated to the cobalt.

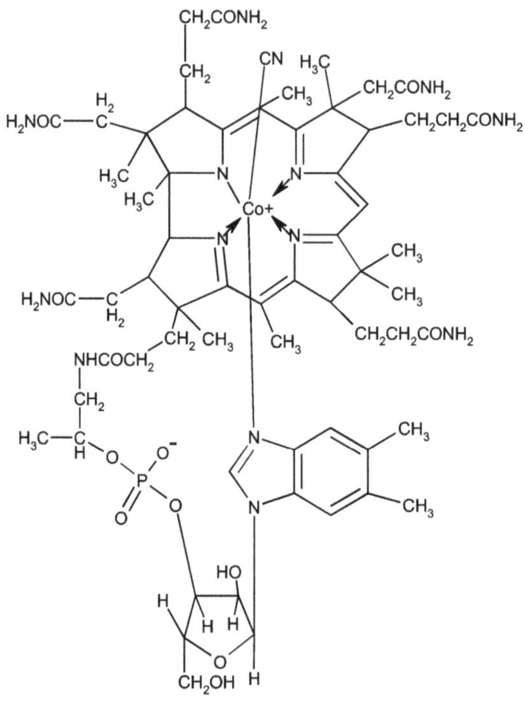

Cyanocobalamin

3. ***Biological functions :***
   (i) In living cell, cyanocobalamin converts to coenzyme, which is responsible for biosynthesis of proteins, succinyl coenzyme A, β-methyl asparate and DNA.
   (ii) Vitamin B_{12} cures neurological disorders resulting from pernicious anaemia.
   (iii) Vitamin B_{12} is responsible for the development of red blood cells.

4. ***Deficiency manifestations :*** The deficiency of vitamin B_{12} causes pernicious anaemia.

Nicotinic acid

1. ***General properties :*** Nicotinic acid was identified and prepared by oxidation of nicotine in 1913. The excellent sources of nicotinic acid are pork, lamb, beef livers, hodg kidneys, yeasts, pork, beef tongue, hearts, wheat germ, peanut meal and green peas. Almost all plants and animals can also synthesize this. Niacin is absorbed readily from the gastrointestinal tract.

   Nicotinic acid occurs as a colorless, odorless, freely water-soluble crystalline solid. It is stable under normal storage conditions and sublimes without decomposition.

2. ***Chemistry :*** Chemically nicotinic acid is pyridine-3-carboxylic acid. It occurs as physiologically active amide derivatives (Nicotinamide or niacinamide).

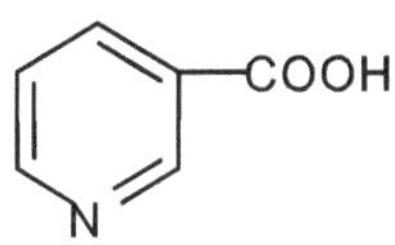

Nicotinic acid

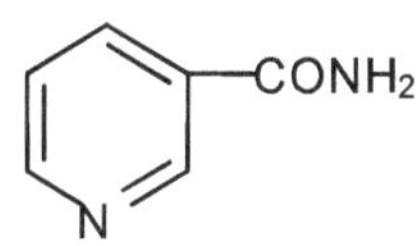

Nicotinamide

3. ***Biological functions :***

   (i) Nicotinamide exists in human and animal tissues as co-enzyme NAD and NADP.

   (ii) It is absorbed from the intestine through the portal vein into general circulation.

   (iii) It is essential for the normal functioning of the skin, intestinal tract and the nervous system.

   (iv) It is used therapeutically, in atherosclerosis, for lowering increased plasma levels of cholesterol.

   (v) The coenzymes of niacinamide, NAD and NADP, play an important role in metabolism by acting as hydrogen and electron transfer events by means of reversible oxidation and reduction.

4. ***Deficiency Manifestations :*** The deficiency of niacin causes a disease called pellagra.

Ascorbic acid or Vitamin C

1. ***Isolation :*** The substance rich in vitamin C is extracted repeatedly with water. To this solution neutral lead acetate is added to precipitate most of the impurities. After filtration, the filtrate is again treated with a lead salt at pH 7.6 to precipitate vitamin C as lead salt, which is removed by filtration. The lead salt of vitamin C is treated with H_2SO_4. When vitamin C goes into solution where as lead is precipitated as $PbSO_4$. After filtration, the filtrate containing vitamin C is concentrated under vacuum and then treated with organic solvents like acetone, alcohol and ether to precipitate impurities. Finally the purified filtrate, when subjected to distillation, yields pure ascorbic acid, which is re crystallized from CH_3OH.

2. ***Synthesis of ascorbic acid :*** L – Lyxose was converted into L (-) xylosone, and xylosone on treatment in an atmosphere of nitrogen with aqueous potassium cyanide containing calcium chloride, gave the β-keto cyanide, which hydrolysis spontaneously into pseudo – L – ascorbic acid. This on heating for 24 hours with 8% HCl at 40^0C – 50^0C, gave a quantitative yield of L(+) – ascorbic acid.

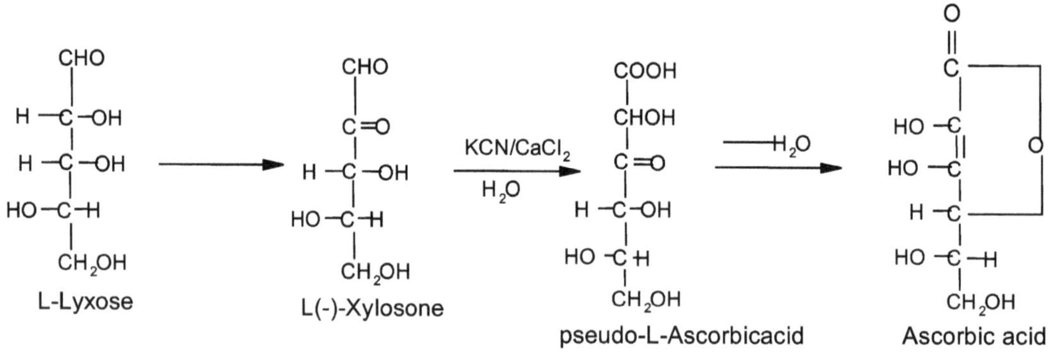

3. ***Biological functions :***
   (i) It involves in oxidation-reduction reactions of the cells.
   (ii) It is responsible for the hydroxylation of steroids, proline and hydroxy proline.
   (iii) Ascorbic acid is required for the metabolism of aminoacids like tyrosine and phenylalanine.
4. ***Deficiency manifestations :*** The deficiency of ascorbic acid causes disease scurvy.

28

STEROIDS

Introduction

Steroids are tetracyclic compounds characterized by the presence of a1,2-cyclopentanoperhydro phenanthrene ring system. They are widely distributed in animals and plants. All the steroids give, among other products, Diel's hydrocarbon on dehydrogenation with selenium at 360°C. If the distillation with selenium is carried out at 420°C, steroids mainly give chrysene and a small amount of picene.

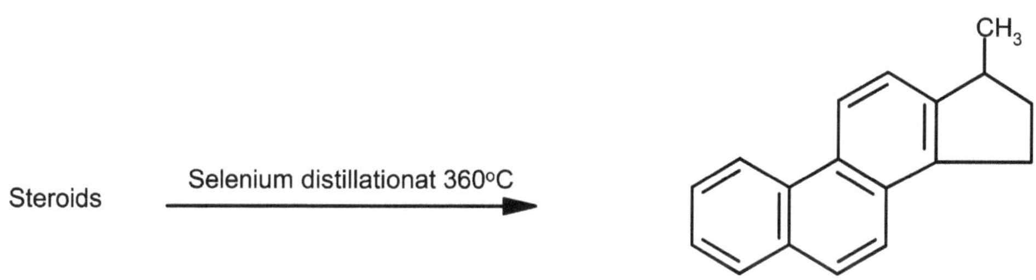

Diel's hydrocarbon

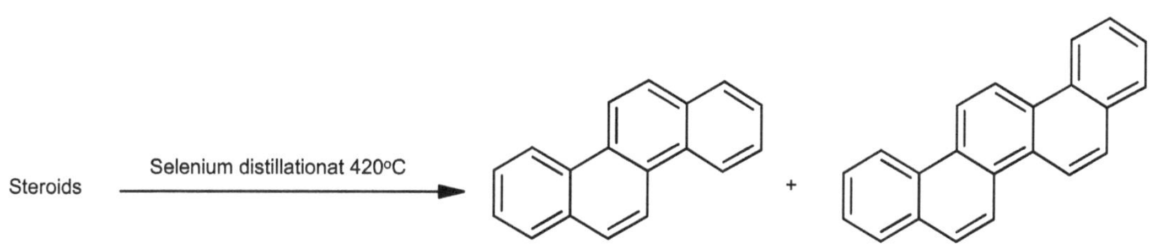

Chrysene

Picene

Classification

Steroids may be classified as:

1. **Sterols :** Sterols contain an alcoholic group. They may be:
   - **A. Phytosterols :** E.g., Stigma sterol
   - **B. Zoosterols :** E.g., Cholesterol, coprostanol
   - **C. Mycosterols :** E.g., Ergosterol.
2. **Bile acids :** E.g.,. Cholic acid, deoxycholic acid

3. **Vitamins :** E.g.,. Ergocalciferol, cholecalciferol
4. **Sex hormones :** They may be
   - A. **Androgens :** E.g., Androsterone, testosterone.
   - B. **Oestrogens :** E.g., Oestrone, oestradiol, oestriol
   - C. **Gestogens :** E.g., Progesterone, pregnanediol.
5. **Corticotrophic hormones :** E.g., Corticosterone, cortisol, cortisone.
6. **Steroidal glycosides :** E.g., Digitoxigenin, sarsapogenin.
7. **Steroidal alkaloids :** E.g., Solanidine, conessine.

Systematic nomenclature of steroids

1. Steroids are the derivatives of cyclopentanoperhydrophenantherene ring system. The four rings are designated with letters A, B, C and D. X-ray analysis and chemical studies have shown that in all naturally occurring steroid hormones the B, C, D ring junctions are trans. Rings A and B are fused either by cis or trans. In normal series of steroids (5α – series) A and B ring junction is cis, where as in 5α -series (allo-steroids) the ring junction is trans. The carbon atoms of this ring system are numbered as shown below.

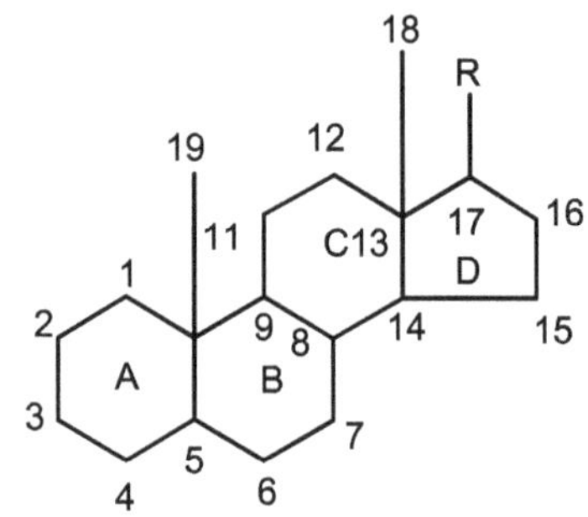

2. The methyl groups at points of ring junction are called angular methyl groups.
3. Groups or substituents that lie above the plane of the molecule i.e., same side as that of angular methyl groups are designated β– substituents. The β– substituents are designated by solid lines.
4. Groups or substituents that lie below the plane of molecule i.e., trans to the angular methyl groups are designated as α - substituents. These substituents are designated by dotted lines. If the configuration of the substituent is unknown, its bond to the nucleus is drawn as a wavy line and is indicated by (ε) symbol.
5. When a methylene group is missing from the side chain, this is indicated by the prefix 'nor' proceeded by the number of the carbon atom which has disappeared. The prefix 'nor' is also used to indicate the loss of an angular methyl group, and in this case nor is proceeded by the number designating that methyl group.

   E.g., : 18-nor, 19-nor.
6. When a ring has been contracted or enlarged, this is indicated by prefixes 'nor' and 'homo' respectively, proceeded by a small capital letters indicating the ring affected.
7. The prefix 'cyclo', proceeded by the numbers of the positions concerned is used to indicate a three membered ring. E.g.,. Cyclopropa [1,2] in cyproterone.
8. When ring-fission has occurred with addition of a hydrogen atom to each new

terminal group, this is indicated by the numbers showing the position of the bond broken, followed by the prefix 'seco'.

9. In systematic nomenclature the nature of R group at position 17 determines the base name of an individual steroid.

E.g.,.

R	Name
-H	Androstane
-H (with –H also replacing – $^{19}CH_3$)	Estrane
- $^{20}CH_2{}^{21}CH_3$	Pregnane
- $^{20}CH(CH_3)^{22}CH_2{}^{23}CH_2{}^{24}CH_3$	Cholane
$^{20}CH(^{21}CH_3)^{22}CH_2{}^{23}CH_2{}^{24}CH_2{}^{25}CH(^{27}CH_3{}^{26}CH_3)$	Cholestane

Cholesterol

1. ***Source :*** Cholesterol occurs as free or as fatty esters in all animal cells, particularly in the brain and spinal cord. The main sources of cholesterol are fish-liver oils, brain and spinal cord of cattle and lanoline.
2. Cholesterol is a colorless crystalline solid. It is insoluble in water and melts at 149°C
3. ***Molecular formula :*** The molecular formula of cholesterol is $C_{27}H_{46}O$.
4. ***Chemistry of cholesterol :*** The structure of cholesterol is elucidated for the following structural features:

   A. Structure of the ring system

   B. Positions of hydroxyl group and double bond

   C. Nature and position of side chain

   D. Positions of angular methyl group

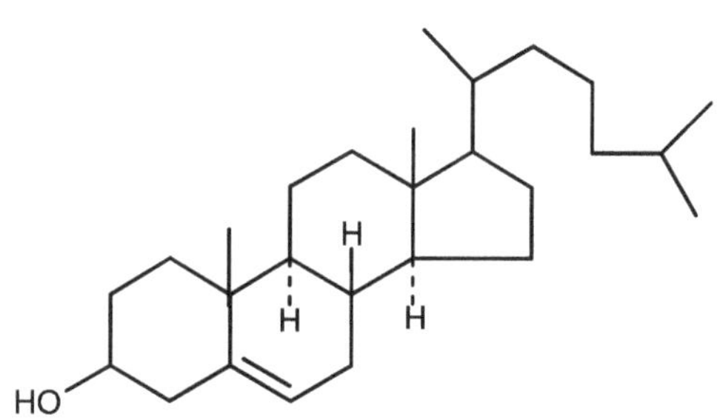

Structure of cholesterol

Biological functions of cholesterol: Cholesterol is important to synthesize steroid hormones. It serves as a membrane component, mostly in the plasma membranes of blood cells. Cholesterol is also used as a diagnostic agent.

Stigmasterol

1. ***Source :*** Sigmasterol is naturally available from soyabean oil.

2. ***Molecular formula*** **:** The molecular formula of stigma sterol is $C_{29}H_{48}O$. It is solid at room temperature and melts at 170°C.

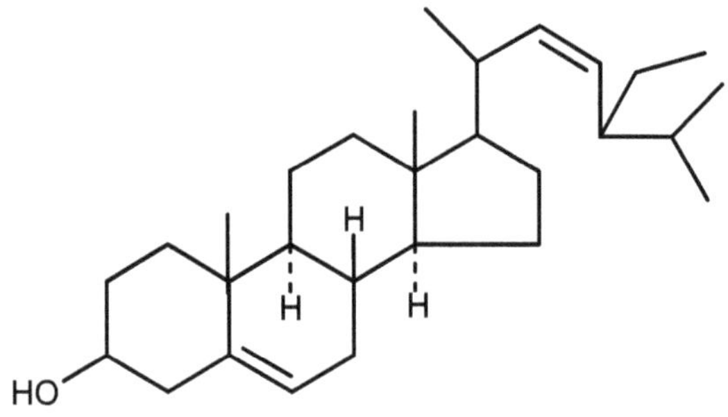

Stigmasterol

3. ***Uses of stigmasterol*** **:**

   (i) Commercially Stigmasterol can be converted to progesterone.

   (ii) Corticosteroids are also synthesized from stigmasterol by microbial conversions.

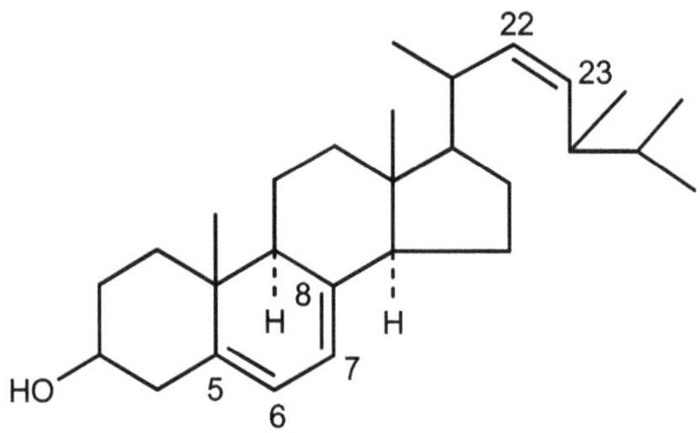

Ergosterol

4. ***Biological functions*** **:** Ergosterol yield ergocalciferol by UV irradiation which has antirachitic properties.

Vitamin D

1. Vitamin D comprises a range of closely related steroidal compounds which possess the property of preventing or curing rickets (anti rachitic vitamin). It is also responsible for bone formation, calcium and phosphorus metabolism. This group has been composed of the following vitamins:

   (i) Vitamin D_1 or calciferol named by medical research council (1931).

   (ii) In 1932, Windaus identified that vitamin D_1 is a molecular compound of calciferol and lumisterol. Hence Windaus renamed the Pure potent component as vitamin D_2, but the medical research council retained the original name calciferol. The chemical society (1951) has proposed the name ergocalciferol.

(iii) Vitamin D_3 (Cholecalciferol).

(iv) Vitamin D_4

Biological functions of ergocalciferol :

(i) Vitamin – D is responsible to increase the availability and retention of calcium and phosphorus and their utilization for proper mineralization of the skeleton.

(ii) It decreases the pH in the lower intestinal tract which helps in increasing the absorption of calcium and phosphorus.

(iii) It is required for the development of bones and normal growth of the body.

Bile acids

1. Bile acids are the hydroxy derivatives of 5 or 5α-cholanic acid which are produced by the metabolism of cholesterol in liver. The bile acids occur in bile, which stored in gallbladder. They exists as sodium or potassium salts of amides with amines like glycine or taurine. E.g.,: Cholic acid, lithocholic acid, chenodeoxy cholic acid.

2. Steroid nucleus : Bile acids on selium distillation at $360^{\circ}C$ yields Diel's hydrocarbon, suggests that steroidal nucleus is present in bile acids.

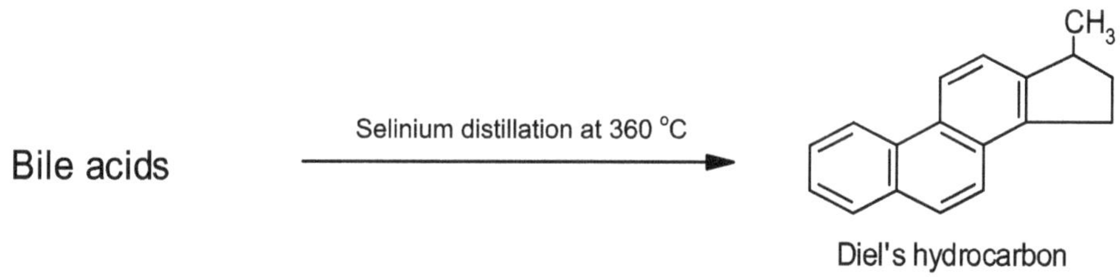

Diel's hydrocarbon

3. They do not consume molecular hydrogens indicating that bile acids are saturated.

4. Bile acids on oxidation do not yield acetone(as in case of cholesterol), hence this indicates that the side chain does not have terminal isopropyl groups.

5. Postion of hydroxyl groups in bile acids: The positions of the hydroxyl groups in the bile acids have been determined by the oxidative degradation.

   E.g., The position of hydroxyl group in lithocholic acid is confirmed by oxidation process. An identical oxidation product was formed by the oxidation of 5β cholestan 3β-ol and lithocholic acid.

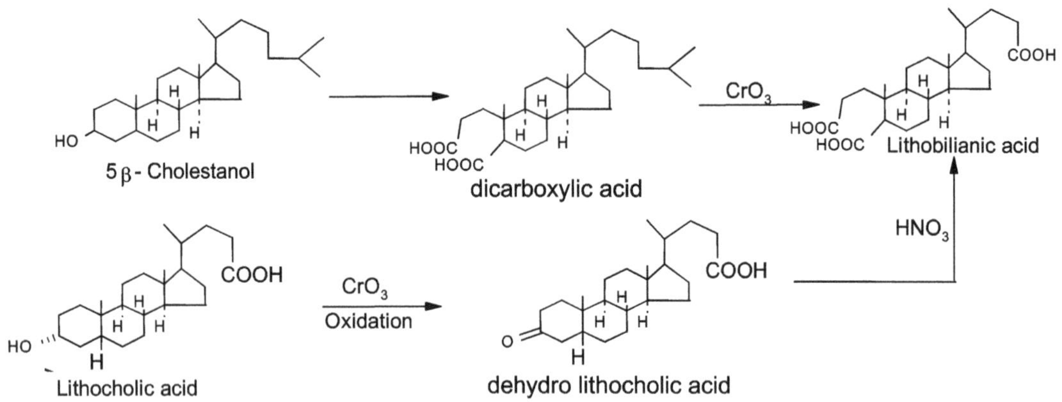

6. All the bile acids can be converted into either 5 or 5 -cholanic acids, hence the bile acids are the hydroxy derivatives of cholanic acids.

7. Biological importamce of bile acids :

   (i) The bile salts are amphiphilic in nature. They form micelles with biliary phospholipids and emulsify the cholesterol in dietary lipids. Thus the bile salts are helpful in digestion and absorption of lipids.

   (ii) Bile acids are administered orally to increase the output of bile.

Steroidal hormones

Introduction

Hormones are chemical messengers. They are organic compounds that are synthesized by the glands and are carried by the blood stream to the target tissues. Many hormones are steroids. Steroidal hormones in mammals are biosynthesized from cholesterol, which in turn is made *In vivo* from acetyl-coenzymeA. The steroidal hormones can be divided into androgens, estrogens, progestins, glucocotricoids and mineralocorticoids.

Androgens

Compounds have both androgenic and anabolic activities are called androgens. Androgens are steroid hormones. They are responsible for the development and growth of male sex organs (androgenic activity), and also influence the increased size and strength of the male (anabolic activity) in comparison to female. Testosterone is the most important androgen in humans and is synthesized by Leydig's cells in the testes and in smaller amounts by the cells in ovary of the female. The FSH and LH of pituitary gland control the secretion of testosterone. The naturally occurring androgens are derivatives of androstane.

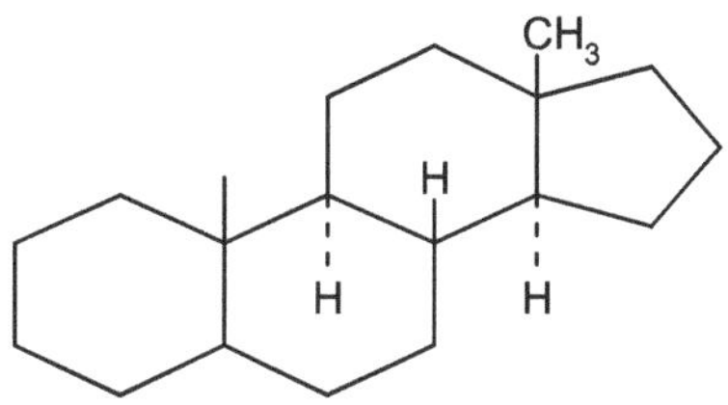

Structure of Androstane

Natural androgens

1. ***Testosterone*** **:**
   (i) Testosterone was isolated from testes. It is colorless crystalline solid melts at 155^{0}C and is optically active.
   (ii) The molecular formula of testosterone is $C_{19}H_{28}O_2$.

Synthesis : The structure of testosterone has been confirmed by its synthesis from cholesterol.

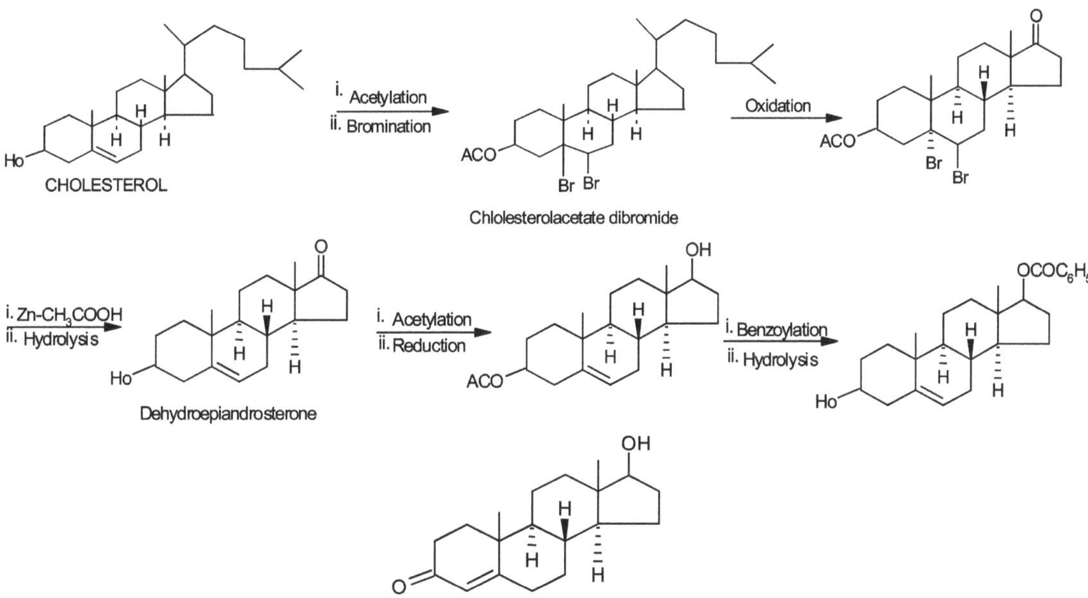

Testosterone

2. ***Androsterone*****:**

Androsterone is an important metabolite of dihydrotestosterone, which is the reduced form of testosterone.

1. ***Source :*** Androsterone occurs in urine, adrenal cortex, human sperm and ovary.
2. Androsterone is crystalline colorless solid, melts at 183^{0}C and shows +94^0 of specific rotation.
3. The molecular formula of androsterone is $C_{19}H_{30}O_2$.

Synthesis of androsterone

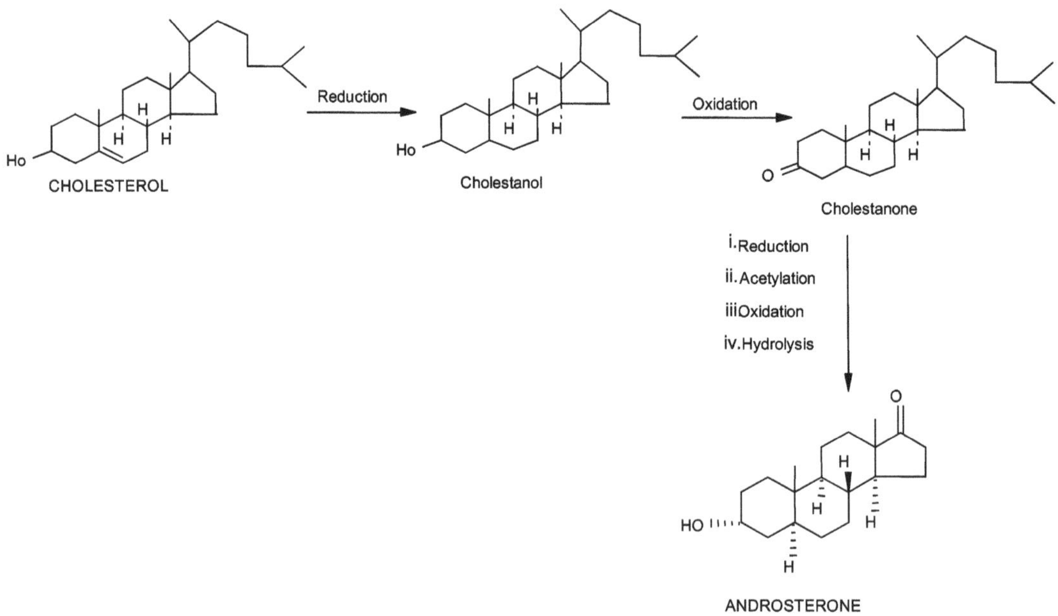

Uses of androgens

1. Androgens are used for substitutional therepy in men with hypogonadism.
2. They have been used to facilitate development of adult masculine characteristics.
3. They are used along with gonadotropins in cryptorchidism.
4. They are also very useful in the treatment of hypopituitarism and Addison's disease, rigidity and impotance.
5. They may also be used to treat endometriosis, cancer of the breast etc.
6. They have been used to increase nitrogen, water retention and to stimulate skeletal muscle growth (anabolic activity).

Synthetic androgens

Several modifications were carried out in the structure of androgens. The aim of chemical modification is to retard the rate of catabolism or to enhance the androgenic potency of each molecule. Three general types of modifications have been particularly useful. They are:

(i) Esterification of the 17β-hydroxyl group with any of several carboxylic acids decrease the polarity of the molecule, makes it more soluble in the lipid vehicles used for injection and hence slows release of the injected steroid into the circulation. E.g., : Testosterone undecanoate.

(ii) Alkylation at the 17α-position also allows androgens to be effective orally, because the alkylated derivatives are slowly catabolised by the liver. E.g., : Fluoxymestrone.

(iii) To separate anabolic and androgenic activities. E.g., : Nandrolone.

The following are various synthetic androgen derivatives:

(i) ***Methyltestostorone :*** It is a semi-synthetic analogue of testosterone and is effective sublingually chemically methytestosterone is 17β-hydroxy 17α-methyl-4-androsten-3-one.

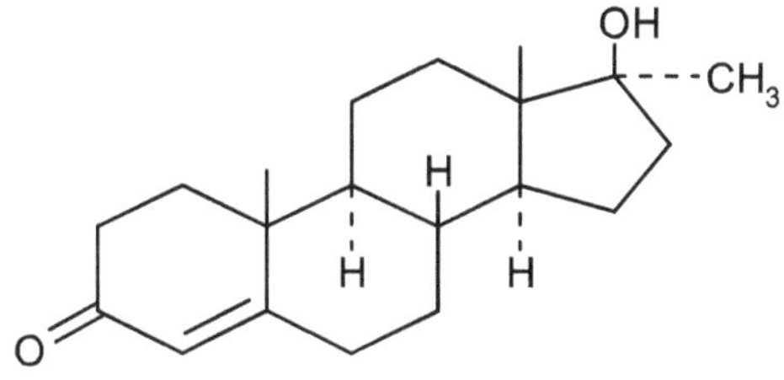

Methyltestosterone

(ii) ***Fluoxymestrone :*** Fluoxymestrone has 9α-fluoro, 11β-hydroxy functional moieties. Chemically it is 9α-fluoro 11,17β-dihydroxy, 17α-metyl 4-androsten -3-one. It is also orally active and is more potent than methyltestosterone.

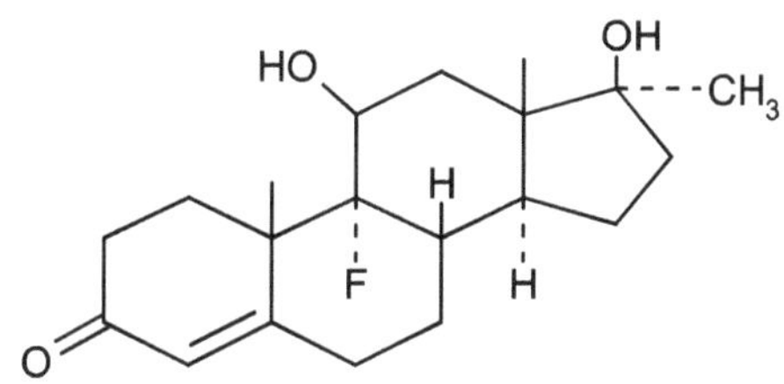

Fluoxymestrone

(iii) ***Nandrolone :*** It is 3-oxo-4-estern-17β-ol. Nandrolone is available as phenylpropionate and decanate esters. They are administered by intra muscular injection. Nandrolone has predominant anabolic but less androgenic activity.

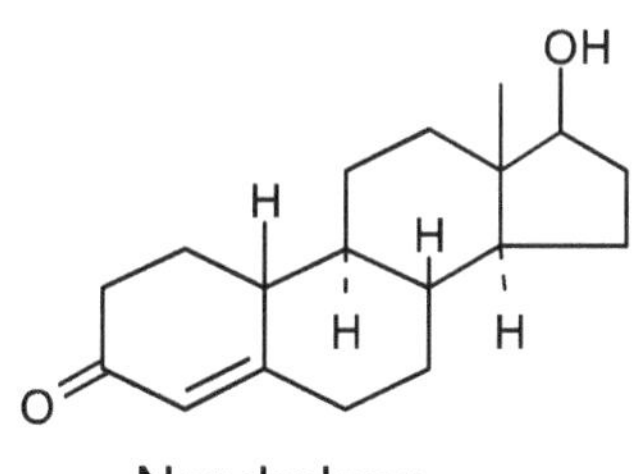

Nandrolone

(iv) ***Methandienone and oxandrolone :*** These are 17α-alkyl derivatives and are orally active. They show increased anabolic/androgenic ratio. Methandienone is different from methyl oxandrolone differs from methyltestosterone by having O in place of CH_2 at 2nd position and no double in between 4 & 5 carbons testosterone in possessing an additional double bond between 1 and 2 positions.

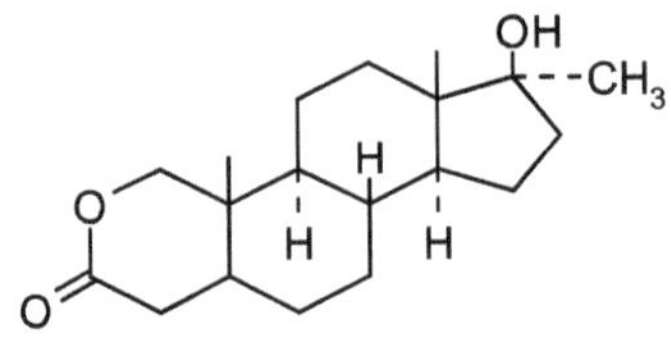

Oxandrolone

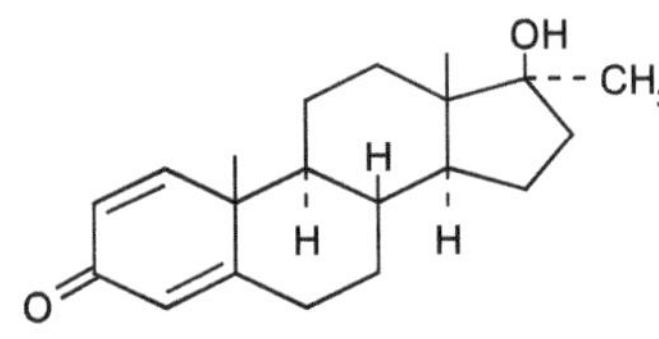

Methandienone

Estrogens

Estrogens are endogenous hormones that are responsible for the control of ovulation, cyclic preparation of reproductive tract for fertilization, implantation and have influence on mineral, carbohydrate, protein and lipid metabolism. Estrogenic activity is shared by many steroidal and non-steroidal compounds.

Introduction : The compounds, which have estrogenic activity, are termed as estrogens. They are of :

1. Natural estrogens: They are produced in females.

   E.g.,: Oestriol, oestrone and oestradiol

2. Synthetic estrogens: They may be steroidal or non- steroidal

   (a) Steroidal synthetic estrogens. E.g.,: Ethinylestradiol, mestranol.

   (b) Non steroidal synthetic estrogens. E.g.,: Stilboestrol, hexoestrol, dienoestrol.

Natural estrogens

Estrone, estriol and estradiol

1. Estrone, estriol and estradiol are steroidal female sex hormones. Estradiol is the main estrogenic hormone formed in the body, whereas estrone and estriol are its metabolic products.
2. Steroid nucleus:These three estrogens yield Diel's hydrocarbon by selenium distillation, hence they possess a steroid moiety.

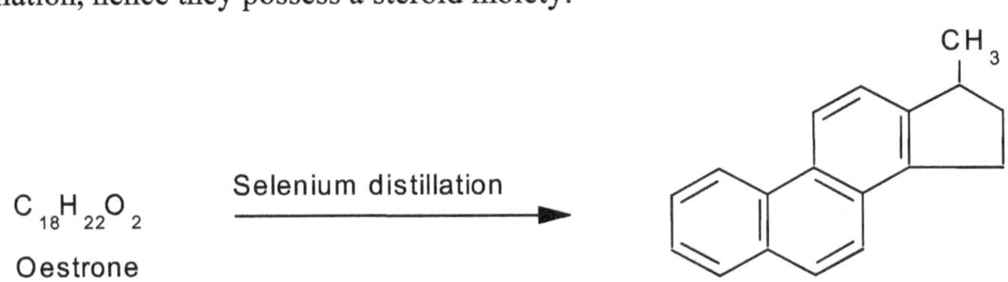

Diel's hydrocarbon

$C_{18}H_{24}O_3$ Oestriol $\xrightarrow{\text{Selenium distillation}}$ 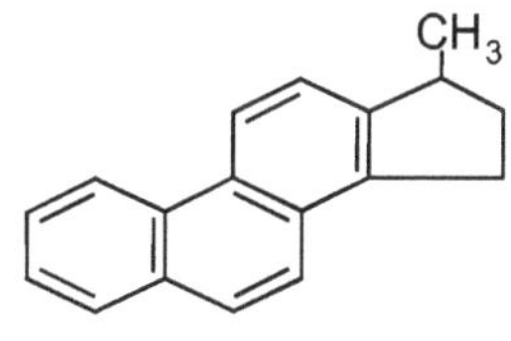

Diel's hydrocarbon

$C_{18}H_{24}O_2$ Oestradiol $\xrightarrow{\text{Selenium distillation}}$ 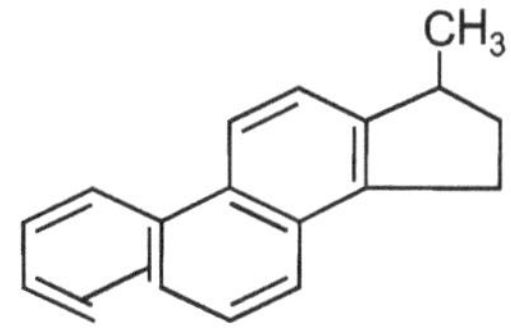

Diel's hydrocarbon

3. They are estrane derivatives and are solid in nature.

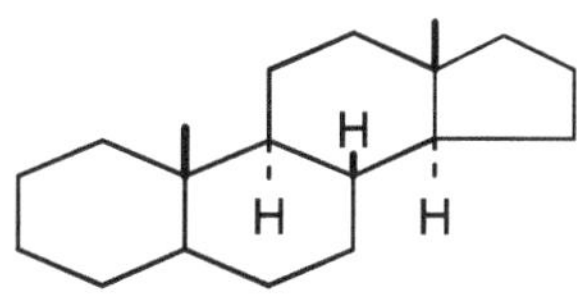

Estrane

4. The molecular formula of estrone, estriol and estradiol is $C_{18}H_{22}O_2$, $C_{18}H_{24}O_3$ and $C_{18}H_{24}O_2$ respectively.

5. The three estrogenic steroids possess one phenolic hydroxyl group, and three double bonds. The presence of three double bonds in ring A to give benzenoid system is supported by ultraviolet absorption spectrum.

$C_{18}H_{22}O_2$
Oestrone

$C_{18}H_{24}O_3$ $\xrightarrow{FeCl_3}$ Blue or Green or Violet colorations
Oestradiol

$C_{18}H_{24}O_2$
Oestriol

6. Oestrone answers for one keto group (formation of oximes), and one phenolic hydroxyl group. Oestriol answers for three hydroxyl groups. One hydroxyl group in estriol was shown to be phenolic, and the other two are secondary alcoholic groups (formation of diketone) present at 16,17 positions as confirmed by x-ray analysis. Estradiol possess two hydroxyl groups i.e., one is phenolic, and the other is alcoholic hydroxyl group at 17-position.

$C_{18}H_{22}O_2$ Oestrone $\xrightarrow{(CH_3CO)_2O}$ $C_{18}H_{22}$. O. $OCOCH_3$ Monoester of estrone

$$C_{18}H_{24}O_3 \xrightarrow{(CH_3CO)_2O} C_{18}H_{22} \cdot (OCOCH_3)_3$$

Triesterof estriol

$C_{18}H_{24}O_2$

$$C_{18}H_{24}O_3 \xrightarrow{(CH_3CO)_2O} C_{18}H_{22} \cdot (OCOCH_3)_2$$

Oestradiol — Diester of estradiol

The phenolic A-ring is the principal structural feature responsible for selective, high affinity binding to estrogenic receptors.

7. All these three estrogens possess one angular methyl group between C and D rings.
8. Finally the structures of natural estrogens can be drawn as:

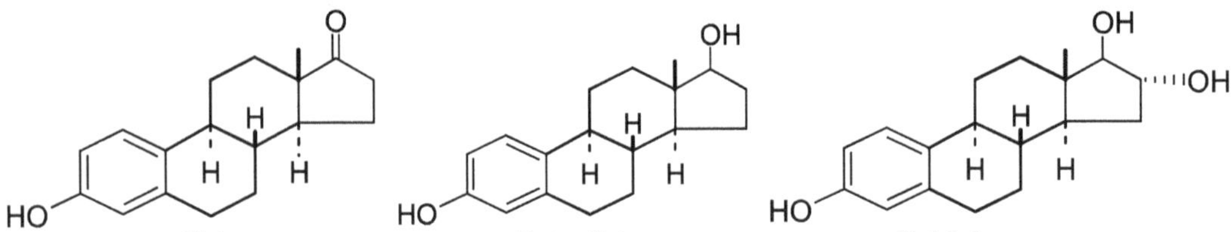

Estrone   Estradiol   Estriol

Inter relationship of natural estrogens :

(i) Estriol, estradiol and estrone are produced naturally in females

(ii) They are estrane derivatives

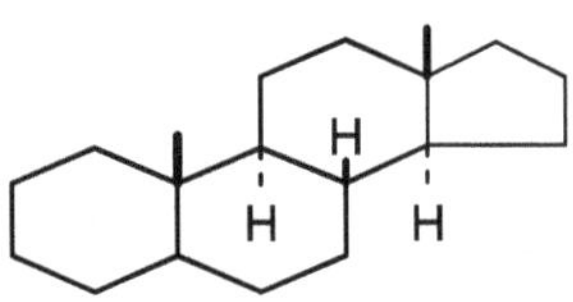

Estrane

(iii) All natural estrogens possess one benzenoid and one phenolic hydroxyl group

(iv) All possess one angular methyl group.

(v) Estrone may be reduced to estradiol (catalytic or Meerwein–Ponndorf–Verley reduction or by lithium aluminium hydride).

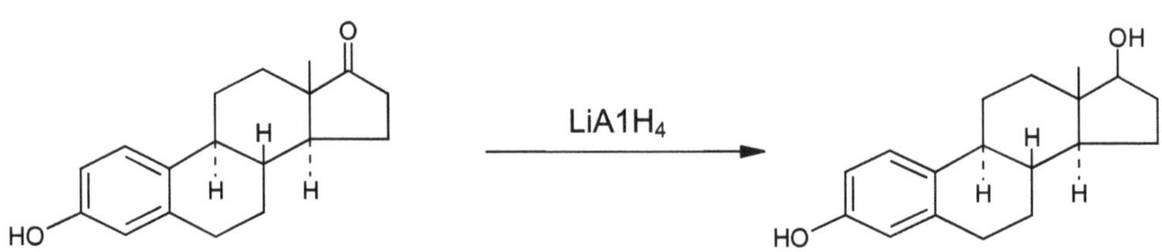

Estrone   Estradiol

(vi) Estrone is formed by heating estriol with $KHSO_4$ (dehydration)

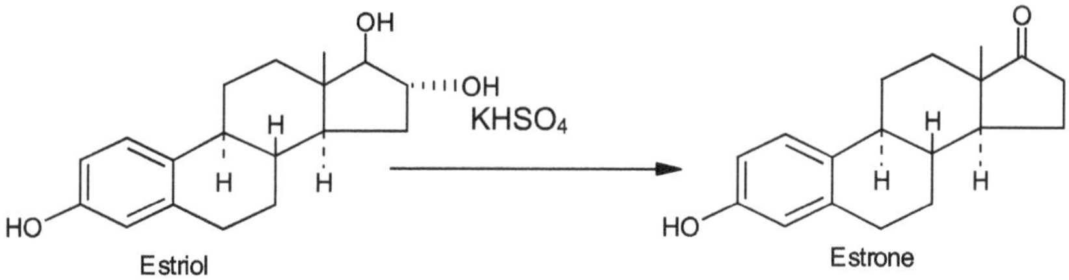

(vii) Estrone may be converted to estriol by the following conversion.

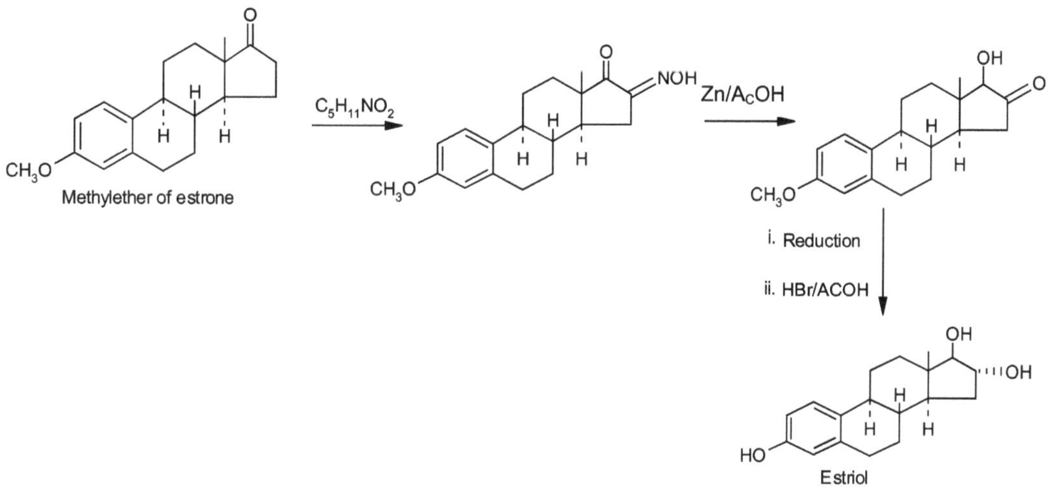

(viii) Estrogens can also be used as hypocholesteremic drugs as they decrease plasma cholesterol.

(ix) They are also used to inhibit the growth of prostatic cancer of men and carcinoma of the breast or carcinoma of reproductive tract of women.

Synthetic steroidal estrogens

1. ***Ethinyl estradiol :*** Ethinyl estradiol is 17α-ethinylestradiol. Ethinyl substitutions at the C-17 position greatly increase oral potency by inhibiting first-pass hepatic metabolism. It is orally active and is equal to estradiol in potency by injection. It is prepared from estrone by the action of potassium acetylide(HC≡CK) in liquid ammonia.

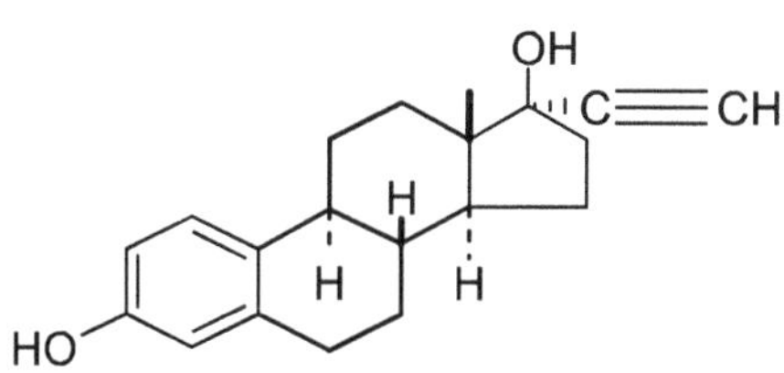

Ethinyl estradiol

Ethinylestradiol is used as the estrogenic compound in oral contraceptives. It is also used to treat menopausal symptoms and carcinoma of prostate.

2. ***Mestranol :*** Mestranol is the 3-methyl ether of ethinyl estradiol. It is prepared by ethinylation of estrone 3-methyl ether.

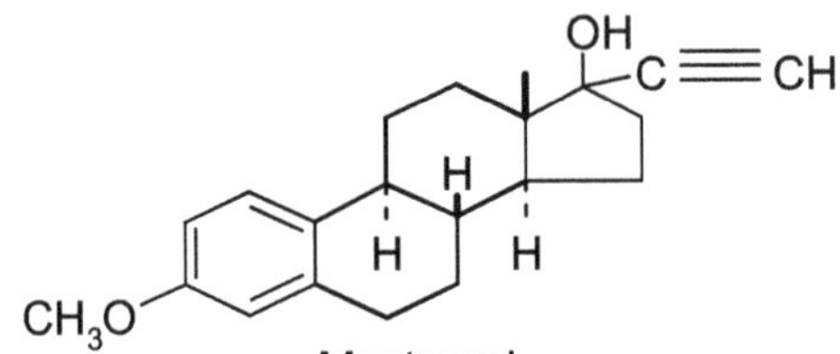

Mestranol

Mestranol is inactive until it is converted to ethinylestradiol in the body. It is used as a oral contraceptive and to treat menopausal symptoms.

3. ***Synthetic non-steroidal estrogens :*** A large number of non-steroidal compounds possessing estrogenic activity were reported. They are inexpensive and are effective orally.

   E.g., : Stilboestrol, hexoestrol, dieoestrol, and benzoestrol.

   (i) ***Stilboestrol :*** It can be synthesized from anethole by the following steps:

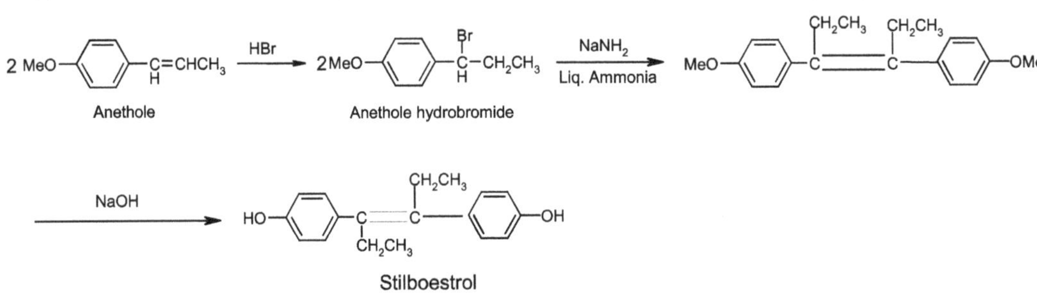

(ii) ***Hexoestrol :*** Hexoestrol is prepared from anethole as:

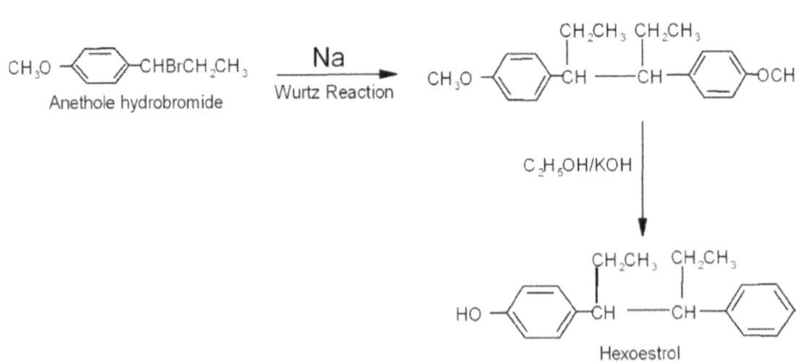

(iii) ***Dienoestrol :*** Dienoestrol differs from hexoestrol in having two double bonds in side chain. It is one-fourth as potent as stiboestrol. Dienoestrol is prepared by pinacol reduction of *p*-hydroxyacetophenone followed by dehydration.

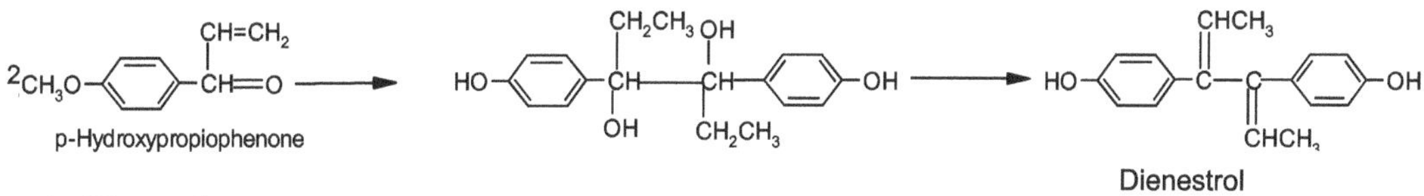

4. ***Uses of estrogens*** **:**

   (i) Estrogens are used as substitutional therapy when menopausal symptoms occur after cessation of ovarian function following ovariectomy or X-ray or radium therapy or in the natural menopause.

   (ii) Estrogens are used in young women in whom there is failure of steroidogenesis.

   (iii) Estrogens are useful in the treatment of atrophic or senile vaginitis, vulvovaganitis or cervicitis resulting from hypoestrogenesis.

   (iv) Estrogens are used as contraceptives because they suppress follicle stimulating hormone release and also inhibit implantation.

Progestogens

Progestogens are steroidal compounds that have biological activities similar to progesterone. Progesterone is the main hormone of corpus leutum or yellow body (corpus luteum is the tissue formed in the human ovary after maturation and rupture of follicle). Progesterone is not orally effective as it is completely metabolized in the liver. Progestogens may be natural or synthetic.

Natural progestogens

Progesterone

1. Molecular formula of progesterone is $C_{21}H_{30}O_2$

2. ***Steroid nucleus*** **:** Progesterone on selenium distillation yields Diel's hydrocarbon. This indicates the presence of steroid nucleus in progesterone.

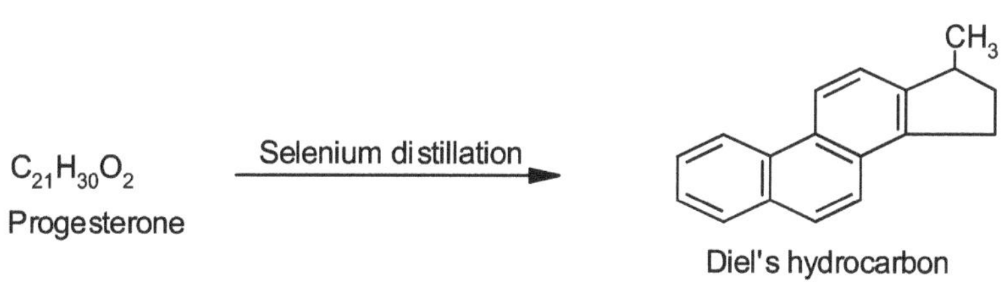

Synthetic progestogens : Several synthetic progestogens have been prepared. They are mostly obtained by partial synthesis from naturally occurring steroids or by total synthesis. All synthetic progestogens are structurally steroids.

(i) ***Ethisterone :*** Ethisterone is 17α-ethynyltestrosterone. It is effective by mouth, preferably sublingually. It is 15 times as active orally as progesterone.

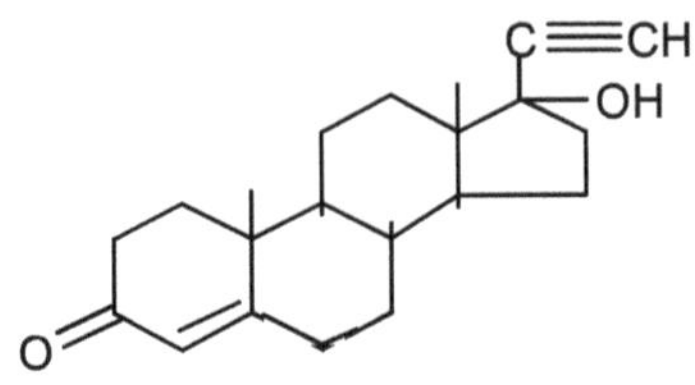

Ethisterone

(ii) ***19-nor pregnane derivatives :*** The various examples of 19-nor steroids are norehisterone, Norethynodrel, lynoesternol and ethynodiol. They are orally effective and more potent to progesterone. Norethisterone is 75 times more potent to progesterone dry oral route. The other two isomers of norethisterone are norethynodrel (3-deoxoderivative), lynoesterol and ethynodiol.

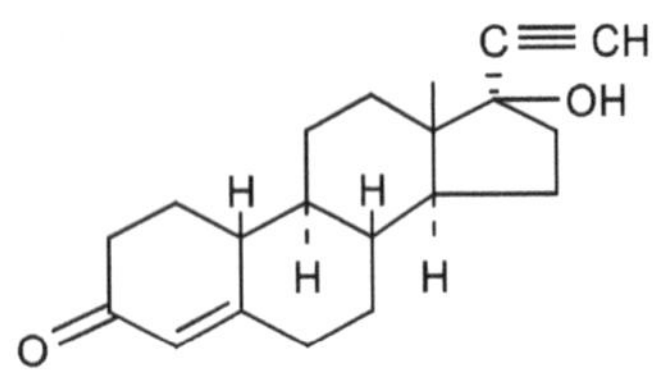

Norethisterone

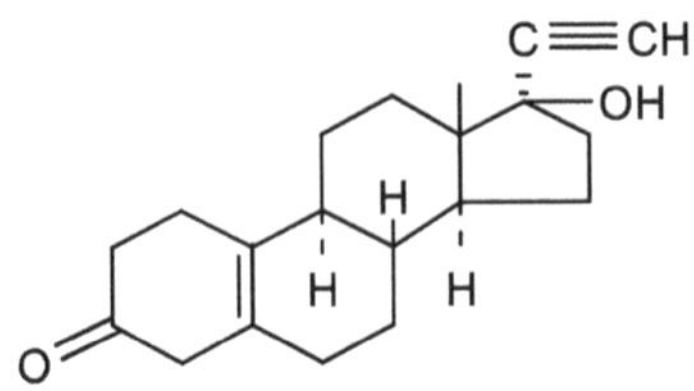

Norethynodrel

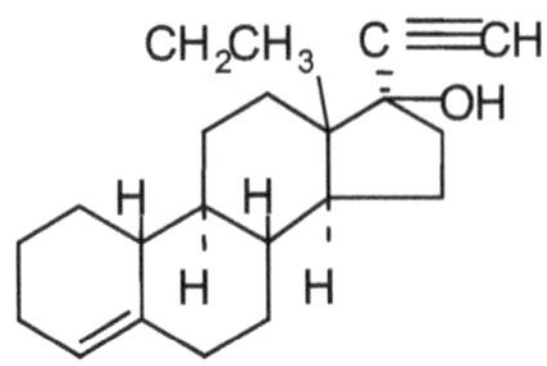

Lynoesterol

(iii) ***17α-acetoxy derivative :*** Medroxylprogesterone, megestrol are 17α-acetoxyl derivatives of progesterone. They have very high oral progestational activity.

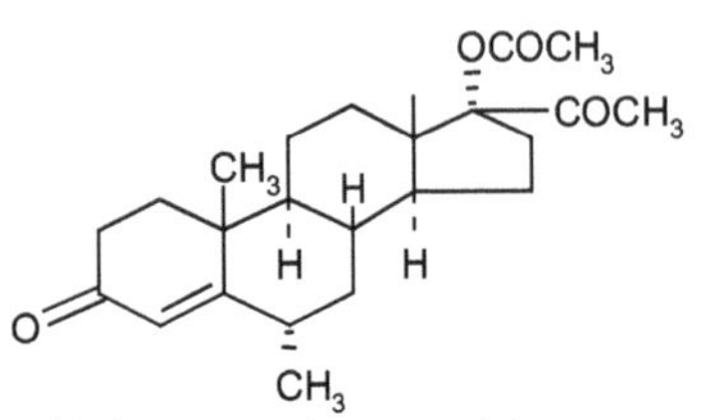

Medroxyprogesterone acetate

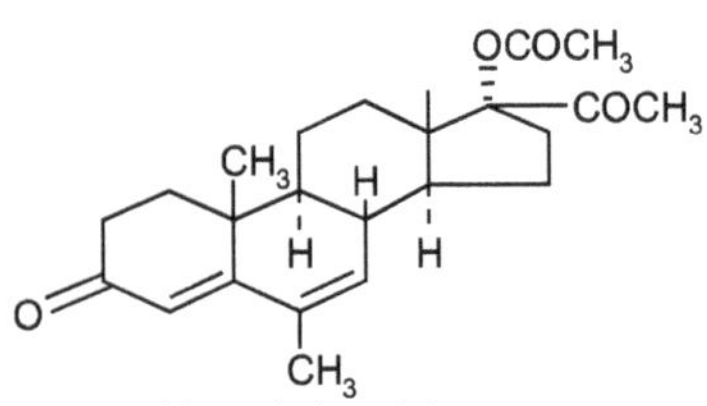

Megestrol acetate

Oral contraceptives : Drugs that decrease fertility by a number of different mechanisms like preventing ovulation, impairing gametogenesis, or gamete maturation or interfering with maturation are called oral contraceptives. Currently interference with ovulation is the most common mechanism for prevention of pregnancy.

Types of oral contraceptives :

1. ***Combination pills :*** Products containing a combination of estrogen and progestin are the most common types of oral contraceptives. The estrogen component suppresses ovulation while the progestin prevents implantation in the endometrium and makes the cervical mucus impenetratable to sperm. The pills are taken for 21 days followed by a 7-day withdrawl period to induce menses. These preparations are highly effective in achieving contraception.

2. ***Progestin pills :*** These pills not contain any oestrogen and further contain progestin in smaller amounts than those used in combined pills. These preparations are less effective than combination pill, may produce irregular menstrual cycles more frequently and prevent conception. Generally these pills contain norethindrone or norgestrol. In addition to pills, injectable forms and repository forms are also available.
3. ***Post coital oral contraceptives :*** These contraceptives contain high-dose of estrogen and are administered within 72 hours of coitus and continued twice daily for 5 days. The estrogen present in these pills is Diethylstilbestrol.

Mechanism of action of oral contraceptives : The mechanism of action of these contraceptives is not completely understood. The estrogen of pills prevents ovulation by suppressing the release of FSH and LH by negative feed back mechanism on FSH-LH from pituitary gland. Progestins also suppress the LH output.

Adrenalcortical hormones : The adrenal glands consist of two distinct parts i.e., the medulla and the cortex. The medulla produces and stores catecholamines(adrenaline) while the cortex secretes corticosteroids or adrenocortical hormones under the control of adrenocoticotrophic hormone. Two categories of adrenocortical hormones produced by adrenal cortex. They are :

(i) ***Glucocorticoids :*** Glucocorticoids influence carbohydrate, protein and lipid metabolism. The glucocorticoids are cortisone, cortisol (hydrocartisone) and corticosterone.

(ii) ***Mineralocorticoids :*** Mineralocorticoids help to control the body's water volume and concentration of electrolytes especially sodium and potassium. E.g.,: Aldosterone.

Cortisone

(i) ***Molecular formula :*** The molecular formula of cortisone is $C_{21}H_{29}O_5$.

(ii) ***α, β - unsaturated carbonyl group :*** Sensitivity of cortisone in alkaline solution and UV absorption spectrum confirms the presence of carbonyl group in cortisone.

(iii) ***Presence of double bond :*** Cortisone reacts with a molecule of bromine to form cortisonedibromide. This confirms the presence of a double bond.

$$\underset{\text{Cortisone}}{C_{21}H_{29}O_5} + Br_2 \longrightarrow \underset{\text{Cortisone dibromide}}{C_{21}H_{29}O_5Br_2}$$

(iv) ***Hydroxyl groups :*** Cortisone possess one primary hydroxyl group and one tertiary hydroxyl group.

(v) ***α-Ketol group :*** Presence of α-ketol group in cortisone is confirmed by reduction of Tollen's or Fehling' reagent.

(vi) ***Oxidation :*** Cortisone on oxidation yields adrenosterone.

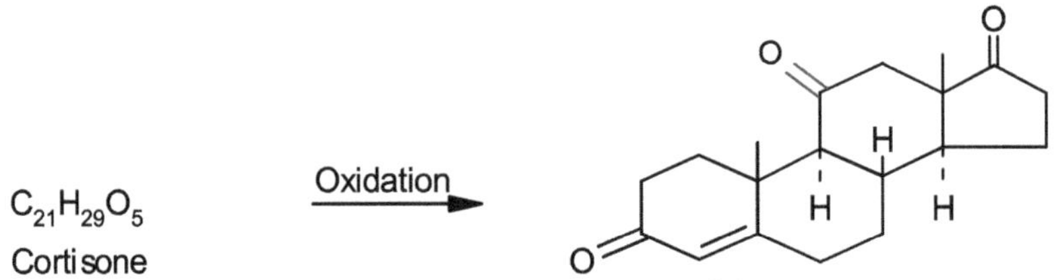

Adrenosterone

(vii) ***Structure of cortisone :*** On the basis of the above facts, the structure of cortisone is written as follows :

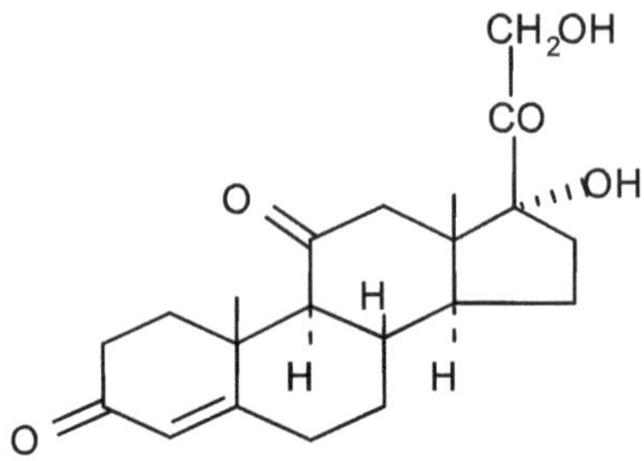

Cortisone

Cortisol

(i) Cortisol is the important adrenocortical hormone which is physiologically more active than cortisone.

(ii) Cortisol secretion is under the control of ACTH of anterior pituitary lobe.

(iii) Structure of Cortisol: The structure of cortisol is same as that of cortisone except the hydroxyl group at C-H instead of a carbonyl group.

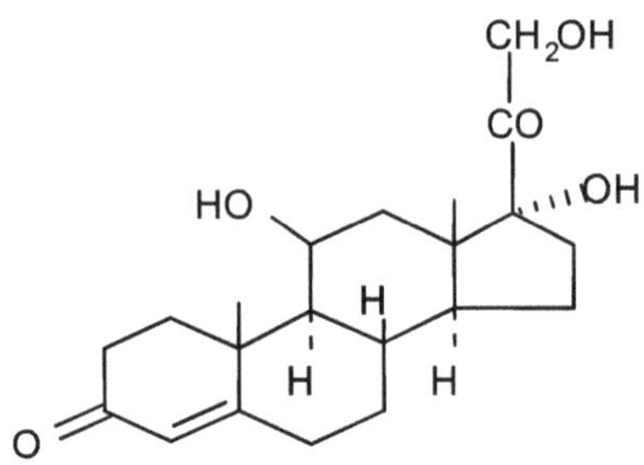

Cortisol

Biological activities of glucocrticoids :

(i) Glucocorticoids exerts influence on carbohydrate, protein and lipid metabolism.

(ii) Glucocorticoids stimulate gluconeogenesis and glycogenesis in the liver.

(iii) They also exert anti-inflammatory action by decreasing cellular protective reactions and by retarding migration of leucocytes into traumatised area.

Aldosterone

(i) Aldosterone is the naturally occurring mineralocorticoid.

(ii) Aldosterone is a colourless crystalline compound. The structure of aldosterone is:

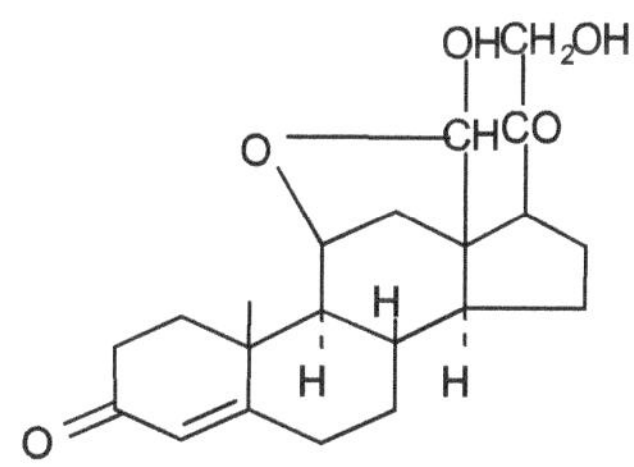

Aldosterone

(iii) Aldosterone has a hemiacetal bridge between 11β-hydroxyl and an 18-aldehyde groups.

(iv) Aldosterone is too expensive to produce commercially, therefore other semisynthetic analogues have taken it's place.

Uses of mineralocorticoids

(i) Mineralocorticoids have greater influence on water and mineral metabolism.

(ii) Mineralocorticoids causes retention of sodium chloride and water and increases excreation of potassium.

Derivatives of corticosteroids

(i) ***Prednisone and prednisolone :*** Prednisone and prednisolone are the modified derivatives of cortisone or hydrocortisone. They are available as prednisone, prednisone acetate, prednisolone, prednisolone acetate, prednisolone pivalates prednisolone sodium phosphate. Prednisone and prednisolone are produced by the introduction of additional double bond between 1 and 2 positions of ring A in steroid nucleus. Chemical method or microorganisms can carry out this modification.

The glucocorticoid and anti-inflammatory activity of these derivatives is enhanced by 3 times to natural hormones.

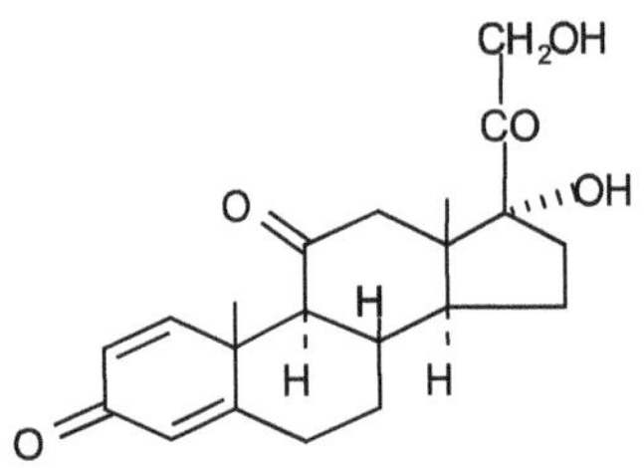

Prednisone

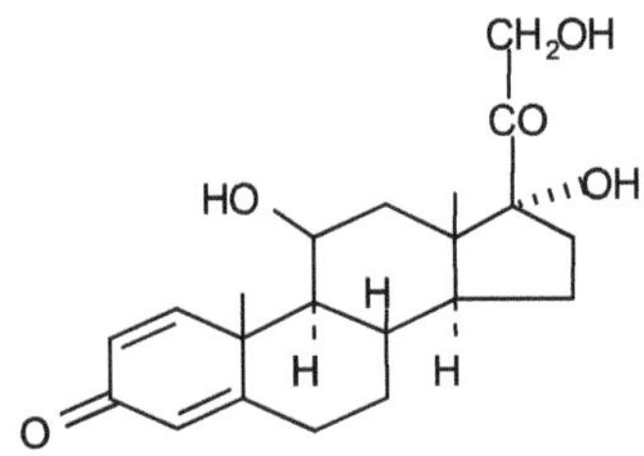

Prednisolone

(ii) ***Betamethasone :*** Betamethasone has the same structure as dexamethasone but the methyl group at 16 positon is in β-configuration. The biological activity and potency are similar to dexamethasone. It is available as betamethasone sodium phosphate, betamethasone valerate.

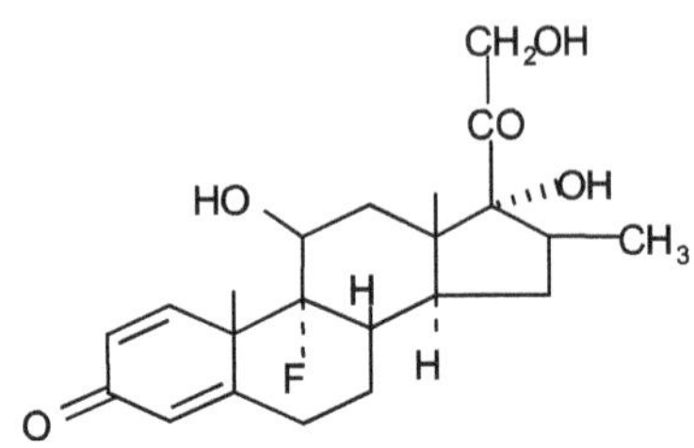

Betamethasone

(iii) ***Triamcinolone :*** Triamcinolone is 9α-hydroxyprednisolone which can be prepared from 9α-fluorohydrocortisone by microbiological oxidation. Introduction of 16α-hydroxyl group eliminates the salt retention activity and reduces anti-inflammatory activity. However, the glucocorticoid and antiinflammatory activities are potentiated by formation of ketal and prevention of intermolecular hydrogen bonding with fluorine atoms.

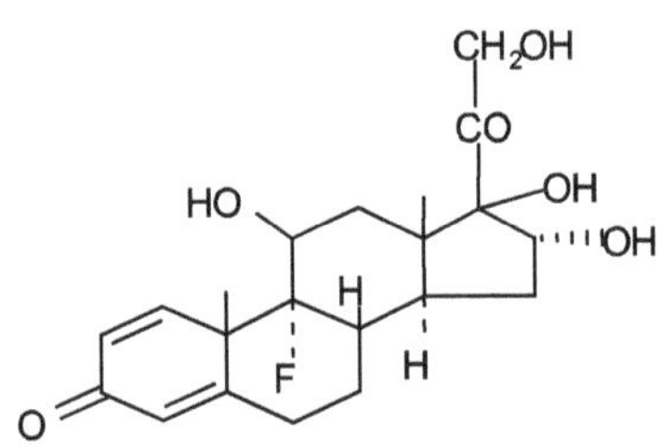

Triamcinolone

(iv) ***Dexamethasone :*** Dexamethasone is a 16α-methyl derivative of prednisolone. It possess 16α-methyl group, 1,2-double bond and 9α-fluoro group. It shows higher glucocorticoid and anti-inflammatory activity (25 times to hydrocortisone) but its mineralocorticoid activity is low.

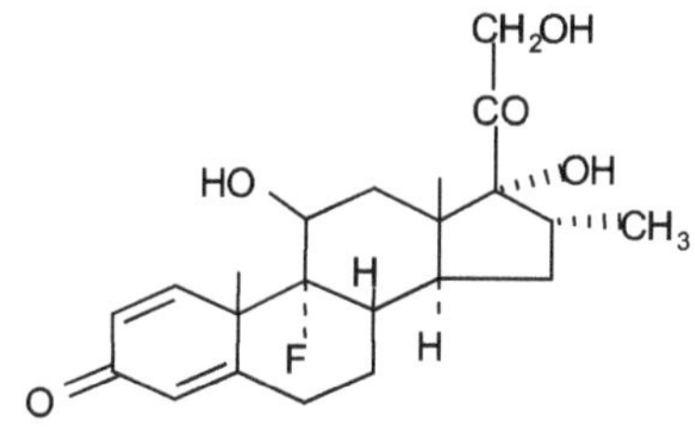

Dexamethasone

(v) ***Fludrocortisone :*** Fludrocortisone is 9α-fluorohydrocortisone. It has 13 times more anti-inflammatory activity to cortisone and equal mineralocorticoid activity to aldosterone.

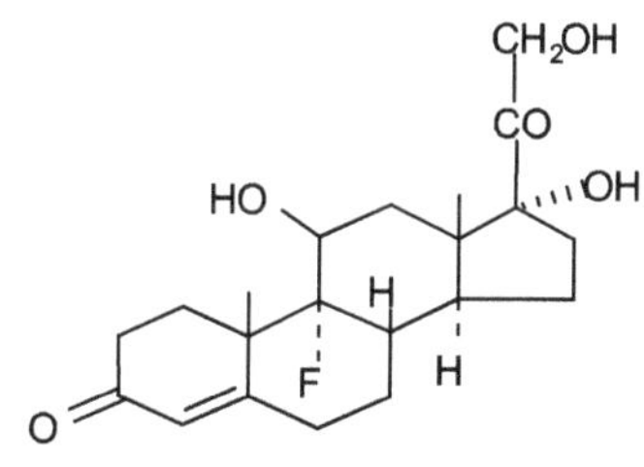

Fludrocortisone

Corticosteroids are also synthesized from stigmasterol by microbial conversions.

ESSAY AND SHORT TYPE QUESTIONS

Chapters 1 to 6

1. Define medicinal chemistry. Explain how medicinal chemistry has interrelationship with other subjects?
2. What are drugs? Explain various routes of drug administration.
3. What are receptors? Discuss various receptors and receptor theories with examples.
4. What are drugs? Explain with examples how drug act.
5. What are drug-receptor interactions? Explain different types of binding forces exist in drug-receptor interactions with examples.
6. Explain different mechanisms of drug actions.
7. Write notes on different sites of drug actions.
8. Discuss the importance of hydrogen bonding, partition coefficient and chelation in relation to biological activity.
9. Enumerate the various physicochemical properties that modulate biological activity and explain any two of them in detail?
10. Enumerate the physicochemical properties that influence biological activity. Give a detailed account of any two of them?
11. Discuss the influence of :

    (a) Bioisosterism (b) hydrogen bonding (c) ionization (d) stereoisomerism on biological activity
12. Discuss the suitable examples the importance of the following in relation to biological activity of drugs :

    (i) Optical isomerism (ii) Partition coefficient.
13. What is bioisosterism? How is it useful in the design of drugs?
14. Giving suitable examples, show how different types of isomerism affects the biological activity of drugs?
15. How does protein binding of drugs affect the biological activity of therapeutic agents?

16. With the help of appropriate examples, elucidate how different physicochemical properties of drug molecules are related to their biological activity?
17. Explain the role of pK_a in the biological activity of drugs.
18. "Biological activity of a drug does not simply depend on its chemical structure but also on its physicochemical properties." Illustrate the above statement with suitable examples.
19. Discuss citing suitable examples how complexation, protein binding and partition coefficient affect biological activity of drugs.
20. What is partition coefficient?
21. What is molar refractivity?
22. What is bioisosterism?
23. What are isosters?
24. (a) Explain the meaning of the terms lead compound and analogue in the context of drug development.
    (b) Outline the general steps in the development of a new drug.
25. State the full wording of the abbreviation 'SAR'. Describe the general way in which SAR is used to develop a drug. Illustrate the answer by reference to the changes in the activities of 4-alkylresorcinols caused by changes in the chain length of the 4-alkyl group.
26. Suggest how the introduction of each of the following groups into the structure of a lead could be expected to affect the bioavailability of the resultant analogue : (a) a sulphonic acid group, (b) a methyl group and (c) a thiol group. Assume that these groups are introduced into the section of the leads structure that does not contain its pharmacophore?
27. Outline the fundamental principle underlying the QSAR approach to drug design.
28. (a) Describe the approach to drug design known as Hansch analysis.
    (b) Phenols are antiseptics. Hansch analysis carried out on a series of phenols with the general structure A yielded the Hansch equation:
29. (a) Describe how the Topliss decision tree is used in drug design.
    (b) What is a major limitation to its use?
30. Outline the basic principle underlying combinational chemistry. What criteria should be satisfied by the building blocks used in a combinatorial synthesis?
31. List the general considerations that should be taken into account when designing a combinatorial synthesis.
32. Outline Merrifield's method of peptide synthesis.
33. State the general factors that need to be considered when designing a drug.
34. Explain the meaning of the terms : (a) Lead compound, (b) dosage form (c) enteral administration of drugs. (d) drug regimen and (e) excipient.

35. Suggest strategies for improving the stability of compound A in the gastrointestinal tract. What could be the general effect of these strategies on the pharmaceutical action of compound A (structure, page 30)?

Chapter - 7

1. Define a chemotherapeutic agent and distinguish it from a pharmacodynamic agent. Explain the terms bacteriostatic, bactericidal and chemotherapeutic index. (12 marks)
2. Give an account of SAR among antibacterial sulphonamides? (4 marks)
3. Write the structure, synthesis and uses of trimethoprim? (4 marks)
4. Give an account of general synthesis and mode of action of antibacterial sulfonamides? (8 marks)
5. Give the classification of sulphonamides with examples. Explain their mechanism of action and toxic effects? (8 marks)
6. Outline the synthesis of (i) Sulphamethoxazole (ii) Sulphadoxine ($4 \times 2 = 8$ marks)
7. Discuss the current status of sulfa drugs in the chemotherapy of bacterial infections? (8 marks)
8. Outline the general synthesis and mode of action of sulpha drugs. Explain how synergism is observed when drugs like trimethoprim are co-administered along with sulfa drugs.
9. Discuss the role of pK_a in the designing of newer sulfonamides? (3 marks)
10. What is crystalluria? How it could be prevented?

Chapter – 8 to 13

1. What are antibiotics? Classify them with examples and discuss the mode of action and therapeutic uses of pencillines? (8 marks)
2. Describe how molecular modification of pencillin molecule led to the development of orally effective penicillins. Give the structures of any three such drugs? (8 marks)
3. Define antibiotics? Classify the various commercially significant pencillins with examples? Discuss the molecular mode of action of beta-lactam antibiotics. Explain the therapeutic of this class of antibiotics? (16 Marks)
4. Write short notes on penicillinase resistant oral pencillins? (8 marks)
5. (a) How are antibiotics classified? Illustrate giving examples?
   (b) Give an account of chemistry and stability of pencillin molecule?
   (c) Outline the synthesis of chloramphenicol.
6. Write notes on : (16 Marks)
   (a) β-Lactam antibiotics
   (b) Macrolide antibiotics
7. Discuss the chemistry of streptomycin? (8 marks)
8. Discuss the SAR of tetracyclines? (8 marks)

9. Outline the synthesis and uses of : (16 marks)
   (a) doxycycline (b) minocycline (c) cefuroxime (d) roxithromycin (e) azithromycin
10. Write notes on polypeptide antibiotics? (8 marks)
11. Write notes on (a) cycloserine (b) lincomycin (c) clindamycin

Chapter - 14

1. Describe mechanism of blood clotting?
2. Discuss how anticoagulants prevent blood clotting?
3. How are Indane dione derivatives synthesized.
4. Write synthesis of warfarin?

Chapter - 15 & 16

1. What is multidrug resistant TB and how it is treated?
2. Classify antimycobacterial agents giving the names and structures of typical examples. Outline the synthesis, mode of action and clinical uses of any three of them? (12 marks)
3. Write a note on the concept of multidrug therapy for mycobacterial diseases? (4 marks)
4. Outline the synthesis, mode of action and clinical uses of (a) paraminosalicylic acid (b) INH (c) Pyrazinamide
5. Give an account of antitubercular antibiotics? (4 marks)
6. What is the current way of treating tuberculosis? What is its status in India? Outline the synthesis and uses of INH and Dapsone?

Chapter - 17

1. Classify antimalarial drugs with examples. Explain their mechanism of action and outline synthesis of one member from each class. (16 Marks)
2. Outline synthesis and uses of chloroquine? (4 Marks)
3. Give an account of antimalarials? (4 Marks)
4. Write the structure, synthesis and uses of amodiaquine?
5. Give an account of antimalarial drugs covering the life history of parasite, clinical symptoms and classification. Describe in detail the status of natural products useful in the treatment of human malarial infections?
6. Explain the mechanism of action and SAR of 9-aminoacridines? (5 Marks)
7. Outline the synthesis of pyrimethamine?
8. Outline the synthesis and clinical uses of proguanil?
9. Write the synthesis, mechanism of action and use of (a) Cycloguanil (b) Chloroquine phosphate. (8 Marks)
10. Show how antimalarial are classified based on (i) their chemical structure and (ii) their type of action giving examples. (8 Marks)

11. Write a note on the use of artemisinine and its derivatives as antimalarial drugs? (5 marks)
12. Write SAR and mode of action of aminoquinoline antimalarials. Write note on the metabolism of proguanil? (8 marks)
13. Outline the synthesis of primaquine and mepacrine? (8 marks)

Chapters 18 & 19

1. Classify the drugs useful in the treatment of amoebiasis giving structures of typical examples for each class. Outline the synthesis of any three such compounds choosing each from a different chemical class? (16 marks)
2. Write explanatory notes on drugs useful in the therapy of helminthic infections? (8 marks)
3. Outline the synthesis and uses of (a) Metronidazole (b) Nitro furantrin? (8 Marks)
4. Write short notes on anthelmentics and antiamoebic agents? (8 Marks)
5. Give an account of anti trypnosomal agents? (8 Marks)
6. Describe the pathophysiological features of human amoebic infections. Classify antiamoebic drugs giving the structures of typical examples for each class. Outline the synthesis and mode of action of tinidazole and diloxanide? (16 Marks)
7. Describe the nature and variety of human helminthic infections. Enlist the various categories of therapeutic agents for treating such infections. Explain the mode of action and synthesis of any three such drugs?
8. Write the structure, chemical name and therapeutic uses of niclosamide, metronidazole? (4 Marks)
9. Outline the synthesis and clinical uses of nitrofurantoin? (4 Marks)
10. Outline the synthesis, mode of action and clinical uses of diloxanide furoate? (4 Marks)
11. Define anthelminties and classify them giving examples. Write the SAR, mode of action and structures of Benzimidazole anthelminties. Write the synthesis of any one official drug? (16 marks)

Chapter - 20

1. Give an account of imidazoles used in therapy of fungal infections? (5 marks)
2. Write briefly on antifungal agents? (8 marks)
3. Classify human fungal infections naming the causative organism enlist the various classes of antifungals and discuss their mechanism of action. Outline the synthesis of clortiziozole and flucytosine?
4. How do you classify antifungal agents? Write the structure, chemical name and uses of any three synthetic antifungal agents. (8 marks)
5. Give an account of antifungal drugs?
6. Outline synthesis of (a) 5-fluorouracil (b) 5-fluorouracli (b) Tolnaftate.

Chapter - 21

1. Enumerate various classes of antiviral chemotherapeutic agents. Explain their mode of action and synthesis of any three such drugs? (16 marks)
2. Write briefly on antiviral agents? (8 marks)
3. Write notes on purines and pyrimidines in the chemotherapy of viral infections? (8 marks)
4. Write structure, chemical name and threpeutic uses of iodoxuridine, Acyclovir. (4 Marks)
5. What are the obstances to effective antiviral chemotherapy? Write notes on (a) Iodoxurine HCl (b) Amantadine HCl
6. Give examples, mode of action and clinical uses of Reverse transcriptase inhibitors (4 Marks)
7. Write short notes on antiviral agents? (4 Marks)
8. Give examples of drugs that act as DNA polymerase inhibitors. Describe their chemistry and threrapeutic uses (8 Marks)

Chapter - 22

1. Give an account of natural products used in cancer chemotherapy? (5 Marks)
2. Discuss the chemistry, SAR and mode of action of alkylating agents? (8 Marks)
3. Outline the synthesis, mode of action and uses of (a) Methotrexate (b) Cyclophosphamide (c) Azathioprine (d) 6-Mercaptopurine (e) 5-Fluorouracil (f) Melphalan
4. What are antineoplastic agents? Classify them with examples. Discuss the mode of action of alkylating agents and write the synthesis of any two anticancer drugs? (16 Marks)
5. Discuss the limitations and problems encountered in the chemotherapy of neoplastic disease. Classify antineoplastics and discuss the mode of action of each class. (16 marks) Outline the synthesis of any two such drugs, selecting each from a different class?
6. Explain the mechanism of action of antimetabolites? (8 Marks)
7. Write short notes on antibiotics used as anticancer agents? (8 Marks)
8. Explain various mechanisms by which antineoplastic drugs at? (8 marks)
9. Outline the synthesis of any two antineoplastic drugs act as antimetabolites? (8 marks)

Chapter - 23

1. What are different drugs used in the treatment of peptic ulcer disease with examples? Explain the mechanism of action and uses of Ranitidine? (8 marks)
2. How do gastric acid secretion controlled? Classify and discuss the various drugs used to treat peptic ulcer. Add a note on proton pump inhibitors? (8 marks)

3. Write short notes on peptic ulcers? (4 marks)
4. Discuss GI tract drugs? (8 marks)
5. Give an account of gastrointestinal agents? (8 marks)
6. Write the synthesis and mode of action of omeprazole? (6 marks)

Chapter – 24 & 25

1. What is primary hypertension? Describe the role of rennin-angiotensin system in the pathogenesis of essential hypertension. What are the important recently used antihypertensive drugs? (8 Marks)
2. Write short notes on the following : (i) Calcium channel blockers
3. What is meant by essential hypertension? Classify antihypertensive drugs giving examples ? Outline the synthesis and mechanism of action of : (a) Nifedipine (b) Atenolol (c) Enalapril (d) Methyldopa
4. Discuss the factors implicated in the origin of essential hypertension. Describe the various categories of therapeutic agents available for its clinical management and indicate their mode of action. Outline the synthesis of Atenolol and captopril?

Chapter - 26

1. Write briefly on diagnostic agents? (8 marks)
2. Write notes on diagnostic agents? (8 marks)
3. Write the structure, chemical name and therapeutic uses of (a) Iopanoic acid (2)
4. Write explanatory notes on dyes used as diagnostic agents?

Chapter - 27

1. Write the structure and uses of the following : (8 marks)

   (i) Cortisone (ii) Progesterone (iii) Estorne (iv) Ergosterol
2. Write short note on :

   (i) Synthetic Oestrogens (ii) Calciferols (8 marks)
3. Outline a method of synthesis of progesterone from diosogenin (8 marks)
4. Give a synthetic scheme for the conversion of diosogenin to progesterone (6 marks)
5. Discuss the relationship between sterols and bile acids. How do you establish that these have common nucleus?
6. Discuss the chemical relationship between oestrone, oestradiol and oestriol and describe the synthesis of oestrone.
7. How is the side-chain (Nature and Position) determined in ergosterol?
8. Write about the interconversion of oestrone, oestradiol and oestriol.

Chapter - 28

1. Write the structure and uses of the following : (a) Riboflavin?
2. Explain various steps involved in the determination of structure of Ascorbic acid.
3. Discuss classification and properties of Vitamins.
4. What are vitamins? Classify them with suitable examples and describe their uses? (6 marks)
5. (a) Define the terms vitamins, provitamins and antivitamins.
   (b) Give an account of chemistry of thiamine.
6. (a) Classify vitamins. Give their structure and uses.
   (b) Write four reactions that go to establish the structure of ascorbic acid.
7. Write the structure, chemical names and uses of the following :
   (a) Thiamine (b) ascrobic acid (c) riboflavine (d) pantothenic acid (8 Marks)

REFERENCES

A.G. Gilman, L.S. Goodman, the Pharmacological Basis of Therapeutics, New York.

A. Kar, Medicinal Chemistry, New Age Publishers, New Delhi, British Pharmacopoeia.

A.M. Beckett and J.B. Stanlake and **Garrel**, Practical Pharmaceutical Chemistry, The Sthalone Press, University of London, London.

A.R. Gennaro, Ed., Remington's Pharmaceutical Sciences, Mack Publications, Pennsylvania.

Abraham, D.J., Ed., Burger's Medicinal Chemistry and Drug Discovery, 6th edition, John wiley and Sons, New York, 2003.

Andriole, V.T., Ed., The Quinolones, 3rd edition, Academic Press, 2000.

Annual Reports in Medicinal Chemistry, September, 30, Elsevier, 2003.

Bently and Driver's Pharmaceutical Chemistry.

Block, J.H. and Beale, J.M., Jr., Wilson and Giswold's Textbook of Organic Medicinal and Pharmaceutical Chemistry, 11th Edition, 2004.

Bryskier, A. and Butzler, J.P., Eds., Antibiotics – Antibacterial and Antifungal Agents, Blackwell Synergy Publishing, 2005.

C. Hansch, Quantitative structure-activity Relationship in drug design, In:drug design, vol-I, chap.2 (Ed., E.J. Ariens) academic press, New York.

Current index of medical specialities (CIMS)

Domagala, J.M., Antimicrob Chemotherapy, Vol. 33, pp. 685-706, 1994.

Fogoros, R.N. Antiarrhythmic drugs, Blackwell, 1997.

G. Thomas, Chemistry for Pharmacy and Life Sciences, Prentice-Hall, New York.

Green, D., Anticoagulants, CRC Press, Boca Raton, 1994.

J.G. Topliss, Quantitative structure-activity relationships of drugs, Academic press, New York.

King, F.D. Lawton, G. and Oxford, A.W., Eds., Progress in Medicinal Chemistry, Elsevier, U.K. 2004.

Marcel Dekkar., New York, Concepts in Drug Metabolism, B. Testa and P. Jenner., V.N. Gogte, Profile in Drug Synthesis, Gokul Publishers, Mumbai.

Martin, Y.C., Kutter, E. and Austel, V., Eds., Modern Drug Research, Marcel Dekker, New York, 1989.

Nelson, M., Hillen, W. and Greenwald, R.A., Eds., Tetracyclines in Biology. Chemistry and Medicine, Birkhauser Verlag, 2001.

Omura, S.Ed., Macrolide Antibiotics – Chemistry, Biology and Practice, 2nd edition, Academic Press, 2003.

Organic drug synthesis-Ledniser mitzsher Vol-1 and 2

P. Parimoo, A text Book of Medicinal Chemistry, CBS Publishers, New Delhi,

Progress in Medicinal Chemistry G.P. Ellis and G.B. West, Butterworth, London.

Rama Rao Nadendla, Pharmaceutical Organic Chemistry (Heterocyclics and Natural Products) by Vallabh Prakasan, New Delhi. Indian Pharmacopoeia.

Rama Rao Nadendla, Principles of Pharmaceutical Organic Chemistry (Revised and Enlarged) by Macmillan India Private Limited.

Reddy, I.K. Chirality in Drug Design and Development, Marcel Dekker, New York, 2004.

Smith, H.J. Introduction to the Principles of Drug Design and Action, Smith and Williams, 3rd edition, CRC Press, Boca Raton, 1998.

The British Pharmaceutical Codex

The Merck Index

United States Pharmacopoeia

Van Zwieten, Anti-hypertensive Drugs, Taylor and Francis, 1997.

Williams, D.A. and Lemke, T.L., Foye's Principles of Medicinal Chemistry, 5th Edition, Lippincott Williams and Wilkins, Philadelphia, 2002.

INDEX

A

D

E

F

M

N

O

P

Q

R

S

T

U

V

W

Z

www.ingramcontent.com/pod-product-compliance
Ingram Content Group UK Ltd.
Pitfield, Milton Keynes, MK11 3LW, UK
UKHW061534190726
13845UKWH00005B/95

9 789386 819710